Signs and Symptoms in
Pediatrics

Third Edition

Walter W. Tunnessen, Jr., M.D.

Senior Vice President
The American Board of Pediatrics;
Clinical Professor of Pediatrics
University of North Carolina at Chapel Hill
School of Medicine
Chapel Hill, North Carolina

with Kenneth B. Roberts, M.D.

Director, Pediatric Teaching Program
Moses Cohn Health System
Greensboro, North Carolina;
Professor of Pediatrics
University of North Carolina at Chapel Hill
School of Medicine
Chapel Hill, North Carolina

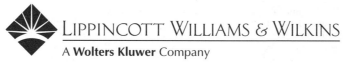

LIPPINCOTT WILLIAMS & WILKINS
A **Wolters Kluwer** Company

Philadelphia · Baltimore · New York · London
Buenos Aires · Hong Kong · Sydney · Tokyo

Acquisitions Editor: Timothy Y. Hiscock
Developmental Editor: Alexandra T. Anderson
Manufacturing Manager: Kevin Watt
Production Manager: Robert Pancotti
Production Editor: Emily Harkavy
Cover Designer: Patricia Gast
Indexer: Linda Van Pelt and Ron Prottsman
Compositor: The PRD Group, Inc.
Printer: Edwards Brothers

Printed in the United States of America

9 8 7 6 5 4 3 2 1

Library of Congress Cataloging-in-Publication Data

Tunnessen, Walter W., 1939–
    Signs and symptoms in pediatrics / Walter W. Tunnessen with
Kenneth B. Roberts. — 3rd ed.
      p.   cm.
    Includes bibliographical references and index.
    ISBN 0-7817-1639-X (alk. paper)
    1. Children—Diseases—Diagnosis. 2. Children—Medical
examinations. 3. Physical diagnosis. 4. Diagnosis, Differential.
I. Roberts, Kenneth B., 1944–   . II. Title.
    [DNLM: 1. Pediatrics handbooks. 2. Diagnosis, Differential—in
infancy & childhood handbooks. WS 39 T926s 1999]
RJ50.T86 1999
618.92′0075—dc21
DNLM/DLC
for Library of Congress   98-51161
                                          CIP

*To my wife, Nancy, and our children, Walter and Anne,
for their support, patience, and understanding.*

*And to the memory of Frank A. Oski, M.D., a wonderful
mentor, an outstanding teacher, an untiring
spokesperson for children, and a sorely
missed friend.*

Contents

Section II. Head

Section III. Ears

Section IV. Eyes

Section V. Nose

Section VI. Mouth and Throat

Preface

The third edition of *Signs and Symptoms in Pediatrics* is a major update of the two previous editions. The focus of the book is to assist the reader in expanding the differential diagnosis for over one hundred presenting signs and symptoms. Almost all chapters have a new section, the most common causes of the sign or symptom, which follows the introduction. This section has been included to direct the attention of the reader to the most likely causes of the problem. The most common disorders, preceded by a diamond, occur most commonly. A list of disorders not to be overlooked, as indicated by a bullet, is also included in most chapters. These are disorders that may not be common causes of a problem, but they are certainly worth remembering and considering in constructing a differential diagnosis.

Although there have not been many new disorders described in the last decade, some have had name changes and others have had their spectrum enlarged, necessitating additions to various chapters. Other disorders have been clarified and better described. Updates to the differential lists were more than the author expected. An attempt has been made to organize each section better and to provide a more helpful approach to a problem. Under each heading in a chapter, the most common causes have been listed first, followed by short descriptive paragraphs.

Two new chapters have been added: Chapter 20, Sudden Infant Death/Apparent Life-Threatening Events; and Chapter 103, Digital Clubbing. In addition, new sections have been added to existing chapters: Excessive Crying to Chapter 9, Irritability; Cyclic Vomiting to Chapter 70, Projectile Vomiting; and Other Color Changes to Chapter 102, Raynaud Phenomenon, Acrocyanosis.

The references and suggested reading sections have been updated. A few classic articles are still referred to, but the new references and suggested readings should help the reader find current information about a particular problem.

Finally, the author recognizes Dr. Kenneth B. Roberts for his contributions to the third edition. It is always helpful to have one's work reviewed, especially by someone with Dr. Roberts' expertise in general pediatrics. He reviewed the entire manuscript and made helpful suggestions.

Walter W. Tunnessen, Jr., M.D.

Preface to the First Edition

Some of us thrive on lists. There is something about a list of diagnostic possibilities that satisfies that quest for thoroughness in our compulsive souls. How this list fetish began is unclear, but the "peripheral brains"—the small pocket notebooks crammed with facts—that all medical students used to carry around may certainly have helped to create the list habit.

Those notebooks have since become obsolete. They are rarely in evidence today. Mine has been replaced by an office file, which is far more capable of holding ever-increasing amounts of information. Without the file I may as well cross the River Styx. When faced with a diagnostic challenge, the file is my refuge. From the file other tributaries arise, clues to solving the diagnostic problems. The other tributaries may comprise journal articles, textbooks, lecture notes, and articles torn from "throw-aways."

What comprises clinical judgment? How do physicians solve diagnostic problems? According to Elstein and colleagues,* the primary factor involved in clinical judgment is recall—the ability to conjure up stored information from the deep recesses of the mind. The amount of information that can be stored in the "cerebral files" is astonishing: The storage capacity of the human mind over a lifetime is far greater than that of any modern computer. It is the retrieval of the information that presents the challenge. This is where lists come in. Many times, review of a list of possible causes for a particular sign or symptom may stimulate the necessary recall. This information can then be combined with probability, other signs, clinical appearance, and so forth to select the most likely cause.

This book is a distillation of lists, designed to help in the retrieval of stored bits of information from the cerebral recesses. For each particular sign or symptom, a list of diagnostic possibilities is offered. The reader may then employ his problem-solving skills to arrive at a tenable diagnosis.

Obviously, there are signs and symptoms other than those presented in this book; only the most common ones, interspersed with some seen less frequently, have been included. (My own experience will undoubtedly be evident in some of the lists as well as in the choice of the signs and symptoms included.) At the end of many chapters, a brief listing of textbooks or journal articles that might be of particular assistance is also included.

This book, then, is intended to act as a catalyst. In combination with information obtained from the history and physical examination, the list of diagnostic possibilities may encourage a release of that stored knowledge that will help the reader arrive at a definitive diagnosis.

Walter W. Tunnessen, Jr., M.D.

---

* Elstein AS, Shulman LS, Sprafka SA. Medical problem solving: an analysis of clinical reasoning. Cambridge: Harvard University Press, 1978.

Preface to the Second Edition

The flavor of the first edition has been retained in the second edition. Differential diagnoses are listed for various presenting symptoms and physical signs. The primary purpose of this book remains unchanged as a stimulator of recall to assist in formulating an appropriate diagnosis. Obviously, recall of previously learned information is not the only mode of problem solving. We must constantly expand our diagnostic horizons. Many disorders, unusual and uncommon, must be considered in a complete differential diagnosis; thus, the lists may sometimes seem slightly unwieldly. Clinical judgment should allow one to separate out the more likely diagnostic possibilities. The more common diagnostic possibilities are listed first.

Three new chapters have been added to this edition: Chapter 41, Chronic Rhinitis/Nasal Obstruction; Chapter 83, Abnormal Vaginal Bleeding; and Chapter 92, Fragile Bones/Recurrent Fractures. In addition, almost 500 new entries have been incorporated into the lists.

I deeply appreciate the feedback from colleagues at all levels—faculty peers, practitioners, house officers, and medical students. Your suggestions and also your additions are always welcomed.

Walter W. Tunnessen, Jr., M.D.

Acknowledgments

Frank A. Oski, M.D., former Professor and Chair of the Department of Pediatrics, John Hopkins University School of Medicine, Baltimore, was the major force behind this book. His untimely death has left a void in pediatrics.

I am also indebted to Lewis A. Barness, M.D., Professor Emeritus and former Chair of Pediatrics, University of South Florida College of Medicine, Tampa, Florida, my pediatric *raison d'etre*.

One cannot overestimate the stimulation by and contributions of the pediatric residents and faculty at the institutions I have had good fortune to be associated with over my career. They have made my profession exciting and fulfilling.

1970–1972: Hospital of the University of Pennsylvania and Children's Hospital of Philadelphia
1972–1986: State University of New York, Upstate Medical Center, Syracuse
1986–1990: John Hopkins University School of Medicine
1991–1995: Children's Hospital of Philadelphia
1995–: University of North Carolina Hospitals
1997–: Duke University Medical Center

SECTION I

General Topics

1

Fever of Undetermined Origin

Next to routine health care, fever is the most common reason why parents bring their children for medical care. While fever is common, prolonged fever is a much less frequent complaint. Prolonged fever is generally defined as a temperature of 38.5°C (101.5°F) or greater of more than 2 weeks' duration. Fever of undetermined origin (FUO) in this section refers to prolonged fever (over 2 weeks) of undiscernible cause despite careful initial evaluation based on history and physical examination. Unlike the classic definition of FUO in adults, fever lasting for 3 weeks after 1 week of hospitalization, there is no standard definition of FUO in children. In this chapter, some general aspects of "fever" are considered first, followed by a list of the most common causes of FUO categorized by frequency of occurrence (1–3).

NORMAL BODY TEMPERATURE

What temperature is normal? Body temperature depends on many factors, including the time of day, where in the body it is measured, and each person's individual "thermostat setting." Like most other clinical measurements, there is a range of normal temperatures. Body temperature is lowest in the early morning and highest in late afternoon, part of the circadian rhythm. Rectal temperatures are higher than oral temperatures by as much as 0.6°C (1°F). Infants and young children generally run higher temperatures than older children. Normal rectal temperatures in children may range from 36.2°C (97°F) to 38°C (100.4°F); normal oral temperatures range from 36.0°C (96.8°F) to 37.4°C (99.3°F). If you ask a parent what constitutes a fever, they will generally state anything over 98.6°F (37.0°C). Everyone thinks this is the normal body temperature, and any elevation over this is a fever. Parents must be taught that "normal" temperatures, 98.6°F (37.0°C), orally, and 99.8°F (37.7°C), rectally, represent mean temperatures; 50% of healthy children will have higher oral or rectal temperatures.

PITFALLS IN ASSESSING FEVER

The thermometer is a fairly crude instrument, whose tolerance of error increases at higher temperature levels; nevertheless, it is certainly more accurate than the hand on the forehead method of temperature assessment. "Low-grade" fever, especially as determined by the latter method, occurring in a child every day after school, should be viewed with suspicion: vigorous physical activity—for example, games such as tag, football, or basketball commonly played on the way home—may temporarily raise body temperature. Temperature measured too soon after meals may similarly give a false impression of fever when it is a reflection of body metabolism generating heat. Anxiety can also produce minor temperature elevations. Over-wrapping with clothing may interfere with normal heat escape. Parents who are unaware of normal temperature range and diurnal variation, may begin monitoring their child's temperature during a febrile illness. They may seek health care evaluation when their child's temperature measures above 98.6°F. This is a relatively common reason for parents, and occasionally doctors, to refer children with "fever of undetermined origin." Evaluation should rule out these physiologic causes of increased body temperature. Before an extensive investigation for FUO is undertaken, the possibility of a child having repeated upper respiratory tract infection (URI) or back-to-back infections of bacterial or viral cause must be considered.

CAUSES OF FUO IN CHILDREN

Common causes of prolonged fever in children differ from those in adults. As noted in the study of Pizzo and colleagues (1), the causes in children over 6 years of age also differ from those in children under age 6. Most cases of prolonged fever in children are not due to unusual or esoteric disorders. The majority represent atypical manifestations of common diseases. Similarly, most children with prolonged fever do not have serious diseases or disorders untreatable by ordinary methods.

The differential diagnosis of FUO may be simplified by the following categorization of possible causes. The percent responsible for each category represents a summary of data from six pediatric series (2).

♦ Infectious Causes (44.6%)

The leading category of causes of FUO in the studies of Pizzo et al. (1), McClung et al. (3), and Steele et al. (4) is infection. The first study attributed infectious causes to 52% of 100 children; the second, to 29% of 99 patients; and the third, to 22% of 109 of the group. A combined list of infectious causes, with the most common first, follows:

"Viral syndrome"	Osteomyelitis
Epstein-Barr Virus Infection	Cat-Scratch Disease
Pneumonia	Lyme Disease
Urinary Tract Infection	Endocarditis
Bacterial Meningitis	Pulmonary Histoplasmosis
Pharyngitis (Chronic)	Salmonella Gastroenteritis
Sinusitis	Malaria
Streptococcosis (Chronic)	Tracheobronchitis
Septicemia	Peritonsillar Abscess
Mycoplasma	Generalized Herpes Simplex
Tuberculosis	Typhoid Fever
Viral Meningoencephalitis	Psittacosis

Acquired immunodeficiency disease should be added to this list.

♦ **Collagen-Vascular Disorders (12.8%)**

Rheumatoid Arthritis
Systemic Lupus Erythematosus
Rheumatic Fever
Henoch-Schönlein Syndrome
Periarteritis Nodosa
Unclassified (includes vasculitides)

♦ **Neoplastic Disorders (5.6%)**

Leukemia
Lymphoma
Reticulum Cell Sarcoma
Neuroblastoma

♦ **Inflammatory Diseases of Bowel (1.6%)**

Crohn Disease
Ulcerative Colitis

♦ **Undiagnosed (10.7%)**

♦ **Resolved (12.6%)**

♦ **Miscellaneous (12.1%)**

The three studies cited in the above breakdown varied considerably in the percentage of patients studied in whom no diagnosis was reached. McClung (3) designated 21% of patients as "no diagnosis established; evidence of resolving disease." Of these patients, nine were thought to have repeated URI. In 3 other patients, recent infectious hepatitis was the probable cause; in another 2 patients, drug fever; and in 4 more, "streptococcal syndromes" were the causes.

For those who desire additional diagnostic stimulation, fuel for roundsmanship, or "I once saw a case of . . . ," the following miscellaneous category is included:

Miscellaneous Causes

Pseudo-FUO. Recurrent self-limited infections may simulate persistent fever.
Factitious. Caused by either child or parents; Munchausen syndrome by proxy.
Drug fever. More common in clinical practice than reported series. Acetaminophen, methylphenidate, and antibiotics are among the most common causes. Chronic salicylate toxicity still must be considered.

Infections

Hepatitis (Anicteric; Chronic Active)
Leptospirosis
Q Fever
Aspergillosis
Tularemia
Ehrlichiosis
Abscesses: Retroperitoneal, intracranial, subphrenic, hepatic, perinephric

Rat-Bite Fever
Diskitis
Tick-Borne Relapsing Fever
Yersinia or *Campylobacter* Enteritis
Syphilis
Brucellosis

Hereditary Disorders

Familial Dysautonomia
Ichthyosis
Familial Mediterranean Fever
Cyclic Neutropenia (recurrent, rather than prolonged)

Ectodermal Dysplasia (Anhidrotic)
Congenital Sensory Neuropathy
Virilizing Adrenal Hyperplasia

Central Nervous System

Altered "Thermostat"   Subdural Hematoma (chronic)

Dehydration

For example, secondary to diabetes mellitus or diabetes insipidus.

Allergy

Other

Kawasaki Disease
Hyperthyroidism
Dermatomyositis
Infantile Cortical Hyperostosis (Caffey Disease)
Syndrome of Periodic Fever, Pharyngitis, and Aphthous Stomatitis (5)
Other Tumors: Retinoblastoma

Behçet Disease
Serum Sickness
Sarcoidosis
Wegener Granulomatosis

Hyperimmunoglobulinemia D Syndrome (6)

This list is not complete; however, remember that most causes of FUO are not unusual, although their presentations may be atypical. In the Pizzo study (1), the history and physical examination suggested or indicated the final diagnoses in 62 of 100 cases. The pattern, height, or duration of fever did not relate to the final diagnosis or the severity of disease with any significance, nor did symptoms such as anorexia, fatigue, weight loss, toxic appearance, or response to antipyretics.

Careful re-examination, attention to detail, review of historical information, and, of course, time are the most helpful tools in differential diagnosis of FUO.

REFERENCES

1. Pizzo PA, Lovejoy FH, Smith DH. Prolonged fever in children: review of 100 cases. *Pediatrics* 1975;55:468–473.
2. Gartner JC Jr. Fever of unknown origin. *Adv Pediatr Infect Dis* 1992;7:1–24.
3. McClung HJ. Prolonged fever of unknown origin in children. *Am J Dis Child* 1972;124:544–550.
4. Steele RW, Jones SM, Lowe BA, Glasier CM. Usefulness of scanning procedures for diagnosis of fever of unknown origin in children. *J Pediatr* 1991;119:526–530.
5. Marshall GS, Edwards KM, Butler J, Lawton AR. Syndrome of periodic fever, pharyngitis, and aphthous stomatitis. *J Pediatr* 1987;110:43–46.
6. Drenth JPH, Boom BW, Toonstra J, et al. Cutaneous manifestations and histologic findings in the hyperimmunoglobulinemia D syndrome. *Arch Dermatol* 1994;130:59–65.

SUGGESTED READING

Jacobs RF, Schutze GE. *Bartonella henselae* as a cause of prolonged fever and fever of unknown origin in children. *Clin Infect Dis* 1998;26:80–84.
Malatack JJ, Long SS. Fever of unknown origin. In: Long SS, Pickering LK, Prober CG, eds. *Principles and practice of pediatric infectious diseases.* New York: Churchill Livingstone, 1997:124–134.
Miller LC, Sisson BA, Tucker LB, Schaller JG. Prolonged fevers of unknown origin in children: patterns of presentation and outcome. *J Pediatr* 1996;129:419–423.
Miller ML, Szer I, Yogev R, Bernstein B. Fever of unknown origin. *Pediatr Clin N Am* 1995;42:999–1015.
Nizet V, Vinci RJ, Lovejoy FH Jr. Fever in children. *Pediatr Rev* 1994;15:127–135.
Saper CB, Breder CD. The neurologic basis of fever. *N Engl J Med* 1994;330:1880–1886.
Simon HB. Hyperthermia. *N Engl J Med* 1993;329:483–487.

2

Hypothermia

Hypothermia refers to the state in which the core body temperature falls below 35°C (95°F). The reduction in temperature reflects a negative balance between heat production, such as a hypometabolic state (e.g., hypothyroidism or starvation), and heat loss when mechanisms to dissipate heat are exaggerated (e.g., evaporation after immersion). The body dissipates heat to the environment by radiation, conduction, evaporation, and convection. The newborn infant, and the premature infant in particular, have a higher surface area to volume ratio than older children and adults, making them at high risk for hypothermia because they may lose heat from their surface faster than their metabolism can generate it. Wet surfaces, as present in the newborn, permit additional heat loss by evaporation.

The immature infant is especially susceptible to the whims of their environment, but all infants are much more likely than older children to have subnormal body temperatures when they incur environmental insults or derangements ranging from hypoxia and infection to metabolic and endocrinologic problems. The causes of hypothermia are grouped into categories reflecting the modes of insult.

◆ Most Common Causes of Hypothermia

Environmental   Infection/Sepsis
Malnutrition

◆ ENVIRONMENTAL FACTORS

Hypothermia may occur rather quickly in newborns, especially those delivered in air-conditioned rooms or those exposed to room temperature before amniotic fluids have been dried off. Immature or sick infants must be maintained in a thermoneutral environment, a critical factor in their survival.

Older infants, children, and adults may become hypothermic when exposed to low temperatures, especially the result of wind chill, immersion in cold or cool water with rapid heat loss, or evaporative heat loss when removed from water, even if the temperature of the water is not cold or cool.

SHOCK

The body temperature may fall dramatically during states of shock. Dehydration, burns, infection, hemorrhage, intestinal obstruction, and trauma may be precipitating causes.

CENTRAL NERVOUS SYSTEM INSULTS

Hypothermia may reflect severe insult to the central nervous system, particularly when the central temperature-regulating mechanism in the hypothalamic area is involved.

Intracranial Hemorrhage or Infarction

Trauma (Including Surgical)

Severe Birth Asphyxia

Tumors

Craniopharyngioma

Hypothalamic disturbances may include hyperthermia or hypothermia, as well as somnolence, hypertension or hypotension, obesity, and inappropriate secretion of antidiuretic hormone. The cardinal signs of this tumor are increased intracranial pressure, visual defects, endocrine dysfuction, and the hypothalamic effects.

Astrocytoma

Cerebral Malformations

Anencephaly

Congenital Absence of the Corpus Callosum (Shapiro Syndrome)

Children with this abnormality may have mild chronic hypothermia or recurrent attacks of hypothermia associated with mutism or coma. Onset of clinical signs may be delayed until childhood or adolescence.

♦ INFECTION

Hypothermia is more likely to occur in infants than in older children.

Meningitis

Encephalitis

Sepsis

Generalized infection, particularly with gram-negative organisms, may significantly lower body temperature.

ENDOCRINE-METABOLIC DISORDERS

Subnormal temperatures or impaired temperature regulation may occasionally occur in endocrine-metabolic disorders, generally the result of reduced metabolic rate and consequent decreased heat production.

Anorexia Nervosa

Addison Disease

Hypothyroidism

Hypopituitarism

Hypoglycemia

In infants hypoglycemia may cause hypothermia, or hypothermia may result in hypoglycemia.

Diabetes Mellitus

Amino/Organic Acidurias

Occasionally, infants with these inborn errors may have hypothermia as part of their tenuous metabolic state.

♦ **ENERGY-PROTEIN UNDERNUTRITION**

In children with kwashiorkor, body temperature may fall below 35°C (95°F) despite a high environmental temperature.

DRUGS

Heavy sedation from drugs may result in subnormal body temperature, generally the result of decreased metabolism.

Alcohol

Narcotics

Substance Abuse

Barbiturates

Phenothiazines

Atropine

Acetaminophen Overdose

MISCELLANEOUS CAUSES

Familial Dysautonomia

This autosomal recessively inherited disorder occurs predominantly in Ashkenazi Jews. In addition to altered temperature regulation, features include decreased or absent lacrimation, emotional instability, relative indifference to pain, postural hypotension, and poor muscular coordination.

Menkes Kinky-Hair Syndrome

Symptoms usually appear in the first few months of life. Major motor seizures, developmental delay, and the characteristic coarse, short, twisted hair are prominent features.

Water Intoxication

Infants fed inappropriately dilute formulas may develop seizures, probably as a result of hyponatremia. Altered sensorium and hypothermia are often present.

Episodic Spontaneous Hypothermia with Hyperhidrosis

An unusual disorder with sudden, and usually short-lived, episodes of hypothermia accompanied by pallor and sweating (1).

REFERENCE

1. Sheth RD, Barron TF, Hartlage PL. Episodic spontaneous hypothermia with hyperhidrosis: implications for pathogenesis. *Pediatr Neurol* 1994;10:58–60.

3

Failure to Thrive

The infant or child who is failing to thrive presents a common diagnostic challenge to all physicians who care for children. The possible causes encompass malfunction in any of the organ systems of the body as well as nutritional, environmental, social, and psychological factors. Failure to thrive (FTT) is defined as deviation of growth away from previously established channels affecting weight more than height (length) and head circumference. It is distinguished from short stature in which height is affected predominantly. FTT is never a diagnosis; it is a symptom.

Some have advocated abandoning the term FTT in favor of growth deficiency, because of the lack of diagnostic specificity of the term (1). Others have stressed that malnutrition is the final common pathway and should, therefore, replace FTT. The term, however, is still ingrained in our medical lexicon and, consequently, it will be used in this discussion.

The index of any textbook of pediatrics may be considered a list of potential diagnoses of disorders associated with FTT. The subsequent lengthy classification, by no means exhaustive, has been designed to reinforce the concept that the possible causes involve all systems. The history and physical examination are by far our most important resources in sorting out the cause of FTT because they may provide evidence that excludes some processes or points to others as causes of this symptom. Of the two, the history will provide the most information. Growth charts are valuable, particularly if sequential records allow multiple points along the growth curve to be plotted. A sudden deviation from an established growth pattern should focus attention on different disorders from those suggested by a curve that demonstrates a continuing deviation or one that has always been below the third percentile for growth. Prenatal onset of growth retardation should suggest causes other than those for postnatal onset FTT. Keep in mind that 3% of the normal population has a growth curve below the third percentile for height or weight.

Despite the fact that the history and physical examination deliver the most useful information, laboratory tests have been relied on too frequently in the differential diagnosis of FTT. Overuse of blood and radiologic imaging tests should be condemned. The yield from these studies is low, the expense is high, and their performance may interfere with careful consideration of the information already at hand. The classic study by Sills (2) demonstrated that of 185 children hospitalized for the evaluation of FTT, only 18% had proven organic diagnoses, but only 1.4% of the laboratory studies performed were of positive diagnostic assistance. In a longitudinal study by Lacey and Parkin in 1974 (3), 82% of children with growth retardation had no evidence of an organic disease. Of 23 children with organic disease, only in 3 was the disease asymptomatic; 1 had probable growth-hormone deficiency, 1 had chronic renal failure, and 1 a chromosomal abnormality. Other studies have reported up to a 50% incidence of organic disease in children with the symptom of FTT. The source of the study populations, however, must be considered. In a referral center, for example, it is more likely that organic causes of FTT will constitute a larger percentage. In a primary-care setting most children have nonorganic causes of FTT. Nonorganic and organic causes of FTT may occur together, producing an additive effect (1). The breakdown into organic and nonorganic groups of FTT needs to be reconsidered. An excellent discussion of the classification dilemma can be found in the article by Zenel (4).

The nonorganic causes of FTT are normal variants and nutritional deprivation. However, children who fall below the third percentile for height because of genetic endowment may be inappropriately labeled as having FTT. Evaluation should include determination of parental and grandparental stature. In these children, the bone age is equivalent to chronologic age. The superb study by Smith and colleagues (5) clearly demonstrates that the deceleration in growth seen after the first 3 to 6 months of life in many infants may reflect the genetic growth factors passed on by their parents. A new growth channel is achieved at a mean age of 13 months. The FTT in older children more often reflects a concern about height than weight. Delayed adolescence (constitutional delay) may be responsible for the shift in growth channels; a history of similar pubertal delay in one of the parents may occasionally be reported. With delayed adolescence, the bone age is appropriate for the height age (the age at which the child's measured height is at the 50th percentile on standard growth curves), but both are less than the chronologic age of the child.

Nutritional deprivation as a nonorganic cause of FTT represents a variety of diagnoses, but all have in common a lack of adequate caloric intake for one reason or another. Worldwide, caloric deprivation on an economic basis is the most common cause of FTT. In the United States, psychosocial factors and feeding problems account for deficient caloric intake. An excellent general outline of "psychosocial FTT" was written by Barbero and Shaheen in 1967 (6). Their diagnostic criteria for "environmental FTT" included the following:

- Weight below the third percentile with accelerated gain during appropriate nurturing. (The height is generally less affected than weight.)
- Developmental retardation with subsequent acceleration of development following appropriate stimulation and feeding.
- No evidence of systemic disease or abnormality. Laboratory investigation is also unrevealing.
- Clinical signs of deprivation that improve in a more nurturing environment. Signs include poor hygiene, cradle cap, diaper rash, and impetigo.
- Significant environmental psychosocial disruption in the family, such as alcoholism, unwanted pregnancies, or marital discord. It is often difficult to extract this kind of information on first contact with the parents.

In addition to these five diagnostic criteria, Barbero and Shaheen (6) described four clinical patterns of environmental FTT. Group I has signs of FTT without obvious symptoms or signs of systemic disease, but with the presence of family discord. Group II has FTT with various clinical manifestations, but these symptoms do not account for the FTT. Group III has FTT associated with signs of abuse. Group IV demonstrates FTT with underlying systemic disease that does not account for the growth disturbance. Examples of Group IV include the infant with a poor start such as a premature infant separated from the mother, or the infant with a cleft lip or congenital heart disease.

With adequate nurturing, in a hospital setting perhaps, the infant begins to thrive. One must be aware that infants with organic FTT may gain weight with similar attention.

Too frequently, the infant with FTT admitted for evaluation is subjected to a multitude of tests that can interfere with adequate nurturing. The infant who undergoes successive radiologic examinations and blood tests during hospitalization may continue to lose weight. Observation, tender care, and stimulation are critical. In the era of managed care, it has become increasingly difficult to admit children with FTT for observation. Consequently, tests are ordered to attempt to "justify" the admission. A difficult task in cases of environmental FTT is finding appropriate support systems for the family.

Psychosocial deprivation, as with any other disorder, has a spectrum of clinical presentations. The most severe and bizarre form is called "deprivation dwarfism." Reversible growth hormone insufficiency may be associated with its macabre symptoms and behavior (7,8).

The reason for the emphasis here on normal variants and nutritional deprivation should be obvious to all who have cared for children in a primary-care setting. These two categories account for most of the children presenting with FTT, perhaps as many as 80%. The myriad of other causes make up a small proportion of the total group. In addition, the organic causes usually have signs and symptoms that direct attention to them. Few of these causes are truly hidden. Nevertheless, the etiologic classification follows.

♦ **Most Common Causes of FTT**

Normal Growth Variants:	**Inadequate Caloric Intake:**
Shifting Linear Growth	Feeding Skills Problems
Familial	Psychosocial

NORMAL VARIANTS

♦ **Shifting Linear Growth During Infancy**

The birth length and weight of infants does not necessarily reflect their growth potential, but relates predominantly to maternal nutrition. Deceleration of growth is seen in the first 3 to 6 months after birth. New growth channels are assumed by 13 months of age (5).

♦ **Familial (Genetic) Factors**

Height and weight are proportionately below the third percentile and follow the growth curves, though below it. The history and physical examinations do not suggest organic disease. Short stature is usually uncovered in the familial history. The bone age equals the chronologic age.

Delayed Adolescence

Children in this group fail to demonstrate the normal pubertal growth spurt until much later in adolescence. History and physical examination are unrevealing except for signs of delayed puberty and perhaps a similar pattern of growth in relatives.

The bone age equals the height age in these adolescents, demonstrating potential for future growth.

NUTRITIONAL DEPRIVATION (INADEQUATE INTAKE)

♦ Caloric Deprivation

This is the most common cause of true FTT. Signs of insufficient or inappropriate intake may be obvious or subtle. A careful feeding history must be obtained. The caretaker may mix formula inappropriately, or dilute formula to stretch feedings, without realizing a deficient caloric intake. Fruit juices may be substituted for higher caloric foods with resultant diminished caloric intake.

♦ Feeding Skills Disorder

Infants who fail to thrive may have various problems that prevent them from obtaining adequate nutrition. They may demonstrate minimally abnormal neurologic features that make feeding by caretakers difficult. Included may be poor appetite, perhaps reflecting a disorder in the regulation of hunger, delayed tolerance for textures, prolonged feeding duration, and difficult feeding behavior (4). These difficulties, which may have been previously determined to be psychosocial in nature, can lead to problems for parents caring for these infants.

♦ Psychosocial Factors

Environmental FTT

This is an important, common cause of FTT, especially in children under 3 years of age. Factors include maternal depression and family disruption. The child's weight is affected before length; head circumference is preserved.

Deprivation Dwarfism

This striking syndrome of FTT is associated with unusual behavior of the child, significant family psychosocial disruption, and endocrinologic aberrations.

Rumination

Characterized by repeated vomiting without gastrointestinal illness. Generally begins during infancy to 15 months.

RENAL DISEASE

Urinary Tract Infection

Even when systemic symptoms are absent, a urine culture should be part of the evaluation in all children with FTT. Vomiting, diarrhea, and unexplained fevers are common presenting symptoms in young infants and children with urinary tract infections.

Renal Tubular Acidosis

Several different types of renal tubular acidosis (RTA) have been described. Proximal RTA may present only with FTT clinically, with hyperchloremic acidosis apparent on laboratory studies. In distal RTA, polyuria, polydipsia, and recurrent episodes of dehydration may also be noted. Hyperchloremic acidosis with a urinary pH that fails to drop below 7.0 is typical.

Acidosis

In addition to RTA, chronic acidosis from any cause may be associated with FTT.

Chronic Renal Insufficiency

Congenital Obstructive Uropathy

Obstructive uropathy may go unnoticed until growth failure becomes evident. Patients with posterior urethral valves may have few symptoms until renal failure occurs.

Malformations or Cystic Disease

Enlarged kidneys or an abdominal mass may be palpable.

Primary Hyperoxaluria (Oxalosis)

Renal failure, nephrolithiasis, and hematuria occur with deposition and excretion of calcium oxalate.

Diabetes Insipidus

Polyuria and a low urinary specific gravity despite dehydration are important clues. There may be episodes of unexplained fever. The origin may be central or renal.

CARDIORESPIRATORY DISEASES

Upper Airway Obstruction

Chronic partial obstruction of the upper airway from enlarged tonsils and adenoids may lead to chronic hypoxemia with resulting pulmonary hypertension and eventually cor pulmonale.

Congenital Heart Disease

Chronic hypoxemia or congestive heart failure may interfere with growth.

Myocardiopathy

Acquired Heart Disease

Endocarditis

Myocarditis

Mulibrey Nanism

An unusual syndrome that features short stature, a characteristic facies, and hepatomegaly secondary to constrictive pericarditis.

Chronic Lung Disease

Cystic Fibrosis

In young infants respiratory or gastrointestinal symptoms may be subtle. Cystic fibrosis must always be considered in an infant who is failing to thrive despite a voracious appetite. Malabsorption is the cause of early FTT; pulmonary contributions to FTT occur later.

Asthma

Severe asthma in young children may interfere with growth for several reasons. Reactive airways disease is common, and its presence may obscure psychosocial causes of FTT. Remember that all that wheezes isn't asthma.

Bronchiectasis

May follow pneumonia or aspiration and occurs in immunocompromised patients.

Bronchopulmonary Dysplasia

The neonatal history is essential for the diagnosis.

GASTROINTESTINAL DISORDERS

Upper Tract Disorders

Cleft Lip or Palate

The severity of the anomaly may interfere occasionally with adequate nutritional intake. Parental reaction to the clefting may also be a factor in FTT. The possibility of other associated defects should be considered.

Esophageal Compression

Vascular rings and other external impingements on the esophagus may lead to difficulty swallowing or the sense of fullness and decreased appetite.

Gastroesophageal Reflux

Severe gastroesophageal reflux (GER) may result in FTT as well as various presentations of this abnormality. Vomiting may or may not be present. Recurrent wheezing, coughing, or pneumonitis, "colic," apneic episodes, and anemia are but a few ways GER may manifest. GER is common; it does not lead to FTT unless associated with severe, chronic esophagitis, leading to a catabolic state.

Hiatal Hernia

The infant or child may have symptoms similar to those of GER. Torsion spasms of the neck (Sandifer syndrome) may be a clue.

Pyloric Stenosis

Projectile vomiting with epigastric distension usually makes this diagnosis obvious.

Celiac Disease

Chronic diarrhea, FTT, and irritability with abdominal distension suggest celiac disease in the differential diagnosis; however, up to 30% of patients have no diarrhea. Flattened villi are found on intestinal biopsy; antigliadin and antiendomysium antibodies are present in the serum.

Pancreatic Disorders

Cystic Fibrosis

Examination of the stool for steatorrhea is indicated in suspected cases. This is the most common cause of malabsorption.

Chronic Pancreatitis

This may be the result of infection or trauma, or, more rarely, pancreatic insufficiency with neutropenia (Shwachman syndrome) may cause FTT.

Food Sensitivity or Intolerance

Expressions include diarrhea, vomiting, and abdominal pain and distension.

Enzymatic Deficiencies

Children with lactase, fructase, maltase-isomaltase, and other enzyme deficiencies generally present with chronic diarrhea.

Hepatic Disorders

Hepatitis

Congenital as well as acquired infections, metabolic disorders, and certain drugs may produce chronic hepatic inflammation.

Cirrhosis

Various disorders, both acquired (inflammatory bowel disese) and inherited (e.g., α-1-antitrypsin deficiency), may result in cirrhosis.

Biliary Disorders

Biliary Atresia

Prolonged and increasing jaundice suggests this diagnosis.

Choledochal Cyst

Inflammatory Bowel Disease

Regional Enteritis

Symptoms other than weight loss, such as diarrhea, fever, abdominal pain, and an abdominal mass, may not be evident. Delayed onset of puberty and growth may be subtle presentations.

Ulcerative Colitis

Diarrhea, often bloody, with tenesmus is characteristic.

Hirschsprung Disease

The chronic constipation may be obscured by intermittent loose stools. Failure to pass meconium in the first 24 hours of life is an important clue.

ENDOCRINE DISORDERS

Thyroid Disorders

Hypothyroidism and hyperthyroidism may both produce FTT.

Growth Hormone Deficiency

May not be noticeable until late in the first year of life when linear growth begins to depend more on growth hormone and the child's growth rate drops off. Hypoglycemic episodes in the neonatal period and micropenis may be early clues.

Adrenal Disorders

Adrenal Insufficiency

Lethargy, fatigue, and increased skin pigmentation with hyperkalemia and hyponatremia suggest this diagnosis.

Adrenocortical Excess (Cushing Syndrome)

This disorder may result from exogenous steroid therapy, a primary adrenal tumor, or a central nervous system problem. The child's growth velocity eventually falls off, but truncal obesity is prominent. This is a cause of short stature rather than FTT.

Diabetes Mellitus

Juvenile onset diabetes mellitus usually develops rapidly. Weight loss is acute.

Parathyroid Disorders

Tetany and seizures secondary to hypocalcemia are common presenting signs.

Sexual Precocity

Early closure of the epiphyses ultimately leads to short stature.

Hyperaldosteronism

Muscle weakness, hypertension, and low serum potassium levels suggest this disorder.

CENTRAL NERVOUS SYSTEM DISORDERS

Chronic Subdural Hematoma

Cerebral Insults

Anoxia

Trauma

Vascular Bleed or Thrombosis

Infection

Degenerative Disorders

Neurologic abnormalities overshadow the FTT.

Diencephalic Syndrome

This striking disorder is usually caused by a tumor in the area of the anterior hypothalamus and results in severe weight loss with euphoria, vertical nystagmus, and papilledema. An increasing head circumference can provide an early clue.

SKELETAL DISORDERS

Chrondrodystrophies

Various disorders have been described but are generally associated with short stature rather than FTT.

Rickets

Vitamin D Deficiency

Enlarged ends of long bones and the chest wall "rosary" may be subtle findings. Infants may present with seizures.

Vitamin D Resistant

Osteopetrosis

Marble bones on radiographic studies, pallor, and splenomegaly may be early findings.

CHRONIC INFECTIONS OR INFESTATION

Human Immunodeficiency Virus

FTT is an increasingly common symptom of acquired immunodeficiency syndrome. Other findings include opportunistic infections, diffuse lymphadenopathy, hepatosplenomegaly, and loss of developmental milestones.

Tuberculosis

Recurrent Infections

Infants with school-age siblings may be subjected to recurrent infections.

INTOXICATIONS

Lead

Mercury

Poisoning is uncommon, but signs are often dramatic including irritability, hypotonia, photophobia, profuse sweating, and erythema of the extremities.

Hypervitaminosis

Vitamin A excess may cause irritability, increased intracranial pressure, and bone pain. Alternative health approaches and "nutrition stores" may result in an increasing prevalence of vitamin excess disorders.

Fetal Exposure

Anticonvulsants

The fetal hydantoin syndrome may include impressive FTT with other phenotypic abnormalities.

Alcohol

Features of the fetal alcohol syndrome may not be striking. Prenatal onset of growth deficiency, microcephaly, short palpebral fissures, and a flat philtrum are best recognized.

METABOLIC DISORDERS

Galactosemia

The combined symptoms of vomiting, diarrhea, jaundice, and FTT in an infant mandate urine examination to detect reducing substance.

Hypercalcemia

May be a result of hyperparathyroidism, but consider in children with subcutaneous fat necrosis who may later develop hypercalcemia.

Amino Acid and Organic Acid Disorders

Recurrent episodes of lethargy, poor appetite, vomiting, seizures, or stupor suggest these disorders.

Storage Disease

Mucopolysaccharidoses

Phenotypic and physical abnormalities suggest the possibility of a storage disorder, particularly coarse features.

Lipidoses

Glycogenoses

Acrodermatitis Enteropathica

Infants present with diarrhea, hair loss, and acral, perianal and perioral psoriaticlike rashes.

Dietary Chloride Deficiency

This disorder has been described in formula manufacturing errors as well as one case of inadequate chloride in breast milk. Additional features include anorexia, hypotonia, metabolic alkalosis, and low serum electrolytes.

CHRONIC ANEMIA

Iron Deficiency Anemia

Children may have many presentations, including pallor, syncope, irritability, lethargy, weakness.

Thalassemia Major

Hepatosplenomegaly is an early and progressive finding.

Sickle Cell Anemia

PRIMORDIAL DWARFISM

The onset of growth failure may be *in utero* or shortly after birth secondary to genetic, infectious, or undetermined insults.

Placental Insufficiency

Chromosomal Disorders

Congenital Infections

Dysmorphogenetic Syndromes

All children with FTT should be examined closely for phenotypic abnormalities that may suggest described syndromes of malformation.

MISCELLANEOUS DISORDERS

Malignancies

Patients with occult tumors occasionally present with FTT before associated symptoms surface.

Vasoactive Intestinal Peptidase-Secreting Tumors

Infants with these tumors present with growth failure, intermittent diarrhea, soiling, and, occasionally, flushing, sweating, and hypertension. The tumors are generally ganglioneuromas and ganglioneuroblastomas.

Reticuloendothelioses

Skin rashes, adenopathy, and bony lesions suggest disorders in this category. Langerhans cell histiocytosis is the most common.

Immune Deficiency Disorders

Recurrent infections, often with unusual organisms that are difficult to control, are common.

Collagen Vascular Disorders

Chronic inflammation may lead to FTT.

Juvenile Rheumatoid Arthritis

Systemic Lupus Erythematosus

Dermatomyositis

Periarteritis Nodosa

Muscular Dystrophy

Failure to thrive may be an early sign of Duchenne muscular dystrophy. Beware of an elevated AST being mistaken for liver disease. A creatine kinase will be elevated.

The list of causes could go on, but expanding would serve no useful purpose. Remember that the first two categories account for perhaps 80% to 90% of causes of FTT in a primary-care setting. Extensive laboratory testing should be avoided. The most effective diagnostic tools are a careful history and physical examination, sequential growth records, determination of parental stature, and evaluation for psychosocial problems.

REFERENCES

1. Bithoney WG, Dubowitz H, Egan H. Failure to thrive/growth deficiency. *Pediatr Rev* 1992;13:453–460.
2. Sills RH. Failure to thrive: the role of clinical and laboratory evaluation. *Am J Dis Child* 1978;132:967–969.
3. Lacey KA, Parkin JM. Causes of short stature; a community study of children in Newcastle-upon-Tyne. *Lancet* 1974;1:42–45.
4. Zenel JA Jr. Failure to thrive: a general pediatrician's perspective. *Pediatr Rev* 1997;11:371–378.
5. Smith DW, Truog W, Rogers JE, et al. Shifting linear growth during infancy: illustration of genetic factors in growth from fetal life through infancy. *J Pediatr* 1976;89:225–230.
6. Barbero GJ, Shaheen E. Environmental failure to thrive: a clinical view. *J Pediatr* 1967;71:639–641.
7. Silver HK, Finkelstein M. Deprivation dwarfism. *J Pediatr* 1967;70:317–324.
8. Powell GF, Brasel JA, Blizzard RM. Emotional deprivation and growth retardation simulating idiopathic hypopituitarism. *N Engl J Med* 1967;276:1271–1278.

4

Tall Stature and Accelerated Growth

Accelerated linear growth and tall stature are much less frequent complaints than is short stature. Most children who grow more rapidly than their peers do so because of their genetic potential. An analysis of familial growth patterns is usually rewarding; however, a careful physical examination should be performed to look for signs of precocious sexual development. An assessment of skeletal maturation by means of radiographs of the hand and wrist should be made. Tall stature is defined as a height of more than 2 standard deviations above the mean for age. Accelerated linear growth is best defined by comparing the rate of growth to normal growth velocity curves.

Early rapid linear growth, particularly if unfounded genetically, may be temporary, due to early maturation. Because of premature closure of the epiphyses in children with early puberty, adult stature may be compromised.

♦ **Most Common Causes of Tall Stature**

    Constitutional (genetic)   Marfan Syndrome

● **Disorders Not to Forget**

    Klinefelter Syndrome   Homocystinuria
    Growth Hormone Excess   Cerebral Gigantism

PHYSIOLOGIC CONDITIONS

♦ Constitutional Factors

Most children who grow rapidly and attain what is perceived as excessive stature usually do so because of genetic predisposition. There is no underlying organic abnormality. The problems that arise are psychological ones: Tall men are accepted readily in society; therefore, tall boys are not usually seen for medical evaluation. Parents, however, are often concerned if their daughters seem to be growing at excessive rates, although this is less true now than a few decades ago.

Familial Rapid Maturation

Affected children grow rapidly early in life and attain full growth and puberty at an earlier age. Their bone age is advanced, corresponding with height age. Their adult height is in the normal range.

Obesity

Children with exogenous obesity often demonstrate accelerated linear growth. Their final adult height is normal.

ENDOCRINE CAUSES

Precocious Puberty

Children with early onset of puberty grow more rapidly than do their peers, but their ultimate height is not excessive. (See Chapter 81, Precocious Puberty.)

Congenital Adrenal Hyperplasia

This inherited disorder should be suspected in any child with excessive linear growth and signs of virilization or ambiguous genitalia. Muscle mass is usually increased and skeletal maturation advanced. If the disorder is not treated, the ultimate adult height is diminished because of early closure of epiphyses.

Hyperthyroidism

There is usually an initial growth spurt in children with untreated hyperthyroidism. Most children present with tachycardia, systolic hypertension, restlessness, weight loss, heat intolerance, tremors, and frequent stools.

Gigantism and Acromegaly

Gigantism occurs if there is excessive secretion of growth hormone before epiphyseal closure. In gigantism and acromegaly, an anterior pituitary tumor is usually responsible; significant enlargement of the hands and feet occurs and the facial features become coarse. The jaw becomes significantly prominent in acromegaly but less so in gigantism. The bone age is not advanced.

Acromegaloidism

A rare disorder characterized by tall stature, excessive growth, and an acromegaly appearance, but without excessive growth hormone or insulinlike growth factor-1. The clinical appearance and manifestations are similar to those of acromegaly and pituitary gigantism.

CHROMOSOMAL ABNORMALITIES

• Klinefelter Syndrome

This syndrome should be considered in males who are relatively tall and slim and have hypogonadism. The limbs tend to be long and the penis and testes small. Gynecomastia occurs in 40% of the cases during adolescence. The karyotype is XXY.

47,XYY Karyotype

There are no diagnostic phenotypic features except for tall stature. Personality disorders seem to be more common.

48,XXYY Males

The phenotype is similar to Klinefelter syndrome, tall and eunuchoidal. Most affected patients are mentally retarded. The testes are small and firm.

Trisomy X (47,XXX Females)

Most affected females have a normal phenotype. Most have normal sexual development. The IQ ranges from 55 to 115, with one-half to two-thirds of girls slightly below normal.

MISCELLANEOUS CAUSES

♦ Marfan Syndrome

Children with this autosomal-dominant disorder have a tendency toward tall stature. Long limbs, arachnodactyly, joint laxity, pectus deformities, subluxation of the lenses, scoliosis, and aortic dilation are characteristic features. The arm span exceeds the height.

● Homocystinuria

The clinical picture in this disorder, inherited as an autosomal-recessive trait, resembles that in Marfan syndrome. Arachnodactyly, pectus deformities, subluxation of lenses, and aortic degeneration are common. The hair tends to be sparse, dry, and light in color. A malar flush is often present. Arterial and venous thromboses are common. Over one-half of affected individuals have mental deficiency.

Multiple Endocrine Neoplasia Syndrome, Type III

Individuals have a Marfanoid habitus, but they do not have accelerated growth. The characteristic features include thick lips, mucosal neuromas, and anteverted eyelids. Medullary thyroid carcinomas and pheochromocytomas often develop in early adolescence.

Beckwith-Wiedemann Syndrome

Infants with this syndrome tend to be large at birth or grow rapidly after the neonatal period. Omphalocele or umbilical hernia and macroglossia are often present. Hypoglycemia is common in the neonatal period. The skeletal age is advanced. Renal or adrenal tumors develop in a significant number of affected infants and children.

● Cerebral Gigantism

Children with cerebral gigantism have significant acceleration of growth in infancy and acromegalic features; macrocephaly and developmental and mental retardation are common. The palate is high and arched, and the face is long with frontal boss-ing, hypertelorism, and an antimongoloid slant to the eyes. The bone age is ad-vanced.

Neurofibromatosis, Type 1

Occasionally, children with neurofibromatosis and central nervous system gliomas may show increased somatic growth.

Lipodystrophy

Children with generalized lipodystrophy have accelerated growth with enlarge-ment of the hands and feet. The loss of subcutaneous tissue creates a muscular appearance. Hepatomegaly with abdominal distension is common. Hyperinsulinemia and insulin resistance are features of the various disorders with lipodystrophy.

Marshall Syndrome

The few cases reported have had accelerated linear growth with failure to gain weight. The bone age is advanced prenatally. The facial appearance is unusual featuring a prominent forehead, elongated skull, shallow ocular orbits, upturned nose, and bluish sclerae.

Patterson-David Syndrome

Birth weight and length are more than 97th percentile, but the weight eventually drops below the third percentile. Affected children have redundant loose folds of skin of the hands and large ears, hands, and feet. In males, the penis is enlarged. A bronzed skin coloration is present. The children have severe mental retardation.

Bannayan-Riley-Ruvalcaba Syndrome

A rare syndrome characterized by macrosomia at birth, with length and weight more than 97th percentile. Growth tends to normalize between 3 and 8 years of age. Macrocephaly, present at birth, continues into adulthood. Mental retardation is present in almost one-half of patients. Almost three-fourths have subcutaneous hamartomas, either lipomas or hemangiomas. Ileal and colonic polyps have been described. Hypotonia is common as are macular hyperpigmented lesions of the glans penis. Inheritance is autosomal dominant.

Weaver Syndrome

This rare syndrome is associated with accelerated growth and prenatal advance-ment of skeletal maturation. The infants described have an unusual appearance characterized by large ears, ocular hypertelorism, mild micrognathia, broad thumbs, and broad forehead. Limited knee and elbow extension and mild hypertonia, with signs of delayed development, are other features.

Proteus Syndrome

A rare disorder in which affected children have asymmetric growth. An unusual thickening of the skin and subcutaneous tissue leads to gyriform convolutions, especially of the feet.

Simpson-Golabi-Behmel Syndrome

Characterized by prenatal onset of striking overgrowth, with ocular hypertelorism, short broad nose, large mouth, and macroglossia. Midline clefts are less common. Macrocephaly continues into childhood. Adults tend to be more than 97th percentile in height. Hypotonia is common. The inheritance is X-linked recessive.

SUGGESTED READING

Frasier SD. Tall stature and excessive growth syndromes. In: Lifshitz F, ed. *Pediatric endocrinology,* 3rd ed. New York: Marcel Dekker, 1996:163–174.

Jones KL. The etiology and diagnosis of overgrowth syndromes. *Growth: Genetics & Hormones* 1994;10:6–10.

Sotos JF. Overgrowth disorders. *Clin Pediatr* 1996;35:517–529.

Sotos JF. Genetic disorders associated with overgrowth. *Clin Pediatr* 1997;36:39–49.

Weaver DD. Overgrowth syndromes and disorders: Definition, classification, and discussion. *Growth: Genetics & Hormones* 1994;10:1–4

5

Anorexia

A brief loss of appetite commonly occurs during acute infections. Prolonged anorexia, accompanied by weight loss or poor weight gain, usually denotes a serious underlying organic or psychological disorder.

The hypothalamus is thought to be the center of appetite control, but the stimuli that influence this control are poorly understood. Nevertheless, the differential diagnosis of anorexia may be simplified by the following categorization into ten groups, including infection and psychosocial factors.

♦ **Most Common Causes of Anorexia**

Parental Expectations   Infections, Acute and Chronic
Response to Stress   Depression
Reflux Esophagitis   Constipation

● **Causes Not to Forget**

Drugs   Crohn Disease
Malignancy   Human Immunodeficiency Virus
Hepatitis   Diencephalic Syndrome

INFECTION

♦ **Acute Infection**

Infection, whether bacterial, viral, or of other types, is the most common cause of acute anorexia in children. Generally, the diminished appetite is short-lived and coincident with the illness.

♦ **Chronic Infection**

Chronic infections may be associated with anorexia over prolonged periods of time, with resulting poor weight gain or weight loss. Pyelonephritis, hidden abscesses, chronic lung infections, tuberculosis, amebiasis, and many other subacute or occult infections may be responsible. Human immunodeficiency virus must not be overlooked.

● **Hepatitis**

Acute and chronic hepatitis from various causes may be associated with anorexia.

PSYCHOSOCIAL FACTORS

♦ Parental Expectations

Some parents may have unrealistic expectations about food consumption by the child, especially the toddler, whose caloric requirements diminish with the deceleration in growth rate normally seen in this age group. The small but normal child may be perceived as anorectic by the parents who want them to grow beyond their genetic capacity.

Parental Pressures

Children may respond to parental over concern about eating by refusing to eat.

♦ Response to Stress

Fear, anger, depression, and mania may result in diminished food intake. Family discord, mealtime disruption and unpleasantness may also affect the appetite.

♦ Psychiatric Disturbances

Anorexia may be present in various forms of mental illness including major depressive disorders, schizophrenia, and paranoid disorders.

Anorexia Nervosa

This striking disorder occurs much more frequently in adolescent girls than boys. Hallmarks in girls include amenorrhea, weight loss, maintenance of or an increase in physical activity, and a distorted body image, in which the child perceives herself to be fat regardless of how thin or emaciated she may be. Onset often follows a change in the child's life such as during trips, separation from the family, or school changes, or an awareness of parental discord. Bradycardia, low blood pressure, and constipation are common. Plasma cortisol levels are usually increased in this disorder, whereas they are decreased in adrenal insufficiency.

Pregnancy

Anorexia and morning sickness may be present in the early months of pregnancy.

Rumination

Characterized by repeated vomiting without gastrointestinal illness. Generally begins during infancy to 15 months.

METABOLIC AND ENDOCRINE DISORDERS

Adrenocortical Insufficiency (Addison Disease)

Adrenocortical insufficiency may be associated with anorexia, fatigue, muscle weakness, postural hypotension, and increased skin pigmentation. The heart rate is generally increased rather than decreased as in anorexia nervosa.

Hypothyroidism

The general demeanor of hypothyroid patients is one of sluggishness, including diminished appetite. Affected children are not generally thin because of decreased metabolic rate.

Diabetes Insipidus

Although affected patients have polydipsia, anorexia is usually present.

Adrenogenital Syndrome

In the salt-losing form in infants, early presenting symptoms are vomiting, weight loss, anorexia, and dehydration.

Lead Poisoning

Chronic plumbism features anorexia with abdominal pain, irritability, and anemia.

Hypercalcemia

Children with hypercalcemia are irritable and anorectic.

Hyperparathyroidism

Symptoms may include nausea, vomiting, abdominal pain, muscle weakness, and polyuria.

Inborn Errors

A number of amino and organic acidurias may have episodes of poor feeding as prominent symptoms.

Pseudohypoaldosteronism

The cause of this unusual disorder is unknown. Biochemically, it is characterized by increased plasma renin and aldosterone levels and renal salt wasting associated with hyponatremia, hyperkalemia, and acidosis. Failure to thrive and lethargy are found in young children.

Hypervitaminosis A

Irritability, pain in the legs and forearms, anorexia, and hepatomegaly are clinical findings.

Dietary Chloride Deficiency

Panhypopituitarism

Polycystic Ovary Syndrome

GASTROINTESTINAL DISORDERS

◆ Constipation

The child with chronic constipation tends to eat less to prevent discomfort elicited by peristaltic activity following meals.

Appendicitis

The anorexia is an early symptom, overshadowed by the abdominal pain.

◆ Esophageal Reflux

Reflux esophagitis should be considered in young children with poor appetites.

Diarrhea

Disorders associated with diarrhea may produce anorexia when the child decreases oral intake to prevent the diarrhea.

Inflammatory Bowel Disease

Ulcerative Colitis

The presenting symptoms are usually bloody diarrhea with pus and mucus and crampy abdominal pain. Anorexia, nausea, and vomiting are later symptoms.

● Regional Enteritis (Crohn Disease)

Chronic inflammation of the bowel and cramps brought on by eating lead to a diminished appetite.

Esophageal Dysfunction

Disordered swallowing may result in anorexia. Achalasia, esophageal strictures, foreign bodies, and tracheo-esophageal fistulas are possible causes.

Liver Failure

Disorders associated with significant acute or chronic insult to the liver may be associated with anorexia.

Obstruction

Distension of the bowel or stomach from obstruction or stenosis may result in anorexia.

Celiac Disease

Anorexia is a common symptom present at the time of diagnosis. Other symptoms include diarrhea, vomiting, abdominal distension, lassitude, weight loss, and irritability.

Superior Mesenteric Artery Syndrome

With significant weight reduction following illness or a prolonged fast, omental fat may be lost, with resulting compression of the duodenum between the superior mesenteric artery and the aorta. The first symptom is often early saiety, and, later, vomiting. Patients may be misdiagnosed as having anorexia nervosa. Imaging studies include delayed emptying of the stomach and dilatation of the duodenum up to the position of the superior mesenteric artery.

Pancreatic Disorders

Pancreatitis and pancreatic pseudo-cyst may be responsible.

Necrotizing Enterocolitis

In the premature infant, refusal to feed may be the first clue.

• MALIGNANCY

Anorexia may be an early sign of an occult malignancy.

CARDIOPULMONARY DISEASE

Congestive Heart Failure

Easy tiring and sweating during feeding is common in infants with congestive heart failure.

Chronic Hypoxemia

Cyanotic congenital heart disease and chronic lung disorders may be associated with anorexia.

Polycythemia

Neonates may present as poor feeders with lethargy and cyanosis.

INFLAMMATORY DISORDERS

Juvenile Rheumatoid Arthritis

Systemic Lupus Erythematosus

Acute Rheumatic Fever

Sarcoidosis

NUTRITIONAL DEFICIENCIES

Iron Deficiency

Anorexia and irritability may be the only symptoms.

Zinc Deficiency

Decreased sensation of taste and smell may lead to anorexia.

Vitamin B$_{12}$ Deficiency

May be seen in children with inborn errors or infants born to mothers with deficient intake of this vitamin during pregnancy.

Kwashiorkor

NEUROLOGIC DISORDERS

Increased Intracranial Pressure

● Diencephalic Syndrome

A tumor in or near the anterior hypothalamus is the usual cause. Children become emaciated and are anorectic; despite their appearance they have a disproportionately happy affect. A vertical nystagmus is often present.

Degenerative Diseases

Neuromuscular Disorders with Defective Swallowing

● DRUGS

A large number of drugs may cause anorexia. The more commonly used drugs include antihistamines, digitalis, antimetabolites, morphine, aminophylline, methylphenidate, amphetamines, diphenylhydantoin, and ephedrine. Alcohol and illicit drugs may be responsible.

MISCELLANEOUS

Renal Failure

Renal Tubular Acidosis

Growth retardation, excessive vomiting, and constipation are additional clues.

Immobilization

Children in traction, casts, or otherwise immobilized may develop hypercalcemia with its attendant problems.

Williams Syndrome

Infants may have hypercalcemia, failure to thrive, irritability, anorexia, a characteristic facies, and heart defects.

SUGGESTED READING

Ulshen MH. Loss of appetite. In: Hoekelman RA, ed. *Primary pediatric care,* 3rd ed. St. Louis: Mosby, 1997:1052–1053.

6

Weight Loss

Growth rates below average for height and weight are common and are related to intrinsic and extrinsic factors, such as genetic potential and an inadequate nurturing environment. Actual loss of weight, unless transient in the course of an acute illness, is a worrisome symptom requiring careful evaluation.

Some of the many disorders that may cause weight loss have been covered in other chapters (see Chapters 3 and 5); this chapter deals primarily with causes of weight loss in children beyond infancy, especially with diseases that may be subtle in presentation.

♦ Most Common Causes of Weight Loss

Infections   Depression
Eating Disorders

● Causes Not to Forget

Inflammatory Bowel Disease   Malignancy
Cystic Fibrosis   Thyrotoxicosis
Chronic Inflammatory Disease   Renal Failure

♦ INFECTION

Acute or chronic infections are the most common causes of weight loss. In acute infections the weight loss is transient, and once the infection clears, the child generally regains the lost weight. Signs and symptoms of acute infections are usually present and recognizable. In chronic infections there may be no obvious signs of illness; a careful evaluation based on history and physical examination may reveal subtle signs and symptoms.

The following chronic infections may be more difficult to detect.

Urinary Tract Infection

Pulmonary Infection

Tuberculosis is less common today.

Abdominal Abscess

Osteomyelitis

Human Immunodeficiency Virus Infection

Must always be considered, even if other symptoms are not present.

GASTROINTESTINAL DISORDERS

Vomiting and diarrhea are obvious symptoms of disturbance that may lead to weight loss. Some disorders, however, may not be associated with blatantly obvious features.

Gastroesophageal Reflux

The reflux may be silent with decreased appetite leading to weight loss.

● Inflammatory Bowel Disease

Although children present with diarrhea, abdominal pain, or rectal bleeding, unexplained weight loss may be the only overt symptom in some. The diarrhea or abdominal cramping may go unnoticed. Early satiety or anorexia may be the prominent symptoms leading to the weight loss. The importance of plotting growth on charts cannot be overstated.

Hepatitis

Chronic hepatitis, resulting in a low-grade smoldering inflammation, may produce anorexia and a general sense of ill health.

Pancreatitis

Recurrent episodes of pancreatic inflammation are generally dramatic but they may pass relatively unnoticed. The location of abdominal pain, usually part of the picture, may vary.

Malabsorption

In addition to fats, carbohydrates and proteins may be poorly absorbed leading to weight loss.

Celiac Disease

This disorder is usually apparent by 3 years of age when the classic triad of steatorrhea, abdominal enlargement, and malnutrition may be noted. Serum antibodies (antigliadin and antiendomysium) are helpful tests.

● Cystic Fibrosis

The abdominal and pulmonary symptoms may not be obvious. If steatorrhea is found a sweat test should be performed.

Constipation

Chronic constipation can affect the appetite and result in decreased appetite with weight loss.

Intestinal Parasites

Giardiasis is a typical parasitic infection that may produce weight loss with a minimum of other symptoms.

Superior Mesenteric Artery Syndrome

Intentional weight loss by dieting or immobilization in a body cast may lead to diminished omental fat, with resultant compression of the duodenum between the superior mesenteric artery and the aorta. The compression creates a sense of early satiety with resultant decreased appetite and weight loss.

PHYSIOLOGIC CAUSES

Dieting

Older children may embark on "fad" diets without their parents knowledge.

Increased Physical Activity

Otherwise healthy-appearing youngsters may lose considerable weight when they are involved in supervised or unsupervised athletic activities. Despite eating their usual or even increased amounts of food at home, weight loss may follow. Despite the weight loss, other symptoms are lacking and they keep up with their peers.

Inadequate Caloric Intake/Malnutrition

EMOTIONAL FACTORS

◆ Depression

Weight loss, loss of interest in activities, and insomnia are warning signals.

◆ Anorexia Nervosa/Bulimia

These problems are more frequent in adolescent girls. Despite the loss of weight they remain active and generally engage in considerable physical activity and exercise. Individuals with anorexia nervosa appear to be superficially interested in food. Those with bulimia binge eat and induce vomiting or take cathartics.

Rumination

Characterized by repeated vomiting without gastrointestinal illness. Generally, this begins during infancy to 15 months.

METABOLIC AND ENDOCRINE DISORDERS

Diabetes Mellitus

Polyphagia, polydipsia, and polyuria are usually present as well.

Addison Disease

Hypoadrenocorticism may mimic anorexia nervosa, but lethargy is a key feature. Skin pigmentation may increase subtly.

• Thyrotoxicosis

The hypermetabolic state may result in weight loss. There may be other signs and symptoms such as tachycardia, tremors, and increased sweating. School disturbances may be part of the picture.

Diabetes Insipidus

Anorexia may accompany the polyuria.

Hypercalcemia

In addition to anorexia, nausea, vomiting, abdominal pain, muscle weakness, and polyuria may be present.

Hypopituitarism

Onset may be later in childhood following encephalitis or as the result of destruction of the hypothalamus by a tumor. The clinical picture may falsely suggest anorexia nervosa.

CARDIOPULMONARY DISEASE

Asthma

Chronic Congestive Heart Failure

Constrictive Pericarditis

Infective Endocarditis

• MALIGNANCY

Occult tumors are often the primary concern of parents whose children are losing weight.

NUTRITIONAL DISORDERS

Iron Deficiency

Anorexia may be a subtle symptom leading to weight loss. Other unusual signs include pagophagia (craving for ice), geophagia (craving for dirt), and the abnormal ingestion of cornstarch.

Zinc Deficiency

Anorexia results from an altered sensation of taste and smell.

NEUROLOGIC CAUSES

Increased Intracranial Pressure

Usually present with other symptoms, especially headache. Pseudotumor cerebri, of various causes, may be subtle and produce anorexia with weight loss. (See Chapter 24, Increased Intracranial Pressure and Bulging Fontanel.)

Degenerative Disorders

Various inherited disorders, such as Wilson disease and Friedreich ataxia, may be associated with weight loss, but neurologic symptoms predominate.

Diencephalic Syndrome

A tumor in or near the anterior hypothalamus is the cause. Despite an emaciated appearance, patients have a happy affect. A vertical nystagmus is often present.

MISCELLANEOUS CAUSES

• Chronic Inflammatory Disease

Patients with connective tissue disorders such as juvenile rheumatoid arthritis and systemic lupus erythematosus may have weight loss as a prominent complaint.

• Renal Failure

Uremia may be subtle.

Drugs

Amphetamines and methylphenidate among other drugs may affect appetite.

Poisonings

Chronic lead and mercury poisonings may cause anorexia and weight loss.

Sarcoidosis

7
Obesity

Obesity is the most common form of malnutrition in the United States. Various studies have found that approximately 10% of prepubertal and 15% of adolescent age groups are obese. Obesity has been defined as a 20% excess of the calculated ideal weight for age, sex, and height. Triceps skinfold thickness measurements have been proposed as a better indicator of obesity than body weight.

Most children (and adults) who are obese have exogenous obesity. In the not-too-distant past, exogenous obesity meant that one simply ate too much. The problem of exogenous obesity is, however, much more complex. Physical activity and genetic influences must be taken into account. Identification of the *ob* gene and its adipocyte specific protein leptin may provide clarification of these relationships in the future. The review by Dietz and Robinson (1) is recommended if your appetite has been whetted.

Perhaps less commonly today than in the past, "glandular" problems are blamed as the cause of obesity. Endocrine causes of obesity are distinctly uncommon and, more importantly, usually can be readily differentiated from exogenous obesity by simple physical examination and an assessment of linear growth. Children with exogenous obesity tend to have an accelerated linear growth, whereas children with endocrine, metabolic, or malformation syndromes are usually short.

♦ **Most Common Causes of Obesity**

Excessive Intake of Calories   Diminished Physical Activity
Genetic Factors

● **Causes Not to Forget**

Prader-Willi Syndrome

EXOGENOUS CAUSES

Most obese children are classified as having exogenous obesity, but there is a great deal of controversy regarding the actual mechanism or mechanisms involved. Implicated in exogenous obesity are the following factors.

♦ **Excessive Intake**

Overeating was previously considered to be the primary cause of obesity, but it is now recognized that an excessive intake beyond caloric requirements is not always operative.

♦ **Diminished Activity**

Failure to utilize the calories taken in results in a gradual increase in fat stores. Forced inactivity, such as after surgery or orthopedic procedures, without a concomitant reduction in calorie intake will result in weight gain.

♦ **Genetic Factors**

The mechanisms involved remain poorly understood, but a familial tendency toward excessive weight is well recognized. In families with obese members, the effects of environment versus those of heredity are still controversial.

ENDOCRINE DISORDERS

Keep in mind that 99% of obesity is related to exogenous causes, as listed previously. The rare disorders associated with obesity are generally associated with short stature, whereas children with exogenous obesity tend to have accelerated linear growth.

Hypothyroidism

This condition is often blamed as the cause of obesity, but seldom is. Evidence of delayed growth with a bone age of less than chronological age separates children with hypothyroidism from those with exogenous obesity.

Hyperadrenocorticism (Cushing Syndrome)

Although most frequently the result of exogenous steroid therapy, hyperadrenocorticism may occur in patients with adrenal tumors or disorders of the hypothalamic-pituitary axis that result in overproduction of adrenocorticotropic hormone. Growth usually decelerates or stops. Truncal obesity, acne, hirsutism, purplish striae, and hypertension are prominent diagnostic clues.

Pancreatic Tumors

Insulinomas may produce hypoglycemia with resultant hyperphagia and secondary obesity. Affected children may be exceptions to the rule regarding metabolic causes of obesity being associated with short stature.

Growth Hormone Deficiency

Fat accumulation, if it occurs, involves the trunk and buttocks.

Hypothalamic Lesions

A number of lesions affecting the hypothalamus may result in hyperphagia and obesity. Injury to the hypothalamus may occur following inflammatory disorders, such as encephalitis, arachnoiditis, sarcoidosis, and tuberculosis, and with craniopharyngiomas, optic gliomas, Langerhans histiocytosis, pituitary tumors, and leukemia.

Central Nervous System Disorders

Hydrocephalus, pseudotumor cerebri, pinealomas, porencephalic cysts, meningeal leukemia, and trauma have been implicated as causes of obesity.

Fröhlich Syndrome (Adipsogenital Dystrophy)

This rare disorder is caused by a hypothalamic tumor resulting in polyphagia, dwarfism, hypogonadism, and optic atrophy.

Polycystic Ovary Syndrome (Stein-Leventhal)

Girls with this syndrome have polycystic ovaries and are overweight. Hirsutism occurs in 50% of those affected. Some girls may show signs of virilization.

Pseudohypoparathyroidism Type 1 (Albright Hereditary Osteodystrophy)

This disorder is characterized by short stature, moderate obesity, mental deficiency, short fourth and fifth metacarpal bones, and variable hypocalcemia and hyperphosphatemia.

Pseudopseudohypoparathyroidism

The physical appearance is that of pseudohypoparathyroidism, but the children are normocalcemic.

CHROMOSOMAL ABNORMALITIES

Klinefelter Syndrome (XXY Karyotype)

In childhood, boys with this abnormality have a tendency toward long limbs and are tall and slim. Only as adults do they become obese, if they have not received testosterone therapy. The testes remain small.

Turner Syndrome (XO Karyotype)

Some girls with the XO karyotype may be short and overweight.

Down Syndrome

• Prader-Willi Syndrome

Hypotonia, bizarre eating habits, hypogonadism, mental deficiency, small hands and feet, and obesity are characteristic. This disorder is most commonly caused by a deletion in chromosome 15, usually of paternal origin.

XXXXY Karyotype

This abnormality may occasionally be associated with obesity. Wide-set eyes, mental deficiency, a low nasal bridge, small penis, hypoplastic scrotum, and limited elbow movement are prominent features.

CONGENITAL OR INHERITED DISORDERS ASSOCIATED WITH OBESITY

Laurence-Moon Syndrome (Bardet-Biedl Syndrome)

Prominent features include truncal obesity, mental retardation, polydactyly and syndactyly, hypogonadism, and retinitis pigmentosa. Height is less than average.

Beckwith-Wiedemann Syndrome

Infants and children with this inherited disorder generally grow excessively and may appear obese. Macroglossia, visceromegaly, an omphalocele or umbilical abnormality, and neonatal hypoglycemia are common.

Carpenter Syndrome

Findings include obesity, mental deficiency, brachydactyly, preaxial polydactyly, and syndactyly. The shape of the skull is usually abnormal secondary to craniostenosis.

Cohen Syndrome

In this rare syndrome, obesity becomes apparent in mid-childhood. Hypotonia, weakness, mental deficiency, a high nasal bridge, narrow hands and feet, and prominent central incisors are present.

Grebe Syndrome

Children with this rare, inherited syndrome have obese and very short limbs, very short fingers, and hypoplastic bones of the arms and legs.

Alström-Hallgren Syndrome

An autosomal recessively inherited disorder whose characteristics include obesity from infancy, progressive loss of vision, and, later, progressive neurosensory hearing loss. Other features include diabetes mellitus, small testes in males, and progressive nephropathy in adults.

MISCELLANEOUS CAUSES

Glycogen Storage Disease, Type I (von Gierke Disease)

Children with this disorder may appear obese. The abdomen is protuberant because of massive hepatomegaly.

Mucopolysaccharidoses

Children with Hurler or Hunter syndrome may appear obese, but striking features of these disorders should make the diagnosis obvious.

REFERENCE

1. Dietz WH, Robinson TN. Assessment and treatment of childhood obesity. *Pediatr Rev* 1993;14:337–344.

SUGGESTED READING

Gortmaker SL, Must A, Perrin JM, Sobol AM, Dietz WH. Social and economic consequences of overweight in adolescence and young adulthood. *N Engl J Med* 1993;329:1008–1012.
Hassink SG, Sheslow DV, de Lancey E, Opentanova I, Considine RV, Caro JF. Serum leptin in children with obesity: relationship to gender and development. *Pediatrics* 1996;98:201–203.

8
Fatigue

Fatigue is characterized by a general state of decreased endurance for or interest in activities and is usually associated with tiredness, irritability, and sleepiness. It is important to characterize the child's or parent's complaint sufficiently to distinguish fatigue from lethargy, weakness, and decreased endurance. While fatigue is a common complaint by teenagers (and about them by their parents!), persistent lethargy, weakness, and decreased endurance are not. Lethargy that appears constant may be due to depression of sensorium, such as might be caused by increased intracranial pressure or drugs/toxins. Weakness, particularly if progressive, suggests a disorder affecting muscles or nerves; decreased endurance may simply be a matter of conditioning but may also reflect limited cardiac (e.g., cardiomyopathy) or pulmonary (e.g., asthma, cystic fibrosis) reserve. This chapter focuses on fatigue.

Physiologic causes of fatigue, such as lack of restorative sleep, excessive exercise, or inadequate caloric intake, or infections are frequently blamed for this symptom. During adolescence, metabolic demands are increased yet sleep is decreased, due to a later bedtime; sleep deprivation is the norm, and fatigue is commonly the result. Caloric insufficiency is more likely a cause of fatigue in young children, because their energy stores are more rapidly depleted. In addition to these physiologic causes, depression should be considered, particularly in adolescents, in whom depression often goes unrecognized. As many as 20% of adults describe themselves as fatigued, of whom about 50% have depression preceding the fatigue.

♦ **Most Common Causes of Fatigue**

Lack of Sleep/Physiologic

Infection: Particularly Epstein-Barr Virus (EBV)

Caloric Deficiency

Depression/Psychologic

Anemia

Excessive Exercise

● **Causes Not to Forget**

Allergies   Pregnancy

Intussusception

The following classification is not a comprehensive one, but is intended to suggest several general categories for consideration in the differential diagnosis of children with fatigue, particularly chronic fatigue.

PHYSIOLOGIC CAUSES

♦ Lack of Sleep or Rest

Particularly a problem in adolescents to whom a late bedtime is considered a rite of passage from "babyhood" but whose rising time is as early or earlier than during childhood. This decrease in restorative sleep is compounded by the increased metabolic demands of growth and physiologic changes.

♦ Excessive Exercise

♦ Insufficient Caloric Intake

Kwashiorkor is the end stage in the spectrum of nutritional deficiency.

Obesity

Overweight children tend to have decreased endurance compared to children of normal weight. Rarely, significantly obese children may have excessive and dangerous periods of somnolence with elevated $PaCO_2$ levels (Pickwickian syndrome).

♦ Anemia

A significant reduction in oxygen-carrying capacity of the blood will result in fatigue. The onset may be insidious.

● Pregnancy

The pregnancy may not be known to the individual or family.

Polycythemia

Neonates with polycythemia are frequently lethargic with cyanosis and feeding problems.

♦ INFECTIOUS CAUSES

Any bacterial, viral, or other infection may be associated with fatigue. The following infections, both acute and chronic, are particularly noteworthy.

♦ Infectious Mononucleosis

This is probably the most commonly suspected cause of fatigue in adolescents. EBV is the usual agent responsible, but other viruses, such as cytomegalovirus (CMV), human herpesvirus 6 (HHV-6), and human immunodeficiency virus (HIV), also may cause a similar syndrome.

♦ Chronic EBV Infection

Recurrent episodes of fever, pharyngitis, malaise, and adenopathy occur in the presence of persistently elevated antiearly antigen. A second syndrome occurs primarily in teenagers who are chronically exhausted. Malignancy is frequently mistaken for this syndrome. Chronic EBV infection is not synonymous with chronic fatigue syndrome, which is usually not associated with persistence of antiearly antigen EBV antibodies.

Hepatitis

Various disorders may cause disruption of liver function. Hepatitis A and B are both relatively common causes. Fatigue may be the initial and the most prominent symptom.

HIV Infection
Tuberculosis

Signs and symptoms other than fatigue may be minimal.

Lyme Disease
CMV Infection

The acquired form must be considered as a cause of seronegative mononucleosis.

Meningitis
Encephalitis
Bacteremia
Histoplasmosis
Toxoplasmosis
Brucellosis

Weight loss, low-grade fever, and back pain are among the subtle symptoms of chronic brucellosis.

Intestinal Parasites

Fatigue may result from interference with various body functions, such as food digestion and absorption or blood loss.

♦ PSYCHOLOGICAL FACTORS

Fatigue is a common presenting symptom of depression, although in many cases other signs and symptoms have been ignored.

● ALLERGY

Allergic individuals commonly seem fatigued. Clinical signs of allergy may be mistaken for other disorders: rhinorrhea and cough for infection, and allergic "shiners" (dark circles under the eyes) for lack of sleep.

Tension-Fatigue Syndrome

Intolerance to certain foods has been suggested to cause various symptoms including recurrent abdominal pain, headaches, and growing pains, in addition to fatigue.

Asthma

Chronic low-grade bronchospasm may be responsible for fatigue. Wheezing may not be clinically evident.

ENDOCRINE DISORDERS

Hypothyroidism

Hyperthroidism

Initial overactivity soon leads to fatigue. Tachycardia, increased sweating, tremor, and systolic hypertension are important clues.

Adrenocortical Insufficiency

Progressive weakness and hyperpigmentation are usually present.

Cushing Syndrome

Adrenocortical excess leads to metabolic changes and fatigue. Obesity and growth retardation are common features.

Primary Aldosteronism

Potassium loss results in muscle weakness and fatigue.

DRUGS

Many kinds of drugs may produce fatigue. Important groups to consider include antihistamines, anticonvulsants, tranquilizers, and opiates.

TOXIC AGENTS

Lead Poisoning

METABOLIC DISORDERS

Hypoglycemia

Fatigue, irrational behavior, irritability, headaches, and seizures may be symptoms of hypoglycemia.

Diabetes Mellitus

Poorly controlled disease results in insufficient fuel for energy and excessive water and mineral losses.

Inborn Errors of Metabolism

Fatigue is rarely recognized because of the generally early age at onset and the presence of more dramatic symptoms such as vomiting, lethargy, convulsions, and coma.

GASTROINTESTINAL DISORDERS

• Intussusception

Primarily seen in infants and children to 3 years of age, this condition is characterized by intermittent episodes of abdominal pain (and drawing up of the legs), diarrhea with currant-jelly stools late in the course, and a "sausage-shaped" mass in the right side of the abdomen. Lethargy and fatigue, described as a "knocked-out" appearance, may also be present and may constitute the major or only sign.

Inflammatory Bowel Disease

Both regional enteritis and ulcerative colitis are frequently associated with impressive fatigue before the onset of other symptoms.

Liver Disease

Fatigue may be an early finding in infectious or metabolic or physiologic disorders that interfere with liver function.

COLLAGEN-VASCULAR DISEASES

Juvenile Rheumatoid Arthritis

Fatigue in children with this disease is frequently more severe than expected with the degree of involvement.

Systemic Lupus Erythematosus

Dermatomyositis

Muscle weakness, pain, and fatigue are early symptoms. Look for erythematous papules (Gottron papules) over the knuckles.

Progressive Systemic Sclerosis

CARDIOVASCULAR DISORDERS

Congestive Heart Failure

Easy fatigability, tachypnea, tachycardia, and dyspnea on exertion are prominent signs.

Pericarditis

Fatigue and dyspnea may precede other physical signs including the friction rub.

Cyanotic Congenital Heart Disease

Cardiomyopathies

Endocarditis

Primary Pulmonary Hypertension

Fatigue and dyspnea are the prominent symptoms.

RENAL DISEASE

Uremia

Anorexia, nausea, vomiting, and fatigue are common symptoms.

Renal Tubular Acidosis

In both early-onset and late-onset forms, fatigue and weakness are common. Growth retardation, anorexia, polyuria, and rickets eventually appear.

MISCELLANEOUS CAUSES

Boredom

May be mistaken for fatigue, particularly in school.

Chronic Fatigue Syndrome

The cause of this oft impugned disorder is still not clear. Many infections have been blamed, including EBV, CMV, herpes simplex virus (HSV), but no direct causal relationship has been found. Some studies have shown an association with neurally mediated hypotension (1).

Pulmonary Disease

Any lung disorder interfering with gas exchange or resulting in chronic inflammation may be associated with fatigue. Children with cystic fibrosis are fatigued, but cough, diarrhea, and other symptoms are more prominent.

Malignancy

Children with leukemia, lymphoma, central nervous system and other solid tumors may manifest fatigability as an early symptom of their disease.

Myasthenia Gravis

Muscle weakness and fatigue are prominent features.

Sleep Apnea-Hypersomnia Syndrome (Tonsillar-Adenoidal Hypertrophy)

The mass of posterior pharyngeal lymphoid tissue may be large enough to compromise air exchange, particularly during sleep. Snoring and retractions during inspiration are usually impressive. Fatigue and lethargy often characterize the waking state.

Familial Periodic Paralysis

Episodic attacks of flaccid paralysis and areflexia, occurring mostly at night, are characteristic. Although the attacks may only last a few hours, fatigue may follow the episodes.

Fibromyalgia

A poorly understood, but well-described disorder, more common in adults. Particular muscles are painful to palpation.

Sarcoidosis

REFERENCE

1. Bou-Holaigah I, Rowe PC, Kan J, Calkin H. The relationship between neurally mediated hypotension and the chronic fatigue syndrome. *JAMA* 1995;274:961–967.

9
Irritability/Excessive Crying

All children, as well as adults, have episodes of irritability at various times for various reasons. Stressful situations, infections, trauma, pain, hunger, and bodily dysfunctions are only a few of the causes. This chapter focuses on causes of irritability that are relatively long lasting; "irritable" here refers to those children who are unable to be soothed.

Infants, who cannot communicate their discomfort, wants, or needs, present a group to whom special attention may need to be directed. Their irritability is usually manifested by excessive or persistent crying. In this age group, disorders associated with the acute onset of crying will also be emphasized.

The tension produced by an unconsolable child often leads to a great deal of family discord and may result in child abuse if the symptom is prolonged. Although psychosocial disruption is a relatively common cause of irritability, particularly in infants, the disruptions may also be produced by the persistent crying of the child; this relationship should be considered in the evaluation. Clues of bodily as well as psychological dysfunction must be sought in the differential diagnosis of irritability.

♦ **Most Common Causes of Excessive Crying and Irritability in Infants**

Hunger	Otitis Media
Infantile Colic	Anal Fissure
Gastroesophageal Reflux	Unrecognized Fracture
Constipation	Drug Withdrawal in Neonates

● **Causes Not to Forget in Infants**

Other Infections: Osteomyelitis; Meningitis; Urinary Tract; Congenital Syphilis

Testicular Torsion	Corneal Abrasion; Foreign Body in Eye
Incarcerated Hernia	Increased Intracranial Pressure
Bowel Obstruction	Urinary Retention
Hair Tourniquet (Digit or Penis)	Shaken Baby Syndrome
Congenital Glaucoma	Milk Protein Allergy

53

♦ **Most Common Causes in Older Children**

Stress	Depression
Mismatched Parental-Child Temperament	Attention Deficit Hyperactivity Disorder
Infections	Migraine

● **Causes Not to Forget in Older Children**

Fractures	Iron Deficiency Anemia
Drugs	Increased Intracranial Pressure
Constipation	Chronic Inflammation: Juvenile Rheumatoid Arthritis, Crohn Disease

BEHAVIORAL AND PSYCHOSOCIAL FACTORS

♦ **Stress**

♦ **Depression**

♦ **Altered Parent-Child Interaction**

The child may be vulnerable to a number of familial disruptions resulting in irritability from a loss of security.

♦ **Mismatch of Temperaments**

The irritable child may not fit into the family structure and personalities.

Marital Discord

● **Battered Child**

Infants who are shaken may show no external signs of abuse. Check for retinal hemorrhages.

Unwanted Child

♦ **Attention Deficit Hyperactivity Disorder**

Hyperactivity and learning disabilities may create frustrations for the child as well as the parents.

Infantile Autism

Autistic children are resistant to changes and may fail to respond to human contact, even from their parents.

♦ **INFECTIONS**

Any infectious process may result in irritability. Generally, the onset is rather acute and the irritability coincident with the duration of the infectious process. A few noteworthy examples are meningitis, encephalitis, otitis media, urinary tract infection, osteomyelitis, acute cerebellar ataxia, measles, diskitis, endocarditis, perianal cellulitis, and the staphylococcal "scalded-skin" syndrome.

SKELETAL DISORDERS

◆ Fractures

Inapparent fractures, especially the "toddler fracture" (a spiral fracture of the lower leg often not detected on radiographs for 1 week to 10 days), may cause the child to be irritable.

● Arthritis

Young children with unrecognized arthritis are usually irritable.

Infantile Cortical Hyperostosis (Caffey Disease)

Onset of symptoms in this rare disorder is before 6 months of age and is characterized by bony swelling, most commonly of the mandible and sternum, but any part of the skeleton may be affected. Soft tissues over the involved bone are usually swollen. The child is often febrile and usually irritable. This disorder has become rare, for unknown reasons.

METABOLIC DISORDERS

Hypoglycemia

Symptoms of hypoglycemia may include restlessness and irritability as well as lethargy, pallor, and seizures.

Hypocalcemia

In addition to irritability, infants are described as "jittery."

Hypercalcemia

Hyponatremia

Water intoxication, for various reasons, is a relatively common cause of hyponatremia.

Hypernatremia

Hypervitaminosis A

Excessive intake of vitamin A may result in irritability, bone pain, and increased intracranial pressure.

Acrodermatitis Enteropathica

Prominent features include skin lesions ranging from bullae to verrucous plaques, especially on the distal limbs, perioral regions, and the perineum, and hair loss and diarrhea. Irritability and emotional disturbances are common along with photophobia, stomatitis, and paronychiae. The average age of onset is 9 months. The serum zinc and alkaline phosphatase are low.

Scurvy

Irritability is the result of bone pain from periosteal bleeding.

Phenylketonuria

If newborn screening has not been done, a quick screening test may be performed by adding a few drops of ferric chloride to an aliquot of urine, producing a blue-green color. Irritability may be seen in infancy.

Gaucher Disease

The juvenile form features gradually increasing dementia during middle or late childhood, often with behavioral changes and irritability, seizures, and extrapyramidal signs. Organomegaly is mild.

Glutaric Aciduria Type I

Infants and young children may present acutely with apnea and retinal and central nervous system bleeding. More commonly they present with dystonia.

Acute Intermittent Porphyria

Symptoms include attacks of neurologic dysfunction, abdominal pain, constipation, sweating, labile hypertension, back or limb pain, and irritability.

Hypophosphatasia

The hypoplastic fragile bones are easily broken, resulting in irritability.

Pompe Disease (Glycogen Storage Disease, Type II)

The heart becomes massively enlarged, and affected children usually die by 1 year of age. Skeletal muscles are also involved. Rock-hard calf muscles in an infant with congestive heart failure may be a clue to this diagnosis.

Pheochromocytoma

During intermittent release of epinephrine and norepinephrine by the tumor, children may be irritable, pale, and sweaty and may vomit and complain of headache along with their hypertension.

Vitamin B₆ (Pyridoxine) Dependency

Symptoms usually develop in the perinatal period and include convulsions, hyper-irritability, hyperacusis, and feeding difficulties.

Tryptophan Malabsorption

A bluish discoloration of the diapers may be noted in infancy. Other features include failure to thrive, unexplained fevers, infections, constipation, and irritability.

Hyperammonemia

Vomiting, lethargy, and coma are associated with increased ammonia levels following protein ingestion. In early stages, however, children may have an agitated delirium. Other manifestations of hyperammonemic disorders are mental retardation and seizures.

Hyperglycinemia, Nonketotic

Lethargy usually appears in the first few days of life with convulsions shortly thereafter. The few children described were microcephalic, severely retarded, and irritable.

Argininemia

Periodic lethargy and irritability have been described in most patients. The onset may be delayed until 2 or 3 years of age or may be within the first 6 months.

Tyrosinemia

The onset is usually between 2 and 7 months of age with fever, irritability, lethargy, failure to thrive, hepatomegaly, vomiting, edema, and ascites. Death usually occurs before 1 year of age.

Pyruvate Carboxylase Deficiency with Lactic Acidemia

Infants are normal at birth, but development is slow. By 1 year of age, failure to thrive, vomiting, irritability, apathy, hypotonia, areflexia, spasticity, and seizures become apparent.

Biotin Deficiency

In addition to irritability, findings include periorificial dermatitis, conjunctivitis, alopecia, and hypotonia.

Argininosuccinic Lyase Deficiency

The subacute form presents a Reye syndromelike picture with vomiting, lethargy, and irritability progressing to coma. Infants have significant hepatomegaly.

Krabbe Disease

Globoid cell leukodystrophy begins acutely at 4 to 6 years of age with restlessness, irritability, and progressive stiffness. Convulsions develop later.

GASTROINTESTINAL DISORDERS

♦ **Constipation**

♦ **Anal Fissure**

Irritability may be associated with defecation in infants. Bright red blood is often present on the stool.

♦ **Gastroesophageal Reflux (Esophagitis)**

A history of regurgitation may be minimal.

● **Bowel Obstruction (Incarcerated Hernia, Volvulus, etc.)**

Gluten-Induced Enteropathy (Celiac Disease)

The classic picture is one of irritability with failure to thrive; stools are greasy, foul-smelling, and bulky. The onset ranges from late infancy to early childhood. A small percentage of children may have constipation. Irritability may be a primary feature.

♦ **Intussusception**

DRUGS, POISONING, AND TOXINS

♦ **Narcotic Withdrawal**

Neonates may demonstrate symptoms of withdrawal from drugs taken by the mother during pregnancy. Irritability, tremors, diarrhea, and a shrill cry are common.

● **Drugs**

Commonly used drugs that may produce irritability include stimulants (theophylline, amphetamines, ephedrine), imipramine, salicylates, and paradoxical effects of depressants (phenobarbital, phenothiazines, and antihistamines).

Lead Poisoning

Carbon Monoxide Poisoning

Fetal Alcohol Syndrome

Phencyclidine Poisoning

Lethargy, ataxia, miosis, a trancelike stare, increased salivation, and hypertension are symptoms in addition to irritability.

Mercury Poisoning (Acrodynia)

Prominent symptoms include irritability, restlessness, anorexia, hypertension, and excessive sweating. A pink macular rash may be seen, or one resembling miliaria.

Scorpion Bite

Restlessness and extreme agitation are common.

Chinese Restaurant Syndrome

Monosodium glutamate is the causative agent. Dizziness, sweating, flushing, headaches, and palpitations are prominent symptoms.

NEUROLOGIC DISORDERS

● **Increased Intracranial Pressure**

Subdural Hematoma or Effusion

◆ **Migraine**

Diagnosis is especially difficult in infants and young children.

Convulsions

Brain Stem Tumors

Even before increased intracranial pressure is evident, irritability may be noted.

Encephalitis

Cerebral Contusions

Infants who are shaken usually show no cutaneous evidence of trauma. Retinal hemorrhages are an important clue.

Neurologic Impairment

Children who are neurologically impaired for various reasons, may be excessively irritable.

Degenerative Diseases

Deterioration of cerebral function may be associated with irritability in several disorders.

Chiari Type 1 Malformation

The more common presenting complaints in children or adults are headache, neck pain, weakness, or ataxia. Infants may present with crying.

HEMATOLOGIC DISORDERS

• Iron Deficiency

Children with iron deficiency may be more irritable than children whose iron stores are sufficient.

Sickle Cell Anemia

Vaso-occlusive crises produce extreme irritability. Dactylitis with the hand-foot syndrome is a relatively common presentation.

Leukemia

Hemolytic-Uremic Syndrome

A hemolytic anemia with thrombocytopenia, hypertension, convulsions, and renal failure may follow a diarrheal illness.

CARDIAC DISEASE

Congestive Heart Failure

Supraventricular Tachycardia

During attacks young children may be fretful.

Endocardial Fibroelastosis

Irritability may precede cardiac symptoms.

Tetralogy of Fallot

During hypoxic attacks, children are anxious and irritable.

Myocardial Infarction

In infancy sweating, circumoral pallor, and irritability may be subtle signs. Older children may have chest pain as a helpful clue.

Anomalous Origin of Coronary Artery

MISCELLANEOUS CONDITIONS

♦ Infantile Colic

Colic is a much-invoked but poorly understood condition characterized by episodes of uncontrollable crying with drawing up of the legs. The cause is uncertain and probably of multiple origins. Colic usually resolves by 3 months of age.

- **Hidden Food Allergy**

  Allergic symptoms may be obvious or at times covert, including unexplained irritability. Allergy is difficult to prove except by elimination of and re-exposure to various food products. Cow milk has been implicated as a cause of "colic."

- **Atopic Dermatitis**

  Pruritus, characteristic of this disorder, makes the child irritable but also elicits the scratching that results in the rash. It is an "itch that rashes." Any chronic pruritic condition may result in irritability.

- **Corneal Abrasions**

  Particularly in infants, the discomfort may manifest as irritability.

- **Glaucoma**

  Infants and children with glaucoma are irritable and have photophobia, tearing, and an enlarged, steamy cornea.

- **Urinary Retention**

  May be the result of posterior urethral valves, constipation, and drugs as well as other causes.

- **Testicular Torsion**

  Includes torsion of the testicular appendix. A bluish, tender dot on the skin of the scrotum above the testicle may be a clue of the latter.

SGA (Small for Gestational Age) Infants

Beginning at a few weeks after birth, SGA infants often seem irritable and cry excessively for hours on end. The irritability may last as long as 9 months.

Respiratory Failure

Increasing agitation may indicate impending respiratory failure.

Spider Bite

Kwashiorkor/Improper or Inadequate Intake

Hyperthyroidism

Deafness

Young children who are deaf may become frustrated and irritable.

Urticaria Pigmentosa (Mastocytosis)

The release of histamine from the mast cells may produce cutaneous flushing and diarrhea accompanied by irritability.

Familial Dysautonomia

Suggestive findings include absent lacrimation, absent filiform papillae on the tongue, recurrent aspiration, unexplained fevers, and postural hypotension. Affected children generally are Ashkenazi Jews.

Lipogranulomatosis

The cardinal feature is discrete, lumpy masses over the wrists and ankles. Hoarseness occurs early; later findings include noisy respirations, restricted joint movement, delayed development, irritability, and recurrent pulmonary infections leading to death.

Smith-Lemli-Opitz Syndrome

Important features include anteverted nares, ptosis, hypospadias and cryptorchidism, syndactyly of the second and third toes, microcephaly, and mental retardation.

DeLange Syndrome

Striking phenotypic features are anteverted nares, hirsutism, downturned corners of the mouth, mottled skin, growling cry, and limb abnormalities.

SUGGESTED READING

Berezin S, Glassman MS, Bostwick H, Halata M. Esophagitis as a cause of infant colic. *Clin Pediatr* 1995;34:158–159.
Listernick R, Tomita T. Persistent crying in infancy as a presentation of Chiari type 1 malformation. *J Pediatr* 1991;118:567–569.
Mendelsohn MJ. Persistent crying and colic. In: Gartner JC Jr, Zitelli BJ, eds. *Common & chronic symptoms in pediatrics.* St. Louis: Mosby, 1997:41–50.
Poole SR. The infant with acute, unexplained, excessive crying. *Pediatrics* 1991;88:450–455.

10

Lymphadenopathy/Lymphadenitis

An enlarged lymph node is usually defined as one that is greater than 1 cm in its largest diameter; however, epitrochlear nodes are considered enlarged if they measure more than 0.5 cm and inguinal nodes if they are more than 1.5 cm in diameter. Lymph nodes are easily palpated in children, particularly because nodal response to a variety of stimuli is rapid and often prolific in children compared to that in adults. Normal children, even newborns, may have small but palpable nodes. The peak of lymphoid tissue development is between the ages of 8 and 12 years. Lymphoid tissue begins to decrease in size during adolescence.

Lymphadenitis refers to inflammation of one or more lymph nodes, usually the result of infection, and is more likely to be localized than generalized. Systemic viral infections are more likely to cause generalized enlargement than any other type of infection. To many parents, however, enlarged lymph nodes suggest a malignant disorder, and they should be carefully reassured when the cause is merely infectious.

Nodes should be carefully palpated to determine consistency and tenderness. Asymmetry of regions containing enlarged nodes should be noted, as should overlying tissue swelling and erythema. The movability of the nodes should also be noted. Fixed nodes or matted nodes have more worrisome associations than freely movable lymph nodes. Sequential measurements of the nodes should be performed if the cause of enlargement is not clear.

In this chapter, lymphadenopathy has been divided into two principal categories, generalized and regional. All infectious causes have not been enumerated. In addition, it would be unnecessarily repetitious to include localized infectious and inflammatory disorders under each regional subsection.

♦ **Generalized Lymphadenopathy: Most Common Causes**

Benign Lymphoid Hypertrophy   Pseudogeneralized
Chronic Skin Irritation (Atopic Dermatitis)   Systemic Infections

● **Causes Not to Forget**

Drug Reactions   Collagen Vascular Disorders

GENERALIZED LYMPHADENOPATHY

♦ Benign Lymphoid Hypertrophy

This is probably the most common cause of lymphadenopathy in children. The enlarged nodes represent a benign response to minor infections, particularly upper respiratory infections.

♦ Pseudogeneralized

Regional adenopathy in several areas, of different causes, such as posterior cervical adenitis from scalp irritation, and axillary or inguinal adenopathy from extremity abrasions or infections, may give the appearance of generalized lymphadenopathy.

♦ Systemic Infections

Generalized lymphadenopathy commonly occurs in a variety of systemic infections, particularly viral. In some cases regional adenopathy may be more prominent.

Bacterial Infection

Sepsis, salmonellosis, scarlet fever, Lyme disease, brucellosis, syphilis, leptospirosis, typhoid fever, and plague may all cause generalized lymph node enlargement.

Streptococcosis

Chronic streptococcal infection in young children may feature excoriative rhinorrhea, prolonged fever, weight loss, and generalized adenopathy.

Viral Infection

Rubella, rubeola, infectious mononucleosis, infectious hepatitis, cytomegalovirus, and enteroviruses are common causes.

Human Immunodeficiency Virus

Special consideration must be given to this infection.

Other Infections

Mycoplasma, tuberculosis, toxoplasmosis, histoplasmosis, malaria, trypanosomiasis, schistosomiasis, and rickettsial diseases may produce nodal enlargement.

Skin Disorders

Chronic irritation of the skin will lead to adenopathy in lymph drainage areas. Children with atopic dermatitis tend to have generalized adenopathy, more prominent with subtle secondary infections.

● **Drug Reactions**

Various drugs may produce generalized lymphadenopathy.

Diphenylhydantoin

Deserves special recognition in this category.

Other Drugs

Aspirin, barbiturates, penicillin, tetracycline, iodides, cephalosporins, sulfonamides, and mesantoin are a few that have been reported to cause nodal enlargement.

● **Collagen-Vascular Diseases**

Juvenile Rheumatoid Arthritis

The adenopathy is more prominent during the acute phase of the illness. The systemic form of juvenile rheumatoid arthritis, Still disease, has more prominent adenopathy.

Systemic Lupus Erythematosus

Malignancies

Acute Stem Cell Leukemias

Neuroblastoma

Occasionally, adenopathy is the first physical abnormality.

Langerhans Cell Histiocytosis

Immunologic Disorders

Acquired Immune Deficiency Syndrome (AIDS)

Prominent features include recurrent, opportunistic infections, failure to thrive, and hepatosplenomegaly.

Serum Sickness

Arthralgias, arthritis, fever, and an urticarial rash occur after sensitization to foreign proteins, often drugs. Serum sicknesslike reactions may occur with hepatitis B infection and antibiotic therapy with cephalosporins, particularly cefaclor.

Autoimmune Hemolytic Anemia

During episodes of hemolysis the lymph nodes may become greatly enlarged but not tender.

Chronic Granulomatous Disease

Children with this disorder have multiple, chronically enlarged nodes that frequently suppurate due to infection with pyogenic organisms.

Wiskott-Aldrich Syndrome

Common Variable Immunodeficiency

Immunoblastic Lymphadenopathy

This disorder occurs mainly in adults; features resemble those of Hodgkin disease. Fever, sweats, weight loss, and hepatosplenomegaly are common; there may be a hemolytic anemia as well as hyperglobulinemia.

Hyper IgE Syndrome

Storage Diseases

Hepatosplenomegaly is also present.

Gaucher Disease

Niemann-Pick Disease

Wolman Disease

Farber Disease

Tangier Disease

Hepatosplenomegaly, large yellowish gray or orange-colored tonsils, and peripheral neuropathy are also found.

Endocrine Disorders

Hyperthyroidism

Adrenal Insufficiency

Miscellaneous Causes

Gianotti-Crosti Syndrome

Papulonodular lesions in an acral distribution, on the face and extremities, adenopathy, and hepatomegaly are common findings. Hepatitis B virus has been suggested as the pathogenic organism, particularly in Europe and Japan, but other infectious agents are responsible in North America.

Sarcoidosis

Chédiak-Higashi Syndrome

In this autosomal recessive disorder there is an increased susceptibility to pyogenic infections. Partial albinism with related ocular signs and progressive hepatosplenomegaly are also found.

Sinus Histiocytosis

This benign disorder is characterized by massively enlarged lymph nodes that appear over a few week's time; the cause is poorly understood. Children under 10 years of age are affected most often. Laboratory findings include anemia, neutrophilia, an increased sedimentation rate, and elevated serum concentration of IgG.

Angiofollicular Lymph Node Hyperplasia

A rare, benign tumor of unknown origin. The plasma cell type can be associated with systemic signs and symptoms: fever, malaise, anemia, hyperglobulinemia, and increased sedimentation rate.

REGIONAL ADENOPATHY

Cervical Region

Viral Infections of the Upper Respiratory Tract

These are the most common causes of cervical adenopathy. The nodes are usually soft and slightly tender.

Other Viral Infections

Patients with infectious mononucleosis, cytomegalovirus infection, rubella, rubeola, varicella, and hepatitis A or B, frequently have prominent cervical nodes, more often posterior than anterior cervical.

Bacterial Infections

The nodes are usually tender; erythema of the overlying skin is frequently seen. Pharyngeal infections, particularly with streptococci, commonly produce cervical adenitis. Staphylococci are often recovered from involved nodes. Patients with diphtheria may present with a "bull-neck" appearance.

Cat-Scratch Disease

The involved nodes are often red and tender and they frequently suppurate. Fever, malaise, and headache follow a kitten scratch by days to weeks. A papule or papulovesicle should be searched for on the skin area that drains to the regional node.

Parasitic Infections

Toxoplasmosis may mimic infectious mononucleosis. Sore throat is not prominent. The lymphadenitis usually involves a solitary lymph node, without systemic symptoms.

Mycobacterial Infections

Tuberculosis

The incidence of scrofula has decreased in recent years. Bilateral nodal enlargement is common.

Atypical Mycobacteria

Nodal enlargement is usually unilateral.

Fungal Infections

Aspergillosis, cryptococcosis, histoplasmosis, and coccidioidomycosis have been implicated.

Mucocutaneous Lymph Node Syndrome (Kawasaki)

Fever, rash, conjunctival injection, fissured lips, and, later, peeling of the finger tips are prominent features. The cervical adenitis is nonsuppurative and generally a single node.

Malignancies

Lymphoma and Leukemia

Adenopathy tends to be bilateral. Nodes are painless and firm.

Hodgkin Disease

Unilateral involvement is typical.

Carcinoma of the Thyroid

Papillary carcinoma of the thyroid is the most common thyroid carcinoma in children. Cervical node enlargement is frequently present. Medullary carcinoma of the thyroid may be associated with multiple endocrine neoplasia syndrome, type IIb. A clue is lumpiness of the lips secondary to neuromas. The children may have a marfanoid habitus.

Lymphangioma or Hemangioma

Generally, these tumors can be distinguished from lymph nodes. Lymphangiomas are soft and easily compressed. Hemangiomas are firmer. Deep hemangiomas may be more difficult to differentiate. They tend to enlarge in the first 6 months of life.

Hand-Schüller-Christian Disease

Cervical node involvement and skull lesions are found.

Sarcoidosis

Adenopathy is generalized, but cervical involvement is most prominent.

Benign Sinus Histiocytosis

Following Immunization

Diphtheria-pertussis-tetanus (DPT) vaccine given in the deltoid muscle may be followed by painless cervical node enlargement.

Suppurative Thyroiditis

Histiocytic Necrotizing Lymphadenitis (Kikuchi-Fujimoto Disease)

Characterized by fever and painless cervical lymphadenopathy. Children may also have weight loss, nausea, vomiting, diarrhea, chills, and diaphoresis.

Occipital Region

Seborrheic Dermatitis

Tinea Capitis

Folliculitis of the Scalp

Pediculosis

External Otitis Media

Roseola

Toxoplasmosis

Tick Bites

Rubella

Preauricular Region

Chronic Eye Infections

Nodal enlargement is seen especially with chlamydia.

Styes or Chalazion

Ear Infections

Infections of the auricle and ear canal may cause preauricular adenopathy.

Adenovirus Infections

Type 3

Symptoms include pharyngitis, conjunctivitis, fever, and enlarged nodes.

Type 8

Epidemic keratoconjunctivitis is associated with a follicular conjunctivitis.

Herpes Simplex Infection

Cat-Scratch Disease

Suppurative preauricular adenopathy may occur if the scratch is near the eye or the inoculum in it.

Tularemia

Eye infection is associated with a suppurative preauricular adenitis.

Submaxillary and Submental Regions

Gingivitis

Dental Infections

Herpetic Gingivostomatitis

Glossitis

Cystic Fibrosis

Submandibular gland enlargement may be mistaken for adenopathy.

Axillary Region

Infection

Bacterial, viral, fungal, or other infection of an upper extremity, lateral chest wall, or breast is the most common cause of tender adenopathy.

Inflammation

Chronic irritation of an extremity, involving either skin or joints, may result in axillary adenopathy. Juvenile rheumatoid arthritis and atopic dermatitis are examples.

Cat-Scratch Disease

Vaccination

BCG vaccine, smallpox, or other immunizations administered in the upper arm may cause axillary node enlargement.

Inguinal Region

Infection

The inguinal nodes drain the lower extremities, genitalia, perineum, buttocks, and lower abdominal wall. Bacterial, viral, fungal, and other infections in any of these areas may cause inguinal node enlargement.

Cat-Scratch Disease

Lymphogranuloma Venereum

Large, matted nodes often suppurate.

Chancroid

A ragged-edged, shallow ulcer on the genitalia precedes the adenopathy.

Rickettsial Infections

Arthropod bites of the lower extremities are a common cause.

Blastomyocosis

Violaceous papules occur at the inoculation site, followed by lymphangitis and lymphadenopathy.

Filiariasis

Repeated infection in this tropical disorder leads to lymphedema and elephantiasis.

Inflammation

Irritation of skin or inflammation of joints may cause nodal enlargement. Diaper dermatitis, mosquito, chigger, or flea bites, and contact dermatitis may be overlooked in the differential diagnosis.

Supraclavicular Region

Left

Nodal enlargement in this area suggests malignant disease arising in the abdomen.

Right

Nodes in this area drain the superior parts of the lungs and the mediastinum; therefore, thoracic disorders are usually responsible for the adenopathy.

DISORDERS THAT MIMIC LYMPH NODES

Branchial Cleft Cyst

These may occur anywhere from the preauricular area to the clavicles. The lesions generally are along the sternocleidomastoid muscle. A small skin opening may overlie the mass.

Thyroglossal Duct Cyst

Located in the midline above the thyroid. Moves up with protrusion of the tongue.

Salivary Gland Enlargement

Thyroid Enlargement

Dermoid

A firm, node with a surface that feels slippery as it is palpated.

Rheumatoid Nodules

Subcutaneous nodules may be associated with rheumatoid arthritis, acute rheumatic fever, and pseudorheumatoid nodules associated with granuloma annulare.

SUGGESTED READING

Barton LL, Feigin RD. Childhood cervical lymphadenitis: a reappraisal. *J Pediatr* 1974;84:846–852.

Chesney PJ. Lymphatic system and generalized lymphadenopathy. In: Long SS, Pickering LK, Prober CG, eds. *Principles and practice of pediatric infectious diseases.* New York: Churchill Livingstone, 1997:134–144.

Lake AM, Oski FA. Peripheral lymphadenopathy in childhood. *Am J Dis Child* 1978;132:357–359.

McCabe RE, Brooks RG, Dorfman RF, Remington JS. Clinical spectrum in 107 cases of toxoplasmic lymphadenopathy. *Rev Infect Dis* 1987;9:754–774.

Margileth AM. Sorting out the causes of lymphadenopathy. *Contemp Pediatr* 1995;12:23–40.

Margileth AM. Lymphadenopathy: when to diagnose and treat. *Contemp Pediatr* 1995;12:71–91.

Zitelli BJ. Lymphadenopathy. In: Gartner JC Jr, Zitelli BJ, eds. *Common & chronic symptoms in pediatrics.* St. Louis: Mosby, 1997:365–380.

Zuelzer WW, Kaplan J. The child with lymphadenopathy. *Semin Hematol* 1975;12:323–334.

11
Edema

Edema refers to the accumulation of fluid in body tissues. Technically, edema is not synonymous with swelling. It refers to increased fluid between and around cells, in the interstitial space, rather than inside the cell (e.g., brain cell swelling, liver cell swelling) or in the so-called third space (e.g., pleural effusion, ascites, fluid in the gastrointestinal tract). The distinction is important, in that accumulation of fluid inside the cell generally results from fluid shifts (e.g., brain cell swelling during treatment of diabetic ketoacidosis) or the cytotoxic effect of a toxin, infectious agent, or trauma (e.g., hepatitis), rather than the pathogenetic mechanisms usually operative in the formation of edema. Third space losses can result from exudative or secretory processes as well as from the usual mechanisms that produce edema.

Edema is generally caused by one (or more) of four pathogenetic mechanisms: (a) increased capillary permeability; (b) decreased oncotic pressure; (c) increased hydrostatic pressure; and (d) impaired lymphatic drainage. It is also important to consider whether the edema is generalized or localized; whether it is acute or chronic; whether inflammation is associated with the swelling; whether there are systemic signs or symptoms of associated disorders; and whether there is a family history of edema.

In this chapter, the most common causes of edema will be considered first. Then the causes will be approached by the pathogenetic mechanism, and, finally, a few pearls to keep in mind will be presented. Remember that the pathogenetic mechanisms may not always be distinct. In some instances, more than one mechanism may be involved, and in some disorders the exact mechanism may be unknown. Other chapters may prove helpful in the discussion of specific areas of edema. (See Chapter 33, Periorbital Edema, and Chapter 64, Ascites.)

◆ Generalized Edema: Most Common Causes

Allergic Reactions   Minimal Change Disease
Allergic Gastroenteropathy   Cystic Fibrosis

● Causes Not to Forget

Menetrier Disease   Congestive Heart Failure

◆ Localized Edema: Most Common Causes

Insect Bites   Localized Infection
Contact Dermatitis

- **Causes Not to Forget**

Sickle Cell Disease	Hand-Foot Syndrome
Henoch-Schönlein Purpura	Serum Sickness
Turner Syndrome	Lymphedema

GENERALIZED EDEMA

Edema Associated with Increased Capillary Permeability

♦ Allergic Reactions

Insect Bites

Hymenoptera stings may result in large areas of swelling and even generalized edema. The lesions are usually pruritic, pink, and have a central punctum.

Ingestants

Reactions to foods and drugs often have urticaria accompanying the swelling. Shellfish and nuts are two of the more common foods producing allergic reactions.

Contact Dermatitis

Depending on the surface area affected, the dermatitis, therefore the edema, may be localized or generalized. Poison ivy may produce facial and extremity swelling suggestive of angioedema, with subtle dermatitis.

Serum-Sicknesslike Reaction

A reaction with urticaria and periarticular swelling, may be associated with many drugs, particularly cefaclor. Infections, particularly hepatitis B may have this type of reaction.

Latex Allergy

Needs to be considered, especially in children with meningomyeloceles.

Inhalants

May produce an angioedema appearance.

Infections

Bacterial infections are more likely to be associated with edema than viral, fungal, or other infectious causes. The distribution of the edema tends to parallel the infection.

Scarlet Fever

The edema may be relatively diffuse, but more likely facial. An erythrogenic toxin is responsible.

Rocky Mountain Spotted Fever

Generalized, nonpitting edema occurs to some degree in all patients. The rash, at first macular, then papular and petechial, appears on the fourth day of the illness, first distally and then centrally. Headache, anorexia, photophobia, and periorbital edema are characteristic features. The Rickettsiae invade and injure the endothelial cells causing a leak of fluid from vessels.

Staphylococcal Scalded Skin Syndrome

The skin is swollen, red, and tender to touch. Perioral and ocular crusting is usually present.

Diphtheria

Rare today, but not to be forgotten. Beware of the child with a mousey odor, serosanguineous nasal discharge, cervical adenopathy, and stridor.

Collagen-Vascular Diseases

Serum Sickness and Serum Sicknesslike Reactions

Characterized by fever, urticaria, edema and arthralgias/periarticular swelling, may occur secondary to infections, injections, or drug ingestion.

Henoch-Schönlein Purpura

May be associated with striking areas of soft-tissue swelling, particularly of the scalp. The acrally located purpuric rash, often with accompanying edema, abdominal pain, arthralgia and periarticular swelling, and nephritis suggest this disorder.

Acute Hemorrhagic Edema of Infancy

Still debated as to whether this is a form of Henoch-Schönlein purpura. Generally, affects children under 2 years of age. The purpuric lesions are acrally located and appear annular or targetoid. Systemic complaints are usually not present. Edema is prominent.

Mucocutaneous Lymph Node Syndrome (Kawasaki)

Often has a brawny edema of the palms and soles in addition to nonpurulent conjunctival injection, cracked, red lips, rashes, and fever lasting longer than 5 days.

Stevens-Johnson Syndrome

Often has significant facial and, occasionally, generalized edema. The associated skin lesions and mucous membrane involvement are most characteristic of the disorder.

Dermatomyositis

Commonly is associated with facial edema. Muscle weakness and the erythematous, scaly patches over the knuckles, knees, and elbows are more characteristic findings.

Allergic Vasculitis

May be accompanied by palpable purpura as well as swelling.

Systemic Lupus Erythematosus

Often has multisystem involvement and various rashes. Photosensitivity should always suggest the possibility of systemic lupus erythematosus. May be responsible for a nephrotic syndrome picture.

Progressive Systemic Sclerosis

May have brawny swelling of the face and extremities. The skin becomes increasingly tight and Raynaud phenomenon is a common finding.

Thrombotic Thrombocytopenic Purpura

Edema may be prominent.

Miscellaneous Causes

Mucopolysaccharidoses

The skin appears coarse and thickened in some forms.

Scurvy

Characterized by easy bruising and bleeding gums.

Beriberi

The result of thiamine deficiency is rare in the United States. Peripheral neuritis and cardiac failure are presenting complaints.

Vitamin E Deficiency

Premature infants deficient in vitamin E may develop edema.

Decreased Oncotic Pressure (Hypoproteinemia)

Renal Disorders

◆ Nephrosis, Minimal Change Disease

Probably the most common cause of generalized edema, not related to allergic reaction, in children.

Nephrotic Syndrome

A wide variety of disorders may be responsible. Characterized by edema, hypoproteinemia, hypercholesterolemia, and proteinuria.

Nephritis

Various types may also cause edema, but usually not as severe as that associated with nephrosis. The urinalysis in nephritis usually contains blood and granular elements as well as protein. Poststreptococcal acute glomerulonephritis is not as common as a few decades ago, but must always be considered in the differential diagnosis. Other bacteria and viruses may also be responsible. Nephritis may be hereditary (Alport), drug induced (particularly methicillin, sulfonamides, and mercurial diuretics), and immune complex related such as with poststreptococcal, but also with subacute bacterial endocarditis.

Gastrointestinal Disorders

◆ Cystic Fibrosis

The most common cause of malabsorption in children and should be high on the list of considerations particularly in breast fed or soy fed infants with edema, anemia, and hypoproteinemia. The infants also demonstrate failure to thrive despite a voracious appetite, mildly elevated liver enzymes, prolonged prothrombin and partial thromboplastin times, and, sometimes, a diffuse scaly rash.

◆ Chronic Allergic Gastroenteropathy

Most often secondary to cow milk protein is the most common exudative enteropathy causing loss of protein. The infants may have intermittent diarrhea and almost always have iron deficiency anemia.

● Transient Protein Losing Enteropathy (Menetrier Disease)

May follow a viral infection, most commonly cytomegalovirus. The children are often mistaken as having nephrosis. The edema resolves spontaneously within weeks to months. Presenting symptoms are anorexia, emesis, or abdominal pain, followed soon by generalized edema.

Protein Losing Gastroenteropathies

May be associated with regional enteritis, ulcerative colitis, constrictive pericarditis, lymphoma, neuroblastoma, and congenital ileal stenosis.

Intestinal Lymphangiectasia

May be part of a generalized congenital abnormality of the lymphatic system, or localized to the gastrointestinal tract. Steatorrhea as well as diarrhea with enteric loss of protein is present.

Trypsinogen Deficiency

May result in the deficiency of other proteolytic enzymes as well. The onset is early and anemia is usually present.

Celiac Disease

The result of gluten-induced enteropathy is most commonly associated with chronic diarrhea, weight loss, abdominal distension, and wasting of the buttocks.

Zinc Deficiency

In low birth weight infants may result in protein deficiency and edema at 1 to 2 months of age.

Pancreatic Pseudocysts

Hypoproteinemia has also been associated.

Miscellaneous Causes

Excessive loss of protein from the gastrointestinal tract may also occur in congenital megacolon, polypoid adenomatosis, bezoars and chronic infections or infestations of the intestinal tract, e.g., *Giardia*.

Liver Disease

May result in edema secondary to poor production of protein.

Cirrhosis

From various causes.

Galactosemia

Jaundice, vomiting, diarrhea, and the presence of reducing substance in the urine of a neonate strongly suggest this disorder.

Hypervitaminosis A

May result in a cirrhotic picture as well as causing bone pain and increased intracranial pressure.

Miscellaneous

Kwashiorkor

The result of deficient protein intake, edema may be a prominent feature.

Marasmus

Severe caloric deficiency, less commonly is associated with edema.

Kawasaki Disease

In addition to vasculitis, the serum albumin level is generally low, sometimes low enough to cause edema.

Increased Hydrostatic Pressure

Increased hydrostatic pressure may be the result of venous hypertension associated with obstruction or poor circulation, or from excessive vascular fluid.

● Cardiac Failure

Is the prototype of a failing pump. Tachycardia, tachypnea, hepatomegaly, and cardiomegaly characterizes cardiac failure. Periorbital edema is most commonly noted before peripheral edema.

Hydrops Fetalis

In the past was most commonly due to Rh isoimmunization, but now has a myriad of possible causes. Isoimmunization to other blood group factors still the most common. Chronic anemia is responsible for the heart failure. A host of nonimmune causes of hydrops fetalis can be found in McGillivray and Hall (1).

Fluid Overload

Most likely to be iatrogenic, particularly following vigorous fluid resuscitation.

Arteriovenous Fistula

High output failure may result. Auscultation of the head and liver should be performed for the presence of bruits.

Venous Thrombosis

The associated edema is usually distal to the obstructed vein. In the newborn, renal vein thrombosis may cause generalized edema. Portal vein thrombosis may result in generalized edema.

Constrictive Pericarditis

Must be considered, particularly in the presence of neck vein distension and hepatomegaly.

Impaired Lymphatic Drainage

Generally speaking, edema associated with impaired lymphatic drainage is localized to either one or more extremities. The edema is rarely generalized. An important problem associated with lymphedema is secondary bacterial infection in the protein enriched edema fluid. Secondary infections result in a worsening of lymphatic drainage.

LOCALIZED SWELLING OR EDEMA

Edema Associated with Increased Capillary Permeability

Allergic Reactions

♦ Insect Bites

The most common cause of localized edema. The lesions are usually pruritic, pink, and have a central punctum.

♦ Contact Dermatitis

Characterized by a rash as well as swelling. Affected areas are usually pruritic and often have linear patterns of involvement. Facial swelling associated with poison ivy dermatitis may mimic angioedema.

Ingestants

Facial edema may be pronounced, including airway compromise.

Inhalants

● Serum Sickness

Periarticular swelling may be prominent. Urticarial lesions are usually present. The swelling usually involves more than one area.

Hereditary Angioedema

Intermittent brawny swelling of the extremities is more common than facial or subglottic swelling. The edema is often precipitated by trauma. Recurrent, crampy abdominal pain is common. The edema usually lasts 24 to 72 hours. Laboratory findings include decreased serum levels of C4 and C1 esterase inhibitor.

Infections

• Cellulitis

Bacterial or viral infections may be responsible. Erysipelas, most commonly secondary to streptococcal infections, is characterized by rapidly expanding swelling, erythema, and pain. Areas involved with herpes simplex and zoster are edematous.

Pertussis

The edema is periorbital and sometimes facial. The paroxysms of cough should alert one to the diagnosis.

Epstein-Barr Virus Infections

Periorbital edema is common, and may be the presenting sign.

Roseola

Periorbital edema may be significant. The rash typically appears after defervesence on the 3rd or 4th day of illness.

Mumps

Parotid swelling is the classic sign, but facial swelling may be prominent. Presternal swelling is an unusual but sometimes prominent finding.

Osteomyelitis

An extremity may be swollen and painful as a result of underlying osteomyelitis.

Collagen Vascular Diseases

• Henoch-Schönlein Purpura

Striking areas of localized edema may be present.

Acute Hemorrhagic Edema of Infancy

Resembles Henoch-Schönlein purpura, but purpuric lesions are annular or targetoid and systemic symptoms are uncommon. Edema is prominent.

Kawasaki Disease

The palms and soles are commonly swollen. The face may appear swollen as well.

Rheumatoid Arthritis

Periarticular swelling is common.

Synovial Outpouchings

A ganglion of the wrist is most common, however, a popliteal cyst, known as a Baker cyst, may create swelling of the leg as well as fullness of the popliteal area.

Miscellaneous Causes

• Sickle Cell Disease

The hand-foot syndrome is characterized by symmetrical, tender swelling of the hands or feet. The children are often febrile, making the separation from infection difficult until the underlying cause is recognized.

Hypothyroidism

Children may have a generalized puffy appearance, particularly around the eyes.

Hyperthyroidism

Pretibial myxedema is rare in children. Tachycardia, tremors, and weight loss suggest this diagnosis.

Pancreatitis

Ascites and extremity swelling may be present. The presentation is usually with abdominal pain.

Eosinophilic Cellulitis

Resembles bacterial cellulitis and usually affects the extremities or trunk. Significant edema and moderate erythema with minimal tenderness and lack of warmth is found. Recurrent episodes are typical. A peripheral eosinophilia of the blood is present.

Episodic Angioneurotic Edema and Hypereosinophilia

An unusual disorder of unknown cause. Recurrent attacks of edema and eosinophilia are typical. Pruritic papules and fever may be present.

Äscher Syndrome

Characterized by recurrent episodes of upper eyelid and upper lip edema, which may result in atrophic slack skin in these areas.

Rosenthal-Melkersson Syndrome

Characterized by recurrent facial and lid edema, furrowed tongue, and facial nerve paralysis.

Caffey Disease

Edema over affected bones (e.g., mandible, sternum) signals the presence of this rare disorder.

Increased Hydrostatic Pressure

Superior Vena Cava Syndrome

The head and neck appear congested.

Failure of Venous Valves

May result in distal swelling, but varicosities are uncommon in children.

Orthostatic Hypertension

Particularly the result of casts, may result in distal swelling.

Reflex Sympathetic Dsytrophy

Although the extremity may not be paralyzed, disuse and poor venous return may result in a cool, blue, swollen extremity.

Paralysis

Dependent extremities may appear edematous.

Tumors

May cause obstruction of venous return resulting in distal swelling.

Hemangiomas

Angiogenic defects may trap platelets and swell, complemented by local edema (Kasabach-Merritt syndrome).

Impaired Lymphatic Drainage

The edema is localized to one or more extremities. Secondary bacterial infections are a common occurrence and worsen the problem.

Lymphangioma

The lesions are usually congenital, but may expand over time.

● Lymphedema Praecox

The result of aplasia or hypoplasia of lymphatics, may manifest at any age, despite the fact that the lymphatic problems have been present since birth.

● Turner Syndrome

The classic presentation is lymphedema of the hands and feet in the neonate. The edema may recur later in life. The other stigmata of this syndrome vary in severity.

Noonan Syndrome

The phenotypic appearance is similar to Turner syndrome, but affects males and females. The lymphedema of the hands and feet is similar to Turner syndrome.

Milroy Disease

Inherited as an autosomal dominant, may present with lymphedema at or shortly after birth.

Meigs Syndrome

Also inherited as an autosomal dominant, usually has the onset of edema around the time of puberty.

Recurrent Lymphangitis

Onset is in childhood or adolescence in this autosomal dominantly inherited disorder. Recurrent infection or inflammation of lymphatic vessels results in edema.

Yellow Nail Syndrome

Is characterized by dystrophic and yellow nails. It too, is inherited in an autosomal dominant fashion. Recurrent pleural effusions, bronchiectasis, and sinusitis may occur.

Distichiasis (Double Row of Eyelashes)

This autosomal dominantly inherited disorder may have the onset of edema at any time from late childhood.

Recurrent Cholestasis

Edema may also be associated. Inherited in an autosomal recessive fashion. The onset is usually in the neonatal period associated with prolonged jaundice. Cirrhosis often develops later in life.

Aagenaes Syndrome

Is a form of idiopathic intrahepatic cholestasis characterized by recurrent episodes of cholestasis associated with lymphedema of the lower extremities.

Lymphangiectasis

Infants with this autosomal dominantly inherited disorder develop edema in infancy. They also have diarrhea, vomiting, hypoproteinemia, chylous effusions, and failure to thrive.

Cerebral Arteriovenous Anomaly

Also inherited in an autosomal dominant fashion, has the onset of edema in late childhood or early adolescence. Pulmonary hypertension is a common accompaniment.

Miscellaneous Disorders with Abnormal Fluid Accumulation:

Idiopathic Chylous Ascites

Chylothorax

Edema with Capillary Hemangiomas

Edema Associated with Congenital Absence of the Nails

Swelling Associated with Constriction from Amniotic Bands

Chylous Reflux Associated with Xanthomatosis

TAR Syndrome (Thrombocytopenia with Aplasia of the Radius)

Dorsal pedal edema may be present.

Infections Associated with Edema

Cat-Scratch Disease

Filiariasis

May result in elephantiasis.

Trichinosis

May be associated with periorbital and pretibial edema, muscle pain, and eosinophilia.

Trauma

Various types may result in damage to lymphatics and resultant lymphedema.

Blunt Force

Burns

Surgical Incisions

Extrinsic Pressure

Tumors

Carcinoid Tumor

An uncommon gastrointestinal tumor associated with recurrent diarrhea and cutaneous flushes.

Retroperitoneal Fibrosis

May be caused by various drugs and other disorders and result in lymphatic obstruction.

MIMICS of EDEMA

A few disorders may suggest edema, but the swelling is nonpitting.

Scleredema

A rare connective tissue disorder of unknown cause sometimes following streptococcal infections. The edema is firm, nonpitting and typically begins in the nape of the neck and spreads to involve the face, shoulders, and trunk. The lower extremities, hands and feet and genitalia are involved in 10% of cases. The face may become masklike.

Scleroderma

The skin appears thickened and often becomes shiny with decreased or increased pigmentation at the borders. Raynaud phenomenon and systemic symptoms are usually present.

Dermatomyositis

The skin may feel indurated. The face often appears swollen or full. Characteristic erythematous papules (Gottron) are found over the knuckles.

Familial Mediterranean Fever

Recurrent episodes of extremity swelling with a cellulitis-like appearance have been reported frequently in this disorder. Fever, peritoneal and pleural pain, and synovitis are present as well.

Myxedema

Hypothyroidism with myxedema is rare in children.

Eosinophilic Fasciitis

An unusual disorder characterized by the rapid onset of scleroderma-like swelling of the distal extremities and the rapid development of contractures. Peripheral eosinophilia is common. The relationship to systemic sclerosis is blurred.

REFERENCE

1. McGillivray BC, Hall JG. Nonimmune hydrops fetalis. *Pediatr Rev* 1987;9:197–202.

SUGGESTED READING

Holmes LB, Fields JP, Zabriskie JB. Hereditary late-onset lymphedema. *Pediatrics* 1978;61:575–579.

Lewis JM, Wald ER. Lymphedema praecox. *J Pediatr* 1984;104:641–648.

Sferra TJ, Pawel BR, Qualman SJ, Li BUK. Menetrier disease of childhood: role of cytomegalovirus and transforming growth factor alpha. *J Pediatr* 1996;128:213–219.

Smeltzer DM, Stickler GB, Schirger A. Primary lymphedema in children and adolescents: a follow-up study and review. *Pediatrics* 1985;76:206–218.

Vereecken P, Lutz R, De Dobbeleer G, Heenen M. Nonpitting induration of the back: Scleredema adultorum. *Arch Dermatol* 1997;133:655–656.

12

Pallor

Parents who seek medical attention for their pale child think of underlying malignancy as the cause, even if they may not state that concern. Physicians think of anemia, because it is probably the most common pathologic cause of pallor. By far the most common causes of pallor, however, are constitutional factors. Pale skin is more likely to be the result of a familial trait or lack of sun exposure, or part of the atopic diathesis, than of a pathologic process.

Pallor has been divided into chronic and acute classifications in this chapter.

♦ **Most Common Causes of Pallor**

Acute	**Chronic**
Infection	Hereditary
Anemia	Lack of Sun
Allergic Reaction	Atopy

● **Causes Not to Forget**

Migraine	Cystic Fibrosis
Hypoglycemia	Edema

CHRONIC PALLOR

Constitutional Factors

♦ **Hereditary (Familial) Trait**

Heredity is the most common cause. Pallor frequently accompanies light hair coloration.

♦ **Lack of Sun Exposure**

Children who live in northern climates during the winter months will have pale skin.

♦ **Atopic Individuals**

Children with a predisposition to allergies or atopic dermatitis often have a striking pallor. Other clinical signs and symptoms of allergic diatheses are usually present, such as allergic "shiner," transverse folds on the lower eyelids, and the allergic salute.

Anemia

In early infancy, pallor may be the presenting sign of transient erythroblasto-penia.

Inflammatory Diseases

Chronic inflammatory diseases are often associated with pallor. The pallor may be due in part to lack of sun exposure, depending on the severity of illness, and may be associated with the anemia of chronic disease. Pallor is a common finding in juvenile rheumatoid arthritis, inflammatory bowel disease, and lupus erythematosus.

● Edema

Disorders that result in edema, such as nephrosis, frequently have associated pallor.

● Cystic Fibrosis

Children with cystic fibrosis commonly demonstrate pallor, unrelated to the severity of the disease.

Juvenile Diabetes Mellitus

Many children with diabetes appear pale, irrespective of disease control.

Uremia

Children with uremia as a result of chronic renal disease have a pallor related partly to their associated anemia. Lethargy, fatigue, anorexia, and weight loss are commonly associated complaints.

Hypothyroidism

Part of the pallor may be related to edema.

Celiac Syndrome

Diarrhea is a more prominent symptom than pallor.

Lead Poisoning

Part may be due to anemia.

ACUTE PALLOR

♦ **Acute Allergic Reactions**

Nausea

Pallor commonly accompanies nausea.

♦ **Acute Anemia**

Acute blood loss or a hemolytic anemia induces pallor.

Syncope

Pallor is pronounced just prior to the loss of consciousness.

Shock

Peripheral vasoconstriction produces a striking pallor in any of the various causes of shock. Poor peripheral perfusion, such as that found in paroxysmal atrial tachycardia, produces a pronounced pallor.

Hypoxia

Disorders causing hypoxia may result in pallor.

♦ **Infection**

Bacteremia

Some infections, particularly those in which bacteremia is found, are likely to be associated with a pallid appearance. Bacteremia caused by gram-negative organisms are more often responsible, though these organisms may also release endotoxins that may cause diffuse vascular dilatation and a hyperemic glow.

Pyelonephritis

Subacute Bacterial Endocarditis

Hypothermia

Vasoconstriction of superficial blood vessels results in pallor.

● **Hypoglycemia**

During episodes of hypoglycemia the child is often pale, sweaty, and nauseated and frequently demonstrates altered behavior.

Intussusception

During the paroxysms of abdominal pain the child often appears pale as if in shock.

Cardiac Disorders

Pallor may be the result of impaired cardiac function. Myocardial infarction as a result of an anomalous left coronary artery or Kawasaki disease are examples.

Neurologic Disorders

Closed Head Injury

Vomiting, pallor, and irritability are common. There may be a history of loss of consciousness.

Cerebral Hemorrhage

Paroxysmal Disorders

● **Migraine**

Headache and visual disturbances are usual in older children. Young children may only have pallor, nausea, and vomiting.

Breath-Holding Spells

Most episodes are associated with cyanosis as the breath is held, but a pallid form has been described in which, after the precipitating event, the child does not cry but suddenly becomes pale and faints.

Psychomotor Seizures

Onset is rarely seen before 10 years of age. Auras, such as anxiety, visceral sensations, olfactory hallucinations, and déjà vu precede the seizure. Following the aura, the child may stare, suddenly stop all activity, stand still, and turn pale and then perform some minor motor acts. There is complete amnesia for these events.

Benign Paroxysmal Vertigo

Recurrent attacks of vertigo are associated with pallor, nystagmus, vomiting, and sweating. There is no loss of consciousness.

Infantile Spasms

Sudden muscular contractions with the head flexed, arms extended, and legs drawn up are characteristic. The infant may become pale, appear flushed, or turn cyanotic during these attacks.

Paroxysmal Atrial Tachycardia

During episodes of tachycardia the infant or child may appear pale.

Acute Rheumatic Fever

Acute Glomerulonephritis

Heavy Sedation

Henoch-Schönlein Purpura

Petechiae and ecchymoses, particularly over the lower extremities, are almost invariably present.

Hemolytic-Uremic Syndrome

A major cause of the pallor is the development of anemia.

Pheochromocytoma

Common symptoms include episodes of headache, sweating, pallor, and palpitations. Hypertension may be chronic or associated with the episodic attacks during release of catecholamines.

Infantile Cortical Hyperostosis (Caffey Disease)

Onset is usually before 6 months of age. Irritability, fever, and soft-tissue swelling over the bony swellings are common findings.

13

Cyanosis

Cyanosis, the bluish color imparted to the skin by unsaturated hemoglobin in capillaries, is often difficult to quantify clinically. At least 5 g of reduced hemoglobin must be present before cyanosis is clinically apparent. Clinical assessment is affected by several factors including skin pigmentation and light source, and also by the acuity of the observer. It may be difficult to decide if the bluish color is peripheral, most commonly from vasoconstriction, or central, a result of true unsaturation of hemoglobin.

Cardiac, pulmonary, and central nervous system disorders usually come to mind first in the differential diagnosis of cyanosis. The differentiation between these three may be aided by the state of alertness of the infant, which may be depressed in central nervous system disorders, and by the degree of tachypnea, which tends to be greater in pulmonary than cardiac causes of cyanosis. The "hyperoxia" test may prove helpful in separating pulmonary disease from cyanotic congenital heart disease. While breathing room air, the arterial oxygen saturation of infants may be depressed to similar levels in heart or pulmonary disorders. If 100% oxygen is administered and the infant is ventilated adequately, cyanotic congenital heart disease is unlikely if the PaO_2 increases above 150 mm Hg. If the PaO_2 fails to increase above 100 mm Hg, cyanotic congenital heart disease is the most likely cause. If the arterial saturation is between 100 and 150 mm Hg, cardiac disease is likely but not certain.

It is important to ascertain that the bluish coloration is not just "skin deep." Blue dye imparted to the skin from fabric, especially that of blue jeans, may initially be mistaken for a potentially serious problem.

♦ **Most Common Causes of Cyanosis**

Cyanotic Congenital Heart Disease
Respiratory Disorders: Asthma, Bronchiolitis, Atelectasis, Croup, Aspiration
Respiratory Depression

● **Causes Not to Forget**

Drugs   Methemoglobinemia
Shock

CARDIAC ABNORMALITIES

♦ **Cyanotic Congenital Heart Disease**

　Tetralogy of Fallot

Transposition of the Great Vessels

Tricuspid Atresia

Truncus Arteriosus

Total Anomalous Pulmonary Venous Return

Pulmonary Atresia or Severe Stenosis with a Ventricular Septal Defect

Severe Aortic Stenosis or Atresia

Ebstein Anomaly

Eisenmenger Complex

A large left-to-right shunt through a ventricular septal defect results eventually in increased obstruction to pulmonary flow, producing a right-to-left shunt.

Atrioventricular Canal

Hypoplastic Left Heart

Preductal Coarctation of the Aorta

The lower extremities appear cyanotic and the upper extremities pink.

Pulmonary Stenosis with a Patent Foramen Ovale

Failure of the Heart as a Pump

Congestive Heart Failure

Congenital Heart Defects

Left-to-right shunts such as in ventricular septal defect, and obstructive lesions to the left ventricle such as in postductal coarctation of the aorta and severe aortic stenosis, may result in congestive failure and cyanosis.

Arrhythmias

Paroxysmal atrial tachycardia, in particular, may result in cyanosis.

Myocarditis

Myocarditis may be of viral origin or associated with inflammatory diseases.

Endocardial Fibroelastosis

Cardiomyopathies

Hypertrophic, dilated, and restricted cardiomyopathies may result in cardiac failure and subsequent cyanosis.

Constrictive Pericarditis

Venous pressure is increased, leading to increased deoxygenation of hemoglobin in the capillaries during stasis.

Heart Block

Severe bradycardia may affect blood flow enough to cause cyanosis.

Atrial Myxoma

Symptoms include the sudden onset of dyspnea, fainting spells, or cyanosis when the tumor obstructs the mitral valve.

DISORDERS AFFECTING THE PULMONARY SYSTEM

Airway Compromise

Upper Airway

Nasal Obstruction

In infants, who are obligate nose breathers, or those with choanal atresia, or even those with nasal obstruction by mucus, cyanosis may be present. Similarly, rebound mucosal swelling from the use of sympathomimetic nose-drop preparations may result in symptoms of airway compromise.

Foreign Body

♦ Croup Syndrome

Laryngotracheitis, acute and spasmodic, may result in severe subglottic narrowing. Various other disorders may mimic croup and cause narrowing of the airway. (See Chapter 59, Stridor.)

Pharyngeal Infections

Retropharygeal abscesses, epiglottitis, pharyngeal diphtheria with pseudomembrane formation, and peritonsillar abscesses may compromise airflow.

Tonsillar-Adenoidal Hypertrophy

Snoring, noisy respirations, and disturbed sleep are the more prominent symptoms.

Vocal Cord Paralysis

Laryngospasm

May be induced by allergic reactions, hypocalcemia, and other disorders.

Glossoptosis

The tongue may fall back and obstruct the airway in infants with micrognathia or poor neuromuscular control.

Angioedema

Tumors

Hemangiomas, papillomas, and lymphangiomas may compromise the airway.

Laryngeal Webs or Cysts

Congenital Goiter

Lower Airway

Foreign Body

♦ **Aspiration**

Inhalation of food or drink or of gastric contents and neardrowning are examples.

Mucus Plugs

Mediastinal Masses

Tracheo-Esophageal Fistula

Vascular Rings

Bronchostenosis

Interference with lung expansion

Pneumothorax and Pneumomediastinum

Pleural Effusions

Severe Abdominal Distension

Lung expansion may be blocked by ascites or abdominal masses; patients with peritoneal irritation may hypoventilate.

Obesity

Profound obesity may compromise pulmonary function (Pickwickian syndrome.)

Severe Scoliosis

Diaphragmatic Hernia

Hypoplastic Lung

Lobar Emphysema

Abnormalities of the Thoracic Cage

Severe pectus excavatum, flail chest following rib fractures, thoracic asphyxiant dystrophies, and the hypophosphatasia syndromes are examples.

Pulmonary Sequestration

Cystic Adenomatoid Malformation

Disorders Affecting the Lung and Small Airways

♦ **Bronchial Asthma**

♦ **Atelectasis**

♦ **Bronchiolitis**

Pneumonia

Respiratory Distress Syndrome

Bronchopulmonary Dysplasia

Cystic Fibrosis

Pulmonary Edema

Bronchospasm

Chemicals or noxious gases may produce spasm.

Hypersensitivity Pneumonitis

Pulmonary Hemorrhage

Idiopathic Pulmonary Hemosiderosis

Pulmonary Fibrosis

Alveolar Proteinosis

Pulmonary Vascular Disorders

Pulmonary Emboli

Pulmonary Thromboses

Persistent Fetal Circulation

Primary Pulmonary Hypertension

Pulmonary Arterio-Venous Malformation

Blood is shunted away from the alveoli, creating a chronic hypoxemic state. Clubbing of the fingers may be a clue.

Oxygen Toxicity

NEUROLOGIC AND MUSCULAR DISORDERS

Central Nervous System Insults

Intracerebral Hemorrhage

Subarachnoid and Subdural Hemorrhages

Cerebral Edema

Meningitis or Encephalitis

- **Drugs**

  Various drugs may cause central nervous system depression or affect the muscles involved in respiration. Narcotics, tranquilizers, muscle relaxants, and anesthetics are but a few.

Disorders Affecting the Muscles of Respiration

Muscular Dystrophy

Pulmonary function may be affected in advanced disease.

Botulism

Myasthenia Gravis

Werdnig-Hoffman Disease

Diaphragmatic Paralysis

Poliomyelitis

DISORDERS AFFECTING THE OXYGEN-CARRYING CAPACITY OF BLOOD

Polycythemia

Cyanosis may be a finding in disorders in which hemoglobin is increased, because the amount of unsaturated hemoglobin is also increased to as much as 5 g/dL.

- **Methemoglobinemia**

  The clue is failure of chocolate colored blood spilled on materials during blood drawing to become red despite high oxygen exposure.

Hereditary

Four types of hereditary methemoglobinemia have been reported, all involving deficiency of cytochrome b 5 reductase. Cyanosis may appear, depending on the type, from birth to adolescence.

Acquired

Exogenous

Various chemicals including nitrites, nitrates, benzocaine, sulfonamides, and aniline dyes may be responsible.

Endogenous

Methemoglobin may develop as a result of alteration in colonic enzymes and intestinal bacteria that result in an accumulation of nitrites. The methemoglobinemia is transient. The endogenous form has been reported with acidosis secondary to severe diarrhea, with dietary protein intolerance, and with renal tubular acidosis.

M Hemoglobins

Five hemoglobin variants, with an autosomal dominant inheritance pattern, have been described. All produce clinical cyanosis. Hemoglobin M can be detected electrophoretically. The cyanosis either is present at birth or appears within 3 to 6 months of age.

Hemoglobins with Low Oxygen Affinity

Six variants have been described, the most common of which is hemoglobin Kansas. Patients have a hemoglobin oxygen saturation of 60% in arterial blood despite a PaO_2 of 100 torr (1).

• SHOCK AND SEPSIS

Blood Loss

Septic Shock

Septicemia

Adrenal Insufficiency

The defect may be congenital or acquired, particularly after withdrawal from exogenous steroid therapy.

PERIPHERAL CYANOSIS

Vasoconstriction

The most common cause of cyanosis is vasoconstriction in response to cold exposure. Vasoconstriction may also occur in response to drugs and in some autonomic nervous system disturbances. (See also Chapter 102, Raynaud Phenomenon, Acrocyanois, and Other Color Changes.)

Deficient Blood Supply

Arterial compromise caused by a thrombus, vasculitis, or disseminated intravascular coagulation or venous stasis from interference with blood return results in cyanosis. Occasionally, after trauma a limb may be cool, cyanotic, and slightly edematous (reflex sympathetic dystrophy).

Acrocyanosis Secondary to Cold Sensitive Antibodies

Agglutination of erythrocytes as they pass through capillaries in cool extremities may result from the presence of antibodies resulting from preceding infections, particularly infectious mononucleosis and mycoplasma pneumonia. The antibodies may persist for months.

MISCELLANEOUS CAUSES

Breath-Holding

Cyanosis may be significant during breath-holding episodes in infants and young children.

Crying

The mechanism of cyanosis apparent during crying is thought to be increased venous pressure resulting in stasis of blood in the capillaries and an increased extraction of oxygen.

Hypoglycemia

Cyanosis is most likely to occur in hypoglycemic infants, perhaps because of right-to-left shunting through a patent foramen ovale and hypoventilation.

Familial Dysautonomia

Infants and children with this disorder have an abnormal response to hypoxia and a decreased sensitivity to hypercapnia.

Superior Vena Cava Syndrome

Swelling of the face, neck, and upper torso may take on a cyanotic or plethoric appearance.

MIMICS OF CYANOSIS

"Acrocyanosis of Levi"

A bluish discoloration may be imparted to the skin, usually of the hands, from new blue jeans. The discoloration can be removed with alcohol swabs.

Argyria, Hemochromatosis

Deposition of metals in the skin may result in discoloration suggestive of cyanosis. The arterial oxygen saturation is normal.

REFERENCE

1. Vichinsky EP, Lubin BH. Unstable hemoglobins, hemoglobins with altered oxygen affinity, and M-hemoglobins. *Pediatr Clin North Am* 1980;27:421–428.

SUGGESTED READING

DiMaio AM, Singh J. The infant with cyanosis in the emergency room. *Pediatr Clin North Am* 1992;39:987–1006.

Driscoll DJ. Evaluation of the cyanotic newborn. *Pediatr Clin North Am* 1990;37:1–23.

Murray KF, Christie DL. Dietary protein intolerance in infants with transient methemoglobinemia and diarrhea. *J Pediatr* 1993;122:90–92.

14

Jaundice

Jaundice, a yellow discoloration of the skin, is the result of the presence of excess bile pigment and reflects a disturbance in the mechanisms for formation or elimination of this pigment. Bilirubin is formed by the breakdown of heme. The causes of jaundice are many, but evaluation should include a blood test to determine whether the bilirubin is of the conjugated or unconjugated form. The presence of large amounts of unconjugated bilirubin in the blood reflects excessive pigment formation from hemolysis or disturbances of the hepatic conjugating mechanisms. Hyperbilirubinemia with the conjugated form is an indication of difficulties in pigment elimination caused by liver parenchymal disease or obstruction of intrahepatic or extrahepatic bile ducts.

In this chapter, causes of jaundice are considered under the two types of hyperbilirubinemia, in which either unconjugated or conjugated bilirubin is present. A category of causes of yellow skin unrelated to jaundice is also included.

♦ **Most Common Causes of Jaundice**

Unconjugated (Newborn)
Physiologic of the Newborn
Breast Feeding Jaundice
Extravascular Blood Reabsorption
Hemolytic Disorders (ABO, G6PD)

Conjugated (Newborn)
Infection [Sepsis/Urinary Tract Infection (UTI)]
Total Parenteral Nutrition
Neonatal Hepatitis

Unconjugated (Infants and Children)
Gilbert Syndrome
Hemoglobinopathy (Sickle Cell)
Red Cell Membrane Abnormalities

Conjugated (Infants and Children)
Infectious Hepatidities
Drugs
Infections (Sepsis, UTI)

● **Disorders Not to Forget**

Acquired Hemolytic Anemias
Chronic Active Hepatitis

Biliary Tract Disorders
Neonatal Hepatitis

HYPERBILIRUBINEMIA WITH UNCONJUGATED BILIRUBIN

Transient Neonatal Jaundice

♦ Physiologic Jaundice

This mild form, common in newborns, has been defined as a total bilirubin serum level of not more than 12 mg/dL and conjugated bilirubin serum level of not more than 1.5 mg/dL. Any of several mechanisms may be involved: a transient deficiency of liver glucuronide transferase; low hepatic levels of the binding protein γ resulting in impaired hepatic uptake of unconjugated bilirubin; decreased intestinal elimination of bilirubin due to lack of intestinal flora necessary to reduce conjugated bilirubin to urobilinogen; a greater rate of production of bilirubin in neonates; and regeneration of free bilirubin from its conjugated form with resorption due to the presence of glucuronidase in the intestinal epithelium (increased enterohepatic circulation). Physiologic jaundice is self-limited, resolving by the end of the first week of life, although it may blend into other causes of jaundice, such as breast milk jaundice, creating an impression of prolonged hyperbilirubinemia.

♦ Breast Feeding Jaundice

Breast fed infants commonly develop jaundice, particularly those not receiving adequate amounts of fluid.

Breast Milk Jaundice

Some mothers' milk contains a hormone that inhibits bilirubin conjugation. In most cases, the inhibition is thought to be caused by a high concentration of saturated free fatty acids or lipoprotein lipase activity in the milk. An increased resorption of bilirubin from the small bowel may also play a role in the pathogenesis. The jaundice usually does not appear before 4 to 5 days of age. Discontinuation of breast feeding results in a rapid reduction of serum bilirubin levels in 36 to 48 hours. Some have wondered whether infants who develop breast milk jaundice actually have Gilbert syndrome.

♦ Gilbert Syndrome

Onset of symptoms is usually late childhood with mild jaundice. Occasionally, the jaundice may be accompanied by vague abdominal pain and nausea. The clinical picture often develops after a fast, such as with surgical procedures, or in response to poor intake associated with an acute illness. The jaundice rarely exceeds 4–5 mg/dL. Bilirubin UDP-glucuronyl transferase activity is less than one half of normal. Inheritance is autosomal dominant.

Immaturity

Prematurely born infants often have more elevated levels of bilirubin than term infants, probably a reflection of a delay in conjugation and excretion of bilirubin.

Intestinal Obstruction

Especially in infancy, intestinal obstruction may result in an increased entero-hepatic circulation. Causes include intestinal atresia, annular pancreas, Hirsch-sprung disease, meconium plug syndrome, pyloric stenosis, and cystic fibrosis.

Lucey-Driscoll Syndrome

The mother's serum contains an inhibitor of bilirubin conjugation; therefore, all of the mother's offspring are affected.

Increased Bilirubin Production

♦ Hemolytic Disorders

Maternal-Fetal Blood Group Incompatibility

Most commonly affected are the Rh and ABO systems. The Coombs test is generally positive.

Red Blood Cell Enzyme Deficiencies

Included are glucose-6-phosphate dehydrogenase, fructokinase, pyruvate kinase, and glutathione peroxidase.

Congenital Disorders

Spherocytosis

Onset of symptoms may be in infancy or later in life, with pallor, abdominal pain, splenomegaly, and, occasionally, an aplastic crisis.

Thalassemia Major

Jaundice is rare, but pallor and hepatosplenomegaly become prominent at a few months of age.

Sickle Cell Anemia

Does not occur in the newborn period because of fetal hemoglobin concentration.

Vitamin E Deficiency

Jaundice related to vitamin E deficiency is most likely to occur in premature infants, especially if acidotic.

Elliptocytosis

Acquired Disorders

Drug-Related Jaundice

Hemolysis may follow the ingestion of various drugs or toxins, including excessive amounts of vitamin K.

Autoimmune Disease

Various diseases may cause hemolytic processes, in which results of Coombs test may be positive. Viral infections and systemic lupus erythematosus are best known examples.

Infantile Pyknocytosis

Pallor, jaundice, hepatosplenomegaly, and the presence of burr cells on peripheral smear are characteristic.

♦ Resorption of Extravascular Blood

In infants increased bilirubin production may be the result of absorption of blood from hematomas (e.g., cephalohematomas, subdural hematomas) or even ingestion of maternal blood during birth.

Polycythemia

Delayed clamping or stripping of the cord or maternal-fetal transfusion may produce polycythemia. The more red cells, the more bilirubin that may be produced as they break down.

Mixed or Undefined Causes

Sepsis

Infection may cause hemolysis as well as cholestasis.

Hypothyroidism

Prolonged jaundice may be the only early clue.

Hyperthyroidism

Infant of a Diabetic Mother

Most infants have polycythemia leading to increased hemoglobin breakdown as well as structural and metabolic instability of the red blood cells.

Dehydration

Hypoxia

Acidosis

Hypoalbuminemia

Premature infants are especially predisposed.

Drugs

Sulfonamides, acetylsalicylic acid, and other drugs may interfere with bilirubin transport.

Hereditary Causes of Defective Conjugation

Crigler-Najjar Syndrome

The hepatic enzyme glucuronide transferase is deficient. Type I, the autosomal-recessive form, is associated with extremely high levels of bilirubin in the neonatal period. Kernicterus often follows. In type II, the autosomal-dominant form, survival into adulthood is the rule, and phenobarbital therapy is effective.

HYPERBILIRUBINEMIA WITH CONJUGATED BILIRUBIN

♦ **Neonatal Hepatitis Syndrome**

Manifestations of neonatal hepatitis may appear at any time after birth. In addition to elevated serum levels of conjugated bilirubin, poor appetite, failure to thrive, and irritability may be seen. Although identifiable causes of neonatal hepatitis have been split away from this group, this syndrome still accounts for a considerable number of cases of neonatal conjugated hyperbilirubinemia and should remain a diagnosis of exclusion.

Biliary Obstruction (Idiopathic Ductal Cholestatic Jaundice)

Cholecystitis

Jaundice, abdominal pain, fever, anorexia, nausea, and vomiting may be presenting signs. The inflammation may follow trauma or be associated with various autoimmune disorders.

Cholelithiasis

Gallstones are much less common in children than adults. Jaundice may be present.

Biliary Atresia

Despite advances in diagnosis and treatment, 90% of the cases remain uncorrectable.

Arteriohepatic Dysplasia (Alagille Syndrome)

The most common form of familial intrahepatic cholestasis. Hypoplastic bile ducts, vertebral arch defects, growth retardation, and other defects are present. Some have a characteristic facies, with a small pointed chin, broad forehead, straight nose, and hypertelorism. This is the syndromic form of disorders with paucity of the bile ducts.

Paucity of Intrahepatic Bile Ducts

Choledochal Cyst

The classic triad of findings includes upper-abdominal pain, jaundice, and an abdominal tumor, the result of cystic dilation of the common bile duct.

Inspissated Bile Syndrome

This syndrome is a rare cause of jaundice today but was more prevalent when severe Rh isoimmunization reactions were more common. Plugging of bile ducts has been suggested as the mechanism; hepatic injury was found in some cases following severe hemolytic disease.

Perforation of Bile Duct

Fibrosing Pancreatitis

Most patients also have abdominal pain, weight loss, steatorrhea, and glucose intolerance.

Primary Sclerosing Cholangitis

A rare disorder, occasionally associated with ulcerative colitis. Hepatomegaly, progressive liver failure, weight loss, and steatorrhea are other features.

Infectious Causes of Cholestatic Jaundice

Bacterial Infections

Jaundice may be the presenting symptom or a common finding in sepsis, pyelonephritis, and other bacterial infections, including liver abscesses and cholangitis. An infant with conjugated hyperbilirubinemia should have a urine culture performed to assure that an occult pyelonephritis is not the cause.

Viral Infections

Viral Hepatitis

Hepatitis A, B, C, CMV, and other forms must be considered.

Coxsackie Virus Infection

Infectious Mononucleosis

Jaundice occurs in 5% to 10% of cases.

Miscellaneous Infection Related Syndromes

Jaundice is usually the result of heptocellular dysfunction associated with the infection. Examples include toxic shock syndrome, Rocky Mountain Spotted Fever, leptospirosis, and Lyme disease.

TORCH Infections

Neonatal hepatitis may follow intrauterine infection with any of a complex of diseases referred to as TORCH—toxoplasmosis, rubella, cytomegalovirus infection, herpes simplex—as well as syphilis.

Fungal Infection

Systemic histoplasmosis may involve the liver.

Parasitic Infestation

Visceral larva migrans caused by *Toxocara canis* or *T. cati* may produce inflammation of the liver with jaundice, hepatomegaly, and a significant eosinophilia. Schistosomiasis may be associated with jaundice.

♦ **Drugs**

Potential hepatotoxins include acetaminophen, acetylsalicylic acid, iron, isoniazid, and vitamin A. Other drugs that appear to cause allergic hepatocellular damage are erythromycin, sulfonamide, oxacillin, rifampin, and halothane. Ethanol, steroids, tetracycline, and methotrexate may all cause jaundice.

Miscellaneous

Chronic Active Hepatitis

This form, more common in adolescent girls, may present as an apparent viral hepatitis, but the jaundice does not resolve when expected. Malaise, fever, weight loss, and other systemic complaints may be present.

Chemical Injury

Carbon tetrachloride exposure may result in hepatic necrosis.

Reye Syndrome

Jaundice may occur during the fatty infiltration of the liver in this disorder, which has disappeared from the scene.

Genetic and Metabolic Disorders

Cystic Fibrosis

Liver involvement includes plugging of periportal canaliculi.

Alpha$_1$-Antitrypsin Deficiency

Onset of symptoms including jaundice and hepatomegaly may be at any age, including the neonatal period. The diagnosis may be made by serum-protein electrophoresis.

Hypopituitarism

May present with conjugated hyperbilirubinemia. Symptoms of hypoglycemia and hypothyroidism may also be present.

Galactosemia

The urine of jaundiced infants should always be tested for reducing substance, before vomiting, diarrhea, failure to thrive, and cataracts develop.

Galactokinase Deficiency

Hyperbilirubinemia and cataracts are the only manifestations. Signs develop later than in galactosemia.

Wilson Disease (Hepatolenticular Degeneration)

Liver dysfunction may occur at any age after infancy. Ceruloplasmin serum levels should be determined in any child with unexplained liver disease.

Hereditary Tyrosinemia

Other features include vomiting, diarrhea, failure to thrive, rickets, renal tubular defects, and hypoglycemia.

Hereditary Fructose Intolerance

Vomiting, diarrhea, and weight loss appear with the introduction of fructose, usually fruits, into the diet.

Niemann-Pick Disease, Type C

Hepatosplenomegaly, failure to thrive, neurologic deterioration, and the presence of cherry red spots on funduscopic examination are characteristic.

Wolman Disease

In infancy, diarrhea and failure to thrive are followed by rapid demise. Adrenal calcification is present on roentgenograms.

Glycogen Storage Disease

Type IV

The cause is a defect in the brancher enzyme. Failure to thrive, jaundice, and hepatosplenomegaly appear in the first 2 months of life, followed by progressive deterioration.

Type III

This form, caused by a defect in the debrancher enzyme, is more benign than type IV. Jaundice and increased serum levels of transaminase may be present.

Zellweger (Hepatocerebrorenal) Syndrome

In the neonatal period the physical appearance is striking; features include high forehead and epicanthal folds. Severe hypotonia, hepatomegaly, and poor appetite are other findings.

Neonatal Hemochromatosis (Iron Storage Disease)

Affected infants have a rapidly progressive course with early death. The majority of newborns develop a conjugated hyperbilirubinemia, with edema, coagulopathy, and respiratory distress in the first few days of life.

Familial Cholestasis Syndromes

Benign Recurrent Intrahepatic Cholestasis

Characterized by recurrent attacks of jaundice, pruritus, anorexia, and weight loss. Recurrent attacks of jaundice with severe pruritus begin in early childhood.

Caroli Disease

Children may have recurrent episodes of abdominal pain, fever, jaundice, and tender hepatomegaly as a result of episodes of cholangitis. The defect is characterized by saccular dilation of the intrahepatic bile ducts.

Recurrent Cholestasis with Lymphedema (Aagenaes Syndrome)

Infants with this syndrome may have prolonged jaundice, often followed by cirrhosis. Pedal edema develops in childhood.

Byler Disease

Loose, fatty stools appear in the first month of life. Jaundice and, then, hepato-splenomegaly develop, followed by cirrhosis and death in childhood.

Syndrome with Growth and Mental Retardation

In addition to findings of hepatosplenomegaly and jaundice, the toes and fingers are short and the skin thick.

Inherited Noncholestatic Syndromes

Dubin-Johnson Syndrome

Jaundice may be noted at birth. A family history of jaundice is often present. The serum bilirubin usually does not exceed 6 mg/dL, of which one third to three fourths is the conjugated form. Constitutional symptoms may include weakness, fatigue, anorexia, nausea, and vomiting. On liver biopsy the hepatic cells are pigmented.

Rotor Syndrome

Findings are identical to those in Dubin-Johnson syndrome, but on liver biopsy there is no pigment in the hepatic cells.

Miscellaneous Disorders

♦ Total Parenteral Nutrition

This has become the most common cause of conjugated hyperbilirubinemia in the newborn intensive care unit. The cause of TPN–associated liver disease is not completely understood. At least 2 weeks of TPN seem to be required.

Neonatal Lupus

Infants of mothers with lupus, Sjögren syndrome, or mixed connective tissue disease, may have cholestatic jaundice in the first few months of life. Most mothers are asymptomatic and undiagnosed.

Hyperthermia

Chromosomal Defects

Infants with Down, Turner, or trisomy 18 syndrome are predisposed to hyperbilirubinemia.

MIMICS OF JAUNDICE

Carotenoderma

A yellow-orange discoloration of the skin may be caused by pigments absorbed from yellow, orange, or red vegetables and fruits. The sclerae of the eyes are not discolored.

Lycopenoderma

A yellowish skin discoloration may also occur following prolonged ingestion of excessive amounts or red pigment in foods, especially tomatoes.

Drugs

Antimalarials such as quinacrine, in particular, may produce a yellow cast.

Sallowness

A sickly yellow hue, which may be seen in the chronically ill.

SUGGESTED READING

Gartner LM. Neonatal jaundice. *Pediatr Rev* 1994;15:422–432.
Hicks BA, Altman RP. The jaundiced newborn. *Pediatr Clin North Am* 1993;40:1161–1175.
Mews C, Sinatra FR. Cholestasis in infancy. *Pediatr Rev* 1994;15:233–240.
Wanek EA, Karrer FM, Brandt CT, Lilly JR. Biliary atresia. *Pediatr Rev* 1989;11:57–62.

15

Recurrent Infections

Parents frequently express concern that their children seem unduly susceptible to infections. Disorders of the immune system are often expected as the cause, but they are, in fact, not common. By far the most likely reason for a young child to have recurrent infections is frequent exposure to pathogens to which the child has not yet developed immunity. Participation in group daycare assures constant bombardment of infectious agents. It is estimated that a normal child endures 100 infections in the first 10 years of life. The average child in the first year of life has eight upper respiratory infections (URIs) alone; because URIs generally last 2 weeks, parents' perception that their infant either has a cold, has just gotten over one, or is about to come down with another one is accurate.

Recurrent infections in a specific anatomic area are due more often to local factors than to a systemic immunodeficiency. Otitis media results when nasopharygeal flora is trapped in the middle ear by Eustachian tube closure. Urinary tract infections may be recurrent in a child with vesicoureteral reflux or in one with a neurogenic bladder, because, in both situations, bacteria that ascend from the perineum to the bladder are not expelled rapidly in the next voiding but are free to multiply in the supportive media of urine. Another example of a localized physiologic process resulting in recurrent infections is asthma as the most common cause of recurrent pneumonia.

A primary immunodeficiency should be considered if a child has had two systemic bacterial infections (sepsis, meningitis, or osteomyelitis), or three serious respiratory (e.g., pneumonia, sinusitis) or bacterial infections (e.g., cellulitis, draining otitis, lymphadenitis) per year (1); an infection with an opportunistic organism; or an unusually severe infection that is normally mild. Unusual reactions to vaccines, recurrent diarrhea, and failure to thrive may also be important clues to immunodeficiencies, as is a history of recurrent severe infections in other family members.

Characteristics of immunodeficiency disorders include: infections with common organisms such as *Candida albicans,* or ubiquitous organisms that are generally nonpathogenic, such as *Pneumocystis carinii;* unusually severe infections; and repeated infections with the same organism, without evidence of immunity, such as recurrent *Neisseria* infections. The pattern of infections provides a clue to the specific abnormality: repeated bacterial infections suggests a disorder of B cell function, whereas repeated viral, fungal, and protozoal infections suggests a disorder of T cell function. Skin and pulmonary infections may be due to a disorder of white cell function; recurrent *Neisseria* infections suggests a disorder of the terminal complement cascade. Physical features may suggest a syndrome, of which immunodeficiency is a part, e.g., a child with eczema, petechiae, and recurrent otitis media may have Wiskott-Aldrich syndrome; children with short-limb dwarfism may have combined immunodeficiency. The family history

may suggest an inherited form of immunodeficiency, such as Bruton agammaglobulinemia. The social history may raise suspicion of vertically transmitted HIV infection.

The prevalence of known immunodeficiencies is about 1 per 100,000 population, excluding IgA deficiency. A better way to keep immunodeficiency as a cause of recurrent infection in perspective is to use the classification of Stiehm of children referred for evaluation of this problem (1). The most common category, accounting for 50% of cases, is the probably well child who is exposed to numerous infectious agents. Category 2, the allergic child, accounts for another 30%; chronic, nonimmunologic diseases, such as cystic fibrosis, asthma, sickle cell disease, diabetes mellitus, urinary tract obstructions, etc., category 3, account for 10%; and, the final 10%, category 4, may truly have an immunodeficiency. Finally, the relative frequencies of the immunodeficiency disorders should be noted. Antibody deficiencies comprise about 50%, combined antibody and cellular immunodeficiencies about 25%, disorders of phagocytic function about 20%, cellular deficiencies 7%, and complement deficiency about 2% of all cases (2).

♦ Most Common Causes of Recurrent Infections

Normal Exposure   Allergic Disorders Mistaken for Infections
Reactive Airways Disease   Anatomic and Physical Problems (Other)

• Cause Not to Forget

Acquired Immunodeficiency Syndrome

♦ PHYSIOLOGIC CAUSES

By far the most common cause of recurrent infections is repeated exposure to infectious agents of an otherwise healthy child. The average child has 6 to 12 infections per year. This number may increase in the child attending school or the preschool child or toddler who attends nursery school or is enrolled in a daycare center. Older siblings may also bring home the infections. An extensive laboratory evaluation is not indicated in these cases, unless the infections are unusual, severe, or prolonged.

♦ ANATOMIC AND PHYSICAL PROBLEMS

Pulmonary Disorders

♦ Bronchial Asthma

Asthma is the most common cause of recurrent "pneumonia." Decreased bronchial lumen and mucus plugs may predispose to repeated infections.

Cystic Fibrosis

Repeated respiratory infections may be prominent before gastrointestinal symptoms and signs appear.

Bronchopulmonary Dysplasia

Foreign Body

Recurrent Aspiration

Gastroesophageal Reflux

Hiatal Hernia

Neuromuscular Disorders

Central nervous system damage causing difficulty in handling secretions or a poor cough reflex should be considered.

Congenital Heart Disease

Conditions causing pulmonary congestion may predispose to infection.

Bronchiectasis

Ciliary Dyskinesia

Tracheoesophageal Fistula

Vascular Ring

Familial Dysautonomia

Tracheal Bronchus

An accessory or aberrant bronchus may lead to recurrent pneumonia and stridor. This anomaly may be associated with Down syndrome.

Asplenia

Children with asplenia are at risk for recurrent pyogenic infections, particularly with *Streptococcal pneumoniae,* including sepsis.

Urinary Tract Obstruction

Repeated infections may be caused by various obstructive disorders such as ureteral stenosis, stones, and ureteral reflux, as well as compression of the urinary system by extrinsic causes such as chronic constipation.

Central Nervous System Disorders

Ventricular Shunts

Skull Fractures

Basilar fractures in particular may be associated with infections.

Midline Sinus Tracts

Mondini Dysplasia

A congenital defect in the formation of the bony and membranous labyrinths of the inner ear. The clinical triad is congenital sensorineural hearing loss, profound vestibular weakness, and recurrent meningitis.

Metabolic Diseases

Diabetes Mellitus

Part of the cause of repeated infections may be poor circulation, but probably more important is impaired leukocyte chemotactic activity. Young infants are particularly prone to gram-negative infections.

Galactosemia

Infants with galactosemia are prone to gram-negative infections, particularly sepsis.

Hematologic Disturbances

Sickle Cell Disease

Functional asplenia develops following repeated infarctions. Defective opsonic function is the likely cause.

Leukemia and Lymphomas

Several factors may be involved including a decreased number of leukocytes and defective phagocytosis.

Neoplasms

Neoplasms may cause obstructive problems as well as defective leukocyte function.

Skin Defects

Atopic Dermatitis

Repeated skin infections are common with staphylococcal or streptococcal organisms.

Burns

Circulatory Compromise

Poor Lymphatic Drainage

Poor Venous Drainage

Anatomic Cardiac Abnormalities

Turbulence in blood flow from various defects may predispose to subacute bacterial endocarditis.

Indwelling Devices

Catheters

Shunts

Includes both cerebrospinal fluid and vascular shunts.

Heart Valves, Patches, etc.

Endothelial Patches

Orthopedic Hardware

DISORDERS OF PHAGOCYTIC FUNCTION

Chemotaxis-Neutrophil Disorders

Most children with neutropenia, defined as less than 1500/mm^3, have a secondary form as a result of infection, drugs, malignancy, or hypersplenism. Bone marrow failure such as aplastic anemia must also be considered. Primary (congenital) neutropenias are relatively uncommon.

Familial Neutropenia (Kostmann Syndrome)

Recurrent, severe infections of early onset, such as omphalitis, abscess formation, and sepsis, are characteristic. The neutropenia may be cyclic.

Cyclic Neutropenia

Cycles of normal neutrophil counts for 3 weeks are followed by 1 week lapses of failure of neutrophils to mature. The course is variable.

Autoimmune Neutropenia of Infancy

Infants may develop an absolute neutrophil count of 0–500/μL, usually associated with monocytosis and eosinophilia. Recurrent fevers and infections are typical. Circulating antibodies to neutrophils are present.

Shwachman Syndrome

Characteristic features are failure to thrive, evidence of pancreatic insufficiency, and neutropenia.

Leukocyte Adhesion Disorder

A family of surface glycoproteins are deficient. The leukocytes are deficient in adhesion related functions such as chemotaxis, phagocytosis, and antibody-dependent cellular cytotoxicity, among others. The disorder is inherited as in an autosomal recessive fashion. Characteristic manifestations in infancy include delayed separation of the umbilical cord, perirectal abscesses, and recurrent staphylococcal and gram-negative bacterial infections. Leukocytosis is common.

Hyper IgE Syndrome (Job Syndrome)

Severe eczema of early onset and almost constant staphylococcal infections are characteristic. Affected children have a coarse facies with a broad nasal bridge. Serum IgE levels are significantly increased.

Chediak-Higashi Syndrome

This uncommon, autosomal recessive inherited disorder is associated with partial oculocutaneous albinism. Affected children have lighter skin and hair than unaffected relatives. Photophobia and nystagmus are common. Neurologic signs include ataxia, seizures, decreased deep tendon reflexes and muscle weakness. A peripheral neutropenia is present with abnormal granules and inclusions in the white blood cells.

Kartagener Syndrome

Chronic or recurrent sinopulmonary and middle ear infections are characteristic. Situs inversus is a finding in about one half of the cases. Dyskinesia of the cilia of respiratory tract is present as is decreased chemotaxis.

"Lazy Leukocyte" Syndrome

Recurrent upper respiratory infections, stomatitis, gingivitis, otitis media, abscesses, and staphylococcal furuncles are common. Peripheral neutropenia with depressed migration of neutrophils is present, but normal mature neutrophils are found in the bone marrow.

Localized Juvenile Periodontitis

Usually occurs in adolescents who have localized areas of periodontitis as a result of impaired chemotaxis.

Neutropenia with Aphthous Stomatitis, Pharyngitis, and Fever

Episodes are recurrent.

Defective Opsonization

This defect occurs after splenectomy and in sickle cell disease. Newborns are deficient in the ability to opsonize coliform bacteria.

♦ Phagocyte Killing

Chronic Granulomatous Disease

Most patients (60%) are boys who have recurrent suppurative and granulomatous lesions, colonized usually by staphylococci, *Escherichia coli, Pseudomonas, Serratia* and *Klebsiella*. Adolescents usually have severe and antibiotic resistant acneiform lesions and seborrheic dermatitis as well. The onset in most cases is by 1 year of age. Hepatosplenomegaly, pneumonitis, and osteomyelitis are also common. Autosomal dominant and recessive forms have also been described.

Myeloperoxidase Deficiency

Chronic moniliasis is common. Severe symptoms are uncommon.

Leukocyte Glucose-6-Phosphate Dehydrogenase Deficiency

Findings are similar to those in chronic granulomatous disease, but infections are less severe.

Glutathione Reductase and Synthetase Deficiencies

DISORDERS OF THE COMPLEMENT SYSTEM

Clq Deficiency

This form has been found in association with severe immunologic deficiency states, especially T cell disorders. Clinical findings include severe wasting, chronic debilitation, chronic candidiasis, and diarrhea. Persistent infections may be caused by various organisms.

C2 Deficiency

In the United States, this is the most frequently described homozygous deficiency of a complement component. In addition to recurrent severe pyogenic infections, affected individuals, both homozygous and heterozygous, are at increased risk of rheumatoid and other autoimmune diseases.

C3 and C5 Deficiencies

Children with deficiencies of these components have had recurrent severe infections such as pneumococcal pneumonia and meningococcal meningitis.

C5 Dysfunction (Leiner Disease)

A generalized seborrhea-like dermatitis, recurrent infections (especially by gram-negative organisms), diarrhea, and failure to thrive are important features.

C6, C7, and C8

Meningococcal and gonococcal bacteremias may be recurrent in families with these deficiencies.

DISORDERS OF ANTIBODY PRODUCTION

Transient Hypogammaglobulinemia

The production of immunoglobulins may be delayed in some infants until 18 to 30 months of age. Recurrent respiratory infections and unexplained fevers are common.

X-Linked Agammaglobulinemia

All classes of immunoglobulins are deficient. Lymphoid tissue, including the tonsils, is hypoplastic. Recurrent, severe, life-threatening pyogenic infections are common after 6 months of age. A rheumatoid arthritis-like picture develops in some patients. Eczematoid skin rashes are common.

X-Linked Hypogammaglobulinemia with Normal or Increased Serum IgM

Infections are similar to those in the form as described, but lymphoid tissue may be enlarged. Neutropenia, thrombocytopenia, hemolytic anemia, and lymphomas are relatively common.

Common Variable Immunodeficiency

Recurrent infections may not begin until late childhood or adulthood. Most immunoglobulin isotypes are present in low levels. Recurrent sinopulmonary infections are the most common presentation. Malabsorption and autoimmune disorders are also common.

Selective IgA Deficiency

This is the most common primary immunodeficiency, but many "affected" children are asymptomatic. Recurrent respiratory infections of upper and lower airways, intractable asthma, chronic diarrhea, autoimmune disorders, and malignancies are common.

IgG Subclass Deficiency

Selective IgG2 and IgG4 deficiencies are most common and associated with infections by pyogenic bacteria.

Selective IgM Deficiency

Recurrent bacteremias, meningitis, and gastrointestinal problems are common.

Secondary Immunodeficiencies

These may occur in malnutrition, during immunosuppressive therapy, in protein losing enteropathies, nephrotic syndrome, and uremia, after splenectomy, and with lymphomas.

Ataxia Telangiectasia

Recurrent sinopulmonary infections with bronchiectasis are most common. The ataxia is progressive, leading to eventual complete debility. Telangiectasia develop gradually, first on the conjunctivae and ears. IgA and IgE deficiencies are common.

Wiskott-Aldrich Syndrome

This is an X-linked recessive disorder characterized by recurrent infections, eczema, and thrombocytopenia. Serum IgM is decreased, but serum IgA and IgE levels are elevated.

Transcobalamin-II Deficiency and Hypogammaglobulinemia

Megaloblastic anemia, granulocytopenia, and thrombocytopenia with absent antibody production are other findings in this rare disease. Large doses of vitamin B_{12} may correct these abnormalities.

DISORDERS OF CELLULAR IMMUNITY

• Acquired Immune Deficiency Syndrome

This disorder has become the most common cause of true immunodeficiency. Symptoms include failure to thrive, chronic diarrhea, recurrent pneumonia, candidiasis, otitis media, and so forth.

DiGeorge Syndrome

The thymus and parathyroid glands fail to develop. Congenital heart disease, an abnormal facies (hypertelorism, micrognathia, low-set abnormally shaped ears, antimongoloid slant to the eyes), and tetany from hypocalcemia are present.

Chronic Mucocutaneous Candidiasis

Chronic candidal infections of the skin, nails, and mucous membranes may be associated with endocrinopathies (especially hypoparathyroidism).

Severe Combined Immunodeficiency

Combined T cell and B cell deficiencies result in early severe recurrent infections, usually before 6 months of age. Diarrhea and pneumonia with failure to thrive are present. Affected children are susceptible to viral infections often with fatal outcomes as well as poliomyelitis following immunization. Inheritance is autosomal recessive (classic Swiss type lymphopenic agammaglobulinemia) or X-linked recessive.

Adenosine Deaminase Deficiency

About one half of children with the autosomal recessive type of severe combined immunodeficiency have absence of this enzyme. Some children have skeletal abnormalities including a rachitic rosary. Another enzyme deficiency, that of nucleoside phosphorylase, has similar findings, but onset of infections may be later (at 6 to 12 months of age).

Nezelof Syndrome

In this cellular immunodeficiency there is a variable degree of normal immunoglobulin synthesis. The cases are sporadic in occurrence. The age at onset of recurrent infections is variable. Eczema, chronic otitis media, and sinusitis are common.

Immunodeficiency with Short-Limbed Dwarfism

Several forms have been described: one with severe combined immunodeficiency; another with cellular immunodeficiency; and a third with humoral immunodeficiency. Redundant skinfolds are found around the neck and large joints.

DRUG-RELATED CAUSES

Corticosteroids

Recurrent infections may be a problem in children taking corticosteroids.

Antineoplastics

Antibiotics

Resistant bacterial infections may develop in some children on chronic antibiotic therapy.

CHRONIC INFECTIONS

Chronic Epstein-Barr Virus (EBV)

An unusual disorder characterized by recurrent episodes of pharyngitis with fever, cervical lymphadenopathy, and malaise. Edema of the eyelids and fingers, arthralgias, and myalgias are often present. Anti-EBV antibody pattern is typical in this syndrome, a persistently elevated anti-early antigen or absent anti-EBV nuclear antigen.

Other

Other infectious agents associated with chronic infections include cytomegalovirus, Coxsackie B virus, toxoplasmosis, parvovirus B19, and mycoplasma.

REFERENCES

1. Stiehm ER. They're back: recurrent infections in pediatric practice. *Contemp Pediatr* 1990;7:20–40.
2. Iseki M, Heiner DC. Immunodeficiency disorders. *Pediatr Rev* 1993;14:226–236.

SUGGESTED READING

Herold BC, Shulman ST. Recurrent infections. In: Stockman JA III, ed. *Difficult diagnosis in pediatrics.* Philadelphia: WB Saunders, 1990:99–115.

Hopp R. Evaluation of recurrent respiratory tract infection in children. *Curr Probl Pediatr* 1996;26:148–158.

Lalezari P, Khorshidi M, Petrosova M. Autoimmune neutropenia of infancy. *J Pediatr* 1986;109:764–769.

Yang KD, Hill HR. Neutrophil function disorders: pathophysiology, prevention, and therapy. *J Pediatr* 1991;119:343–354.

Zitelli BJ. Recurrent infections. In: Gartner JC Jr, Zitelli BJ, eds. *Common & chronic symptoms in pediatrics.* St. Louis: Mosby, 1997:381–397.

16

Unusual Odors as Clues to Diagnosis

With increasing reliance on laboratory findings for diagnosis, the art of clinical diagnosis using the physical senses may be neglected. In particular, the physician's sense of smell may not be used to full advantage.

Certain disorders may produce characteristic odors of body, sweat, urine, or breath. Many of these disorders are rare, but a quick and accurate diagnosis based on odor will make the physician "smell like a bed of roses."

UNUSUAL BODY OR URINE ODOR

Foods

Asparagus and garlic are examples of foods that may impart their distinctive odors.

Drugs

Various drugs may produce strong "medicinal" odors of the urine and occasionally of the skin. The odors from ampicillin and its derivatives are most pungent and occur frequently in children.

Lotions, Body Oils, Perfumes

Poor Hygiene

Foreign Body

Nasal foreign bodies are perhaps the best known cause of pervasive foul body odor; even the clothing may be permeated. A unilateral nasal discharge should always suggest a nasal foreign body. Vaginal foreign bodies, and, much more rarely, foreign bodies in the external ear canal may also produce a generalized odor, known as bromhidrosis.

Skin Disturbances

Disorders of the skin, such as some forms of ichthyosis, keratosis follicularis (Darier disease), or any disorder resulting in significant thickening and fissuring, may be associated with an unusual body odor. Ulcers or other necrotic skin lesions or tumors may also produce a generalized foul odor.

124

Typhoid Fever

An odor of freshly baked bread is said to be emitted by patients with this disease.

Urinary Tract Infection

An ammoniacal odor may be prominent in infection by urea-splitting bacteria.

Fish Odor Syndrome

This familial disorder inherited in an autosomal recessive fashion, should be considered in patients with body odor. The cause is impaired N-oxidation of excreted trimethylamine in the urine (1).

Phenylketonuria

The odor is often described as mousey, musty, or horselike. If neonatal screening for this disorder were omitted, diagnosis may be based on the clinical features of developmental delay, fair complexion, microcephaly, eczema, and seizures.

Maple Syrup Urine Disease

Infants often present in the first week or two of life with decreased appetite, vomiting, acidosis, seizures, coma, and the characteristic urine odor. A milder form may present with intermittent episodes of ataxia, vomiting, and lethargy in apparently healthy children. The disorder is caused by a defect in metabolism of branched-chain amino acids.

Isovaleric Acidemia (Sweaty Sock Syndrome)

This disorder, resulting from a defect in leucine catabolism, is characterized by recurrent vomiting, acidosis, and coma. (Another enzyme defect, green acyl dehydrogenase, has been reported in some cases to produce the same odor. The infants, who had poor appetite, vomiting, seizures, and severe acidosis, died within a few months of age.)

Glutaric Acidemia Type II

Both fatty acid and amino acid metabolism are affected in this disorder. Findings are variable and range from profound hypoglycemia to metabolic acidosis without ketosis, cardiomyopathy, and the smell of sweaty feet.

Oasthouse Urine Disease

A yeastlike odor is produced in this rare defect in methionine absorption. The two patients described had white hair, convulsions, and attacks of hyperpnea.

Hypermethioninemia

Three siblings between the ages of 2 and 8 weeks developed a fishy smell along with lethargy and irritability. All died of infection within a few months.

Beta-Methylcrotonyl CoA Carboxylase Deficiency

Only a few cases of this disorder, associated with the smell of cat urine, have been described. Poor appetite and lethargy are findings in early infancy.

Rancid Butter Syndrome

Hypermethioninemia and hypertyrosinemia were found in three siblings who developed poor appetite, irritability, seizures, and coma in the first few months of life along with the offensive odor.

Schizophrenia

A pungent body odor has been described in patients with schizophrenia, apparently caused by the presence of trans-3-methyl-2-hexanoic acid in the sweat (2). Others have not confirmed this finding. It may be the former were children with a genetic condition with central nervous system manifestations.

Scurvy

The sweat is said to smell putrid.

Gout

Although a medical rarity in children, gout is said to produce a characteristic odor.

UNUSUAL BREATH ODORS

Tonsillitis

Infection of tonsils and adenoids with any infectious agent may produce an abnormal odor. Some experienced clinicians feel that Group A beta-hemolytic streptococcal infections have a characteristic odor.

Gingivitis/Poor Dental Hygiene

Infection of the gingiva produces a pungent breath odor. Decaying food particles between the teeth are a common cause of bad breath.

Acetone

A fruity odor is found in ketoacidosis, whether produced by short-term starvation, diabetes, or other disorders that result in the increased use of lipids as fuel, or salicylates.

Uremia

An ammoniacal smell is often noticeable on the breath of patients with uremia.

Hepatic Failure

The fetor hepaticus of liver failure resembles musty fish or raw liver.

Intestinal Obstruction

The odor is feculent.

Lung Abscess

Anaerobic organisms produce a foul breath odor.

Diphtheria

A mousey odor may be present.

Mitochondrial Acetoacetyl-CoA Thiolase Deficiency

A fruity odor is present in this disorder characterized by intermittent severe acidosis, ketosis, hematemesis, melena, vomiting, and diarrhea.

Cytosolic Acetoacetyl-CoA Thiolase Deficiency

A rare disorder characterized by mental retardation, ketosis with a fruity odor, hypotonia, ataxia, and coma.

Tyrosinemia

Individuals with this disorder are also said to have a yeastlike odor. The disease is characterized by hepatorenal failure, failure to grow, ascites, and coagulopathy.

REFERENCES

1. Ayesh R, Mitchell SC, Zhang A, Smith RL. The fish odour syndrome: biochemical, familial, and clinical aspects. *BMJ* 1993;307:655–657.
2. Mace JW, Goodman SI, Centerwall WR, et al. The child with unusual odor. *Clin Pediatr* 1976;15:57–62.

SUGGESTED READING

Hayden GF. Olfactory diagnosis in medicine. *Postgrad Med* 1980;67:110–118.
Henkin RI. Body odor. *JAMA* 1995;273:1171–1172.
Liddell K. Smell as a diagnostic marker. *Postgrad Med J* 1976;52:136–138.
Replogle WH, Beebe DK. Halitosis. *Am Fam Physician* 1996;53:1215–1218.
Rizzo WB, Roth KS. On 'being led by the nose': rapid detection of inborn errors of metabolism. *Arch Pediatr Adolesc Med* 1994;148:869–872.

17

Excessive Sweating

Children who sweat excessively do so most frequently in response to exercise, in reaction to stress, or with fever. Sweating allows the individual to lose heat by the evaporation of water (sweat) from the body surface. Failure to sweat and reduce body temperature may result in heat stroke. This subsequent classification enumerates common and uncommon causes of excessive perspiration. Keep in mind mercury poisoning (acrodynia) in any child with profuse sweating.

PHYSIOLOGIC CAUSES

Exercise

Increased Environmental Temperature/Humidity

Fever

Excessive Clothing Covering

Obesity

Emotional Stimuli

The increased perspiration may be generalized or localized, especially in the axillae or on the perineum, forehead, and palms of the hands and soles of the feet.

Gustatory Stimuli

The forehead, upper lip, and cheeks may show an increase in perspiration accompanying the ingestion of certain foods, especially spicy and hot ones.

Breathholding and Sleep Apnea

Individuals with these symptoms often have associated increased sweating at night associated with the episodes.

SWEATING WITH INFECTION

During Defervescence

Excessive sweating is most likely to occur as the body temperature falls toward normal, during infections or inflammatory diseases.

Chronic Illnesses

Pulmonary Tuberculosis

Night sweats are a classic sign of active pulmonary tuberculosis, but this is an uncommon cause of excessive sweating in children.

Brucellosis

Although in acute infection the symptoms are variable, constitutional symptoms include fatigue, vague muscle aches, headaches, fever, and hyperhidrosis.

Malaria

ENDOCRINE AND METABOLIC DISORDERS

Hypoglycemia

In the newborn, symptoms include tremors, sweating, cyanosis, poor appetite, and apneic episodes. In older infants and children, pallor, staring episodes, and abnormal behavior, as well as sweating and tachycardia, may be findings. The symptoms are caused by catecholamine secretion as a physiologic response to hypoglycemia.

Hyperthyroidism

Tremor, fatigue, tachycardia, elevated systolic blood pressure, and hyperhidrosis are common signs.

Pituitary Gigantism or Acromegaly

Increased perspiration is common, probably secondary to hypermetabolism.

Pheochromocytoma

Episodic elevations of the blood pressure are a classic sign, but headaches, sweating, pallor, and palpitations are the most common symptoms.

Phenylketonuria

Infants and children with untreated phenylketonuria are reported to sweat excessively.

Citrullinemia

DRUGS AND TOXINS

Salicylate Intoxication

Fever, sweating, vomiting, and hyperpnea are common.

Narcotic Withdrawal

This possibility must be considered in infants with tremors, irritability, increased appetite, and sweating.

Organophosphate Poisoning

Symptoms depend on the severity of the exposure. Excessive salivation, lacrimation, and sweating are common. Muscle cramping, anxiety, vomiting, diarrhea, and bronchospasm may also be seen.

Acrodynia

In mercury poisoning, the gradual onset of irritability, anorexia, and low-grade fever is followed by generalized erythema, or a miliarial-like rash, profuse sweating, photophobia, and hypotonia, and painful, peeling fingers. Profuse sweating should always suggest this possibility.

Emetics

Ipecac may cause sweating as well as its desired effect.

Insulin Overdose

Carbon Monoxide Poisoning

CARDIOVASCULAR DISORDERS

Congestive Heart Failure

In infants the more prominent signs include tachycardia, tachypnea, hepatomegaly, and dyspnea. Sweating is most common about the head and neck.

Syncope

Pallor, sweating, and restlessness may precede syncopal episodes.

Raynaud Phenomenon

Sweating of the involved hands and feet commonly accompanies the color change.

Cluster Headaches

The headaches are severe and often short-lived but recur frequently during attacks. Conjunctival injection, tearing, nasal stuffiness, facial flushing, and sweating accompany the attacks.

Myocardial Infarction

Although infarctions are rare, disorders such as Kawasaki syndrome may produce coronary occlusion. Chest pain, syncope, hypotension, and tachycardia are other features.

NEUROLOGIC DISORDERS

Spinal Cord Lesions

Following cord disruption, stimulation of the affected limbs causes a mass reaction with spasm and sweating.

Benign Paroxysmal Vertigo

The recurrent attacks of vertigo are short-lived and associated with pallor, nystagmus, and, often, significant sweating.

Reflex Sympathetic Dystrophy

Sweating may occur in the involved extremity.

Diencephalic Syndrome

Infants with tumors in the diencephalon (usually optic gliomas) sweat excessively; failure to thrive, nystagmus, and a happy affect are other features.

Subacute Sclerosing Panencephalitis

In the terminal stages, profuse sweating may occur.

Auriculotemporal Syndrome

A unilateral facial flush and sweating, the result of disruption of the auriculotemporal nerve, may accompany food intake .

Hydrocephalus

Sweating has been described as one of the associated signs.

MISCELLANEOUS CAUSES

Atopic Disposition

Children with atopic dermatitis and allergic conditions may sweat excessively.

Respiratory Failure

Increased sweating is a clinical index of the degree of failure.

Juvenile Rheumatoid Arthritis (JRA)

Children with JRA are frequently noted to perspire excessively, even without fever.

Lymphoma, Leukemia

Occult tumors, especially lymphomas and leukemia, may be associated with excessive sweating.

Mushroom Poisoning

Some mushrooms contain muscarine leading to cholinergic symptoms of sweating, salivation, lacrimation, and diarrhea.

Familial Dysautonomia

In this rare autosomal recessive disorder, there may be many unusual responses such as difficulty in swallowing, repeated aspiration and infection, absent lacrimation, blotchy skin, temperature swings, emotional lability, relative indifference to pain, and excessive sweating.

Familial Periodic Paralysis

Episodic attacks of flaccid paralysis and areflexia occur most commonly at night. The attacks last a few hours and then subside. Increased thirst and sweating may precede the attacks.

Carcinoid Syndrome

The malignant carcinoid syndrome is rare in children. The classic features include right-sided valvular heart disease, sudden flushing of the skin, frequent watery stools, and asthmatic attacks.

Chédiak-Higashi Syndrome

Prominent features of this rare inherited disorder include areas of depigmented skin, photophobia accompanying ocular albinism, decreased lacrimation, hepatosplenomegaly, increased susceptibility to infection, and progressive granulocytopenia. Large inclusions are seen in the cytoplasm of white blood cells.

Thrombocytopenia with Aplasia of the Radius (TAR) Syndrome

Children with this syndrome have been noted to have increased sweating.

Pyridoxine Deficiency

Sweating, especially of the head, has been reported in this rare vitamin deficiency.

Vasoactive Intestinal Peptide Secreting Tumor

Infants usually present with growth failure, intermittent diarrhea and, occasionally, flushing, sweating, and hypertension. Tumors are usually ganglioneuromas and ganglioneuroblastomas.

Episodic Spontaneous Hypothermia with Hyperhidrosis

This unusual combination has been described in a number of children. Some have had agenesis of the corpus callosum. It has been postulated that specific serotonin dysfunction in the anterior hypothalamic extrapyramidal shivering mechanism is central to the pathogenesis.

SUGGESTED READING

Sheth RD, Barron TF, Hartlage PL. Episodic spontaneous hypothermia with hyperhidrosis. *Pediatr Neurol* 1994;10:58–60.

18

Polydipsia

Polydipsia, or excessive thirst, is a rather uncommon symptom in childhood. Polyruria, excessive urine production, almost always follows. Nuclear centers in the ventromedial and anterior hypothalamus integrate signals that alter water ingestion. Some drugs may alter thirst, and psychological factors may also have a profound effect.

The underlying causes of polydipsia that come to mind first include diabetes mellitus and diabetes insipidus. Diabetes mellitus is probably the most common organic cause of polydipsia; however, other symptoms, particularly weight loss and polyuria, generally outweigh the increased thirst as the primary complaint. Psychogenic polydipsia (also called hysterical or primary polydipsia or compulsive water drinking) is probably underrated in frequency, especially after one considers the organic disorders listed below.

◆ Most Common Causes of Polydipsia

Psychogenic Polydipsia   Diabetes Mellitus
Diabetes Insipidus

● Disorders Not to Forget

Hypercalcemia   Sickle Cell Anemia
Renal Tubular Acidosis   Hypokalemia

◆ PSYCHOGENIC POLYDIPSIA

Affected children are compulsive water drinkers and may have other neurotic traits such as immature behavior. Social history is important. Water deprivation usually increases urine osmolality, but if the polydipsia has been present for some time, urinary concentrating ability may be compromised, making the diagnosis difficult to confirm.

NEUROGENIC POLYDIPSIA

Lesions of the hypothalamus may cause excessive thirst without a deficiency of antidiuretic hormone, and may be mistaken for psychogenic polydipsia.

METABOLIC-ENDOCRINE CAUSES

◆ Diabetes Mellitus

Polydipsia is usually fairly abrupt in onset, with progression to weight loss and acidosis. In suspected cases, the urine can be quickly checked for glucose.

● Hypercalcemia

Several disorders including vitamin D intoxication and malignancies may produce hypercalcemia with resultant hyposthenuria and polydipsia. Anorexia, constipation, lethargy, failure to thrive, and renal stones may be present. In hyperparathyroidism, repeated bone fractures or deformities may also be findings.

◆ Diabetes Insipidus

Antidiuretic hormone production is deficient due to destruction of the neurohypophysis or hypothalamic lesions from various causes including histiocytosis, trauma, infection, cysts, tumors, leukemia, and sarcoidosis. Water deprivation fails to increase urine osmolality. This form of diabetes insipidus responds to vasopressin therapy.

● Hypokalemia

11 β-Hydroxysteroid Dehydrogenase Deficiency (Pseudohyperaldosteronism)

Onset occurs in early childhood with failure to thrive, polyuria, and polydipsia, secondary to hypokalemia, and severe hypertension.

Bartter Syndrome

Growth failure, polydipsia and polyuria, constipation, and episodes of fever and dehydration may be seen as early as 2 months of age. Symptoms are secondary to severe hypokalemia caused by excessive aldosterone secretion. The blood pressure is normal.

Primary Hyperaldosteronism

Polydipsia and polyuria are part of the picture produced by hypokalemia. Causes include aldosterone-secreting adenomas and bilateral micronodular adrenocortical hyperplasia. Hypertension is present.

Pheochromocytoma

All patients have hypertension at some time although usually paroxysmal. During attacks of hypertension, symptoms of headache, palpitations, sweating, vomiting, and pallor may be present.

Neuroblastoma and Ganglioneuroblastoma

Catecholamines may be secreted by these tumors, resulting in hypertension, flush, pallor, polydipsia and polyuria, and diarrhea.

Cystinosis

Onset of symptoms is in the first year of life, with irritability, slow growth, anorexia, polydipsia and polyuria, constipation, and heat intolerance. Photophobia, cherubic facies, and decreased pigment of hair and skin are other findings, as well as glucosuria with hyperglucosemia.

RENAL CAUSES

• Sickle Cell Anemia

Hyposthenuria is thought to be secondary to sludging of sickle cells in the renal medulla and an impaired countercurrent mechanism. Polydipsia follows the resultant water loss from the kidneys.

• Renal Tubular Acidosis

This clinical syndrome has multiple causes and should be considered in children with dehydration and constipation with polyuria. In infants, vomiting, failure to thrive, anorexia, and lethargy are common. Laboratory findings include hyperchloremic acidosis, hypokalemia, and an alkaline urine with low specific gravity.

Nephrogenic Diabetes Insipidus

This form is seen principally in boys; inheritance is probably X-linked, although girls may be affected. This possibility must be considered in a child with hypertonic dehydration who continues to excrete urine of low specific gravity. Failure to thrive, repeated bouts of dehydration, and fever are common manifestations. Vasopressin therapy is ineffective.

Interstitial Nephritis

Renal parenchymal inflammation may occur for no apparent reason. In these cases, onset of polyuria and polydipsia is at 3 to 4 years of age, but most cases are diagnosed in the teens with the development of hypertension. Known causes of interstitial nephritis include analgesic abuse, nonsteroidal anti-inflammatory drugs, mercury poisoning, methicillin reaction, diphenylhydantoin, and sulfonamides.

Medullary Cystic Disease of Kidney (Nephronophthisis)

There may be a history of polyuria and polydipsia beginning at 2 to 6 years of age. Growth failure and rickets may be present; anemia and renal failure occurs later. Inheritance is autosomal recessive.

MISCELLANEOUS CAUSES

Congestive Heart Failure

Hypertension

Renin-induced hypertension and secondary angiotension II production may cause polydipsia.

Increased Salt Intake

Verapamil

An infant who developed polydipsia after treatment with verapamil has been described. The polydipsia stopped on discontinuation of the drug.

SUGGESTED READING

Horev Z, Cohen AH. Compulsive water drinking in infants and young children. *Clin Pediatr* 1994;33:209–213.
Leung AK, Robson WL, Halperin ML. Polyuria in childhood. *Clin Pediatr* 1991;30:634–640.

19

Sleep Disturbances

Interference with normal sleep patterns is relatively common in children. Fortunately, most of these disturbances are benign and are commonly precipitated by changes in the child's routine. Suggestions for evaluation and management of common sleep problems in infants and young children may be found in the articles by Blum and Carey (1) and Ferber (2).

Nightmares and difficulty in falling asleep may follow daytime stresses, activities, and excitement. Genuine serious psychological problems manifesting as sleep disturbances are much less common in children than in adults.

DISTURBANCES IN NORMAL SLEEP PATTERNS

Night Wakening

This common phenomenon occurs around 9 months of age, and it may follow an illness or just appear. Virtually all infants wake during the night, but most are able to settle themselves back to sleep. Those who do not return to sleep and cry for assistance are labeled as having night awakening.

Nightmares

This is a common sleep disturbance during which the child usually awakes in terror from a dream. The disturbing incident is remembered and the child is oriented after the event. Nightmares often occur following disturbances in routines during the day.

Night Terrors (Pavor Nocturnus)

In this uncommon disorder, most prevalent in mid-childhood, an intense anxiety reaction with physical signs such as screaming, agitation, hallucinations, sweating, and tachycardia occurs. The child appears awake but does not recognize surroundings. The episode lasts a few minutes; the child falls back to sleep and does not remember the event.

Bronchial Asthma

In some children, the onset of attacks during sleep causes repeated wakening accompanied by anxiety.

138

Airway Obstruction

Frequent episodes of wakening and sleeplessness are common in upper-airway obstruction.

Gastroesophageal Reflux

Milk Intolerance

In a group of 146 children less than 5 years of age, referred to a sleep clinic for continual waking and crying during sleep, 10% normalized their sleep patterns when cow milk was removed from the diet (3).

Sleepwalking (Somnambulism)

Sleepwalking may occur in up to 5% of children. The eyes are open, but the child seems not to recognize the environment. Motor skills are clumsy. The duration is usually only a few minutes, and the child has amnesia for the event, which often follows a stressful event during the preceding day. The incidence increases in families where there is a history of this disorder.

Sleeptalking (Somniloquy)

Usually the child does not wake but may awaken others with the talking, which often accompanies sleepwalking.

Pinworms

In infected young girls, the pinworm may crawl out of the anus during the night and migrate forward onto the hymenal ring. The associated irritation may awaken the child.

Nocturnal Seizures

Tonic-clonic motor activity may waken others in the household. Other clues include incontinence or injuries to the tongue from biting.

DISTURBANCES CAUSING EXCESSIVE SLEEPINESS

Depression

Depressed individuals, including children, are often lethargic and sleep excessively although restlessly. Maternal depression may be a factor in young children.

Drugs

Various drugs may cause excessive sleepiness including antihistamines, anticonvulsants, analgesics, and opiates.

Airway Obstruction

Some children with enlarged tonsils and adenoids or those who have a falling back of the tongue (glossoptosis) during the pharyngeal muscular relaxation of sleep may have excessive lethargy, snoring, and episodic periods of apnea.

Head Trauma

Increased Intracranial Pressure

Migraine

Prolonged episodes of sleep may occur following episodic attacks of migraine.

Narcolepsy

This disorder is uncommon in childhood; attacks usually begin after age 15. The characteristic feature is an uncontrollable, episodic change in consciousness, usually of short duration (less than 15 minutes), commonly associated with a sudden loss of muscle tone (cataplexy), sleep paralysis, and, much less commonly, states of auditory or visual hallucinations.

Postencephalitic Disturbances

Hypoglycemia

Hypothyroidism

Pickwickian Syndrome

Excessively obese individuals may experience hypercapnia and excessive sleepiness due to respiratory insufficiency.

Kleine-Levin Syndrome

This rare disorder has been described in boys over 10 years of age, who have episodes of excessive sleep lasting for days to weeks. They may awake intermittently and eat excessively.

DIFFICULTY FALLING ASLEEP

Anxiety

Children may have difficulty sleeping because of fears or emotional stimulation or following parental discipline, or, particularly in older infants and toddlers, because of fear of separation from parents.

Depression

Overstimulation

Young children need a period of relaxation prior to bedtime.

Curiosity

Activity in the environment may make it difficult to sleep.

Hyperthyroidism

This condition is a rare cause of insomnia.

OTHER DISTURBANCES

Sleep Myoclonus

Sudden, single, generalized jerks as the child is falling to sleep are common and benign.

Sleep Apnea

Short periods of apnea (less than 10 seconds) are common in infants. Children with narcolepsy and upper-airway obstructive disorders may also have apneic episodes. Prolonged episodes of sleep apnea may be a cause of sudden infant death syndrome.

REFERENCES

1. Blum NJ, Carey WB. Sleep problems among infants and young children. *Pediatr Rev* 1996;17:87–92.
2. Ferber R. Sleeplessness, night awakening, and night crying in the infant and toddler. *Pediatr Rev* 1987;9:69–82.
3. Kahn A, Mozin MJ, Rebuffat E, Sottiaux M, Muller MF. Milk intolerance in children with persistent sleeplessness: a prospective double-blind crossover evaluation. *Pediatrics* 1989;84:595–603.

SUGGESTED READING

Lozoff B, Zuckerman B. Sleep problems in children. *Pediatr Rev* 1988;10:17–24.

20

Sudden Death/Apparent Life-Threatening Events

The sudden unexpected death of an infant or child is as devastating for the family as it is for the pediatrician who has taken care of the child. Sudden infant death syndrome (SIDS) has received considerable attention over the years with thousands of postulated causes for the catastrophe. This chapter will not attempt to reiterate the literature on the subject; rather, the focus will be on causes of sudden death or apparent life-threatening events (ALTEs) that may prove important for family counseling in cases of death, or, possibly, the prevention of both events.

In 1991 the National Institute of Child Health and Human Development defined SIDS as "the sudden death of an infant under 1 year of age that remains unexplained after a thorough case investigation, including performance of a complete autopsy, examination of the death scene, and review of the clinical history" (1). SIDS primarily affects infants between 1 and 6 months of age (95%), with 85% between 2 and 4 months of age (1). The campaign to have infants sleep supine instead of prone (Back to Sleep) has been associated with decreases of as high as 50% in the rate of SIDS in some countries. Various other risk factors for SIDS are well known, including maternal smoking, both during and after pregnancy, native American heritage, and soft bedding. A challenge, delicate in the individual case, is to determine if child abuse is the cause.

ALTEs were defined by the National Institutes of Health Consensus Development Conference in 1986, as "an episode that is frightening to the observer and is characterized by some combination of apnea (central or occasionally obstructive), color change (usually cyanotic or pallid but occasionally erythematous or plethoric), marked change in muscle tone (usually marked limpness), choking, or gagging. In some cases the observer fears that the infant has died" (2). This terminology should replace "near-miss SIDS" because it implies an association between the two conditions, which may be misleading. The risk of subsequent infant death among infants who have an ALTE is probably 1% to 2%, although the severity of the ALTE may increase this percentage (2).

Although the causes of sudden death or ALTE in infants may be different than those in older children and adolescents, there is some overlap; consequently, the differential diagnosis has been combined in this chapter.

♦ **Most Common Causes**

Sudden Death in Infants	Sudden Death in Older Children
SIDS	Long QT Syndrome
Asphyxia	Myocarditis
Long QT Syndrome	Hypertrophic Cardiomyopathy
Child Abuse (Suffocation)	Drugs/Cocaine

♦ **ALTE**

Gastroesophageal Reflux	Respiratory Syncytial Virus
Seizure	Pertussis
Obstructive Sleep Apnea	

● **Causes of SIDS or ALTE Not to Forget**

Sepsis Associated with Asplenia	Fatty Oxidation Disorders
Passive Inhalation of Crack Cocaine Smoke	Botulism
Child Abuse (Suffocation)	

♦ **IDIOPATHIC SIDS**

Despite adequate autopsy examination and other investigation, about 85% of sudden deaths in infants remain unexplained. Maternal smoking during pregnancy is a major risk factor.

OTHER CAUSES OF SIDS/ALTE IN INFANTS

♦ **Child Abuse**

This remains an important cause of infant death. Suffocation may be very difficult to distinguish from SIDS. A history of recurrent apnea, cyanosis, or seizures may be obtained. A history of siblings with sudden death or similar symptoms may be obtained. The shaken baby syndrome must be considered as well.

♦ **Asphyxia**

May occur with prone sleeping with or without soft bedding. Rebreathing of CO_2 may play an important role.

Aspiration

Gastroesophageal reflux is very common in infants; apnea with aspiration with or without coughing may be responsible. Laryngeal chemoreceptors may be stimulated with minute amounts of aspirate. The role of gastroesophageal reflux in SIDS is controversial. Other causes of pharyngeal incoordination may also be responsible.

● **Passive Inhalation of Crack-Cocaine Smoke**

Aerosolized crack cocaine may induce arrhythmias in infants; body levels are low.

Cardiac Causes in Infants

Cyanotic Congenital Heart Disease

Sudden death is usually due to ductus-dependent lesions.

Arrhythmias

♦ Long Q-T Syndrome

A prolonged QT interval may be a significant cause of sudden death in infants (3).

Wolff-Parkinson-White Syndrome

CARDIAC CAUSES IN OLDER INFANTS, CHILDREN, AND ADOLESCENTS

Sudden unexpected death has been defined as death caused by cardiac arrest up to 6 hours after the initial onset of symptoms or collapse in individuals who have not been previously recognized to have cardiovascular disease.

♦ Myocarditis

Accounts for about one third of cardiac causes of sudden death. Group B coxsackieviruses are the most common cause of myocarditis.

♦ Hypertrophic Cardiomyopathy

Diagnostic findings usually are not apparent until late childhood or adolescence. A familial history of sudden death should be sought; syncope may be an early symptom. Unfortunately, the first sign of this disorder is often sudden death. This disorder is the leading cause of death among young athletes.

Blunt Chest Trauma

A blow to the sternum or over the heart may induce an arrhythmia.

Dilated Cardiomyopathy

May be familial or may follow myocarditis.

Atherosclerotic Coronary Artery Disease

Occasional cases occur in adolescents; risk factors for coronary artery disease should be sought. In the second decade, familial dyslipidemias are responsible.

Kawasaki Disease

May result in persistent coronary artery aneurysms and subsequent occlusion and myocardial infarction. Most deaths occur within 2 months of onset of the illness, but the initial illness may have not been diagnosed. Myocardial infarction may occur years later.

Pulmonary Vascular Hypertension

May be primary or associated with heart disease.

Congenital Coronary Artery Abnormalities

Ectopic origin of either the right or left coronary artery in the sinus of Valsalva is most common.

Aortic Dissection

Children with Marfan syndrome are at risk, but dissections are most common in the fourth decade of life.

Congenital Heart Disease

After Repair

Children who have had reparative surgery for tetralogy of Fallot and transposition of the great arteries run risks of sudden death, usually from conduction abnormalities. Other repaired cardiac disorders are also at risk for arrhythmias.

Never Repaired

Aortic stenosis and tetralogy of Fallot are best known.

Mitral Valve Prolapse

A rare cause in children under 20 years of age; arrhythmias may be responsible.

Cardiac Tumor

Myxomas or rhabdomyosarcoma may obstruct outflow and precipitate conduction abnormalities.

Ebstein Anomaly of Tricuspid Valve

Associated with supraventricular and ventricular arrhythmias.

Arrhythmogenic Right Ventricular Dysplasia

May be responsible for up to one third of episodes of ventricular tachycardia. This is a rare disorder whose presenting symptoms may include sudden death, syncope, and arrhythmias.

Arrhythmias

Are probably the common pathway leading to sudden death in most of the previously listed disorders. Primary disorders descriptions follow.

♦ **Congenital Long QT syndrome**

The hereditary forms may occur with (Jervell and Lange-Nielsen, autosomal recessive) or without (Romano-Ward, autosomal dominant) neurosensory deafness. Some speculate that nearly one half of the yearly sudden deaths in children are the result of these syndromes (4).

Wolff-Parkinson-White Syndrome

Small risk of sudden death in children.

METABOLIC DISORDERS

● **Fatty Acid Oxidation Disorders**

In one study, 5% of cases previously diagnosed as SIDS were considered to have been caused by these disorders (5). Suspicion should be raised at autopsy with findings of fatty infiltration of the liver or muscles. Analysis of fatty acids, glucose level, and carnitine concentrations can be performed on liver samples at autopsy.

Glutaric Aciduria Type 1

May be mistaken for the shaken-baby syndrome because of the presence of subdural hematomas and retinal hemorrhages. If not diagnosed early, progressive dystonia occurs because of degeneration of the putamen.

Acyl-Co-A Dehydrogenase Deficiencies

Medium, long, short, and very long chain acyl-Co-A dehydrogenase deficiencies may produce the similar effects with sudden unexpected deaths.

Carnitine Transporter Deficiency

Most patients described have episodes of fasting hypoglycemia (less than 2 years of age) or progressive cardiomyopathy. Diffuse microvesicular fatty infiltration of the liver and myocardium at autopsy should raise the suspicion of fatty oxidation disorders.

Mitochondrial Carnitine-Acylcarnitine Translocase Deficiency

Fatty infiltration of the liver and muscle is apparent at autopsy. Hypoketotic hypoglycemia is present with low levels of carnitine.

♦ DRUGS

Tricyclic Antidepressants

Sudden death has been described in children treated with desipramine and imipramine.

♦ Cocaine

Causes coronary artery constriction, myocardial ischemia, and arrhythmias.

Ingestions/Poisonings

Many drugs may cause sudden life-threatening events if taken in large doses. The ingestion may be accidental or deliberate.

Glue Sniffing

INFECTIONS

♦ Pertussis

An association between epidemic pertussis and SIDS has been described.

♦ Respiratory Syncytial Virus

Apnea may be the presentation of respiratory syncytial virus bronchiolitis.

Other Acute Infections

Sepsis, severe pneumonia, and meningitis are examples. There are almost always clues of a preceding infection. A child with asplenia offers no clinical clues; overwhelming pneumococcal sepsis and sudden death may occur.

MISCELLANEOUS

Apnea as a manifestation of an ALTE has many central and obstructive causes. All will not be listed. Most have preceding symptoms and signs that should suggest the possibility of a problem.

♦ Seizures

Sudden death is rare in seizures, but ALTE may be caused by convulsions.

Breathholding

History should separate this event from other pathologic conditions.

♦ Obstructive Sleep Apnea

When snoring stops, complete obstruction may have occurred.

Hypoglycemia

Various causes may be responsible.

Foreign Body

Obstruction of the airway may be the cause.

Acute Cerebral Hemorrhage

Hydrocephalus

Apnea has been described as a presentation of unsuspected hydrocephalus.

Pulmonary Embolus

• Botulism

Infants may seem to become ill suddenly with airway compromise, especially if early signs of botulism are ignored. Constipation, ptosis, lethargy, poor feeding, and poor tone usually precede respiratory distress.

Addison Disease

An infection or other stress may be life threatening in a child with adrenal insufficiency.

Anorexia Nervosa/Bulimia

May result in prolonged QT interval, electrolyte abnormalities, and bradycardia.

Williams Syndrome

Sudden death is a more common complication than previously recognized. Biventricular outflow obstruction and coronary artery stenosis may lead to decreased cardiac output, myocardial ischemia, and arrhythmia.

Rett Syndrome

QT interval abnormalities appear as affected girls age.

Dandy-Walker Syndrome

Sudden death is an uncommon but well-recognized occurrence. May be related to vascular compromise rather than uncal or tonsillar herniation.

Arnold-Chiari Malformation

Vocal cord paralysis may occur suddenly, creating a life-threatening situation.

Central Hypoventilation Syndrome (Ondine's Curse)

Infants become apneic during sleep.

REFERENCES

1. Gilbert-Barness E, Barness L. Sudden infant death: a reappraisal. *Contemp Pediatr* 1995;12:88–107.
2. Brooks JG. Apparent life-threatening events. *Pediatr Rev* 1996;7:257–259.
3. Schwartz PJ, Stramba-Badiale M, Segantini A, et al. Prolongation of the QT interval and the sudden infant death syndrome. *N Engl J Med* 1998;338:1709–1714.
4. Ackerman MJ, Schroeder JJ, Berry R, et al. A novel mutation in KVLQT1 is the molecular basis of inherited long QT syndrome in a near-drowning patient's family. *Pediatr Res* 1998;44:148–153.
5. Boles RG, Buck EA, Blitzer MG, et al. Retrospective biochemical screening of fatty acid oxidation disorders in postmortem livers of 418 cases of sudden death in the first year of life. *J Pediatr* 1998;132:924–933.

SUGGESTED READING

Carroll JL, Loughlin GM. Sudden infant death syndrome. *Pediatr Rev* 1993;14:83–93.
Carroll JL, Marcus CL, Loughlin GM. Disordered control of breathing in infants and children. *Pediatr Rev* 1993;14:51–65.
Kanter RJ. Syncope and sudden death. In: Garson A Jr, Bricker JT, Fisher DJ, Neish SR. *The science and practice of pediatric cardiology,* 2nd ed. Baltimore: Williams & Wilkins, 1998:2169–2199.
Liberthson RR. Sudden death from cardiac causes in children and young adults. *N Engl J Med* 1996;334:1039–1044.
McCaffrey FM, Braden DS, Strong WB. Sudden cardiac death in young athletes: a review. *Am J Dis Child* 1991;145:177–183.
Southall DP, Plunkett CB, Banks MW, Falkov AF, Samuels MP. Covert video recordings of life-threatening child abuse: lessons for child protection. *Pediatrics* 1997;100:735–760.
Taylor JA, Sanderson M. A reexamination of the risk factors for the sudden infant death syndrome. *J Pediatr* 1995;126:887–891.

SECTION II

Head

21

Headache

Headache is a common complaint in children. In most children, episodes are short-lived and infrequent so that medical advice is not sought; children with persistent or recurrent headaches are the ones usually brought for evaluation. Headaches come in all "shapes and sizes." Certain features of headache can often be helpful in identifying a specific cause. One of the most practical ways of classifying headaches is by their pattern. Rothner (1) has divided the patterns into five categories: acute generalized, acute localized, acute recurrent, chronic progressive, and chronic nonprogressive. In this chapter, headaches will be divided into these categories as a way of approaching the differential diagnosis of this problem, with the most common causes listed first in each category.

In the evaluation of recurrent or persistent headache in children, the history is especially important and should include information about location, severity, associated symptoms, duration, and usual time of onset. A family history of migraine may be obtained, but headaches may also be the learned somatic expression of anxiety or stress in the family. Also keep in mind that migraine headaches may occur in conjunction with other types of headaches, creating some difficulty in defining a typical pattern.

Unfortunately, not all causes of headaches have a typical pattern, and specific characteristics of headache may be associated with several disorders. The atypical presentation in particular poses a greater diagnostic challenge.

Many parents consider that a brain tumor is the most likely cause of their child's headache, although they are usually reluctant to voice this fear. Fortunately, brain tumors are not common. Anticipation and dismissal of this concern after a thorough examination can be an important therapeutic intervention.

♦ **Most Common Causes of Headaches**

Acute	**Chronic**
Tension	Tension
Fever (Febrile Illness)	Migraine
Otitis Media	Depression
Exertion	
Head Trauma	

• **Causes Not to Forget**

Central Nervous System Bleed	Sinusitis
Temporomandibular Joint Dysfunction	Increased Intracranial Pressure

ACUTE GENERALIZED HEADACHE

♦ Fever

Generalized dilatation of cranial arteries is the most common cause of headaches, particularly in acute infectious diseases. Fever associated with chronic systemic disease may also be responsible for recurrent headaches secondary to vascular dilatation.

♦ Exertion

Particularly in adolescents during intense physical activity.

Hyperventilation

Chest tightness, dizziness, numbness and tingling of arms and legs, and carpopedal spasm may be other findings.

Central Nervous System Infections

Meningitis and encephalitis are usually associated with headache. Children with Rocky Mountain spotted fever generally have severe frontal headaches.

Hypoxia and Hypercapnia

Vasodilatation is the cause.

Hypoglycemia

Decreased Intracranial Pressure

Headache may follow lumbar puncture.

Anemia

With severe anemia, compensatory increased blood flow may lead to vasodilatation.

Seizures

In convulsive disorders, headache is present most commonly in the postictal state, although occasionally as an aura that may mimic migraine. Vascular dilatation is the probable cause.

Electrolyte Disturbances

A variety of conditions may lead to inappropriate antidiuretic hormone secretion. Hyponatremia may be associated with nausea, delirium, incoordination, and seizures.

Drugs

Amphetamines, for example, may cause headaches as well as irritability, insomnia, and loss of appetite and weight. Nitrates and nitrites produce vasodilatation, which can cause headache.

Metabolic Acidosis

Acute Intracranial Bleed

Epidural Hematoma

Aneurysm

One fifth of patients may have a history of recurrent headaches; cranial nerve palsies may be other findings. Coarctation of the aorta and polycystic disease of the kidneys are found in 25% of patients with aneurysms. Unfortunately, the usual presentation is sudden; severe headache, confusion, vomiting, and loss of consciousness are associated with massive subarachnoid bleeding.

Arteriovenous Malformation

Arterial Inflammation

Systemic lupus erythematosus and subacute bacterial endocarditis are examples. Other systemic clues may be present.

Carbon Monoxide Poisoning

Headache and vertigo are early symptoms; with continued exposure, bounding pulse, vomiting, dilated pupils, dusky skin, and convulsions may develop. Ask about home heating and other ill family members.

Hypertension

This is not as common a cause in children as often thought. Headache may be present on awakening and increases with activity. Renal causes of increased blood pressure are most frequent.

Cerebral Venous Sinus Thrombosis

Initial symptoms may be mild and suggest a functional disorder. Headache, nausea, vomiting, photophobia, blurred vision, diplopia, and lethargy may be present. Birth control pills have been implicated in some cases.

ACUTE LOCALIZED HEADACHES

Aural Disorders

Acute otitis media, serous otitis media, and mastoiditis are more likely to have localized complaints.

Sinusitis

Sinusitis may be infectious or allergic. Rhinorrhea, sinus tenderness, nasal congestion, and fever may be present. Pain is often retro-orbital, accentuated on eye movement. The headaches may also be chronic, nonprogressive.

♦ Trauma

Headache may last for days or, rarely, for years following a concussion.

Dental Problems

Caries or abscesses may manifest as headache rather than local pain. Malocclusion of teeth or grinding of teeth during sleep (bruxism) may also cause headache.

● Temporal Mandibular Joint Dysfunction

May also be responsible for recurrent, chronic headaches.

Ocular Disorders

Headache may be an early co-complaint in glaucoma or uveitis. "Eye strain" is most often a manifestation of stress rather than a primary eye disorder.

Occipital Neuralgia

Pain is usually unilateral and can be induced by palpation over the occiput or second cervical vertebra; it results from root compression due to malformation of the joint space between the first and second cervical vertebrae with intermittent subluxation.

ACUTE RECURRENT HEADACHES

Migraine

The classic pattern is paroxysmal, unilateral headache with preceding visual aura and nausea or vomiting, as well as a family history. In children, however, paroxysmal symptoms overshadowing the headache may be present. Cyclic vomiting, ataxia, hemiparesis, abdominal pain, and diplopia may suggest other disorders. Headache may become a prominent complaint later. A history of motion sickness may be a clue.

Sinusitis

Cluster Headache

An unusual migraine variant in children. Severe, short-lived, retro- or periorbital pain often associated with signs of sympathetic overactivity on the ipsilateral side of the face.

Chronic Paroxysmal Hemicrania

Recurrent episodes of unilateral headaches without nausea or vomiting. Responds dramatically to indomethacin.

MELAS Syndrome

Mitochondrial encephalomyopathy, lactic acidosis, and strokelike episodes (MELAS) is characterized by recurrent attacks of prolonged migrainous headache and repeated vomiting in childhood, partial epileptic seizures (33%) with recurrent bouts of epilepsia partialis continua or convulsive status epilepticus, and repeated cerebral infarctions, ultimately leading to cortical blindness, cortical deafness, and dementia. Serum lactate and pyruvate are increased.

CHRONIC PROGRESSIVE HEADACHE

- **Increased Intracranial Pressure**

Headaches are produced by traction on pain-sensitive structures. (See Chapter 24, Increased Intracranial Pressure and Bulging Fontanel, for additional causes.)

Brain Tumor

The head pain is generalized but often more severe in the occiput; it is most frequently present early in the morning on arising but may last all day. Vomiting before arising without nausea and increased pain on position change or with coughing may develop later. Papilledema and complaints of diplopia, weakness, and numbness may be other features.

Pseudotumor Cerebri

Excessive vitamin A ingestion (as in acne therapy), outdated tetracycline usage, and hypoparathyroidism may be causes.

Withdrawal From Steroids

May result in increased intracranial pressure.

Oral Contraceptives

Hydrocephalus

Intoxications with Cerebral Edema

Lead poisoning should be considered.

Subdural Hematoma

Brain Abscess

Symptoms depend on the child's age and on the size and location of the abscess and include headache, fever, lethargy, and seizures, as well as focal neurologic deficits.

Vascular Malformation

Meningeal Irritation From Leukemic or Tumor Infiltration

Basilar Impression

Invagination of margins of the foramen magnum result in posterior displacement of the odontoid and compression of the spinal cord and brain stem. Ataxia, stiff neck, head tilt, nystagmus, and cortical tract signs may occur.

Sarcoidosis

CHRONIC NONPROGRESSIVE HEADACHES

♦ **Tension and Stress**

These headaches usually appear in late afternoon; the ache is located posteriorly in and around the neck muscles and is described as "tight." Pain fluctuates with stressful situations but does not interfere with recreation. These are most common in adolescents.

♦ **Depression**

Associated symptoms include loss of appetite, sleep disturbances, inability to concentrate, and failure to participate in activities.

Environmental Factors

Heat, humidity, noxious fumes, and noise have all been implicated. Tension may be a common factor, because muscle contraction is the pathogenetic mechanism.

Allergy

Allergy may cause the tension-fatigue syndrome with headache. A past history of milk or other allergies suggest this possibility. An elimination diet, especially of milk, chocolate, and eggs, is worthwhile, in suspected cases.

Obstructive Sleep Apnea

Children who develop intermittent obstruction of their upper airway during sleep may wake in the morning with a headache, probably the result of chronic hypoxemia and hypercapnia with vascular dilatation. Snoring with obstructive-type breathing patterns may be a clue.

Conversion

Vivid descriptions of the head pain may be given. There may be other somatic complaints, frequently associated with an indifferent attitude.

Mimicry

Headaches may be a common expression of frustration or stress in the family. A parent or other family member may be a role model.

Temporal Mandibular Joint Dysfunction

Malingering

Postconcussion

The headaches may last for weeks or even years following a concussion.

REFERENCE

1. Rothner AD. Headache. In: Swaiman KF, ed. *Pediatric neurology, principles and practice,* 2nd ed. St. Louis: Mosby, 1994:219–226.

SUGGESTED READING

Honig PJ, Charney EB. Children with brain tumor headaches. *Am J Dis Child* 1982;136:121–124.
Ling W, Oftedal G, Weinburg W. Depressive illness in childhood presenting as severe headache. *Am J Dis Child* 1970;120:122–124.
McIntre SC. Recurrent and chronic headaches. In: Gartner JC Jr, Zitelli BJ. *Common and chronic symptoms in pediatrics.* St. Louis: Mosby, 1997:51–62.
Prensky AL. Migraine and migrainous variants in pediatric patients. *Pediatr Clin North Am* 1976;23:461–471.
Rothner AD. A practical approach to headaches in adolescents. *Pediatr Ann* 1991;20:200–205.
Singer HS, Rowe S. Chronic recurrent headaches in children. *Pediatr Ann* 1992;21:369–373.

22

Macrocephaly

Macrocephaly is defined as a head circumference that is greater than two standard deviations above the mean for age, sex, race, and gestational age. In infancy, the most common cause of an enlarged head is hydrocephalus produced by various lesions. It is important to remember, however, that the head being measured may be a "chip off the old block." In other words, the child's macrocephaly may reflect a familial trait. Measurements of the head circumference of the parents and other family members are an essential part of evaluation.

Head enlargement in older children may be due to a chronic pseudotumor cerebri; signs of increased intracranial pressure will predominate, however. In cranial and skeletal dysplasias, other prominent somatic features assist in defining the cause of the macrocephaly and related problems.

Macrocephaly may also be the result of an increase in brain substance rather than of increased intracranial pressure or thickness of the skull. In addition to familial or primary forms of increase in brain substance, metabolic disorders, neurocutaneous syndromes, and other disorders must be considered in the differential diagnosis.

♦ **Most Common Causes of Increased Head Size**

Familial   Hydrocephalus (Various Causes)
Benign Subdural Effusions   Achondroplasia
Pseudotumor Cerebri   Neurofibromatosis

DISORDERS ASSOCIATED WITH HYDROCEPHALUS

Malformations with Obstruction

Arnold-Chiari Malformation

This anomaly accounts for 40% of cases of hydrocephalus in infants and children. Obstructive hydrocephalus results from the herniation of the lower brain stem through an enlarged foramen magnum.

Aqueductal Stenosis

Stenosis of the cerebral aqueduct is responsible for about 20% of cases of hydrocephalus in children; however, hydrocephalus may develop at any time from birth to adulthood and may be associated with other malformations including spina bifida. In a few cases, sex-linked recessive inheritance has been reported.

Dandy-Walker Syndrome

The fourth ventricle becomes greatly dilated and acts as a cyst; onset of symptoms may be delayed until after infancy. Presenting signs include a bulging occiput, nystagmus, ataxia, and cranial nerve palsies.

Malformation of the Vein of Galen

In addition to enlarging head size, the infants have intracranial bruits and may develop congestive heart failure as a result of shunts in the aneurysm.

Holoprosencephaly

Failure of division of the cerebral hemispheres is usually associated with midline facial defects. Hydrocephalus is rare; microcephaly is more common.

Aqueductal Gliosis

Obstruction of the aqueduct is a result of an inflammatory response to an infection or hemorrhage.

Infections

Rubella, cytomegalovirus, toxoplasmosis, and syphilis are the most frequently recognized congenital infections. Mumps may cause this problem in older children.

Perinatal Hemorrhage

Intraventricular hemorrhage, especially in hypoxic premature infants, or vascular malformations or trauma may result in obstruction to cerebrospinal fluid flow.

♦ **Communicating Hydrocephalus**

Normal absorption of the cerebrospinal fluid may be impaired in various disorders. This form accounts for 30% of childhood hydrocephalus.

Intracranial Hemorrhage

Bacterial Hemorrhage

Bacterial or Granulomatous Meningitis

Obstruction of Vein or Sinuses

Any number of disorders that result in an increased intracranial venous pressure may cause diminished cerebrospinal fluid absorption.

Diffuse Meningeal Malignant Tumors

Rarely, lymphomas or leukemias produce this problem.

Excess Cerebrospinal Fluid Secretion: Choroid Plexus Papilloma

Head enlargement is usually not seen until after infancy, with signs of increased intracranial pressure.

Tumors

Neoplasms

Various primary and metastatic tumors may cause increased intracranial pressure and head enlargement. Headache and vomiting are the most constant signs.

Arteriovenous Malformations

As the lesions enlarge, obstruction of cerebrospinal fluid flow may occur. Cranial bruits and unexplained congestive heart failure are possible associated findings.

Cysts

Porencephalic cysts may enlarge to produce a clinical picture resembling that of hydrocephalus. Because the cysts are usually unilateral, focal neurologic problems are common.

Brain Abscess

An abscess generally causes acute symptoms, and its clinical course is rarely prolonged enough to result in head enlargement.

Leptomeningeal Melanosis

Usually associated with large congenital cutaneous nevi.

Hydranencephaly

The cerebral tissue is minimal and replaced by a sac filled with cerebrospinal fluid. Infants with this disorder appear normal at birth but then have progressive head enlargement. Primitive reflexes persist. Hypertonia, hyperreflexia, and later, decerebration follow.

◆ DISORDERS ASSOCIATED WITH PSEUDOTUMOR CEREBRI

Various disorders may cause increased intracranial pressure without obstruction of cerebrospinal fluid flow. If the disorders are longstanding, some increase in head circumference may be seen. Symptoms of increased intracranial pressure predominate the clinical picture, however.

Lead Poisoning

Drug Reactions

The most frequently implicated drugs are tetracycline, sulfonamides, penicillin, nalidixic acid, and oral contraceptives.

Corticosteroids (Administration or Withdrawal)

Cyanotic Congenital Heart Disease

Hypoparathyroidism

Hypervitaminosis or Hypovitaminosis A

Adrenal Insufficiency

Galactosemia

INTRACRANIAL HEMORRHAGE

Subdural Hematoma

Chronic subdural collection of fluid may produce slowly progressive head enlargement, seizures, developmental delay, and sometimes anemia. Subdural effusions may develop following meningitis.

Intraventricular or Subarachnoid Hemorrhage

Symptoms are almost invariably acute. Head enlargement may develop in infants following hemorrhage as a result of aqueductal stenosis or diminished cerebrospinal fluid absorption.

SKELETAL AND CRANIAL DYSPLASIAS

♦ Achondroplasia

In short-limbed dwarfism, head enlargement is secondary to increased brain size. Hydrocephalus may be a complication.

Anemia

Any severe chronic anemia may result in skull enlargement secondary to bone marrow expansion. Beta-thalassemia major is best recognized for this phenomenon.

Osteogenesis Imperfecta

Brittle bones, bowing of the legs, blue sclerae, and wormian bones of the skull are classic features.

Rickets

Findings include frontal and parietal bossing, epiphyseal enlargement, bowing of the legs, and swelling of the costochondral junctions. The skull may have the feel of a ping-pong ball (craniotabes).

Craniosynostosis

The head may appear enlarged because of a distortion of shape.

Cleidocranial Dysostosis

There is congenital absence or hypoplasia of the clavicles. The skull is soft at birth; fontanels are large, and sutures remain open. Short stature is a common finding.

Proteus Syndrome

Other features include asymmetric rapid growth, macrodactyly, and an unusual thickening of the skin and subcutaneous tissues.

Metaphyseal Dysplasia

Progressive enlargement of the skull, hypertelorism, and a broad flat nose are characteristic. Cranial nerve deficits may occur secondary to obliteration of foramina by bony overgrowth.

Osteopetrosis

There is early onset of generalized bone sclerosis with thickening of the skull, delayed development, cranial nerve deficits, pancytopenia, and occasionally hydrocephalus.

Hyperphosphatasia

Bowed tubular bones, flared ribs, a protruding sternum, and significant dwarfism are characteristic.

Conradi Syndrome (Chondrodystrophia Calcificans Congenita)

Scoliosis, cataracts, asymmetrical limb shortening, joint contractures, short stature, and stippled epiphyses on roentgenograms are found.

Marshall Syndrome

In this rare disorder, linear growth and skeletal maturation are accelerated; other features are prominent eyes, blue sclerae, and motor and mental delay.

Camptomelic Dwarfism

This is a prenatal growth deficiency characterized by significantly bowed legs, a flat facies, macrocephaly, and many other skeletal anomalies.

Craniofacial Dysostosis

Premature synostosis of the lambdoid suture and the posterior part of the sagittal suture results in a prominent forehead and a flat occiput. Short stature, hypoplastic supraorbital ridges, and micrognathia are other features.

Hallermann-Streiff Syndrome

The children are small but the head appears enlarged, secondary to parietal and frontal bossing. The nose and facies appear "pinched." The eyes are small and cataracts are usually present.

Greig Cephalopolysyndactyly Syndrome

An autosomal dominantly inherited syndrome, which also features polydactyly of the hands and feet, broad thumbs, and hypertelorism.

Thanatophoric Dysplasia

Characterized by short limbed dwarfism and a small rib cage that results in respiratory insufficiency.

Trisomy 9p Syndrome

Affected children are severely developmentally delayed and have growth, skeletal, and facial abnormalities.

Hypochondroplasia

The facial features and limbs are less involved than in achondroplasia.

Robinow Syndrome

This condition has also been called the "fetal face syndrome" because of the disproportionately large cranium. Midface hypoplasia, a short upturned nose, short forearms, and genital hypoplasia are other features.

Pycnodysostosis

Findings include short stature, frontal and occipital skull prominence, delayed closure of the anterior fontanel, and wormian bones.

Kenny Syndrome

This syndrome is a rare cause of growth retardation with delayed closure of the anterior fontanel, hyperopia, episodic hypocalcemic tetany, internal cortical thickening, and medullary stenosis of tubular bones. Intelligence is normal.

Osteopathia Striata and Cranial Sclerosis

This is a rare autosomal dominant disorder in which striae replace the normal appearance of trabecular bone.

Macrocephaly, Hypertelorism, Short Limbs, Hearing Loss, and Developmental Delay

Affected children also have sparse anterior scalp hair, downslanting palpebral fissures, and a short nose with a broad flat nasal bridge and anteverted nares.

X-Linked Recessive Nephritis with Mental Retardation, Sensorineural Hearing Loss, and Macrocephaly

May be a clinical variant of Alport syndrome.

Simpson-Golabi-Behmel Syndrome

Characterized by striking prenatal onset of overgrowth, ocular hypertelorism, short broad nose, large mouth, and macroglossia. Midline clefts are less common. Macrocephaly continues into childhood. Adults tend to be taller than the 97th percentile in height. Hypotonia is common. The inheritance is X-linked recessive.

Acrocallosal Syndrome

Features include significant developmental delay, hypoplastic or absent corpus callosum, postaxial polydactyly of the hands and feet, hypotonia, and hypertelorism.

FG Syndrome

Affected males have the postnatal onset of macrocephaly. They are mentally retarded, hypotonic with delayed motor development, and have a prominent fore-head with frontal hair upsweep. Their thumbs and great toes are broad.

INCREASE IN BRAIN SUBSTANCE

Primary Megalencephaly

Macrocephaly may be familial without associated anomalies. Measurement of the head circumference of other family members is mandatory.

Metabolic Diseases

Tay-Sachs Disease

Macrocephaly may be a feature in children surviving beyond about 2 years of age. Hypertonia, hyperreflexia, psychomotor retardation, and blindness, are earlier findings.

Glutaric Aciduria Type I

The association of progressive macrocephaly, dystonia, and bilateral arachnoid cysts seems to be diagnostic of this disorder. An intercurrent illness may precipitate the dystonia and hypotonia. Acute episodes of ketoacidosis with hypoglycemia and hyperammonemia with hepatomegaly and coma may occur.

Mucopolysaccharidoses

Both Hurler and Hunter syndromes are characterized by progressive mental retardation and coarse features. Macrocephaly is occasionally seen in the Maroteaux-Lamy syndrome, as well as coarse features, stiff joints, and hepatosplenomegaly, but without mental retardation.

Metachromatic Leukodystrophy

Several forms occur; age of onset is variable. Progressive neurologic and mental deterioration are present in all.

Canavan Disease (Spongy Degeneration of Central Nervous System)

Megalencephaly is striking. Onset is between 3 and 9 months of age with initial hypotonia and progressive dementia followed by spasticity and blindness.

Alexander Disease (Infantile Leukodystrophy)

Deterioration begins in the first year of life, with progressive psychomotor retardation, seizures, spasticity, and macrocephaly.

Generalized Gangliosidosis

Coarse features, joint stiffness, and hypotonia are present in early infancy.

Methylmalonic Acidemia

Microcephaly or macrocephaly may be seen in the vitamin B_{12}-responsive form, characterized by difficulty in nursing, vomiting, failure to thrive during the neonatal period, and episodic metabolic acidosis.

Maple Syrup Urine Disease

Macrocephaly is an uncommon feature. In the first few weeks of life, the infants have seizures, episodes of opisthotonos, and intermittent hypertonia, followed usually by an early death.

Neurocutaneous Syndromes

♦ **Neurofibromatosis I**

Multiple café au lait spots and, later, neurofibromas in the skin are key features. Cranial enlargement may be due to hydrocephalus or intracranial tumors as well as an increase in brain substance.

Tuberous Sclerosis

Hypopigmented macules and shagreen and ashleaf patches precede the development of adenoma sebaceum on the face.

Sturge-Weber Syndrome

Port-wine stains of the face, particularly those involving the upper eyelid and forehead, may be associated with ipsilateral cerebral hemangiomatosis.

Klippel-Trénaunay-Weber Syndrome

Unilateral hemangiomatoses, varicosities, and bony overgrowth are characteristic.

Hypomelanosis of Ito

Swirled hypopigmentation is the cutaneous finding. Skeletal, developmental and other defects are variable. Chromosomal mosaicism is usually found.

Cutis Marmorata Telangiectatica Congenita

Macrocephaly has been described. The skin lesions give a reticulated vascular appearance.

Bannayan-Riley-Ruvalcaba Syndrome

Characterized by megalencephaly, delayed motor development, hamartomas, usually lipomas or hemangiomas, an unusual distribution of tan spots involving the glans penis in males, and increased amounts of intracellular lipid in muscle cells. These infants are large at birth. Hypotonia as a feature should suggest possible carnitine deficiency.

Disseminated Hemangiomatosis

Basal Cell Nevus Syndrome

Multiple nevi (actually hamartomas) increase with age. Basal cell carcinomas are a major problem. Other features include a square jaw, tiny pits in the skin of the palms and soles, rib and vertebral anomalies as well as multiple jaw cysts.

Miscellaneous Syndromes

Cerebral Gigantism (Soto Syndrome)

There is excessive somatic growth during the first few years of life. Children are usually large at birth, have acromegalic features including large hands and feet and a large jaw, and are mentally retarded.

Beckwith-Wiedemann Syndrome

Characteristic features include macroglossia, an omphalocele or umbilical anomaly, macrosomia, and, often, severe hypoglycemia in the neonatal period. Affected children are at risk for development of Wilms' and other tumors.

Histiocytosis X

Children with Hand-Schuller-Christian disease may appear to have macrocephaly.

Weaver Syndrome

Few cases have been reported. Features include macrosomia, camptodactyly, an unusual facies, and accelerated skeletal maturation.

Fetal Alcohol Syndrome

Although most affected children have microcephaly, a few with enlarged cranial vaults have been described.

♦ BENIGN SUBDURAL EFFUSION IN INFANTS

The development of computed tomography has allowed identification of children with rapid head growth who appear to have areas of cortical atrophy resembling those seen with subdural effusions. Features include some ventricular enlargement, wide cerebral sulci, large sylvian cisterns, prominent interhemispheric fissures, and decreased density over the cerebral convexities. In some infants, initial developmental delay disappears with time.

SUGGESTED READING

DeMyer W. Megalocephaly and megalencephaly. In: Swaiman KF, ed. *Pediatric neurology: principles and practice,* 2nd ed. St. Louis: Mosby, 1994:208–218.

Jones KL. *Smith's recognizable patterns of human malformation*, 5th ed. Philadelphia: WB Saunders, 1997.

Powell BR, Budden SS, Buist NR. Dominantly inherited megalencephaly, muscle weakness, and myoliposis: a carnitine-deficient myopathy within the spectrum of the Ruvalcaba-Myhre-Smith syndrome. *J Pediatr* 1993;123:70–75.

Robertson WC Jr, Chun RWM, Orrison WW, et al. Benign subdural collections of infancy. *J Pediatr* 1979;94:382–385.

Sandler AD, Knudson MW, Brown TT, Christian RM Jr. Neurodevelopmental dysfunction among children with idiopathic megalencephaly. *J Pediatr* 1997;131:320–324.

Strassburg HM. Macrocephaly is not always due to hydrocephalus. *J Child Neurol* 1989;4:32–40.

23

Microcephaly

Microcephaly describes a small head, and a small head generally denotes a small brain, because it is brain growth that produces head enlargement. (A notable and perhaps the only exception is microcephaly secondary to craniosynostosis.) There is some disagreement about the clinical definition of microcephaly. The criterion of a head circumference more than two standard deviations below the mean for age, sex, and gestational age has been used; measurements three or more standard deviations below the mean have also been recommended.

There seems to be a linear relationship between head size and intellectual capacity: The smaller the head, the less likely intelligence will be normal. Some children with microcephaly may be exceptions to this rule, but the association cannot be ignored in the differential diagnosis.

Primary microcephaly is caused by anomalous development of the brain during the first 7 months of gestation. Familial factors, congenital infections, chromosomal abnormalities, syndromes of dysmorphogenesis, anatomic defects of the brain produced by insults to the fetus during early gestation, drugs, and toxins, and metabolic disorders, as well as craniosynostosis, are the most common causes. Secondary microcephaly follows injuries to the growing rather than to the developing brain; these include anoxia, trauma, and hypoglycemia occurring any time in the last 2 months of gestation or during early infancy.

The lists of dysmorphogenetic syndromes and chromosomal abnormalities are exceptionally long; undoubtedly, they are not comprehensive but they are offered as an aid to additional evaluation of these disorders, in which distinctions may be subtle. Although the possible causes of microcephaly are many, most are rarely seen in clinical practice. It is important to measure the head size of all family members, and to obtain a careful history of the gestational period, including maternal infections and drug or alcohol ingestion. In the infant who does not have an unusual phenotype or evidence of premature closure of the cranial sutures, serologic tests for congenital infections may be in order.

♦ **Most Common Causes of Microcephaly**

Genetic (Familial)
Drugs or Toxins (Fetal Alcohol)
Chromosomal (Trisomies)

Congenital Infections (including Human
　Immunodeficiency Virus)
Hypoxic-Ischemic Encephalopathy

♦ GENETIC OR FAMILIAL MICROCEPHALY

Autosomal Dominant Form

The microcephaly is generally not as severe as in the autosomal-recessive form. Affected children may have receding or small foreheads, upslanted palpebral fissures, and prominent ears.

Autosomal Recessive Form

The phenotype is usually striking. Height is less than normal, the forehead inclines acutely, and the chin may be hypoplastic and the nose and ears prominent; the scalp may be furrowed. Spastic diplegia and seizures are frequently present. Severe mental retardation occurs in most cases.

♦ CONGENITAL INFECTIONS

Intrauterine infections with rubella, cytomegalovirus, toxoplasmosis, herpes simplex, syphilis, human immunodeficiency virus, coxsackievirus, varicella, and others may result in microcephaly. Many infants may have other signs and symptoms in the newborn period including thrombocytopenia, low-birth weight, hepatosplenomegaly, and jaundice. Some infections, however, are subclinical and manifest as psychomotor retardation, microcephaly, or deafness later.

SECONDARY MICROCEPHALY

Several insults to the growing brain may occur prior to delivery or in the early neonatal period.

Meningitis

Birth Trauma

♦ Hypoxic-Ischemic Encephalopathy

Severe Dehydration

Hypoglycemia

♦ Acquired Immune Deficiency Syndrome

♦ DRUGS AND TOXINS

Fetal exposure to drugs or toxins ingested by the mother or to which the mother was exposed may affect brain growth.

Fetal Alcohol Syndrome

Growth deficiency, microcephaly, short palpebral fissures, and maxillary hypoplasia are characteristic. This is a significant cause of microcephaly.

Fetal Hydantoin Syndrome

Growth deficiency, large fontanel, hypertelorism, cleft lip and palate, hypoplastic distal phalanges, and coarse hair are among the many features.

Fetal Trimethadione Syndrome

Midfacial hypoplasia, short upturned nose, upslant to eyebrows, broad nasal bridge, and cleft lip and palate may be seen.

Aminopterin Syndrome

Growth deficiency, hypoplasia of facial bones, upswept frontal scalp hair, micrognathia, and short limbs are found.

Irradiation

Exposure to ionizing radiation during the first two trimesters may cause interference with brain growth.

Methadone

Carbon Monoxide Poisoning

CRANIOSYNOSTOSIS

Premature closure of sutures usually occurs in utero. Only 10% of cases are associated with dysmorphic syndromes. The shape of the skull depends on which sutures are closed.

CHROMOSOMAL ABNORMALITIES

Many chromosomal aberrations are associated with anomalous brain development. Usually many phenotypic abnormalities are present, some of which are listed with each defect.

Down Syndrome

The most common of the chromosomal defects is associated with a mild microcephaly.

♦ Trisomy 18 Syndrome

Features include hypertonia, failure to thrive, prominent occiput, short sternum, congenital heart disease, micrognathia, and limited hip abduction.

♦ Trisomy 13 Syndrome

The triad of microphthalmia, cleft lip and palate, and polydactyly suggests this defect. Literally hundreds of other anomalies have also been reported.

Cri du Chat Syndrome

A weak, catlike cry in an infant with microcephaly, hypertelorism, growth failure, microphthalmia, and hypotonia suggests this syndrome.

18 p Syndrome

Low-birth weight, webbed neck, lymphedema, shield chest, short stature, hypertelorism, ptosis, epicanthal folds, strabismus, and stubby hands are prominent features.

19 q Syndrome

Low-birth weight, midfacial dysplasia, carp-shaped mouth, atretic ear canals, long finger tips, and hypotonia are characteristic.

11 q Partial Trisomy

Features include short nose with a long philtrum, growth retardation, micropenis, micrognathia, and congenital heart disease.

4 p Syndrome

Retardation, hypertelorism, downward-slanted palpebral fissures, cleft palate, beaked nose, and a carplike mouth are seen.

14 q Distal Partial Trisomy

Normal birth weight, hypertonia or hypotonia, high forehead, epicanthal folds, low-set ears, micrognathia, and camptodactyly are findings.

14 q Proximal Partial Trisomy

Features are low-birth weight, seizures, hypertonia, low anterior hairline, hypotelorism or hypertelorism, low-set and malformed ears, and a short neck.

13 q Syndrome

Broad nasal bridge, low-set abnormal ears, ptosis, and microphthalmia are characteristic.

Triploidy

Incidence is rare. Variable features include very low birth weight, coloboma, and cutaneous syndactyly.

21 Monosomy

Low-birth weight, prominent nose, wide nasal bridge, large and low-set ears, microcephaly, micrognathia, and hypertonia are the features.

22 Monosomy

Low-birth weight, seizures, hypotonia, ptosis, and hypertelorism are found.

SYNDROMES OF DYSMORPHOGENESIS

Smith's Recognizable Patterns of Human Malformation offers a wellspring of information on syndromes, including a listing of those with microcephaly.

Pierre Robin Syndrome

This triad of cleft palate, micrognathia, and glossoptosis may be seen in other disorders.

Smith-Lemli-Opitz Syndrome

Infants demonstrate failure to thrive with anteverted nostrils, ptosis, cryptorchidism, and hypospadias.

Prader-Willi Syndrome

Hypotonia, hypogonadism, short stature, obesity, and small hands and feet characterize this syndrome.

Williams Syndrome

Microcephaly is mild, with short stature, prominent lips, a hoarse voice, and, often, cardiac abnormalities.

De Lange Syndrome

Severe mental retardation, a growling-like cry, long philtrum, anteverted nares, hirsutism, and deformities of the extremities are common.

Cockayne Syndrome

Infants appear normal for the first year but then become dwarfed. The face appears thin, with a prominent nose and deep-set eyes; other features include neurologic deficits, cataracts, and a photosensitive dermatitis.

Hallermann-Streiff Syndrome (Oculomandibulofacial Syndrome)

Short stature, microphthalmia, cataracts, micrognathia, sparse hair, and a small, pinched nose are common.

Focal Dermal Hypoplasia (Goltz Syndrome)

Hypoplastic areas of skin with protrusions of fat, reddish streaks, papillomas, sparse hair, deformities of fingers, and short stature are characteristic.

Rubinstein-Taybi Syndrome

Features include broad thumbs and toes, often with angulation, retardation, a beaked nose, and downward slant to palpebral fissures.

Seckel Syndrome (Bird-Headed Dwarfism)

Features include significant growth deficiency, prominent nose, low-set malformed ears, and dislocated hips.

Laurence-Moon-Biedl Syndrome

Obesity, mental deficiency, polydactyly and syndactyly, hypogonadism, and retinitis pigmentosa are common.

Fanconi Syndrome (Pancytopenia)

Hypoplastic or absent thumb, short stature, hyperpigmentation, and the later development of pancytopenia are characteristic.

Meckel-Gruber Syndrome

The key feature is a posterior encephalocele. Polydactyly, microphthalmia, micrognathia, and a short neck are frequently present.

Langer-Giedion Syndrome (Trichorhinophalangeal Syndrome)

Mild microcephaly with large protruding ears and a large bulbous nose is characteristic. Cone-shaped epiphyses appear in the hands at age 3 or 4 years.

Bloom Syndrome

Short stature, facial telangiectasia, light photosensitivity, and microcephaly of variable degree are features.

De Sanctis-Cacchione Syndrome

Growth deficiency, mental deterioration, sun sensitivity, and hypogonadism are found.

Johanson-Blizzard Syndrome

Deafness, retardation with hypoplastic alae nasi, and hypothyroidism are characteristic.

Coffin-Siris Syndrome

Features include hypotonia, mild microcephaly, sparse scalp hair, and hypoplasia or absence of the fifth finger and toenails.

Rhizomelic Chondrodysplasia Puncata

Proximal shortening of extremities with stippled epiphyses on radiographs, flat facies, and low nasal bridge are characteristic.

Roberts Syndrome

There is severe retardation with significant deformities of the extremities.

Cerebrocostomandibular Syndrome

Severe micrognathia and rib deformities with pronounced respiratory difficulties are findings.

Cerebrooculofacioskeletal Syndrome

Sloping forehead, cataract, microphthalmia, narrow palpebral fissures, large ears, scoliosis, and kyphosis are features of this syndrome.

Craniofacial Dysostosis with Diaphyseal Hyperplasia

Findings include premature craniosynostosis, exophthalmos, maxillary hypoplasia, hypertelorism, strabismus, short stature, and short hands.

Craniofacial Dyssynostosis

Features are a prominent forehead and a small, flat (or bulging) occiput due to premature closure of the lambdoid and posterior part of the sagittal sutures.

Craniooculodental Syndrome

Affected children have a low hairline, nasal septum deviation, brachydactyly, ptosis, facial asymmetry, and beaked nose.

Dubowitz Syndrome

Low-birth weight, sparse hair, high sloping forehead, flat supraorbital ridges, broad nasal bridge, and ptosis are characteristic.

Dyggve-Melchior-Clausen Syndrome

Findings include short-trunk dwarfism, protruding sternum, barrel chest, restricted joint mobility, and flat vertebral bodies.

Ectrodactyly and Ectodermal Dysplasia with Clefting

Absence of fingers or hand clefts, cleft lip or palate, and sparse scalp hair are the findings.

Angelman Syndrome

Affected children have jerking movements and a pleasant laughing demeanor with retardation and seizures, sometimes called the Happy Puppet syndrome.

Leprechaunism (Donohue Syndrome)

Prenatal growth and adipose tissue deficiency are characteristic, as well as thick lips, wide eyes, hirsutism, and genital enlargement.

Megalocornea and Mental Retardation

Short stature, hypotonia, ataxia, seizures, and enlarged corneas are features.

Microphthalmus with Digital Anomalies

One or both eyes are small, the ears are misshapen, and rudimentary sixth digits are present.

Oculodentoosseous Dysplasia

Features include a thin nose with hypoplastic alae nasi, microcornea, syndactyly of fourth and fifth fingers, and enamel hypoplasia.

Opticocochleodentate Degeneration

Optic atrophy and deafness occur with spastic quadriplegia.

Orocraniodigital Syndrome

Bilateral or unilateral cleft lip, thumb anomalies, and curvature or syndactyly of the toes are characteristic features.

Osteoporosis and Pseudoglioma

Recurrent fractures from minor injuries and blindness from retinal detachment are problems.

ANATOMIC DEFECTS SECONDARY TO EARLY INSULTS TO THE DEVELOPING BRAIN

Agenesis of Corpus Callosum

Two forms are seen: In one, patients have seizures with mild to moderate mental retardation. In the X-linked form, severe retardation and seizures are found.

Holoprosencephaly

Failure of development of the forebrain leads to midface abnormalities that may range in severity from cyclopia to hypotelorism. Midfacial defects such as hypotelorism or clefting deformities suggest the possibility of serious problems in brain development.

Schizencephaly (Schizencephalic Porencephaly)

Clefts are placed symmetrically within the cerebral hemispheres; there are profound neurologic and developmental defects, with symmetric spastic and rigid quadriparesis and seizures.

Macrogyria

The gyri of brain are too few and are coarse. Neurologic deficits tend to be lateralized.

Polymicrogyria

There are small, numerous gyri. The clinical picture is one of retardation, spasticity, or hypotonia with active deep tendon reflexes.

Lissencephaly (Miller-Dieker Syndrome)

The cortex of the brain is smooth and lacks sulci. Spastic quadriplegia with severe retardation and seizures is present.

METABOLIC DISORDERS

Maternal Diabetes Mellitus

Infants of diabetic mothers may have microcephaly if the mother's diabetes has been poorly controlled.

Phenylketonuria

Features include mental retardation, seizures, and imperfect hair pigmentation. Vomiting and irritability are frequent in the first few months of life. The skin is rough and dry.

Maternal Phenylketonuria

Growth retardation, both before and after birth, microcephaly, and severe intellectual delay are common.

Citrullinemia

Infants may appear normal for a few months and then have severe vomiting with coma and seizures; a rapidly fatal course is the rule.

Maple Syrup Urine Disease

Infants usually die in the first few weeks. Opisthotonos, respiratory irregularities, and seizures are common.

Hyperglycinemia

Profound retardation and seizures are present from the time of birth.

Glycogen Synthetase Deficiency

Hepatomegaly, lethargy, and poor weight gain are the result of a severe neonatal hypoglycemia.

MISCELLANEOUS DISORDERS

Incontinentia Pigmenti

This hereditary disorder is seen predominantly in females. Vesiculobullous linear skin lesions are present at birth or appear shortly thereafter, followed by verrucous lesions and then hyperpigmented swirls. Seizures, cataracts, and dental and renal abnormalities may also be found.

Riley-Day Syndrome (Familial Dysautonomia)

Recurrent aspiration, absent lacrimation, unexplained fevers, absent deep tendon reflexes, and insensitivity to pain are among the unusual features of this syndrome.

Beckwith-Wiedemann Syndrome

Microcephaly is occasionally seen, in striking constrast to the postnatal gigantism; associated findings include an omphalocele or umbilical anomaly, macroglossia, and visceromegaly.

Myotonic Dystrophy

Microcephaly is sometimes a feature of this disorder of difficulty of muscle relaxation. Infants are usually hypotonic. The facies is immobile.

Shwachman Syndrome

Pancreatic insufficiency and leukopenia are prominent features.

SUGGESTED READING

DeMyer W. Microcephaly and microencephaly. In: Swaiman KF, ed. *Pediatric neurology: principles and practice*, 2nd ed. St. Louis: Mosby, 1994:206–208.
Haslam RHA, Smith DW. Autosomal dominant microcephaly. *J Pediatr* 1979;95:701–705.
Jones KL. *Smith's recognizable patterns of human malformation*, 5th ed. Philadelphia: WB Saunders, 1997.

24

Increased Intracranial Pressure and Bulging Fontanel

Increased intracranial pressure may be of sudden onset with characteristic symptoms or may develop gradually and be relatively asymptomatic. The symptoms often depend on the age of the child. The rigidity of the cranial container plays a major role in dictating what signs and symptoms may be present. Infants with open cranial sutures and fontanels often differ in their manifestations of increased pressure from children with a rigid cranial vault.

In the older child who complains of headaches and has papilledema, the diagnosis of increased intracranial pressure is almost assured. In the infant, who may not be able to express the presence of headache, signs and symptoms suggesting increased intracranial pressure include irritability, colic, head-holding, and, of course, a tense or bulging fontanel. Nausea, vomiting, strabismus, personality changes, head enlargement, and lethargy progressing to coma may be part of the clinical picture and all are important clues in the differential diagnosis. Dilation and poor reactivity of pupils to light is critical and specific sign of increased intracranial pressure suggesting impending brain herniation, while depressed consciousness is the most sensitive sign of critically elevated intracranial pressure.

In this chapter, increased intracranial pressure and bulging fontanel are considered together, because most of the disorders listed may produce a bulging or tense fontanel, if it is open.

♦ **Most Common Causes**

Hydrocephalus   Pseudotumor Cerebri (Idiopathic)
Hypoxic-Ischemic Injury   Meningitis/Encephalitis
Trauma

● **Causes Not to Forget**

Brain Tumor   Intracranial Hemorrhage
Diabetic Ketoacidosis

♦ HYDROCEPHALUS

Several disorders may cause ventricular enlargement as a consequence of increased pressure of the cerebrospinal fluid (CSF). Most cases are secondary to obstruction of the normal flow and egress of the CSF. In young infants, in addition to progressive cranial enlargement, other symptoms include irritability, poor feeding, and developmental delay in severe cases. The scalp veins may appear distended, and, eventually, the disproportion between the size of the face and the head becomes apparent. The fontanel may bulge later. Older children, with closed cranial sutures, demonstrate the usual signs of increased intracranial pressure.

SPACE-OCCUPYING LESIONS

● Brain Tumor

Presenting signs are often the result of increased intracranial pressure. Headache and vomiting are the most constant signs. Increasing head size occurs in longstanding cases. Convulsions are rarely a part of the picture. Spinal cord tumors and, much less commonly in children, metastatic tumors, particularly neuroblastoma, may also be causes.

● Intracranial Hemorrhage

In the neonate, hemorrhage is usually due to birth trauma or anoxia, though it need not occur immediately following delivery.

Intraventricular Hemorrhage

Decreased movement and tone, seizures, and a decreasing hematocrit with a tense fontanel are suggestive signs.

Cerebral Hemorrhage

Diffuse parenchymal bleeding with secondary brain swelling may produce signs similar to those seen with intraventricular hemorrhage.

Subarachnoid Hemorrhage

Lacerations of the tentorium or falx in newborns, trauma in children of any age, or a ruptured aneurysm may be the initiating event. Symptoms are generally sudden in onset.

Subdural Hemorrhage

Changes in consciousness, vomiting, convulsions, papilledema, and retinal hemorrhages may be found. In young children, child abuse should be considered. If there is no external evidence of trauma, a shaking insult may have produced the bleeding. Children with chronic subdural hematomas may present with slowly progressive head enlargement, seizures, developmental delay, and sometimes anemia.

Brain Abscess

Early symptoms are nonspecific. Most children have no fever. This diagnosis must be considered in the child with cyanotic congenital heart disease, or with a primary infection such as mastoiditis, who develops headaches, vomiting, and convulsions, followed by localized neurologic signs.

INFECTIOUS CAUSES

♦ Meningitis

A bulging fontanel in a sick child demands examination of the CSF.

♦ Encephalitis

Roseola

Bulging of the fontanel occasionally occurs during this common infection.

Shigella

Central nervous system symptoms including convulsions and increased intracranial pressure may precede the development of diarrhea.

Infectious Mononucleosis

Lyme Disease

Mastoiditis

May result in transverse sinus thrombosis and a presentation of increased pressure.

Cerebral Malaria

Most children with cerebral malaria have increased intracranial pressure, thought to be secondary to increased blood volume of the brain.

Cysticercosis

The larval form of the pork tapeworm may invade the central nervous system resulting in seizures and signs of increased intracranial pressure.

Guillain-Barré Syndrome

The development of an ascending paralysis or paresis suggests this possibility.

Poliomyelitis

Other Infections

Several infections may cause increased intracranial pressure, the mechanism of which is unclear: otitis media, paranasal sinusitis, ethmoiditis, upper-lobe pneumonia, and pyelonephritis.

ENDOCRINE CAUSES

Hyperthyroidism

Hypoparathyroidism

Repetitive convulsions, particularly at the time of fever, may be the presenting sign. Tetany may be the primary sign in older children.

Pseudohypoparathyroidism

Affected children have short stature with short hands, especially the fourth and fifth metacarpals, a round face, and sometimes intracranial calcifications visible on radiographs.

Addison Disease

Hypoadrenocorticism is another rare cause of increased pressure. Vomiting, muscle weakness, increased skin pigmentation, or patches of vitiligo may be seen.

Hypothyroidism

Ovarian Dysfunction

The cause of the increased pressure is unclear; it is most frequently present in adult women (1).

CARDIOVASCULAR CAUSES

Congestive Heart Failure

The cause is probably increased venous pressure.

Dural Sinus Thrombosis

Ear, pharyngeal, or sinus infections or, in some cases, trauma or tumor invasion may cause the thrombosis.

Hypertensive Encephalopathy

Obstructed Vena Cava

Obstruction is by an intrathoracic mass. Blockage of venous return produces increased venous pressure.

HEMATOLOGIC DISTURBANCES

Polycythemia

Polycythemia may result in cerebral infarction and swelling or dural sinus thrombosis.

Anemia

Severe iron-deficiency anemia has been described as a cause.

Leukemia

Central nervous system involvement may produce pressure symptoms.

METABOLIC CAUSES

• Diabetic Ketoacidosis

Irreversible cerebral edema is a feared complication of diabetic ketoacidosis.

Electrolyte Disturbances

Water intoxication secondary to inappropriate antidiuretic hormone secretion may result from a number of disorders.

Hepatic Encephalopathy

Uremia

Galactosemia

Hypophosphatasia

In severe cases, the fontanel may be large and tense and the skull soft. Anorexia, vomiting, and irritability are other prominent symptoms. Serum alkaline phosphatase levels are low.

Osteopetrosis

As a cause of increased intracranial pressure, osteopetrosis is rare. The bones become sclerotic and thickened. Head enlargement, hepatosplenomegaly, pancytopenia, and multiple cranial nerve palsies are highly suggestive findings.

Maple Syrup Urine Disease

DRUGS AND TOXINS

Tetracycline

Infants on tetracycline therapy may develop increased intracranial pressure by an unknown mechanism after only a few doses. This phenomenon occasionally occurs in adolescents being treated for acne with this drug.

Other Antibiotics

Nalidixic acid, gentamicin, and sulfonamides have been implicated.

Steroid Withdrawal

Steroid Therapy

Oral Contraceptives

Hypervitaminosis A

High doses of vitamin A may cause an increased intracranial pressure picture. The vitamin may have been taken for the treatment of acne, ichthyosis, or other skin disorders. The ingestion of polar bear liver, which has a high vitamin A content, is a favorite "roundmanship" cause.

Lead Encephalopathy

The prodrome of lead poisoning may have been overlooked. This possibility should always be considered in the child with pica who has central nervous system signs and symptoms.

Aluminum Toxicity

Infants receiving aluminum containing phosphate binders may develop an osteo-dystrophy with delayed closure of the fontanel, poor muscle tone, and a ricket-like picture.

MISCELLANEOUS CAUSES

◆ Brain Contusions

Injury to brain tissue may result in tissue swelling and increased pressure.

◆ Idiopathic

The most common cause of pseudotumor cerebri.

◆ Hypoxic-Ischemic Injury

Diffuse brain swelling, a result of cytotoxic edema, may follow insults to the brain.

Water Intoxication

Dilution of formula may result in hyponatremia, seizures, and increased intracranial pressure.

Iron Deficiency

Craniosynostosis

Coronal synostosis, as seen in Crouzon syndrome, may produce signs of increased intracranial pressure and a bulging fontanel.

Status Epilepticus

Cerebral edema associated with the seizures results in increased pressure.

Rapid Brain Growth During Refeeding Following Starvation/Malnutrition

This finding has been reported after nutritional improvement in cystic fibrosis.

Chronic Pulmonary Disease

Hypercarbia, with resultant cerebrovascular dilatation is felt to be the pathogenetic mechanism.

High Altitude Brain Edema

Obesity

Following DPT and DT Immunizations (2)

Hypovitaminosis A

Vitamin B$_2$ (Riboflavin) Deficiency

Food or Drug Allergies

Congenital Subgaleal Cyst Over the Anterior Fontanel

Lupus Erythematosus

Sarcoidosis

Reye Syndrome

REFERENCES

1. Hagberg B, Sillanpää M. Benign intracranial hypertension. *Acta Paediatr Scand* 1970;59:328–339.
2. Gross TP, Milstien JB, Kuritshy JN. Bulging fontanelle after immunization with diphtheria-tetanus-pertussis vaccine and diphtheria-tetanus vaccine. *J Pediatr* 1989;114:423–424.

SUGGESTED READING

Bergman I. Increased intracranial pressure. *Pediatr Rev* 1994;15:241–244.
Finberg L. Why do patients with diabetic ketoacidosis have cerebral swelling, and why does treatment sometimes make it worse? *Arch Pediatr Adolesc Med* 1996;150:785–786.
Harris G, Fiordilisi I. Physiologic management of diabetic ketoacidemia: a 5-year prospective pediatric experience in 231 episodes. *Arch Pediatr Adolesc Med* 1994;148:1046–1052.
Williams RS. CPC: otitic hydrocephalus. *N Engl J Med* 1986;318:1322–1328.

25

Enlarged Anterior Fontanel

An enlarged anterior fontanel may indicate increased intracranial pressure or any of several disorders affecting calcification and development of the calvarium. In conditions with increased intracranial pressure, the head circumference usually is enlarged as well.

The first step in the evaluation of an apparently enlarged anterior fontanel is measurement for comparison with the range of normal size consistent with age. Popich and Smith (1) developed a graph of anterior fontanel size based on measurements of normal newborn infants. The fontanel size was calculated as length plus width divided by 2. In the infants measured, anterior fontanel size ranged from 0.6 to 3.6 cm, with a mean of 2.1 cm. These measurements are recommended as limits of normal size in newborns, with 0.6 cm defined as two standard deviations below and 3.6 cm as two standard deviations above the mean. The mean anterior fontanel measurement during the first year of life may be found in *Smith's Recognizable Patterns of Human Malformation* (2). Note that black newborns have significantly larger anterior fontanels than white newborns, mean 2.67 cm (3).

♦ **Most Common Causes of Enlarged Anterior Fontanel**

Increased Intracranial Pressure   Down Syndrome
Achondroplasia   Congenital Hypothyroidism
Rickets

♦ **INCREASED INTRACRANIAL PRESSURE**

Any disorder resulting in increased intracranial pressure may produce an abnormally large anterior fontanel. (See Chapter 24, Increased Intracranial Pressure and Bulging Fontanel.)

SKELETAL DISORDERS

♦ **Achondroplasia**

Short stature, short limbs, and a large head with a prominent forehead and depressed nasal bridge are characteristic features.

Osteogenesis Imperfecta

Affected children usually are short in stature and have a history of multiple bone fractures. The sclerae are bluish. In infants, there is a soft feel to the skull caused by wormian bones, as well as a large fontanel.

♦ Rickets

In addition to the large fontanel there may be frontal and parietal bossing. Other findings include bowed legs, enlarged epiphyses, prominent costochondral junctions, and scoliosis. The rickets may be vitamin D deficient or dependent.

Apert Syndrome (Acrocephalosyndactyly)

Inheritance is autosomal dominant; craniosynostosis with a short anteroposterior diameter, a high forehead and flat occiput, flat facies with hypertelorism, and syndactyly of fingers and toes are findings.

Cleidocranial Dysostosis

This disorder, with autosomal-dominant inheritance, features partial to complete aplasia of the clavicles, brachycephaly with frontal bossing, wormian bones of the skull, late dentition, and irregular finger length.

Hypophosphatasia

This rare disorder, characterized by hypoplastic fragile bones, bowed lower extremities, short ribs with a rachitic rosary, and defective dentition, is inherited as an autosomal-recessive trait.

Pyknodysostosis

Features include short stature, osteosclerosis with a tendency to fracture, frontal and occipital prominence, a persistent anterior fontanel with delayed suture closure, wormian bones of the skull, and irregular teeth.

Kenny Syndrome

The main findings are short stature, myopia, and a late closure of the fontanel.

Lenz-Majewski Hyperostosis

This rare disorder features cutis laxa, large fontanels, and syndactyly at birth. Affected children do not thrive. The bones become dense.

CHROMOSOMAL ABNORMALITIES

♦ Down Syndrome

Trisomy 13 Syndrome

Trisomy 18 Syndrome

7 p Duplications

Large anterior fonatanel may be the most characteristic feature of this chromosomal abnormality. Other findings include micrognathia, choanal stenosis/atresia, large low-set ears, cardiac septal defects, joint hyperextensibility, dislocations and contractures, and gastrointestinal and genital defects.

Shprintzen Syndrome

Large anterior fonatanels have been described in a few patients with this syndrome, the result of a deletion of chromosome 22q11, the same region as DiGeorge syndrome.

ENDOCRINE DISORDERS

◆ **Hypothyroidism**

In addition to a large fontanel other findings include an immature facies, macroglossia, umbilical hernia, dry skin, neonatal jaundice, and constipation. These features may not be prominent in the neonate. An enlarged posterior fontanel should suggest this diagnosis.

CONGENITAL INFECTIONS

Rubella

The classic major abnormalities, in various combinations, are deafness, microcephaly, congenital heart disease, psychomotor retardation, and cataracts.

Syphilis

DRUGS AND TOXINS

Fetal Hydantoin Syndrome

Infants born to mothers who are taking this anticonvulsant may manifest several dysmorphogenic abnormalities including failure to thrive, cleft lip or palate, hypoplastic nails, hypertelorism, broad nasal bridge, and mental deficiency.

Aminopterin-Induced Malformation

Exposure of the fetus to this folic acid antagonist results in severe hypoplasia of facial and skull bones, micrognathia, and clubfoot.

DYSMORPHOGENETIC SYNDROMES

Beckwith-Wiedemann Syndrome

Russell-Silver Syndrome

Prenatal onset of growth deficiency with short stature, small triangular facies, short incurved fifth fingers, and occasionally limb asymmetry are characteristic features.

Rubinstein-Taybi Syndrome

A large anterior fontanel is occasionally seen in this syndrome in which the main features are short stature, broad thumbs and great toes, antimongoloid slant to the palpebral fissures, and cryptorchidism.

Hallermann-Streiff Syndrome (Oculomandibulofacial Syndrome)

Small stature, brachycephaly with frontal and parietal bossing, micrognathia, cataracts, a small thin nose, and hypoplastic teeth are found.

Zellweger (Cerebrohepatorenal) Syndrome

There is significant hypotonia from birth, as well as a high forehead, flat occiput, redundant skin of the neck, hepatomegaly, and an early death.

Robinow Syndrome (Fetal Face Syndrome)

Mild-to-moderate short stature, macrocephaly, frontal bossing, hypertelorism, small upturned nose, long philtrum, short forearms, and hypoplastic genitals are findings in this disorder inherited as an autosomal-dominant trait.

Cutis Laxa

Inheritance is autosomal recessive; in affected children, loose skin creates a "bloodhound" appearance. Short stature and laxity of joints are other features.

Progeria

In this rare but striking syndrome, early onset of premature aging is seen, with alopecia, loss of subcutaneous fat, and short stature.

VATER Association

This group of anomalies may occur in various combinations: vertebral defects, ventricular septal defect, anal atresia, tracheoesophageal fistula, and radial dysplasia.

Opitz-Frias Syndrome

Swallowing problems with recurrent aspiration, stridor, a weak hoarse cry, hypertelorism, and hypospadias are characteristic findings.

MISCELLANEOUS CAUSES

Malnutrition

Hydranencephaly

The head is enlarged at birth with a large fontanel. The skull vault is thin, and primitive reflexes are preserved. Transillumination verifies the diagnostic suspicion.

Intrauterine Growth Retardation

Term newborns, who are small for gestational age, may have large anterior fontanels, particularly if their epiphyseal ossification is delayed (4).

Mucopolysaccharidoses

A large fontanel is most likely to be found in Hurler syndrome (type I mucopolysaccharidosis).

Hyperpipecolic Acidemia

Additional features include developmental delay, hypotonia, and retinopathy with visual impairment.

REFERENCES

1. Popich GA, Smith DW. Fontanels: range of normal size. *J Pediatr* 1972;80:749–752.
2. Jones KL. *Smith's recognizable patterns of human malformation*, 5th ed. Philadelphia: WB Saunders, 1997;767.
3. Faix RG. Fontanelle size in black and white term newborn infants. *J Pediatr* 1982;100:304–306.
4. Philip AGS. Fontanel size and epiphyseal ossification in neonates with intrauterine growth retardation. *J Pediatr* 1974;84:204–207.

26

Delayed Closure of Anterior Fontanel

The anterior fontanel generally closes by 12 to 18 months of age; however, there is great variability in the size of fontanels and their time of closure in normal children. In a study of closure times, no significant differences were found in the size and time of closure of the anterior fontanel between term and preterm infants or between sexes (1). Closure of the anterior fontanel was noted at 3 months after term in 1% of infants, at 12 months in 38%, and at 24 months in 96% (1). The median age of closure was found to be 13.8 months in term infants.

In Chapter 25, disorders associated with a large fontanel were presented. Delayed closure of the anterior fontanel is subsequently seen in many of these disorders. Descriptions of conditions associated with a large fontanel as well as delayed closure are not repeated here. Many of the disorders associated with delayed closure have dysmorphic features that should facilitate their recognition.

♦ **Most Common Causes of Delayed Closure of the Anterior Fontanel**

Normal Variation   Increased Intracranial Pressure
Congenital Hypothyroidism   Down Syndrome
Primary Megalencephaly   Rickets

♦ **INCREASED INTRACRANIAL PRESSURE**

In addition to causing an enlarged anterior fontanel, increased intracranial pressure generally results in delayed closure of the anterior fontanel. (See Chapter 24, Increased Intracanial Pressure and Bulging Fontanel.)

SKELETAL DISORDERS

Achondroplasia

Osteogenesis Imperfecta

♦ **Vitamin D Deficiency Rickets**

Vitamin D Resistant Rickets

Bony changes similar to those in rickets are found but are unresponsive to treatment with vitamin D. Additional findings are hypotonia, growth deficiency, susceptibility to fractures, and hypocalcemia.

Cleidocranial Dysostosis

Apert Syndrome (Acrocephalosyndactyly)

Campomelic Dysplasia

Prenatal growth deficiency is prominent, along with bowing of the tibiae with unusual dimples at the area of maximal bowing.

Oto-Palato-Digital Syndrome, Type II

Achondrogenesis-Hypochondrogenesis, Type II

Acrocallosal Syndrome

Associated with hypoplastic or absent corpus callosum. Seizures, polydactyly of the hands and feet, and severe mental retardation are among the findings.

Antley-Bixler Syndrome

Multiple abnormalities are found including cranial synostosis, midfacial hypoplasia, dysplastic ears, radiohumeral synostosis, and joint contractures.

Hypophosphatasia

Pyknodysostosis

Schinzel-Giedion Syndrome

In addition to other dysmorphic features, the metopic suture is widely open to the nasal root.

Kenny Syndrome

Lenz-Majewski Hyperostosis

This rare disorder features cutis laxa, large fontanels, and syndactyly at birth. Affected children do not thrive. The bones become dense.

Stanesco Dysostosis

In this unusual form of dwarfism, features include a thin skull, shallow orbits, and a small mandible.

CHROMOSOMAL ABNORMALITIES

♦ **Down Syndrome**

Trisomy 13 Syndrome

Trisomy 18 Syndrome

ENDOCRINE DISORDERS

♦ **Hypothyroidism**

DRUGS AND TOXINS

Fetal Hydantoin Syndrome

Aminopterin-Induced Malformation

Aluminum Toxicity

Infants receiving aluminum-containing phosphate binders may develop an osteo-dystrophy with a bulging fontanel, poor muscle tone, and a ricketlike picture.

DYSMORPHOGENETIC SYNDROMES

Russell-Silver Syndrome

Rubinstein-Taybi Syndrome

Occasional late closure may be seen.

Hallermann-Streiff Syndrome (Oculomandibulofacial Syndrome)

Zellweger Syndrome (Cerebrohepatorenal Syndrome)

Robinow (Fetal Face) Syndrome

Cutis Laxa

Occasional late closure may occur.

Progeria

VATER Association

Occasional late closure may occur.

Aase Syndrome

Triphalangeal thumbs, congenital anemia, narrow shoulders, and mild growth deficiency are features.

Melnick-Needles Syndrome

Infants fail to gain well; physical findings include exophthalmos, full cheeks, micrognathia, significant malocclusion, and large ears.

Conradi-Hunermann Syndrome

Occasional late closure may occur. Features include mild-to-moderate growth deficiency, asymmetrical limb shortening downslanting palpebral fissures, and frequently scoliosis.

Otopalatodigital Syndrome

Late closure of the anterior fontanel is occasionally seen. Prominent findings are frontal prominence, hypertelorism, small nose and mouth, broad distal digits, conduction deafness, and mild mental retardation.

Saethre-Chotzen Syndrome

MISCELLANEOUS CAUSES

♦ Primary Megalencephaly

Macrocephaly may be familial without associated anomalies. Measurement of the head circumference of other family members is mandatory. The macrocephaly may be related to idiopathic hydrocephalus.

Malnutrition

Congenital Syphilis

REFERENCE

1. Duc G, Largo RH. Anterior fontanel: size and closure in term and preterm infants. *Pediatrics* 1986;78:904–908.

SUGGESTED READING

Jones KL. *Smith's recognizable patterns of human malformation*, 5th ed. Philadelphia: WB Saunders, 1997.

27

Early Closure of Anterior Fontanel

The conditions associated with delayed closure of the anterior fontanel are considerably more numerous than those associated with early closure. What constitutes early closure? The definition is not clear, but if the anterior fontanel is no longer palpable at 3 to 4 months of age, additional investigation should be considered. In some children, radiologic examination discloses that the fontanel is still open despite clinical evidence to the contrary. If the fontanel is truly closed, the following conditions should be considered in the differential diagnosis.

NORMAL VARIATION

Although the median age of closure of the anterior fontanel in term infants is 13.8 months, closure as early as 3 months of age may still be a normal variation (1). Subsequent head growth must be closely monitored.

MICROCEPHALY

Abnormal brain development may be accompanied by microcephaly and early fontanel closure. Causes of failure of development include prenatal and postnatal insults.

CRANIOSYNOSTOSIS

Idiopathic Causes

Hyperthyroidism

Premature closure has been reported in idiopathic hyperthyroidism as well as with the administration of excessive amounts of thyroid hormone in replacement therapy.

Hypophosphatasia

In this rare inherited disorder, skeletal changes are similar to those in rickets. Hypercalcemia is frequently found, the serum alkaline phosphatase is low, and excessive amounts of phosphoethanolamine are excreted in the urine. The fontanel closure may be early or late.

Rickets

Craniosynostosis may occur in as many as one third of cases of rickets.

Hyperparathyroidism

A few cases of premature fontanel closure have been described in this disorder. Hypercalcemia, generalized bone rarefraction, and failure to thrive suggest hyperparathyroidism in infancy.

REFERENCE

1. Duc G, Largo RH. Anterior fontanel: size and closure in term and preterm infants. *Pediatrics* 1986;78:904–908.

28

Parotid Gland Swelling

The normal parotid gland is not palpable. Before widespread immunization, enlargement of this salivary gland was most commonly due to infection by mumps virus, the symptoms of which were usually well recognized, even by most laymen.

In some cases, swelling of the parotid is recurrent, and careful evaluation of the amount and nature of the glandular secretions is required. Secondary or recurrent infections often develop in glands with deficient saliva production. "Wind parotitis," swelling of the gland as a result of air forced into Stensen's duct, may be mistaken for recurrent infections.

◆ Most Common Causes of Parotid Swelling

Infection: Mumps, Parainfluenza	Human Immunodeficiency Virus
Wind Parotitis	Strictures of Parotid Ducts
Sjögren Syndrome	Idiopathic

◆ WIND PAROTITIS

Air may be forced into the parotid duct and cause glandular swelling, especially in children learning to play wind instruments or blowing up balloons. More rarely, the child may learn how to force air into Stensen's duct as an attention-getting device.

INFECTION

Viral Infections

◆ Mumps

Mumps is the most common and easily recognized cause of parotid gland swelling. The gland is usually tender to touch, but the overlying skin is not erythematous. There is some debate about whether mumps parotitis can be recurrent.

◆ Parainfluenza Types 1 and 3

Parainfluenza types 1 and 3 are probably the second most common causes of acute parotitis.

♦ **Acquired Immune Deficiency Syndrome**

Chronic parotid swelling may be part of the picture usually characterized by recurrent infection and poor growth, the result of human immunodeficiency virus.

Other

Viruses implicated less commonly include coxsackieviruses A and B, echoviruses, varicella, cytomegalovirus, influenza A and B, Epstein-Barr, herpes simplex virus 1, and lymphocytic choriomeningitis virus.

Bacterial Infections

Acute Suppurative Infections

These infections are most frequently seen in neonates or infants under 1 year of age and in those with debilitating diseases. *Staphylococcus aureus* is the most common pathogen, but Streptococcus species are second most common. In the neonatal period gram-negative organisms are most common. The gland is tender and red and there may be significant systemic symptoms. In some cases, pus can be expressed from Stensen's duct. Suppurative parotitis is often associated with dehydration, immunosuppression, or ductal obstruction.

Abscess of Parotid Gland

Other Infections

Cat-Scratch Disease

Granulomas may develop in the parotid gland following scratches about the face. Facial swelling due to preauricular lymphadenitis may simulate parotid gland disease.

Tuberculosis

As a cause of swelling, tuberculosis is uncommon. Infection is not as acute as with viral and bacterial causes. *Mycobacterium tuberculosis* is, however, the most common cause of granulomatous parotitis.

Actinomycosis

Swelling is usually the result of direct extension from infection elsewhere.

Tularemia

Swelling is part of the uveoparotid syndrome.

Brucellosis

Histoplasmosis

Consider this possibility particularly if hilar adenopathy is present.

CHRONIC OR RECURRENT SIALADENITIS

Nonobstructive, Intermittent Sialadenitis

♦ Idiopathic Causes

Enlargement is usually unilateral. It is associated with mild pain and lasts 1 to 2 weeks. The recurrences resolve at puberty.

Benign Lymphoepithelial Lesion

Decreased salivary flow and stasis due to changes in the salivary ducts predispose the gland to recurrent inflammation. The lesion generally occurs in children over 5 years of age. The swelling is recurrent, may be slightly tender, and is nonerythematous. The diagnosis is confirmed by sialography, which shows punctate sialectasia. This lesion has been thought to represent a localized form of Sjögren syndrome.

Functional Hypersecretion

This is a rare cause of enlargement.

Allergic Reactions

The presence of eosinophilic plugs in the parotid duct with swelling has been documented in allergic reactions. In a significant number of patients, there are other allergic symptoms. The onset of the swelling is sudden and it lasts hours to several days.

Drug Sensitivities

Iodides in drugs or food are the best-known cause of parotid swelling from drugs. Other medications that may cause swelling are rarely used in children. Phenothiazines in large doses may cause xerostomia (dry mouth) and repeated infections, resulting in swelling.

TUMORS

Hemangioma

The swelling is soft and nontender. There may be a bluish hue to the overlying skin. When the infant cries, the swelling may become more tense.

Lymphangioma

The swelling tends to be more diffuse than with hemangiomas and not confined to a specific salivary gland.

Mixed Tumor

This form is the most common of the benign tumors and is first seen as a firm, painless mass.

Pleomorphic Adenoma

Mucoepidermoid Tumor

This is the most common of the malignant tumors. The usual presenting feature is a firm, mobile mass in the parotid fascia. A sudden growth of a mass or facial nerve palsy raises the suspicion of malignancy.

Acinic Carcinoma

Rhabdomyosarcoma

METABOLIC AND ENDOCRINE DISORDERS

Endocrine Disturbances

The parotid enlargement seen with endocrine disturbances is benign, slowly progressive, painless, and lacking inflammation.

Hypothyroidism

Cushing Syndrome

Enlargement is due to fatty infiltration.

Metabolic Disorders

Diabetes Mellitus

Salivary gland swelling as a result of diabetes is unusual in childhood.

Starvation

Parotid hypertrophy is the cause and it may be secondary to hypoproteinemia.

Anorexia Nervosa/Bulimia

If starvation is severe enough, salivary gland hypertrophy may occur.

Postnecrotic Cirrhosis

OBSTRUCTIVE ENLARGEMENT

♦ Strictures

Strictures may be congenital or secondary to poor oral hygiene, dental or external trauma, recurrent infection, or calculi. The swelling usually occurs suddenly with eating and is painful. Secondary infection is common. Sialography is diagnostic.

Calculi

Calculi rarely occur in the parotid gland. Symptoms are the same as in strictures. Calculi occur more commonly in teenagers than in younger children and may follow recurrent infection.

MISCELLANEOUS CAUSES

Cystic Fibrosis

Parotid enlargement rarely occurs, but the submaxillary gland is enlarged in 90% of affected children.

Autoimmune Disorders

♦ Sjögren Syndrome

Dry mouth and eyes are characteristic. The swelling may be related to intermittent blockage of the parotid duct by mucus plugs or to repeated infection. The swelling may be bi- or unilateral, painful or painless.

Mixed Connective Tissue Disease

Children with this disorder have various symptoms of various connective tissue disorders.

Systemic Lupus Erythematosus

Recurrent swelling may occasionally be the initial clue.

Sarcoidosis

Swelling of the parotid gland occurs in less than 10% of the cases of sarcoidosis. The swelling is firm, painless, and often nodular. Heerfordt syndrome is an unusual form characterized by febrile uveitis and parotitis, preauricular swelling, and occasional paralysis of the facial nerve.

Impaction of Stensen Duct with a Food Particle

Starch Eating

DISORDERS THAT MIMIC PAROTID SWELLING

Lymphadenopathy

Masseter Muscle Hypertrophy

Hypertrophy may occur as a result of teeth grinding, while awake or sleep. In some cultures, such as that of the Alaskan Eskimo, hypertrophy is normal and is associated with a diet of foods requiring prolonged chewing.

SUGGESTED READING

Ericson S, Zetterlund B, Ohman J. Recurrent parotitis and sialectasis in childhood. *Ann Otol Rhinol Laryngol* 1991;100:527–535.

Kessler A, Handler SD. Salivary gland neoplasms in children: a 10 year survey at the Children's Hospital of Philadelphia. *Int J Pediatr Otorhinolaryngol* 1994;29:195–202.

Nassimbeni G, Ventura A, Boehm P, Guastalla P, Zocconi E. Self-induced pneumoparotitis. *Clin Pediatr* 1995;34:160–162.

29

Facial Paralysis/Weakness

Facial paralysis or weakness is a relatively uncommon problem in general pediatric practice. Bell palsy is the most common cause of acquired facial palsy and is labeled as idiopathic, although increasing evidence supports an association with infection (1). As many as one third to two thirds of cases of facial palsy are labeled as Bell palsy. Otitis media may be associated with a transient facial weakness and accounts for about 10% of causes of this problem, while Lyme disease is the most common cause of facial palsy in some areas of the United States. It is important not to mistake hypoplasia of the depressor anguli oris muscle for facial palsy.

The causes of facial nerve paralysis or weakness may be broken down into three major categories (2). Postnatal acquired causes are the most common. Birth trauma accounts for the majority of perinatal acquired causes, but the paralysis may, in fact, not be traumatic in origin. New evidence suggests that the problem may have occurred in utero (3,4). The third category is congenital, which represents developmental errors occurring during embryogenesis.

♦ **Most Common Causes**

Bell Palsy   Otitis Media
"Traumatic," Birth or Later   Congenital (Developmental)

● **Causes Not to Forget**

Lyme Disease   Brain Stem Glioma
Hypoplasia of Depressor Anguli Oris Muscle
  (Simulates Facial Palsy)

POSTNATAL ACQUIRED FACIAL NERVE PARALYSIS

Idiopathic Causes

♦ **Bell Palsy**

This is an acute onset facial palsy, without evidence of other cranial nerve involvement or brain stem dysfunction. The exact pathogenetic mechanism is unclear, but the paralysis is thought to follow vasospasm of the blood vessels supplying the facial nerve, leading to edema and resultant loss of function. Onset is usually sudden and often following a viral infection. Paralysis is usually unilateral and may be complete or partial. Ear pain may be an early symptom. Vertigo, loss of taste, and hyperacusis may also occur. There is increasing evidence, mostly serologic, for an etiologic role for viruses and, perhaps, other infections. It is likely that an immunologic response associated with infection triggers a cranial or generalized polyneuropathy resulting in facial nerve compression, degeneration, and paralysis (1).

Melkersson Syndrome

This hereditary syndrome is characterized by recurrent facial paralysis that is often bilateral, relapsing, and familial, angioneurotic edema, especially of the lips, and, in some cases, a furrowing of the tongue. Facial swelling is much more common, with facial paralysis occurring in only one third of cases.

Infectious Disorders

● Lyme Disease

Lyme disease is the most common cause of facial palsy in some parts of the United States.

♦ Otitis Media, Acute

Acute otitis media may produce a transient palsy, treated best with antibiotics and a myringotomy.

Guillain-Barré Syndrome

Up to one third of patients with this ascending peripheral neuropathy have a facial paralysis. Bilateral facial nerve palsy is often associated with Guillain-Barré syndrome.

Gradenigo Syndrome

This is the name given to petrositis with cranial nerve involvement. Chronic otitis media may result in suppuration of the apex of the petrous portion of the temporal bone, resulting in sixth and seventh nerve paralysis. Fever, ear pain, and chronic otorrhea may be present.

Meningitis

Encephalitis

Various encephaliditides may result in facial palsy, including varicella, mumps, rubella, poliomyelitis, and other enteroviral infections.

Mastoiditis

Incidence is much less today than in the preantibiotic era. The auricle may be pushed forward, and the mastoid area is swollen and tender.

Brain Abscess

Central paralysis may occur, but this sign is overshadowed by central nervous system signs and symptoms.

Herpes Zoster Oticus (Ramsay Hunt Syndrome)

This disorder is much more common in adults. Severe, deep-seated ear pain followed by the appearance of vesicles on the tympanic membrane, in the external auditory canal, or on the auricle is characteristic.

Osteomyelitis of Temporal Bone

Mumps Parotitis

Rarely, facial weakness occurs during mumps.

Miscellaneous Infections

Varicella-zoster virus, *Mycoplasma pneumoniae* infection, Epstein-Barr virus, tuberculosis, tetanus, trichinosis, and syphilis are examples.

♦ TRAUMATIC

Facial Trauma

Injuries to the facial nerve may occur from accidents or missiles. The injury may also be the result of surgical injury.

Skull Fracture

Temporal bone fracture may result in a delayed paralysis. Cochlear function is lost in a large percentage of cases.

Acute Nose-Blow Palsy

Forceful blowing of the nose with occlusion of the external auditory canal has been reported (5).

Odontoid Dislocation

May cause compression of the posterior vertebral artery and result in cranial nerve abnormalities including facial weakness and decreased gag reflex.

METABOLIC DISORDERS

Hypothyroidism

Hyperparathyroidism

Idiopathic Infantile Hypercalcemia

Osteopetrosis

Overgrowth of bone may compress cranial nerves. Bones are brittle; the head is square; and anemia, blindness, and deafness develop.

Diabetes Mellitus

Diabetes is a rare cause in children.

Uremia

TUMORS AND NEOPLASIA

● Gliomas of Brain Stem

Facial paralysis may be a presenting complaint. Sixth nerve palsy, with or without headache and ataxia, is common.

Acoustic Neuroma

A neuroma rarely produces paralysis and is rare in children. Suggestive symptoms include unilateral progressive hearing loss, unilateral tinnitus, and intermittent vertigo or unsteadiness.

Leukemia

Metastatic Tumors

Neuroblastoma may be a cause in children.

Eosinophilic Granuloma, Teratoma, Hemangioma, Rhabdomyosarcoma

Paralysis may result when the middle ear is involved.

Neurofibromatosis

Parotid Gland Tumors

Facial Nerve Tumors

A slowly progressive paralysis results.

MISCELLANEOUS CAUSES

Vascular Lesions

Thrombosis of the carotid artery or of the middle cerebral or pontine branches of the basilar artery may produce paralysis. Aneurysms may also be responsible, but in both lesions, central nervous system signs are evident.

Intracerebral Arteriovenous Malformation

Hypertension

Facial paralysis is an uncommon finding in severe hypertension.

Polyarteritis Nodosa

Postictal Paralysis

Paralysis is brief if it occurs.

DPT Immunization Reaction

Increased Intracranial Pressure

Drug Reactions

Vincristine is best known.

Myasthenia Gravis

Myotonic Dystrophy

Ptosis, immobile facies with eventual facial muscle atrophy, and muscle weakness with myotonia are found.

Nemaline Myopathy

Kawasaki Disease (Mucocutaneous Lymph Node Syndrome)

Henoch-Schönlein Purpura

Compression of the seventh nerve from edema has been reported.

Iron Deficiency

Facial nerve palsy has been described in iron deficient individuals.

Sarcoidosis

Facial paralysis is the most common neurologic complication of sarcoidosis. It is generally associated with parotid swelling and, less commonly, with uveitis.

PRENATALLY/PERINATALLY ACQUIRED FACIAL NERVE PARALYSIS

♦ **Traumatic**

Facial paralysis not uncommonly is believed to be a result of trauma during the birth process, either a result of pressure on the peripheral portion of the facial nerve during forceps application, by the maternal sacral promontory, or occasionally by bone fragments in skull fractures. New evidence questions whether birth trauma is the cause.

Intracranial Hemorrhage

Congenital Rubella Infection

Thalidomide Embryopathy

CONGENITAL FACIAL NERVE PARALYSIS

◆ Congenital (Atraumatic)

New evidence questions whether many infants with facial palsy formerly assigned as traumatic are truly developmental (3). No association was found between the development of permanent congenital facial palsy and recognized risk factors for birth injury (4). Intrauterine rather than traumatic etiology is suggested.

• Hypoplasia of the Depressor Anguli Oris Muscle

Asymmetric movements of the face, noted especially on crying, may suggest facial nerve paralysis, but in fact there is a congenital absence or hypoplasia of this muscle. The forehead wrinkles, the eyes close, and nasolabial folds appear equal. A high incidence of congenital anomalies may be associated with this syndrome, including cardiac, renal and musculoskeletal.

Goldenhar Syndrome (Oculoauriculovertebral Dysplasia)

Multiple facial anomalies, with hemifacial microsomia, small or atretic ears, and epibulbar dermoids, are characteristic.

Congenital Facial Paralysis (Möbius Syndrome)

Absence of seventh nerve nuclei, usually evident at birth, is bilateral and associated with bilateral involvement of the sixth nerve. The face is expressionless, the eyes do not close completely, and the infant drools constantly. Mental retardation is frequent.

Temporal Bone Malformation

A unilateral paralysis may result.

Supranuclear Facial Nerve Lesion

This lesion is associated with anoxia before or during birth. The lower half to two thirds of the face is affected on the side opposite the lesion.

Freeman-Sheldon Syndrome (Craniocarpotarsal Dystrophy)

Masklike facies with a small mouth gives a "whistling face" impression; the chin is dimpled and the tongue is small.

Schwartz-Jampel Syndrome

Myotonia with a masklike face, joint motion limitation, and short stature are findings.

Oromandibular-Limb Hypogenesis Spectrum

Cranial nerve palsies, including the Möbius sequence, are included in this spectrum of disorders that may include tongue and limb abnormalities, among others.

REFERENCES

1. Morgan M, Nathwani D. Facial palsy and infection: the unfolding story. *Clin Infect Dis* 1992;14:263–271.
2. Orobello P. Congenital and acquired facial nerve paralysis in children. *Otolaryngol Clin North Am* 1991;24:647–652.
3. Shapiro NL, Cunningham MJ, Parikh SR, Eavey RD, Cheney ML. Congenital unilateral facial paralysis. *Pediatrics* 1996;97:261–265.
4. Laing JH, Harrison DH, Jones BM, Laing GJ. Is permanent congenital facial palsy caused by birth trauma? *Arch Dis Child* 1996;74:56–58.
5. Onundarson PT. Acute nose-blow palsy: a pneumatic variant of sudden facial paralysis [Letter]. *N Engl J Med* 1987;317:1227.

SUGGESTED READING

Franco SM, Tunnessen WW Jr. Congenital hypoplasia of the depressor anguli oris muscle. *Arch Pediatr Adolesc Med* 1996;150:325–326.
Grundfast KM, Guarisco JL, Thomsen JR, Koch B. Diverse etiologies of facial paralysis in children. *Int J Pediatr Otorhinolaryngol* 1990;19:223–239.
Rathore MH, Friedman AD, Barton LL, Dunkle LM. Herpes zoster oticus. *Am J Dis Child* 1991;145:722–723.

SECTION III

Ears

30
Earache

Earache, or otalgia, is a common symptom in the pediatric age group. Earache in most cases is the result of acute middle ear infections or chronic accumulations of fluid in the middle ear. Otitis externa is more common in the summer months. Self-induced trauma to the ear canal or tympanic membrane occurs more frequently than generally thought; children (and adults) stick all sorts of matter into their ear canals.

In this chapter causes of otalgia are divided into two groups: disorders involving the ear primarily, and those in which ear pain is referred from disease in another region, particularly those innervated by cranial nerves with ties to the ear.

♦ Most Common Causes of Earache

Acute Otitis Media	Serous Otitis Media
Otitis Externa	Acute Pharyngitis
Temporomandibular Joint Dysfunction	Ear Trauma

PRIMARY OTALGIA

External Ear

♦ Otitis Externa

The pain associated with infection of the ear canal is intensified by pulling on the auricle. *Pseudomonas aeruginosa* is the most common pathogen.

♦ Ear Trauma

The ear canal or auricle may be injured by self-induced trauma with sticks, paper clips, and similar objects used to scratch the ear or remove cerumen, or by falls, blows, and other forms of trauma.

Furuncle or Abscess

Furuncles or abscesses of the external canal are exquisitely painful.

Foreign Body

Irritation and pain may result from the presence of foreign material in the canal.

Impacted Cerumen

Occlusion of the ear canal by cerumen may cause loss of hearing and, occasionally, ear pain.

Cellulitis

The auricle may become acutely red, tender, and swollen owing to a bacterial infection. Frequently an external otitis has preceded the cellulitis.

Chronic Eczema

Pruritus of the auricular skin induces chronic rubbing with resulting irritation. Fissuring of the auricle and canal may occur and secondary infections are common.

Herpes Simplex

The finding of grouped vesicles suggests this infection.

Herpes Zoster

Painful vesicles may be present on the auricle and in the external canal.

Bacterial Chondritis

Penetrating trauma (e.g., earrings) or punctures, may introduce bacteria and consequent infection.

Relapsing Polychondritis

Recurrent attacks of inflammation of the auricular cartilage is characteristic of this condition, which is rare in children. It is usually bilateral, and the auricle becomes swollen, red, and quite tender.

Middle and Inner Ear

♦ Acute Otitis

This is by far the most common cause of ear pain. The tympanic membrane is dull, often bulging, and sometimes erythematous; the usual landmarks are obscured.

♦ Serous Otitis Media

Fluid in the middle ear may cause intermittent acute sharp or dull aching pain. Hearing is often diminished. Ear "popping" or cracking sensations may be reported.

Eustachian Tube Obstruction

Swelling of the lining tissues of the eustachian tube by infection or allergies may prevent equalization of air pressure between the middle ear and the environment. Serous otitis media may follow longstanding obstruction.

Barotrauma

Sudden changes in air pressure cause acute ear pain.

Bullous Myringitis

Vesicles, often hemorrhagic, may be noted on the tympanic membrane.

Mastoiditis

Untreated middle ear infection may extend to the mastoid air cells. The mastoid area becomes swollen, erythematous, and tender to touch. The pinna may be pushed out and forward away from the head.

Bell Palsy

A deep earache may accompany acute peripheral facial nerve paralysis.

Leukemia/Lymphoma

Involvement of the nasopharynx may result in obstruction of the eustachian tubes, producing serous effusions and otalgia.

Other Tumors

Angiomas, rhabdomyosarcomas, and other tumors may result in eustachian tube dysfunction.

Temporal Bone Neoplasms

Tumors are a rare cause of ear pain. Embryonal rhabdomyosarcoma may be associated with excruciating ear pain with hearing loss and tinnitus.

Petrositis

Infection of the petrous ridge, secondary to otitis media, may cause a sixth nerve palsy by entrapment of the nerve. Facial nerve paralysis is less frequent.

SECONDARY OTALGIA

Pain is referred.

Pharyngeal Lesions

♦ **Acute Pharyngitis**

Tonsillitis

Peritonsillar abscess may cause ear pain.

Retropharyngeal Abscess

Following Tonsillectomy or Adenoidectomy

Nasopharyngeal Fibroma

This lesion occurs most commonly in adolescent boys. The presenting symptoms are usually recurrent nose bleeds and unilateral or bilateral nasal obstruction.

Oral Cavity Lesions

Acute Stomatitis or Glossitis

Dental Problems

Dental abscesses and impacted maxillary molars may produce referred ear pain.

Laryngeal and Esophageal Causes

Laryngeal Ulceration

Esophageal Foreign Body

Difficulty in swallowing and throat pain are much more common symptoms than ear pain.

Gastroesophageal Reflux

Rarely, reflux may be so forceful that esophagitis and pain referral to the ear occur.

Cricoarytenoid Arthritis

Rarely, a child with juvenile rheumatoid arthritis may develop hoarseness, stridor, a feeling of fullness in the throat, and referred ear pain.

MISCELLANEOUS CAUSES

♦ **Temporomandibular Joint Dysfunction**

Suspect in children who have recurrent facial or ear pain for which no etiology can be determined. Pain may be reproduced by having the individual open the mouth widely and then bite forcefully.

Postauricular Lymphadenopathy

Pain is localized to the area of the adenopathy.

Sinusitis

Mumps

Ear pain may precede or accompany overt parotid gland swelling.

Acute Thyroiditis

The thyroid is usually enlarged and tender to palpation.

Temporomandibular Arthritis

Pain associated with arthritis of this joint rarely is referred to the ear.

SUGGESTED READING

Belfer ML, Kaban LB. Temporomandibular joint dysfunction with facial pain in children. *Pediatrics* 1982;69:564–567.

Gibson WS Jr, Cochran W. Otalgia in infants and children—manifestation of gastroesophageal reflux. *Int J Pediatr Otorhinolarygnol* 1994;28:213–218.

31

Hearing Loss and Deafness

Early profound deafness is present in 4 to 11 per 10,000 children born in the United States, some 2,000 to 4,000 annually. If acquired causes of hearing loss are added to this number, it becomes readily apparent that deafness is a major problem for various health, educational, and social reasons. Unfortunately, recognition of deafness or hearing loss often occurs relatively late, compounding the difficulties for the child and the family. Some states now mandate hearing tests for all newborn infants, and other states are considering whether to do so.

The list of possible causes of hearing loss and deafness in this chapter is long in order to illustrate the many types of disorders that should be considered in the differential diagnosis in children. Too often during evaluation little attempt is made to uncover the precise cause of a hearing disability; or, when children have other abnormalities, testing for hearing loss may be delayed or not done at all. The monograph *Genetic and Metabolic Deafness* by Konigsmark and Gorlin (1) is a literal treasure of such disorders. The hereditary causes are too numerous to include in this chapter. Careful physical examination of the deaf child may reveal characteristics suggestive of one of these hereditary conditions. Some of the major abnormalities of hereditary nature associated with deafness are listed in this chapter as headings, for example, deafness with anomalies of the external ear, deafness associated with eye disorders, and so forth.

Genetic causes of hearing loss can be attributed to at least 50% of the cases (2). Of genetic causes, about one third are sporadic. A careful family history is important to disclose possible hereditary causes. Some of the better known genetic causes of deafness associated with other abnormalities include the syndromes of Pendred, Usher, Jervell and Lange-Nielsen, Waardenburg, and Alport.

Acquired causes of severe profound deafness account for approximately one half of all cases. Excluded from this group are the most common causes of acquired hearing loss, serous otitis media and purulent otitis media. These disorders usually result in a transient conductive hearing loss, usually of a mild nature. Chronic infections may lead to permanent damage. Fraser (3), in a review of thousands of cases of deafness in children, estimated that deafness in close to 10% is perinatally acquired (associated with prematurity, cerebral palsy, and hyperbilirubinemia), and that in another 25% deafness is postnatally acquired (following meningitis, viral infections, and head trauma).

Rapin (4) lists three main etiologic categories for severe to profound hearing loss: genetic, acquired, and malformative, the major causes of which are included under the most common causes.

♦ **Most Common Causes of Severe Profound Deafness**

Acquired	Genetic	Malformative
Congenital Cytomegalovirus Infection	Autosomal Recessive	Treacher Collins Syndrome
Prematurity	Autosomal Dominant	Goldenhar Syndrome
Bacterial Meningitis	X-Linked	Hemifacial Microsomia
Head Trauma		
Acoustic Trauma		
Drug Ototoxicity		

ACQUIRED CAUSES OF HEARING LOSS

Prenatally Acquired Deafness

Congenital Infections

♦ Cytomegalovirus Infection

Infections may be asymptomatic or symptomatic. Congenital cytomegalovirus is probably the most common cause of acquired deafness. The deafness may not be present at birth but may appear later in childhood.

Rubella

Epidemic rubella was a leading cause of deafness.

Toxoplasmosis

Deafness is rare but retinal changes are common.

Herpes Simplex

Varicella

Syphilis

Formerly, prenatal infection was an important cause of deafness.

Exposure to Drugs Taken By Mother

Streptomycin

Quinine

Chloroquine

Trimethadione

Thalidomide

Perinatally Acquired Deafness

Usually the deafness is not an isolated finding. Associated abnormalities include cerebral palsy, epilepsy, blindness, and mental retardation.

♦ **Prematurity**

Perhaps as many as 2% of premature infants suffer some hearing loss. Several factors may be involved, including hereditary predisposition, anoxia during birth, trauma, drugs, and possibly incubator noise.

♦ **Drugs**

Aminoglycosides are best known, but many others, including vancomycin and furosemide may affect hearing.

Kernicterus

The classic signs of kernicterus—shrill cry, opisthotonos, and spasticity followed by hypotonia—may not have been obvious in the neonatal period. Deafness is usually detected much later. Hyperbilirubinemia has been implicated in some cases, but there may have been many factors involved.

Hypoglycemia

Anoxia and Hypoxia

♦ **Trauma**

Deafness may be a result of hemorrhage or skull fractures, especially of the temporal bone.

Meningitis and Encephalitis

Deafness Acquired in Infancy or Childhood

Otitis Media/Eustachian Tube Dysfunction

Serous fluid collections in the middle ear are the most common cause of transient hearing loss in children. Chronic infections may cause permanent damage to the inner ear, with perforations and cholesteatoma formation. Mastoid infection resulting in hearing loss is less commonly seen today.

Other Infections

Mumps

Mumps most commonly causes unilateral hearing loss.

Measles

Rubella

Poliomyelitis

Scarlet Fever

Infectious Mononucleosis

Varicella

Herpes Zoster

Adenovirus

Diphtheria

Influenza

♦ **Meningitis**

Acute bacterial or tuberculous meningitis is an important cause of deafness. All children should have hearing evaluations following these infections.

♦ **Trauma**

Deafness may follow head trauma, from destruction of the middle ear by hemorrhage, ossicular dislocation, or severance of the acoustic nerve by fractures.

♦ **Acoustic Trauma**

Noise injury from prolonged or sudden loud noise may also result in deafness. Moderate deafness is becoming increasingly common in individuals exposed to loud music.

♦ **Drugs**

Various drugs have been implicated as causes of hearing loss including vancomycin, kanamycin, gentamicin, neomycin, furosemide, quinine, streptomycin, cisplatin, nortryptyline hydrochloride, and naproxen.

Acetylsalicylic Acid

The ingestion of excessive amounts of aspirin is an important cause of transient deafness.

Tumors

Acoustic Neuromas

These tumors generally occur in young adulthood but may occur in childhood. Type II neurofibromatosis is an autosomal dominantly inherited disorder that features acoustic neuromas.

Cholesteatomas

Meningiomas

Other

Histiocytosis X, neuroblastoma, and leukemia may invade the temporal bone and result in hearing loss.

Obstruction of the Auditory Canal

Cerumen, foreign bodies, and polyps may cause obstruction with hearing loss.

Cogan Syndrome

The diagnostic triad is interstitial keratitis, bilateral sensorineural hearing deficit, and nonreactive serologic tests for syphilis. Other systemic symptoms include headaches, arthralgias, myalgias, fever, abdominal pain, and aortic insufficiency.

Psychogenic Deafness

CONGENITAL CAUSES OF DEAFNESS

Occurrence is sporadic.

Turner Syndrome

Klippel-Feil Sequence

The clinical picture is a short neck with a low hairline and limited movement of the head. The cervical vertebrae are malformed and often fused. Deafness is associated in about 30% of cases.

Dysplasias of the Inner Ear

A number of inner ear malformations have been described, including Michel, Mondini, and Scheibe.

Trisomies

Deafness has been associated with Down syndrome and trisomies 13, 18, and 22.

◆ Goldenhar Syndrome (Oculoauriculovertebral Dysplasia)

Microtia, hemifacial microsomia, and hemivertebrae are present.

Frontonasal Dysplasia

Features include median cleft face, hypertelorism, and cleft palate.

Langer-Giedion Syndrome (Trichorhinophalangeal Syndrome)

Affected infants have mild postnatal growth deficiency, large protruding ears, and a bulbous nose.

De Lange Syndrome

Frontometaphyseal Dysplasia

Features include a pronounced supraorbital ridge, pointed chin, and wasting of muscles of the arms and legs with contraction of fingers, as well as conductive hearing loss.

Congenital Perilymphatic Fistula

CHARGE Association

HEREDITARY DEAFNESS

Deafness without associated abnormalities

In the following descriptions, the inheritance pattern is indicated in brackets as appropriate: AD = autosomal dominant; AR = autosomal recessive; X = sex-linked; XR = sex-linked recessive.

♦ **Congenital Severe Deafness**

[AD]

Progressive Deafness

[AD] Onset of mild high-tone hearing loss is in childhood, progressing slowly to moderate to severe deafness.

Unilateral Deafness

[AD] Deafness is usually severe and may be bilateral.

Low-Frequency Hearing Loss

[AD] Early onset of hearing loss in low frequencies is followed by high-tone loss in later life.

Mid-Frequency Hearing Loss

[AD] Progressive mid-frequency loss begins in childhood.

Otosclerosis

[AD] Otosclerosis is one of the most common causes of hearing loss in the elderly. There is variable penetration of the trait. Onset is in the second or third decade.

♦ **Congenital Severe Deafness**

[AR] In one series, 26% of cases of profound childhood deafness was the result of recessive inheritance.

Early-Onset Sensorineural Deafness

[AR] Hearing loss becomes severe by 6 years of age.

♦ Congenital Moderate Hearing Loss

[AR] This form is noted usually when the child first starts school.

Congenital Sensorineural

[X] Severe deafness is the rule.

Early-Onset Sensorineural Deafness

[X] Deafness is severe.

Moderate Hearing Loss

[X] Hearing loss is slowly progressive and moderately severe.

Hereditary Meniere Disease

[AD and AR] Vertiginous attacks are a common finding.

Atresia of External Auditory Canal and Conductive Deficits

[AD]

Deafness Associated with External Ear Malformations

Preauricular Pits

Lop Ears

Most children with lop ears do not have hearing deficits.

Microtia

Cup-shaped ears

Deafness Associated with Eye Disorders

Cataracts

Examples are Cockayne and Marshall syndromes and Norrie disease.

Retinitis Pigmentosa

Usher, Refsum, Laurence-Moon-Biedl syndromes, plus others with neurologic defects.

Myopia

Myopia occurs particularly with skeletal deformities or hypertelorism.

Optic Atrophy

Optic atrophy occurs with juvenile diabetes mellitus and polyneuropathy.

Iris Dysplasia

Corneal Degeneration

Deafness Associated with Skeletal Disorders

Noonan Syndrome

The phenotype resembles that of Turner syndrome, but the defect is nonchromosomal.

Osteogenesis Imperfecta

Cranial Synostosis

Crouzon; Apert.

♦ Facial Bone Hypoplasia

Treacher Collins.

Poly- or Syndactyly

Orofaciodigital; ectrodactyly.

Bony Overgrowth

Osteopetrosis; craniodiaphyseal dysplasia; van Buchem sclerosteosis; Stickler syndrome; craniometaphyseal dysplasia; Camurati-Engelmann disease.

Joint Fusion

Proximal symphalangism, with mitral stenosis; Wildervanck syndrome (deafness with Klippel-Feil deformity and Duane syndrome).

Dwarfism

Cockayne, Weill-Marchesani; Kniest; metaphyseal dysostosis; spondyloepiphyseal dysplasia, diastrophic dwarfism; Fanconi syndrome.

Deafness Associated with Disorders of the Integument

Waardenburg Syndrome

This autosomal dominant condition may account for 2% of cases of congenital deafness. Prominent findings include heterochromia (25%), white forelock (20%), lateral displacement of the medial canthi and lacrimal puncta, broad nasal root (75%), and congenital unilateral or bilateral hearing loss, mild to severe (50%).

LEOPARD Syndrome

This is also an AD inherited disorder. Frecklelike skin lesions are the classic finding; hearing loss occurs in 50% of the cases. Cardiac abnormalities (pulmonary stenosis or subaortic stenosis) electrocardiographic abnormalities (including conduction defects), growth retardation, and occasionally, hypogonadism, delayed puberty, and cryptorchidism are other findings.

Neurofibromatosis

Hearing loss due to acoustic neuromas develops in the second or third decade, in type II.

Albinism

Piebaldism

Vitiligo

Anhidrosis

Knuckle Pads

Nail Dystrophies

Alopecia

Twisted Hair (Pili Torti)

Ichthyosis

Includes Refsum syndrome with polyneuritis, mental retardation, and cerebellar ataxia.

Deafness Associated with Renal Disease

Alport Syndrome

This is an autosomal-dominant disorder in which progressive nephritis (hematuria and proteinuria) begins in the first or second decade. Deafness begins by about 10 years of age. Changes in the ocular lenses have been described. This syndrome may account for up to 1% of cases of congenital deafness.

Branchio-Otorenal Syndrome

An autosomal dominantly inherited disorder with branchial fistulas, anomalies of the ear, and renal abnormalities, both structural and functional.

Other Nephritides

Renal Tubular Acidosis

Renal Hypoplasia

Deafness Associated with Central Nervous System Disease

Acoustic Neuroma

Sensory Neuropathy

Ataxia

Bulbar Palsy

Myoclonic Epilepsy

Mondini Dysplasia

A developmental arrest during embryogenesis of the inner ear. Commonly associated with deafness and a propensity to develop meningitis secondary to communications between the middle ear and the subarachnoid space.

Deafness Associated with Metabolic and Endocrine Disorders

Thyroid

Pendred Syndrome

Sensorineural hearing loss and goiter, with Mondini dysplasia of the inner ear.

Johanson-Blizzard Syndrome

Congenital Hypothyroidism

Mucopolysaccharidoses

Most children with Hurler (type I) and Hunter (type II) syndromes and some with other forms of this disorder, have deafness.

Mannosidosis

Progressive Lipodystrophy

Wilson Disease

Miscellaneous Causes

Cardioauditory Syndrome of Jervell and Lange-Nielson

This autosomal recessive disorder is characterized by deaf mutism, a prolonged Q-T interval with Stokes-Adams syncope, and sudden death.

Sickle Cell Anemia

Otodental Dysplasia

REFERENCES

1. Konigsmark BW, Gorlin RJ. *Genetic and metabolic diagnosis.* Philadelphia: WB Saunders, 1976.
2. Marazita ML, Ploughman LM, Rawlings B, Remington E, Arnos KS, Nance WE. Genetic epidemiological studies of early-onset deafness in the US school-age population. *Am J Med Genet* 1993;46:486–491.
3. Fraser GR. *The causes of profound deafness in childhood.* Baltimore: Johns Hopkins University Press, 1976.
4. Rapin I. Hearing disorders. *Pediatr Rev* 1993;14:43–49.

SUGGESTED READING

Chan KH. Sensorineural hearing loss in children. *Otolaryngol Clin North Am* 1994;27:473–486.
Coplan J. Deafness: ever heard of it? Delayed recognition of permanent hearing loss. *Pediatrics* 1987;79:206–213.
Fowler KB, McCollister FP, Dahle AJ, Boppana S, Britt WJ, Pass RF. Progressive and fluctuating sensorineural hearing loss in children with asymptomatic congenital cytomegalovirus infection. *J Pediatr* 1997;130:624–630.
Konigsmark BW. Hereditary childhood hearing loss and integumentary system disease. *J Pediatr* 1972;80:909–919.

32

Tinnitus

Tinnitus is the sensation of a noise or ringing in the ear. It is a relatively uncommon symptom in the pediatric age group and is almost never a verbalized complaint in young children.

In this section, the causes of tinnitus have been divided into nonpulsatile and pulsatile types: Nonpulsatile tinnitus is a steady, uninterrupted noise, whereas pulsatile tinnitus usually has a rhythmic quality, often coinciding with the heart beat. The most common cause of tinnitus is hearing loss.

♦ **Most Common Causes of Tinnitus**

Nonpulsatile	Pulsatile
Hearing Loss	Serous Otitis Media
Noise Injury	Cerumen
Physiologic	Physiologic
Drugs	

NONPULSATILE TINNITUS

♦ **Hearing Loss**

Tinnitus may be the first symptom of hearing loss, especially of sensorineural causes. The hearing loss generally begins in the high tones and may be detectable only by an audiometric examination.

Perforation of Tympanic Membrane

Physiologic Tinnitus

In extremely quiet rooms some people may note the presence of a noise in their ears.

♦ **Drug-Induced Tinnitus**

Various drugs with ototoxic properties may produce tinnitus; the most frequently recognized are kanamycin, gentamicin, streptomycin, neomycin, and quinine. Tinnitus is a sign of salicylate toxicity and is sometimes used in determining the salicylate dosage in therapy for chronic diseases such as arthritis. Arsenic poisoning may also cause tinnitus secondary to cochlear damage.

♦ **Noise Injury**

A sudden loud blast or exposure to loud background noise over a period of years may produce tinnitus. The tinnitus is a warning of impending hearing loss.

Convulsive Disorders

Tinnitus may be an aura, preceding the onset of the seizure.

Migraine

In rare cases tinnitus may precede the headache phase of attacks of migraine.

Acoustic Neuroma

Tinnitus may precede or accompany the hearing loss associated with this and other lesions of the cerebellopontine angle. The tinnitus and hearing loss are unilateral.

Meniere Disease

Attacks of labyrinthitis of sudden onset are characterized by vertigo, a distorted hearing loss, and often a roaring tinnitus. Nausea is constant, and vomiting is common.

Functional Tinnitus

Tinnitus may be a subjective complaint. If the noise description is bizarre, a psychiatric problem should be considered.

Hypoxia and Ischemia

Episodes of decreased blood and oxygen supply to the cells in the organ of Corti may result in tinnitus.

Labyrinthine Concussion

Tinnitus may follow a head injury.

Temporomandibular Joint Dysfunction

Tinnitus may accompany temporomandibular joint disorders.

Brain Stem Tumors

Perilymph Fistula

An abnormal communication between the inner and middle ear should be considered in any child with progressive sensorineural hearing loss, especially if they also have intermittent dizziness or imbalance.

PULSATILE TINNITUS

♦ Serous Otitis Media

Conductive hearing loss secondary to fluid or acute or chronic infections of the middle ear is the most common cause of pulsatile tinnitus.

♦ Cerumen

Occlusion of the external ear canal by cerumen or a foreign body may result in tinnitus.

♦ Physiologic Causes

Compression of the ear on a pillow may occlude the external canal and produce a pulsatile tinnitus.

Foreign Bodies

Hair, grains of sand or stone, and other foreign bodies may scratch the tympanic membrane, causing tinnitus.

Hypertension

Pulsatile tinnitus may fluctuate with the blood pressure elevation.

Patent Eustachian Tube

This is an uncommon cause in children. The eustachian tube may remain open, particularly while the person is upright, resulting in rushes of air into the middle ear during respiration. The breath sounds may be heard with a stethoscope placed in the external auditory canal. Causes include sudden weight loss, adhesions around the nasopharyngeal opening secondary to adenoidectomy, and paralysis of the fifth nerve.

Glomus Jugulare Tumor

This benign but locally invasive tumor arises from tissue in the middle ear histologically similar to that of carotid and aortic bodies. The earliest symptom is a pulsatile tinnitus.

Intracranial Arteriovenous Fistula

The bruit may also be heard by the examiner's stethoscope.

Aberrant Internal Carotid Artery

In this rare congenital abnormality, the artery lies on the medial wall of the middle ear and may be seen as a bluish mass behind the tympanic membrane.

Carotid Artery Lesions

Turbulence in the carotid artery produced by internal lesions or severe stenotic lesions may result in a pulsatile tinnitus.

Palatal Myoclonus

The muscles of the palate may undergo rhythmic contractions, producing a clicking sound in the ear. The clicking may be heard by placing a stethoscope over the auditory canal.

Functional Tinnitus

SUGGESTED READING

Cody DTR, Kern EB, Pearson BW. *Diseases of the ears, nose and throat.* Chicago: Year Book Medical Publishers, 1981.

SECTION IV

Eyes

33

Periorbital Edema

Periorbital edema may be a reflection of local or systemic disorders. Often the cause of the swelling is obvious, either from accompanying local findings or from systemic signs and symptoms. Many disorders that cause edema in other parts of the body (see Chapter 11) may also cause swelling of the tissues around the eye, because of the looseness of subcutaneous tissues and the redundancy of skin.

♦ **Most Common Causes of Periorbital Swelling**

Unilateral	**Bilateral**
Conjunctivitis	Allergy
Contact Dermatitis	Hypoalbuminemia
Sinusitis	Urticaria/Angioedema
Orbital or Periorbital Cellulitis	Drug Reaction
Insect Bite	Roseola
	Infectious Mononucleosis

● **Cause Not to Forget**

Hemangioma

INFLAMMATORY CAUSES

♦ **Conjunctivitis**

Various types—bacterial, viral, chlamydial, and chemical—may be responsible.

♦ **Contact Dermatitis**

Erythema of the skin, usually with pruritus and some scaling, may be present. Other areas of dermatitis are often present.

♦ **Sinusitis**

There may be tenderness over the sinuses, but the infection may be "silent."

◆ Orbital and Periorbital Cellulitis

Signs of infection are present: fever, erythema, and pain. Both types require parenteral antibiotic therapy. Orbital cellulitis is associated with proptosis and decreased extraocular muscle movement. The ethmoid sinus may be the initial site of infection.

Atopic Dermatitis

Chalazion or Stye

The swelling is at the lid margin in the meibomian gland.

Dacryocystitis

The swelling and tenderness are greatest below the lid margin at the side of the nose.

Cat-Scratch Disease

Preauricular adenopathy is associated with the swelling, which is usually unilateral. A history of contact with cats, usually kittens, should be sought.

Dental Abscess

Toothache may not be present, but there may be pain when the affected tooth is tapped. Dental radiographs will support this diagnosis. The swelling may wax and wane.

Erysipelas

This is a rapidly expanding cellulitis secondary to group A streptococcal infection. Children usually have fever and other signs of toxicity.

Herpes Zoster

Vesicles develop in a dermatome distribution and do not cross the midline. When the cornea is involved, serious damage to the eye often results. Beware of lesions at the tip of the nose, as they indicate eye involvement.

Vaccinia

The edema is secondary to a local lesion caused by autoinnoculation.

Tularemia

The swelling is nearly always unilateral. Small yellowish white areas of necrosis occur in the upper conjunctival folds. The preauricular glands are swollen. A history of contact with rabbits is common.

Iridocyclitis

Periorbital swelling is associated with the acute form; eye pain, photophobia, and flushing of ciliary vessels are present. The pupil is small.

Cavernous Sinus Thrombosis

Affected children are acutely ill; proptosis develops. The disorder may follow a facial infection, bacterial meningitis, or severe dehydration.

Myiasis

The swelling increases as the fly larva develops.

Anthrax

The swelling is painless. An ulcer with a central eschar develops. Patients usually have a history of contact with animal hides.

Syphilis

NONINFLAMMATORY CAUSES

Angioedema

◆ Drug-Induced Swelling

Swelling may follow the administration of antibiotics, aspirin, barbiturates, or other drugs.

◆ Allergic Reaction to Foods

Other Allergens

Inhalants and contactants are examples.

Hereditary Form

The swelling is often precipitated by trauma. A familial or personal history of recurrent extremity swelling, abdominal pain, or (most serious) laryngeal edema should be sought.

Serum Sickness

Symptoms include urticaria, arthritis or arthralgia, and fever.

Foreign Proteins from Parasites

The intestinal infestation may be occult. Stool examination for ova and parasites is required in suspected cases.

Acute Glaucoma

Features include pain, photophobia, lacrimation, and a steamy large cornea.

SYSTEMIC DISORDERS

See also Chapter 11, Edema.

Renal Diseases

Causes include acute glomerulonephritis and nephrosis.

Protein Losing Enteropathy

The presentation of low levels of serum albumin, the result of enteropathy, from cystic fibrosis, milk protein allergy, or Ménétrier disease, may be subtle periorbital swelling.

Thyroid Disorders

Puffiness of eyelids, often subtle, is a common feature of acquired hypothyroidism. Hyperthyroidism may be associated with a prominence of the eyes and the deposition of mucopolysaccharides in the orbit leading to exophthalmos and eyelid swelling.

Cardiac Disease

Swelling of soft tissues occurs early in congestive heart failure.

Collagen-Vascular Disease

Swelling may be seen especially with dermatomyositis, lupus erythematosus, and scleroderma.

Localized Scleroderma

Periorbital edema has been described as the presenting finding in a case with coup de sabre linear scleroderma of the scalp.

INFECTIOUS DISEASES

♦ Infectious Mononucleosis

Eyelid edema is common and often impressive in mononucleosis.

♦ Roseola

Scarlet Fever

Pertussis

Rocky Mountain Spotted Fever

Kawasaki Disease

Malaria

Potts Puffy Tumor

Osteomyelitis of the frontal bone.

Measles

Trichinosis

Periorbital swelling may be an early manifestation; muscle pain and eosinophilia may be significant.

Trypanosomiasis

Painless edema of the eyelid is a classic sign of acute trypanosomiasis or Chaga disease.

Onchocerciasis (Filariasis)

Diphtheria

TRAUMATIC CAUSES

Injuries

A history and signs of trauma are diagnostic.

♦ **Insect Bite**

A papule is present at the site of the bite.

Foreign Bodies

Corneal pain and lacrimation are usually present. Retained foreign body of the lid may also produce swelling.

TUMORS AND MALIGNANCIES

• **Hemangiomas**

Lymphangiomas

Neuroblastoma

Metastatic neuroblastoma has a propensity for the orbit. Ecchymoses and proptosis are usually present.

Leukemia

Pallor, lymphadenopathy, and splenomegaly are clues. Leukemic cells may infiltrate the eyelids and orbital tissues.

Neurofibromas

Café au lait macules and the familial history suggest this possibility.

MISCELLANEOUS CAUSES

Melkersson-Rosenthal Syndrome

This condition is characterized by recurrent facial and lid edema, furrowed tongue, and facial nerve paresis.

Vasociliary Syndrome (Charun Syndrome)

Unilateral lid edema, conjunctivitis, rhinorrhea, and in some cases, keratitis are primary features. Pain is a prominent symptom.

Blepharochalasis Syndrome

Characterized by recurrent attacks of upper eyelid edema, usually bilateral, lasting for a few days. Repeated attacks lead to stretching of the skin and the levator muscle resulting in ptosis.

Dermatochalasis (Cutis Laxa)

Lax skin of the upper eyelids may hang over the lid margins simulating swelling.

Subcutaneous Emphysema

This disorder may follow fractures of the sinuses. Palpation of the swelling elicits a crackling sensation.

Superior Vena Cava Syndrome

Periorbital puffiness, especially in the morning, is often the first sign.

Sickle Cell-Hemoglobin C Disease

An orbital infarction crisis is characterized by the rapid onset of exophthalmos, significant edema of the eyelids, and a severe, localized headache.

Rifampin Toxicity

A striking red discoloration of the skin occurs in addition to facial and periorbital edema.

Ascher Syndrome

Characterized by recurrent episodes of upper eyelid and upper lip edema. May result in atrophic, slack skin of these areas.

Caffey Disease (Infantile Cortical Hyperostosis)

This unusual disorder, which begins in infants under 6 months of age, may be associated with periorbital edema if the bones around the orbit are involved with the periostitis.

SUGGESTED READING

Nield LS. Milk intolerance presenting solely as periorbital edema. *Clin Pediatr* 1995;35:265–267.
Weiss AH. The swollen and droopy eyelid. *Pediatr Clin North Am* 1993;40:789–804.

34
Ptosis

Ptosis, or drooping of one or both eyelids, is not a common pediatric complaint or finding. Nevertheless, this sign cannot be ignored for it may be a subtle presentation of a number of serious disorders. A careful examination of the child may disclose other diagnostic clues, such as muscle weakness or involvement of other cranial nerves. The age at onset of the condition is particularly important because several conditions associated with ptosis are congenital. Often, the ptosis is more prominent when the child is tired; photographs of the child as an infant may be helpful. A familial history of ptosis is also important to uncover genetic causes. In some cases, the eyelid may appear ptotic because of reduced orbital volume.

The causes of ptosis include disorders featuring a maldevelopment of the muscles that raise the eyelids or those that are a result of damage to the motor nerves that innervate the muscle. Cranial nerve III innervates the levator palpebrae muscle, the muscle responsible for most of the action of the eyelid. A smooth muscle in the lid is innervated by the sympathetic nervous system, while the frontalis muscle, innervated by cranial nerve VII, indirectly raises the eyelid by raising the brow.

◆ Most Common Causes of Ptosis

Congenital Ptosis	Acquired
Idiopathic	Myasthenia Gravis
Horner Syndrome	Migraine
Noonan Syndrome	Botulism
Fetal Alcohol Syndrome	Hemangioma of Lid
Smith-Lemli-Opitz Syndrome	Horner Syndrome

CONGENITAL PTOSIS

◆ Idiopathic Congenital Ptosis

Most often unilateral. Superior rectus palsy may coexist. It is usually the result of abnormal development of the levator muscle of the eyelid or the branch of the third nerve that innervates it.

Genetic Trait

Most often bilateral; inherited as an autosomal dominant. Some weakness of the superior rectus muscle may be present.

Traumatic Origin

If unilateral, the ptosis may be secondary to birth trauma or an intracranial third cranial nerve lesion.

Marcus-Gunn Phenomenon

In this condition, also called the jaw-winking syndrome, opening of the mouth or movement of the jaw laterally causes elevation of the ptotic eyelid. A misdirected cross-innervation between the oculomotor and pterygoid nerves is thought to be the cause. The disorder may be inherited as an autosomal-dominant trait.

Hereditary External Ophthalmoplegia

In this rare disorder, there is total paralysis of extraocular eye movements; other findings include bilateral ptosis, convulsions, ataxia, mental impairment, and retinitis pigmentosa.

Möbius Syndrome

Affected children usually have bilateral facial paralysis and sixth cranial nerve palsy. The face is expressionless; ptosis is not always present.

Syndromes and Chromosomal Abnormalities

Congenital ptosis is part of a host of other findings in these disorders. For additional definition, *Smith's Recognizable Patterns of Human Malformation* (1), from which the following list was modified, is recommended.

Chromosomal Disorders

Turner syndrome, Trisomy 18 syndrome, aniridia-Wilms' association, deletions of 3p, 11q, 13q, and 18p, and duplications of 10q and 15q may be associated with ptosis.

◆ Fetal Drug Exposure

Alcohol, hydantoin, and trimethadione have been implicated.

◆ Inherited Syndromes

Aarskog syndrome, familial blepharophimosis, Börjeson-Forssman-Lehmann syndrome, cardio-facio-cutaneous syndrome, Dubowitz syndrome, Escobar syndrome, Freeman-Sheldon syndrome, Kabuki syndrome, Killian/Teschler-Nicola syndrome, Marden-Walker syndrome, Noonan syndrome, Schwartz-Jampel syndrome, pachydermoperiostosis, Saethre-Chotzen syndrome, Crouzon syndrome, Apert syndrome, **Smith-Lemli-Opitz syndrome,** Fanconi pancytopenia, and the craniooculodental syndrome.

Syndromes of Unidentified Etiology

The Coffin-Siris and Rubinstein-Taybi syndromes are examples.

NEUROMUSCULAR DISORDERS

◆ Myasthenia Gravis

Ptosis is the most common presenting sign. Other findings include diplopia, facial weakness, dysphonia, weakness of arms or legs, external ophthalmoplegia, and respiratory difficulties. Increased weakness generally develops during the day.

◆ Migraine

Unilateral ptosis or a complete third nerve palsy may be seen in ophthalmoplegic migraine. Paralysis usually lasts only a few hours, but with repeated attacks it may persist for weeks or months or even become permanent.

◆ Horner Syndrome

Ptosis is mild; there may be unilateral miosis, enophthalmos, and absence of facial sweating due to involvement of cervical sympathetic ganglion.

Cluster Headache

Is associated with severe eye pain, ptosis, pupillary change, injection of the conjunctiva, and unilateral rhinorrhea on the same side as the pain.

Myotonic Dystrophy

Congenital ptosis may precede involvement of other muscle groups or generalized myotonia (failure of relaxation of voluntary muscles). The distinctive "hatchet face" (sharp facial features) is eventually produced by facial muscular atrophy. In infants, hypotonia, weak sucking reflex, elevated diaphragm, and arthrogryposis may be present as well as facial weakness.

Hydrocephalus

Ptosis may be present. Other findings include a large forehead and head circumference and a tense fontanel (if open); there may be a unilateral or bilateral sixth nerve palsy.

Oculomotor Nerve Involvement

Trauma, intracranial aneurysms, diabetes mellitus, and other disorders may affect the third nerve. Ocular muscle palsy as well as ptosis is present. The eye is displaced outward and downward with impaired adduction and elevation.

Dermatomyositis

In addition to skin changes and muscle weakness, there may be extraocular muscle myositis with ptosis.

Ocular Muscular Dystrophy

Onset of symptoms of this autosomal-dominant condition is generally delayed until late childhood or adulthood. Findings include diplopia, ptosis, and strabismus, as well as weakness of facial muscles, particularly of the upper face.

Oculopharyngeal Dystrophy

Has an onset in adulthood with ptosis and dysphagia.

Myotubular (Centronuclear) Myopathy

Ptosis and weakness of the extraocular muscles are characteristic. Progressive weakness of limb girdle and neck muscles is most prominent during acute respiratory illnesses but may have been present from birth.

Tension Pneumothorax

A case is described in which the tension pneumothorax resulted in a unilateral Horner syndrome.

Sinusitis

A pansinusitis has been described as causing compression of the oculomotor nerve branch to the levator muscle.

POISONING

◆ Botulism

Ptosis may be an early sign. Progressive neurologic symptoms include blurring of vision, impaired pupillary reaction to light, diplopia, difficulty in swallowing, respiratory difficulties, and paralysis.

Lead, Arsenicals, Carbon Monoxide, and Dichlorodiethylsulfide

Ptosis may be part of the clinical picture.

LESIONS OF THE EYELID

Ptosis may be the result of local inflammation, edema, styes, tumors, conjunctival scarring, deposition of amyloid, or trauma.

TUMORS

Orbital Tumors

Orbital tumors, primary or metastatic, may be associated with ptosis.

◆ Hemangioma or Sturge-Weber Syndrome

Involvement of the lid may cause ptosis.

Neurofibromatosis

A plexiform neuroma of the upper lid is the cause.

Neuroblastoma

Rhabdomyosarcoma

Intracranial Tumors Affecting the Third Nerve

Pinealoma

Paralysis of upward gaze is the classic localizing sign. Bilateral ptosis may be the presenting symptom. Signs of increased intracranial pressure eventually follow.

INBORN ERRORS OF METABOLISM

Carnitine Deficiency

Myopathic facies with ptosis may be present, but extraocular muscle movement is normal. Other findings are progressive muscular weakness, greater in the proximal muscles, and impaired liver function.

Abetalipoproteinemia

Abdominal distension and steatorrhea begin after 1 to 2 months of age. By 7 or 8 years of age, ataxia, muscle weakness, and awkward gait have developed. Affected children eventually lose visual acuity, deep tendon reflexes, and vibratory and position sense, and develop nystagmus.

Tangier Disease

Ptosis may be present in this disorder characterized by hepatosplenomegaly and significant orangish-yellow tonsillar enlargement with a variable peripheral neuropathy.

MISCELLANEOUS CAUSES

Cutis Laxa

Excessive skin folds may simulate ptosis.

Contact Lens

The lens may embed in the soft tissues of the superior fornix.

Addison Disease

Cushing Syndrome

Thiamine Deficiency

Onset in infancy is characterized by anorexia, vomiting, lethargy, pallor, ptosis, edema of the extremities, and cardiac failure.

Vitamin E Deficiency

Hyporeflexia is the initial sign. Ptosis and mild ataxia occur later.

Familial Posterior Lumbosacral Fusion

Blepharochalasis Syndrome

Recurrent attacks of short-lived edema eventually lead to stretching of the skin of the eyelids and levator muscle resulting in ptosis.

REFERENCE

1. Jones KL. *Smith's recognizable patterns of human malformation*, 5th ed. Philadelphia: WB Saunders, 1997.

SUGGESTED READING

Weiss AH. The swollen and droopy eyelid. *Pediatr Clin North Am* 1993;40:789–804.

35

Strabismus

The term strabismus comes from the Greek word meaning "a squinting." It refers to an imbalance of movements of the eyes causing a lack of parallel movements; a misalignment of the eyes. Strabismus has been estimated to occur in about 4% of children younger than 6 years of age (1). Because 30% to 50% of children with strabismus will develop secondary visual loss (amblyopia), it is important to detect and treat the problem as early as possible. Keep in mind that infants are rarely born with aligned eyes. It may be difficult to adequately assess eye alignment until 3 months of age.

There are various types of strabismus, named according to the direction of the abnormal eye movement, including esotropia (turning in), exotropia (turning out), and hypertropia and hypotropia (upward and downward, respectively). Some classifications divide strabismus into nonparalytic (concomitant) causes, which are most common in children, and paralytic (nonconcomitant) causes that comprise most of the cases with onset in adulthood.

Probably 50% of cases of strabismus in children are hereditary. The exact anatomic cause is unknown. In this chapter, the causes of strabismus have been divided into three main groups: congenital, acquired, and those associated with syndromes. If the cause of strabismus in a child older than 3 months is not apparent, an ophthalmologist should be consulted for additional evaluation.

♦ **Most Common Causes of Strabismus**

Pseudostrabismus

Infantile or Congenital Esotropia

Visual Deprivation: Retinoblastoma and
    Cataracts

Accomodative Esotropia

Childhood Exotropia

● **Causes Not to Forget**

Botulism

Increased Intracranial Pressure

Trauma

Congenital Third Nerve Palsy

CONGENITAL STRABISMUS

♦ **Pseudostrabismus**

In young infants and children, a broad, flat nasal bridge and epicanthal folds may create a false impression of strabismus. The reflection of light on the corneas from a source held 2½ to 3 feet in front of the child is symmetrically placed, however.

True Congenital Strabismus

Nonparalytic esotropia or exotropia may be noted before 6 months of age. Esotropia is much more common than exotropia; both are frequently genetically determined. The cause of this problem, which accounts for a large percentage of cases of childhood strabismus, is unclear.

Infants Born to Drug Dependent Women

A 24% prevalence of strabismus was found in infants born to drug abusing mothers (2).

Duane Syndrome

This hereditary disorder features decreased abduction of one or both eyes. The palpebral fissure widens on attempted abduction and narrows on adduction.

Möbius Syndrome

In this unusual disorder there is hypoplasia or agenesis of several cranial nerve nuclei. The face is masklike because of facial paralysis; sixth nerve palsies are also present. Several other deformities may also be found.

Brown Syndrome

An inability to elevate the eye, especially pronounced in medial gaze.

Strabismus Fixus

This is a rare disorder involving both medial rectus muscles, which are taut. The eyes cannot be abducted past the midline.

Double Elevation Palsy

This is a congenital weakness of both the superior rectus and inferior oblique muscles. The eye cannot be rotated upward.

Congenital Familial External Ophthalmoplegia

In this autosomal-dominant disorder, bilateral ptosis with partial to complete paralysis of the external ocular muscles causes affected children to walk with the chin held up.

- **Congenital Third Nerve Paralysis**

Paralysis is usually unilateral. Ptosis, hypotropia, and exotropia are found. The palsy has been observed to occur in families.

Congenital Fourth Nerve Palsy

Creates weakness in the superior oblique muscle. An "ocular" torticollis may result as the child tries to minimize double vision.

Central Nervous System Insults

Various insults to the developing central nervous system, whether hypoxic, vascular, or infectious, may result in strabismus, as well as other signs such as microcephaly and cerebral palsy.

ACQUIRED STRABISMUS

Accommodative Strabismus

Strabismus occurs during visual accommodation and may be due to hyperopia or high accommodation/convergence ratios or both. Refractive errors, particularly hyperopia, are common. This form usually develops between 1½ to 4 years of age and may be hereditary; it accounts for about one third of all esotropias. Amblyopia commonly occurs.

- ◆ **Childhood Exotropia**

This is the most common divergent strabismus in childhood. One eye will drift outward when the child is fixating at a distance. Onset is generally between infancy and 4 years of age.

- ◆ **Interference with Foveal Vision**

Eye disorders such as cataracts may prevent fusion of sight on the fovea, resulting in strabismus.

Tumors

Tumors involving the orbit, either primary or metastatic, as well as primary eye tumors, such as retinoblastoma, may cause strabismus. Exophthalmos and hemorrhages of retina, conjunctivae, and lids may suggest orbital tumors. A white pupillary reflex is the most common sign of a retinoblastoma. Intracranial tumors may cause increased intracranial pressure or entrap the ocular nerve, with resulting strabismus.

- **Increased Intracranial Pressure**

Any cause of increased intracranial pressure may affect cranial nerves, especially the sixth, resulting in strabismus. (See Chapter 24, Increased Intracranial Pressure and Bulging Fontanel.) Many children with hydrocephalus have sixth nerve palsies. Children with meningomyelocele have a high incidence of strabismus related to hydrocephalus.

Orbital Injury

Fracture of orbital bones may cause entrapment of eye muscles, so that full range of movement is impossible. The eye often appears sunken, and the palpebral fissure is narrowed.

● Head Trauma

Neuromuscular Disorders

● Botulism

Ptosis, diplopia, and difficulty in swallowing usually precede other signs of progressive weakness.

Myasthenia Gravis

Ocular complaints and signs are often early findings. Ptosis, ophthalmoplegias, and facial weakness, especially if intermittent, suggest this disorder.

Benign Sixth Nerve Palsy

This painless palsy typically develops 1 to 3 weeks after an upper respiratory infection, and begins to improve in 3 to 6 weeks. If improvement does not occur, concern should turn toward an intracranial lesion.

Guillain-Barré Syndrome

Ocular Myopathy

Progressive, symmetrical external ophthalmoplegia with ptosis, occasionally involving the facial muscles, appears in infancy to late adulthood. A familial history is positive in most cases.

Multiple Sclerosis

Childhood onset is unusual. Neurologic signs and symptoms are often rapid in onset but initially may regress quickly.

Miller-Fisher Syndrome

This rare disorder is characterized by the acute onset of ophthalmoplegia, ataxia, and hyporeflexia, and often follows an upper respiratory infection. Some feel it is a variant of Guillan-Barré syndrome.

Acquired Postganglionic Cholinergic Dysautonomia

This rare disorder of unknown cause is characterized by bilateral internal ophthalmoplegia, lack of tears, saliva and sweat, atony of the bowel and bladder, and normal adrenergic function. It may appear at any age.

Vascular Disorders

Cerebral Hemorrhage

Ophthalmoplegic Migraine

Strabismus is an unusual occurrence in migraine. Third nerve palsy most frequently occurs 6 to 24 hours after the onset of the migraine attack.

Infections

Strabismus may occur in various infections including encephalitis, meningitis (bacterial and tuberculous), measles, diphtheria, poliomyelitis, and other enteroviruses. Orbital cellulitis usually results in loss of full ocular mobility, whereas periorbital cellulitis does not. Gradenigo syndrome is a sixth nerve palsy resulting from entrapment of this nerve as it crosses the petrous ridge in children with chronic otitis media.

Drugs and Toxins

Strabismus has been described in lead and other heavy metal poisonings and also with the use of tricyclic antidepressants.

Miscellaneous Causes

Orbital Myositis

The onset of acute rectus palsy is accompanied by eye pain and, usually, some swelling of the eyelid and ptosis (3).

Endocrine Disorders

An ocular myopathy may occur with thyrotoxicosis and diabetes mellitus, but these rarely cause strabismus in children.

Metabolic Disorders

Transient strabismus may occur during episodes of hypoglycemia.

Cyclic Esotropia

Esotropia is cyclic, coming and going in 48-hour cycles. Seizures, personality changes, excessive sleepiness, and increased urination have been reported in some patients.

DYSMORPHOGENETIC SYNDROMES WITH STRABISMUS

Strabismus is a feature in a rather large number of syndromes. In some, anatomic abnormalities of the orbits are the cause, but in most cases the exact cause is unknown. (For more detailed information, *Smith's Recognizable Patterns of Human Malformation* is recommended (4).)

Albright Hereditary Osteodystrophy	Apert Syndrome
Cri du Chat Syndrome	Down Syndrome
Fanconi Syndrome	Fetal Alcohol Syndrome
Fetal Hydantoin Syndrome	Goltz Syndrome
Hemifacial Microsomia	Incontinentia Pigmenti
Laurence-Moon-Biedl Syndrome	Marfan Syndrome
Noonan Syndrome	Onychodystrophy and Deafness
Osteopetrosis	Pierre Robin Syndrome
Prader-Willi Syndrome	Pseudohypoparathyroidism
Rubinstein-Taybi Syndrome	Smith-Lemli-Opitz Syndrome
Williams Syndrome	Trisomy 18 Syndrome
Turner Syndrome	18 p-Syndrome
18 q-Syndrome	5 p-Syndrome

REFERENCES

1. Lavrich JB, Nelson LB. Diagnosis and treatment of strabismus disorders. *Pediatr Clin North Am* 1993;40:737–752.
2. Nelson LB, Ehrlich S, Calhoun JH, Matteucci T, Finnegan LP. Occurrence of strabismus in infants born to drug-dependent women. *Am J Dis Child* 1987;141:175–178.
3. Pollard ZF. Acute rectus muscle palsy in children as a result of orbital myositis. *J Pediatr* 1996;128:230–233.
4. Jones KL. *Smith's recognizable patterns of human malformation*, 5th ed. Philadelphia: WB Saunders, 1997.

36

Nystagmus

Nystagmus is defined as rhythmic oscillations of the eyes occurring involuntarily. In general, the eyes move together in the same direction. Neurology and ophthalmology texts describe various types of nystagmus such as pendular, jerky, vertical, and downbeat; these designations may offer some help in localization of the causative lesion. It is important not to confuse the searching eye movements associated with blindness or severe visual impairment, or opsoclonus, a peculiar type of chaotic, jerky, rapid eye movement, for nystagmus.

This chapter presents an overview of causes of nystagmus, rather than a comprehensive listing. The most common causes include disorders affecting central vision, drugs, hereditary conditions, and disorders affecting the vestibular apparatus of the ear. Neoplasms, particularly those involving the brain stem, must always be included in the differential diagnosis.

♦ **Most Common Causes of Nystagmus**

Congenital	**Acquired**
Poor Central Vision	Poor Central Vision
Albinism	Acute Cerebellar Ataxia
Optic Nerve Hypoplasia	Drugs
Fundus Abnormalities	Intracranial Neoplasms
Primary Congenital Nystagmus	Spasmus Nutans

CONGENITAL NYSTAGMUS

Disorders that generally present in the first 6 months of life.

♦ **Ocular Causes**

Nystagmus is secondary to poor central vision. If a child is born blind or becomes blind before the age of 2 to 3 years, nystagmus usually follows. The eye movements are random and not rhythmic, often called searching. Some children may develop nystagmus after visual loss up to 6 years of age. Defective vision acquired later in childhood or in adult life is not associated with nystagmus unless macular vision is affected. Congenital nystagmus may be associated with structural abnormalities of the globe, opacities affecting the transmission of images, retinal abnormalities, and abnormalities of the afferent visual pathways (1). For a more complete listing of disorders that may affect vision, and in doing so result in nystagmus, see Chapter 40, Loss of Vision and Blindness.

Down Syndrome

Congenital Cataracts

Clouding of the Cornea

Chorioretinitis

♦ **Albinism**

Generalized Albinism

Inheritance pattern is autosomal recessive.

Ocular Albinism

This disorder is inherited as a sex-linked recessive trait. Affected boys may have light skin and hair, decreased visual acuity, photophobia, and nystagmus.

Aniridia

Congenital Optic Atrophy

Optic Atrophy of Early Onset

Septo-Optic Dysplasia

This is a congenital optic nerve hypoplasia with a midline brain defect, usually associated with hypopituitarism. Hypoglycemia may be a clue in the neonatal period. Growth retardation, recurrent hypoglycemia, seizures, and diabetes insipidus may appear.

Coloboma

Retinal Detachment

Retinal Infections

Toxoplasmosis and cytomegalic inclusion disease are examples.

Vitreous Consolidation, Hemorrhage

Macular Abnormalities

Leber Congenital Amaurosis

A severe form of congenital blindness inherited as an autosomal recessive disorder.

Total Color Blindness

Findings in this autosomal-recessive condition include poor vision, prominent photophobia, nystagmus, and normal or near-normal fundi.

Rod-Cone or Cone-Rod Dystrophy

Hereditary Nystagmus

A familial history is often present; inheritance may be autosomal dominant or sex-linked recessive. Nystagmus either is present at birth or appears shortly thereafter. The nystagmus is horizontal, not vertical, and may be associated with bobbing of the head; it tends to lessen with age.

Congenital Jerking Nystagmus

This horizontal nystagmus is more pronounced in one direction of gaze than in the other. The nystagmus may interfere with vision so that the child will turn the head to achieve the position with least nystagmus.

Drug Use

Includes maternal use of hydantoin and alcohol.

Hypothyroidism

Hyperbilirubinemia

Cortical Blindness

♦ **Primary Motor Congenital Nystagmus**

LATENT NYSTAGMUS

This form is often associated with strabismus but is not apparent on examination unless vision in one eye is occluded. It must be considered when a child's binocular vision is much better than monocular vision.

ACQUIRED NYSTAGMUS

♦ **Drugs and Toxins**

Anticonvulsants

Barbiturate and hydantoin intoxication are well-known causes of nystagmus.

Antihistamines

Alcohol

Lead Poisoning

Codeine

Salicylates

Bromides

Nicotine

Quinine

♦ SPASMUS NUTANS

This poorly understood disorder, with an onset at between 4 and 18 months of age, is characterized by the triad of nystagmus, head nodding, and torticollis. These signs may not all be present at the same time; they disappear usually within months and invariably by 2 years of age. It is important to look for other neurologic signs suggestive of an intracranial neoplasm.

DISORDERS AFFECTING THE VESTIBULAR SYSTEM

Tumor

Neoplasms and other tumors of the brain stem or upper spinal cord may involve the vestibular nuclei and associated tracts, causing nystagmus.

Trauma

The most common cause is head trauma, especially with fracture of the petrous portion of the temporal bone. Vertigo is a common accompanying symptom.

Labyrinthitis

Labyrinthitis is an uncommon cause of nystagmus in children but may follow middle ear infections. Vertigo usually accompanies the nystagmus.

Benign Paroxysmal Vertigo

Attacks of vertigo are brief but recurrent, with an onset before 5 years of age. After the attack the child appears normal. Nystagmus may be present during the episodes.

Arnold-Chiari Malformation

With a type I defect, the onset of symptoms may be delayed until late childhood or adolescence. Symptoms may include headache, neck pain, and ataxia.

Basilar Impression

In this skeletal malformation, inherited as an autosomal-dominant trait, pressure on the medulla and upper cervical spinal cord produces neck stiffness, progressive leg weakness, head tilt, and a short neck; occasionally, nystagmus may be seen.

♦ **OTHER NEUROLOGIC DISORDERS**

♦ **Acute Cerebellar Ataxia**

There is an acute onset of truncal ataxia followed by extremity involvement. The cause is unclear, but there appears to be an association with viral illnesses.

Brain Tumors

Tumors in various locations may produce nystagmus. Signs of increased intracranial pressure, headache, vomiting, diplopia, strabismus, and papilledema are often present.

Encephalitis

Tuberculous Meningitis

Demyelinating and Degenerative Disorders

A wide variety of disorders may have nystagmus as an associated feature. Friedreich ataxia, Pelizaeus-Merzbacher disease, ataxia telangiectasia, metachromatic leukodystrophy, and multiple sclerosis are but a few.

Ataxic Cerebral Palsy

Hypotonia, nystagmus, dysmetria, and a wide-base gait are characteristic.

Ocular Muscle Paresis

Nystagmus may occur in the affected eye when the direction of gaze requires action by the paretic muscle.

Cerebellar Abscess

Coordination disturbances, ataxia, and dysmetria, with signs of increased intracranial pressure, are common.

Extradural Hematoma

This injury most commonly follows a severe blow to the occiput. There are persistent diminished consciousness, headache, vomiting, stiff neck, and in some cases, nystagmus, ataxia, and cranial nerve palsies.

OPSOCLONUS

Opsoclonus is a condition characterized by nonrhythmic, chaotic, rapid eye movements that often occur in bursts. This special type of movement has received most notoriety for its association with occult neuroblastoma in young children. Polymyoclonus is present as well (dancing eyes, dancing feet). In adults and older children it may be seen as a consequence of postinfectious encephalopathy.

MISCELLANEOUS DISORDERS

Maple Syrup Urine Disease

Hyperpipecolaemia

In the few cases described, hepatomegaly and hypotonia were present. A horizontal nystagmus is usually apparent by 1 year of age.

Hypervalinemia

Mental and physical retardation, recurrent vomiting, and nystagmus are prominent symptoms.

Trembling Chin Syndrome

This inherited disorder is characterized by episodes of chin trembling that may be associated with nystagmus.

Scorpion Bite

PHYSIOLOGIC TYPES OF NYSTAGMUS

End-Position Nystagmus

This type occurs in normal children on extreme lateral gaze.

Optokinetic Nystagmus

This type may be induced when a series of objects is followed across the field of vision.

Evoked Vestibular Nystagmus

Rotation of the body or irrigation of the ear with cold or warm water can induce this type.

REFERENCE

1. Repka MX. Common pediatric neuro-ophthalmologic conditions. *Pediatr Clin North Am* 1993;40:777–788.

SUGGESTED READING

Brodsky MC, Baker RS, Hamed LM. *Pediatric neuro-ophthalmology.* New York: Springer, 1996.

37

Cataracts

Cataracts, or opacities of the lens, are not a common pediatric problem; nevertheless, they occur frequently enough that a differential diagnosis is warranted. Although 1 of every 250 newborn infants may have a congenital cataract, most are benign, especially in premature infants, and may disappear over time (1). A large number of syndromes may have cataracts as a feature, along with dysmorphic features. The reader may want to consult Jones' text *Recognizable Patterns of Human Malformation* for additional syndromes (2). The pediatrician should work in concert with the ophthalmologist, particularly in attempting to uncover any recognizable etiologic pattern.

The clinical presentation of a cataract depends on the size, location, and age at presentation. A white reflex, leukocoria, is the most common sign. Clinical signs such as a strabismus, nystagmus, and a lack of visual attention suggest that vision has been impaired (ambylopia).

In most cases, cataracts are hereditary or sporadic, not associated with other underlying problems. In a review of 97 children with primary cataracts who were born between 1954 and 1986 and presented to a visually impaired program in British Columbia, prenatal infection was responsible for the cataracts in 36%, idiopathic in 31%, hereditary in 23%, and various syndromes and metabolic disorders in 10% (3). In this chapter, an overview of disorders in which cataracts may develop is given first, according to frequency and the classification just presented. Then causes are grouped according to the age at which the cataracts are most likely to appear; however, there is often some overlap among age groups. In some disorders, the cataracts may be present at birth, or they may not appear until much later; whereas, in others, cataracts may not appear until late childhood or adolescence.

◆ Most Common Causes of Cataracts

Sporadic   Hereditary
Prematurity   Corticosteroids
Down Syndrome

● Causes Not to Forget

Retinoblastoma   Congenital Rubella
Galactosemia

♦ HEREDITARY CONDITIONS

From 10% to 25% of congenital cataracts have been reported to be hereditary. Autosomal-dominant inheritance is most common. These cataracts occur as an isolated finding, unlike those associated with syndromes listed below.

♦ SPORADIC OCCURRENCE

Another one third of all congenital cataracts are sporadic in occurrence and are not associated with other systemic abnormalities.

CONGENITAL INFECTIONS

The cataracts may be present at birth or appear later in the first year of life.

● Rubella

Maternal rubella infection was the first (reported in 1941) and is the most widely recognized cause of congenital cataracts in this group. The most common associated defects are growth retardation, microcephaly, deafness, and congenital heart lesions. Congenital rubella has become a less common cause in the United States and Canada.

Varicella

Maternal varicella in the first trimester of pregnancy may result in low-birth weight, cortical atrophy with seizures, cicatricial skin lesions, and atrophic limbs in the affected infant.

Herpes Simplex, Toxoplasmosis, Cytomegalovirus Infection

Variable sequelae of these infections include growth retardation, mental retardation, hydrocephalus, microcephaly, cerebral calcifications, chorioretinitis, jaundice, hepatosplenomegaly, and petechiae.

Other Infections

Cataracts have been reported following maternal infection during pregnancy with rubeola, poliomyelitis, influenza, hepatitis, infectious mononucleosis, syphilis, and smallpox.

♦ CATARACTS ASSOCIATED WITH PREMATURITY

Transient cataracts may be noted in low-birth weight infants. Generally, they appear during the second week of life and disappear over a 4-month period.

CATARACTS PRESENT AT BIRTH

Primary Persistent Hyperplastic Vitreous

White pupillary reflex is present; the defect is usually unilateral. The eye is microophthalmic.

Smith-Lemli-Opitz Syndrome

Cataracts are occasionally present. Key features include microcephaly, anteverted nose, ptosis of eyelids, micrognathia, and, in males, cryptorchidism and hypospadias.

Hallermann-Streiff Syndrome (Oculomandibulofacial Syndrome)

Cataracts are a primary feature of this disorder characterized by short stature, a small thin nose, micrognathia, and sparse hair.

Norrie Syndrome

In this X-linked recessive disorder, congenital microphthalmia, retinal dysplasia, and cataract are often associated with mental retardation and sometimes deafness.

Cerebrooculofacioskeletal Syndrome

Affected children have microcephaly, sloping forehead, cataracts, microphthalmia, large ears, scoliosis, hip dislocation, and flexion contractures.

Trisomy 13 Syndrome

Cataracts have rarely been described in this chromosomal disorder associated with myriad other abnormalities. Microcephaly, cleft lip or palate, scalp defects, apneic episodes, and cardiac abnormalities are important features.

Trisomy 18 Syndrome

Cataracts are unusual in this trisomy. Infants are generally of low-birth weight and have low-set ears, micrognathia, a short sternum, and cardiac defects.

Treacher Collins Syndrome

Antimongoloid slant of eyes, malar hypoplasia, malformed ears, and deafness are prominent findings. Cataracts are uncommon.

Pierre Robin Syndrome

Micrognathia, cleft soft palate, and glossoptosis create neonatal feeding and breathing difficulties. Cataracts are uncommon.

Rubinstein-Taybi Syndrome

Broad thumbs and great toes with downward slanting palpebral fissures and a beaked nose are common features. Cataracts are rare.

Goldenhar Syndrome (Oculoauriculovertebral Dysplasia)

Auricular deformities, malar hypoplasia, macrostomia, and, occasionally, epibulbar dermoids are present. Cataracts are uncommon.

Craniosynostosis

Cataracts have been rarely reported in Apert syndrome and Crouzon syndrome.

Osteogenesis Imperfecta

Cataracts are rarely seen in this syndrome characterized by brittle bones of the skull.

CATARACTS PRESENT AT BIRTH OR OF LATER ONSET

◆ Down Syndrome

Cataracts are a relatively common finding. On slit-lamp examination, most children with Down syndrome are found to have cataracts, but they generally do not become clinically apparent until after age 10 years.

Turner Syndrome

Approximately one third of affected girls may develop cataracts at some time. Key features include short stature, webbed neck, cardiac anomalies, and lymphedema of the hands and feet in the neonatal period.

Noonan Syndrome

The phenotype is similar to that in Turner syndrome but without an abnormal karyotype. The heart defect is right-sided, pulmonic stenosis, rather than left-sided as in Turner syndrome.

• Galactosemia

Vomiting, diarrhea, jaundice, hepatosplenomegaly, and failure to thrive are important features. Cataracts tend to develop early.

Galactokinase Deficiency

Cataracts are the only known manifestation. They may rarely be present at birth but generally appear in the first decade.

Lowe Syndrome (Oculocerebrorenal Syndrome)

Hypotonia, hyporeflexia, short stature, mental retardation, and cataracts are the characteristic findings. Renal tubular acidosis, proteinuria, and aminoaciduria are common.

Conradi Syndrome (Chondrodystrophica Calcificans Congenita)

Associated features include asymmetrical shortening of long bones, a flat nasal bridge, and the diagnostic feature of stippled epiphyses on roentgenographic examination.

Incontinentia Pigmenti

This condition, primarily seen in girls, is characterized by linear vesiculobullous lesions at birth that become verrucous, then flatten out, and are later replaced by hyperpigmentation. Seizures and dental anomalies are also common.

Peters Anomaly

In addition to the cataract, the anomaly includes thinning of the posterior aspect of the cornea and iridocorneal adhesions attached to the edges of the leukoma.

Cerebrohepatorenal (Zellweger) Syndrome

Affected infants have severe neonatal hypotonia with a narrow facies, hepatomegaly, and cardiac anomalies, and usually die in the first year.

Marinesco-Sjögren Syndrome

Mental retardation, ataxia, and cataracts are primary features.

Anhidrotic Ectodermal Dysplasia

Lack of sweating with sparse hair, missing teeth, and thick lips create a striking appearance.

Shafer Syndrome

Disseminated cutaneous follicular hyperkeratosis, retardation, short stature, microcephaly, cicatricial alopecia, and thick nails accompany the congenital cataracts.

Clouston Syndrome

This syndrome is characterized by thick dyskeratotic palms and soles; areas of hyperpigmentation over the knuckles, elbows, and axillae; sparse hair; absent or dysplastic nails; retardation; and short stature.

Warburg Syndrome

This is an autosomal recessive disorder with many ocular anomalies including megalocornea, coloboma, microophthalmos, as well as central nervous system defects: agyria, cerebellar dysplasia, encephalocele, and hydrocephalus.

CATARACTS WITH ONSET IN EARLY INFANCY

Retrolental Fibroplasia

Neonatal Hypercalcemia

Niemann-Pick Disease

Symptoms begin in the first year of life and include persistent early jaundice, enlarging abdomen, and psychomotor retardation. Seizures, hypotonia, a cherry red retinal spot, and hepatosplenomegaly may be found. Cataracts are common.

Mannosidosis

This defect is characterized by macroglossia, hepatosplenomegaly, hypotonia at birth, repeated infections, and lens opacities.

Otooculomusculoskeletal Syndrome

Some cases in children with early deafness, cataracts, muscular atrophy, and growth retardation have been described.

CATARACTS WITH ONSET IN LATE INFANCY OR EARLY CHILDHOOD

• Retinoblastoma

Cataract is secondary to tumor involvement.

Aniridia

All or part of the iris is absent at birth. Cataracts occur in two thirds of cases. Sporadic cases have been associated with Wilms' tumor, hemihypertrophy, and genitourinary tract anomalies. A syndrome of aniridia, mental retardation, and other anomalies, which features a chromosome 11p 13 deletion, has a 50% incidence of Wilms' tumor.

Hurler Syndrome

Gradual development of coarse features, with stiff joints, visceromegaly, retardation, and corneal clouding is seen. Corneal opacities may also be seen with other mucopolysaccharidoses, including Hunter-Scheie syndrome, Maroteaux-Lamy, Scheie syndrome, Morquio syndrome, and mucopolysaccharidosis VII.

Cockayne Syndrome

Onset of symptoms is delayed until after the first year of life. Short stature, neurologic defects, a photosensitive dermatitis, deafness, and cataracts are found.

Rothmund-Thomson Syndrome

The clinical picture includes an unusual cutaneous atrophy, with a reticulated appearance, telangiectasia, alopecia, and nail and dental defects.

Refsum Disease

A peripheral neuropathy with motor weakness, cerebellar ataxia, and retinitis pigmentosa is usually found. Some affected children develop an ichthyotic skin disorder, and almost one half have cataracts. The cerebrospinal fluid protein is increased.

Osteopetrosis

Thick, dense bone results in obliteration of cranial nerve foramina, pancytopenia, and usually, early death.

Maroteaux-Lamy Syndrome

Growth deficiency becomes apparent by 3 years of age. Coarse facies, mild joint stiffness, macrocephaly, and macroglossia are present, but affected children are not retarded.

Stickler Syndrome

Features include a flat facies, midfacial hypoplasia, myopia, a marfanoid habitus, prominence of large joints, and, in rare cases, cataracts.

Congenital Retinal Degeneration (Leber Disease)

Signs of poor vision are noted shortly after birth. Pupillary reflexes are minimal or absent. Nystagmus, cataracts, strabismus, pigmentary stippling of the fundus, and optic atrophy may occur.

Alstrom Syndrome

Only three cases have been reported. Obesity develops in infancy along with nystagmus, photophobia, progressive visual impairment, and cataracts.

Deafness, Myopia, Cataract, and Saddle Nose

This is another rarely described combination of defects.

CATARACTS WITH ONSET IN LATE CHILDHOOD OR ADOLESCENCE

Diabetes Mellitus

Hypoparathyroidism

Muscle aches, tetany, dry skin, patchy alopecia, and, occasionally, increased intracranial pressure may be signs.

Pseudohypoparathyroidism and Pseudopseudohypoparathyroidism

Affected children have a short, stocky build with a round facies, short hands, bowing of legs, and the characteristic shortened fourth and fifth metacarpals.

Myotonic Dystrophy

In this disorder inherited as an autosomal dominant trait, myotonia, muscle wasting, and immobile myopathic facies are features; cataracts are found on slit-lamp examination.

Sex-linked Ichthyosis

Alport Syndrome

Familial nephritis and nerve deafness are findings; cataracts may develop later.

Prader-Willi Syndrome

Features include hypotonia, short stature, mental retardation, small hands and feet, and later obesity. Cataracts are rare.

Marshall Syndrome

This is a variant of anhidrotic ectodermal dysplasia with features of saddle nose, myopia, and the late appearance of cataracts.

Cerebrotendinous Xanthomatosis

Slowly progressive cerebellar ataxia with myoclonus or spasticity, xanthomas of tendons, and bilateral cataracts are features.

Basal Cell Nevus Syndrome

Multiple basal cell carcinomas develop later in adolescence; jaw cysts, vertebral defects, and, occasionally, cataracts may be found.

Weill-Marchesani Syndrome

Short stature, myopia, ectopic lens, spherophakia, and brachydactyly are findings.

Nail-Patella Syndrome (Arthro-Onychodysplasia)

The patellae are absent or hypoplastic; renal abnormalities develop later.

Fabry Disease (Angiokeratoma Corporis Diffusum)

Attacks of burning pain of the hands and feet begin in childhood. Angiectases are noted on the skin at about 10 years of age, and corneal opacities may develop.

Wilson Disease (Hepatolenticular Degeneration)

Cataracts rarely develop. The initial clinical picture may suggest a hepatitis, a hemolytic anemia, portal hypertension, or dystonia.

Marfan Syndrome

Cataracts may develop secondary to dislocated lenses.

Homocystinuria

The phenotype of children with this aminoaciduria may resemble that of Marfan syndrome. Cataracts may occur secondary to a dislocated lens.

Werner Syndrome

Onset is usually in early adulthood with signs of premature aging. Cataracts develop later.

Head Banging

A bizarre association of cataracts in children who are habitual head bangers has been reported.

Retinitis Pigmentosa

This disorder may be seen in several other syndromes or may occur without other systemic features. A progressive loss of night vision and constricted visual fields are the first symptoms. Cataracts may develop.

CATARACTS WITH VARIABLE ONSET (AT ANY AGE)

◆ Atopic Dermatitis

Anterior subcapsular cataracts are common in children with eczema but are rarely significant.

◆ Trauma

An important cause of acquired cataracts.

Glaucoma

Cataracts may develop in the presence of increased intraorbital pressure.

Retinal Detachment

Ionizing Radiation

Endophthalmitis

Inflammation of various layers of the eye may cause cataract formation.

Hemolytic Anemias

Cataracts are rare but have been reported to occur in hereditary spherocytosis and glucose-6-phosphate dehydrogenase deficiency.

Scleroderma

Laurence-Moon-Biedl Syndrome

Cataracts are rare. Features include mental retardation, obesity, hypogenitalism, polydactyly, and retinitis pigmentosa.

Cataracts Secondary to Intraocular Inflammatory Disease

Cataracts may develop during the course of intraocular inflammation. Juvenile rheumatoid arthritis, tuberculosis, sarcoidosis, syphilis, Behçet syndrome, and the Vogt-Koyanagi syndrome are included in this group of disorders.

Varicella

Cataracts may develop rapidly when they follow acquired infection.

DRUG-INDUCED CATARACT

♦ **Corticosteroids**

Prolonged treatment with systemic steroids almost invariably results in the formation of posterior subcapsular cataracts. Topical and inhaled steroids may also result in cataract formation.

Chlorpromazine

The condition is reversible on withdrawal of the drug.

Ergot

Vitamin D in Excessive Doses

Other Drugs

Cataracts have been reported to occur with these drugs or chemicals: triparanol, dinitrophenol, and naphthalene.

REFERENCES

1. Potter WS. Pediatric cataracts. *Pediatr Clin North Am* 1993;40:841–853.
2. Jones KL. *Smith's recognizable patterns of human malformation,* 5th ed. Philadelphia: WB Saunders, 1997.
3. Pike MG, Jan JE, Wong PKH. Neurological and developmental findings in children with cataracts. *Am J Dis Child* 1989;143:706–710.

SUGGESTED READING

Calhoun JH. Cataracts in infancy. *Pediatr Rev* 1988;9:227–233.
Kohn BA. The differential diagnosis of cataracts in infancy and childhood. *Am J Dis Child* 1976;130:184–192.

38
Unequal Pupils

Anisocoria, or unequal pupils, may be physiologic or indicative of underlying disease of the eye or central nervous system (CNS). It may be difficult at times to decide which eye is the one with the abnormal response—the larger or the smaller. Associated signs and symptoms are important, and usually the expertise of an ophthalmologist is required for the complete evaluation. The inequality may be familial. Before embarking on an extensive search for CNS or ophthalmic causes, it is important to recognize that 20% of the population have some degree of anisocoria. Old photographs may prove more helpful than new scans!

♦ **Most Common Causes of Unequal Pupils**

Normal Variation	Drugs
Anisometropia	Amblyopia
Blindness	

NORMAL VARIATION

Unequal pupil size is apparent in about 20% of the population.

♦ **Familial Trait**

One form of anisocoria is inherited as an autosomal dominant trait. Other members of the family should be examined.

♦ **Sporadic Occurrence**

Mild degrees of anisocoria are common and of no pathologic significance.

PRIMARY EYE DISORDERS

♦ **Anisometropia**

When the visual acuity of the eyes is different, the more myopic eye may have a larger pupil.

♦ **Amblyopia**

Failure of binocular fusion results eventually in suppression of the visual image from one eye. The pupils may appear unequal.

♦ **Blindness**

Disorders causing blindness may result in unequal pupillary size.

Iritis

Inflammation of the iris, ciliary body, or uveal tract causes reduction in reactive capacity of the iris and inequality of pupils.

Ocular Trauma

The pupil may be mydriatic following trauma.

Corneal Abrasion

Keratitis

Inflammation of the cornea, from various causes, produces dilation of limbic vessels and a flush around the cornea. Herpes simplex virus is a common pathogen.

Cataract

Any opacity of the cornea, lens, or vitreous may result in pupil inequality.

Glaucoma

Pupillary size may vary as a result of increased intraocular pressure. The cornea is enlarged and sometimes "steamy," and the eye is photophobic with increased lacrimation.

CNS DISORDERS

Horner Syndrome

This syndrome is characterized by miosis, ptosis, and decreased facial sweating on the affected side. The affected pupil constricts on exposure to light but fails to dilate fully in darker conditions. In children, the most common cause is a birth injury affecting the brachial plexus; in these cases the affected iris may be hypopigmented. Several other lesions may cause Horner syndrome including lesions with systemic effects, such as tumors, hemorrhage, and syringobulbia; neck lesions such as from trauma, cervical ribs, and enlarged cervical nodes; and mediastinal lesions, including tumors, aortic aneurysms, and thyroid adenomas.

Hutchinson Pupil

The dilated pupil results from third nerve compression, usually caused by an expanding supratentorial lesion such as tumor or hematoma. Decreasing levels of consciousness are usually found as intracranial pressure increases.

Adie Pupil (Tonic Pupil)

The pupil reacts slowly or not at all to light, and in a delayed manner to accommodation of near gaze, and it redilates slowly. A distinctive feature of this condition is constriction following administration of methacholine chloride (Mecholyl). Adie pupil may occur in women up to 30 years of age for unknown reasons, sometimes with depressed knee- and ankle-stretch reflexes; with lesions of the ciliary ganglion, often attributed to viral infections such as varicella or herpes zoster, and with familial dysautonomia (Riley-Day syndrome).

Encephalitis and Meningitis

Unequal pupils may occur during CNS infections. The pupils are usually miotic.

Migraine

Third nerve palsy may accompany migraine attacks.

Epilepsy

Rarely, unilateral mydriasis may be found following seizures.

Multiple Sclerosis

Unequal pupil size may occur as one of the signs of this disorder, which is rare in children.

Parinaud Syndrome

The pupil does not react to light, but does to accommodation. Associated findings include paresis of upward gaze, eyelid retraction, and nystagmus. The syndrome is indicative of mid brain dysfunction, usually hydrocephalus or a pineal-area tumor.

DRUGS AND TOXINS

♦ Drugs

Miotic or mydriatic and cycloplegic drugs may cause anisocoria. Beware of atropine aerosolized in the treatment of asthma. Scopolamine in patches, used in children undergoing chemotherapy to help reduce emesis, may be touched and then rubbed into the eye.

Toxins

Organophosphates that get in the eye may result in anisocoria that lasts for months.

SUGGESTED READING

Harley RD. *Pediatric ophthalmology*, 2nd ed. Philadelphia: WB Saunders, 1983.
Liu GT. Abnormalities of the pupil: when should you worry? *Contemp Pediatr* 1995;12:83–98.

39

Proptosis and Exophthalmos

The forward protrusion of an eye or eyes is a relatively uncommon finding in the pediatric age group. Orbital cellulitis is the most common cause of proptosis of acute onset, usually secondary to an ethmoid sinusitis. In cases with gradually increasing degrees of exophthalmos, orbital masses—particularly neoplasms—must be considered. Neuroimaging has greatly assisted in the evaluation of the proptotic eye, but the history and physical examination remain the most important elements in the successful delineation of the problem.

♦ **Most Common Causes of Proptosis**

Orbital Cellulitis   Vascular Tumors
Dermoid Cysts   Hyperthyroidism
Rhabdomyosarcoma   Neuroblastoma

● **Causes Not to Forget**

Leukemia   Lymphangioma
Craniosynostosis   Optic Nerve Glioma
Retinoblastoma

INFECTION

♦ **Orbital Cellulitis**

This infection is most commonly the result of acute ethmoiditis; however, it may follow trauma or the spread of local infection. Periorbital cellulitis, which is far more common, does not cause true proptosis. Extraocular movements are lost in orbital cellulitis but not in periorbital cellulitis.

Osteomyelitis of Orbit

Orbital Tuberculosis

Periostitis may produce proptosis. Ocular tuberculosis is more common and may be associated with ocular protrusion.

ENDOCRINE

◆ Hyperthyroidism

Hyperthyroidism is a relatively common cause of proptosis, more frequent in adolescents than in younger children. Affected women outnumber men with this disorder, which may be present at any age, including at birth. Tachycardia, irritability, nervousness, and tremors are common.

NEOPLASIA

Primary Orbital Tumors

◆ Dermoid Tumor

This is the most common benign orbital tumor; it is congenital but presenting signs may appear at any age. An external component may be visible.

◆ Rhabdomyosarcoma

Rhabdomyosarcoma is the most common malignant orbital tumor and must be considered in any eye rapidly becoming proptotic.

● Optic Nerve Glioma

This tumor may be associated with proptosis and unilateral visual loss.

Teratoma

The tumor is obvious at birth.

● Retinoblastoma

Proptosis is rare; a white pupillary reflex and strabismus are much more common signs.

Lacrimal Gland Tumors

These tumors are a rare cause of proptosis.

Juvenile Xanthogranuloma

Surprisingly, the yellowish skin nodules that are a characteristic finding with this tumor are rarely associated with those affecting the orbit.

Metastatic and Secondary Tumors

◆ Neuroblastoma

Metastatic neuroblastoma must be considered in any young child who presents with the spontaneous development of purpura of the eyelids with or without proptosis.

Neurofibromatosis

The skin should be examined carefully for café au lait spots. The eye may be pulsating. Optic gliomas are also common in this disorder.

- ### Leukemia

Langerhans Cell Histiocytosis

Children with the Hand-Schüller-Christian syndrome often have proptosis, which may be a sole finding without clinically apparent diabetes insipidus or punched-out bony lesions on radiographs.

Hodgkin Disease

Lymphoma

Metastatic Sarcomas

Juvenile Angiofibroma of the Nasopharynx

This locally invasive tumor usually produces epistaxis or symptoms of nasal obstruction.

Intracranial Tumors Involving the Orbit

VASCULAR DISTURBANCES

- ### Vascular Tumors

Deep hemangiomas and vascular malformations may involve the orbit and create a proptotic eye as they enlarge during infancy and early childhood.

Sturge-Weber Syndrome

The ipsilateral facial hemangiomatosis may involve orbital structures, creating glaucoma or a proptotic eye.

- ### Lymphangioma

The associated masses are usually non-compressible.

Cavernous Sinus Thrombosis

Signs and symptoms usually develop rapidly. The third cranial nerve runs through the cavernous sinus. The lids are edematous, there is paresis of extraocular movement, and the eye is injected.

Carotid-Cavernous Sinus Fistula

A progressive exophthalmos, ophthalmoplegia, secondary glaucoma, retinal edema, and unilateral headaches are associated findings.

♦ **S-C or SS Disease**

Rapid onset of exophthalmos may be seen in an orbital infarction crisis. A severe, localized headache and significant edema of the eyelids are also found.

BONY DISTURBANCES

● **Craniosynostosis**

Early closure of sutures may cause shallow orbits and prominent eyes. Apert and Crouzon syndromes are typical examples.

Encephalocele

Protrusion of brain tissue through a defect in the orbital vault may occur.

Metaphyseal Dysostosis

Bony overgrowth of the orbits may cause proptosis and optic atrophy as the optic foramina close.

Osteopetrosis

In this lethal disorder, the bones become dense and obliteration of the marrow leads to pancytopenia.

McCune-Albright Syndrome

Key features are fibrous dysplasia of bone, pigmented skin patches, and precocious puberty. Unilateral proptosis rarely occurs.

Rickets

Hypertelorism

In severe hypertelorism the eyes may appear proptotic.

Progressive Diaphyseal Dysplasia (Engelmann Disease)

Leg pain and muscle weakness are the most prominent presenting features of this autosomal dominant disorder.

Infantile Cortical Hyperostosis (Caffey Disease)

Onset is invariably before 6 months of age. Soft-tissue edema is prominent over the involved bones.

HEMORRHAGE

The following conditions may cause proptosis as a result of orbital hemorrhage.

Trauma

Fracture of the orbital floor may result in exophthalmos, diplopia, and superior maxillary pain.

Hemophilia

Scurvy

SYNDROMES WITH PROPTOSIS OR PROMINENT EYES

Incontinentia Pigmenti

An orbital mass may occur as one of the many systemic effects of this disorder, in which skin lesions are prominent during infancy.

Möbius Syndrome

Facial diplegia is the most prominent finding.

Progeria

Turner Syndrome

Seckel Syndrome (Birdheaded Dwarfism)

Leprechaunism

Leopard Syndrome

Pyknodysostosis

MISCELLANEOUS CAUSES

Collagen-Vascular Diseases

Proptosis may occur as part of the vasculitis in periarteritis nodosa and systemic lupus erythematosus.

Sarcoidosis

Orbital granulomas may cause proptosis.

Cystic Fibrosis

Unilateral proptosis has been reported as an early sign of cystic fibrosis.

Orbital Myositis

Congenital Hydrocephalus

Foreign Body in Orbit

Myasthenia Gravis

Acrodynia

In mercury poisoning, symptoms of hypotonia, irritability, photophobia, recurrent erythematous rashes, and profuse sweating overshadow proptosis if it occurs.

Crohn Disease

An orbital pseudotumor has been described in inflammatory bowel disease.

PSEUDOPROPTOSIS

High Myopia

Infantile Glaucoma

Contralateral Fractures, Ptosis, or Microophthalmia

SUGGESTED READING

Harley RD. *Pediatric ophthalmology*, 2nd ed. Philadelphia: WB Saunders, 1983.
Shields JA, Bakewell B, Augsburger JJ, Donoso LA, Bernardino V. Space-occupying orbital masses in children. *Ophthalmology* 1986;93:379–384.
Taylor D. *Pediatric ophthalmology*. Boston: Blackwell Scientific, 1990.

40

Loss of Vision and Blindness

Although the evaluation of subnormal vision in children requires the aid of an ophthalmologist, the physician who cares for children should have a good general knowledge of causes of loss of vision and blindness in order to approach the problem systematically. The referring physician can supply valuable information disclosed by the history and physical examination that may provide important diagnostic clues. It is important to determine if the visual loss occurred suddenly, is unilateral or bilateral, affects a visual field, or is associated with other systemic findings.

No attempt has been made in this chapter to enumerate all of the possible causes of subnormal vision. Ophthalmologic textbooks are better suited for that purpose. The aim of the following classification is to present general categories of visual loss that serve as a guide in evaluation.

◆ **Most Common Causes of Loss of Vision**

Sudden	Congenital	Acquired
Traumatic	Optic Nerve Atrophy	Retinopathy of Prematurity
Migraine	Cataracts	Genetic
Optic Neuritis	Albinism	Traumatic
Hysterical		Optic Nerve Gliomas

SUDDEN LOSS OF VISION

◆ **Trauma**

Loss of vision is most apt to occur after trauma to the occiput. The visual loss is sudden and complete, but vision usually returns in a matter of hours.

◆ **Migraine**

Vision may become blurred or distorted or may be characterized by the appearance of flashing lights; the loss may occasionally be complete. The visual loss may last minutes or hours. Headache, nausea, and vomiting are common but not always present. Ophthalmoplegias occur in some cases. The attacks tend to be repetitive.

◆ **Optic Neuritis**

Unilateral or bilateral optic or retrobulbar neuritis are relatively common causes of sudden loss of vision. The optic disc is usually swollen, and retinal vessels are engorged. Although the condition is usually painless, there may be localized pain above the eye. Systemic signs of other disease are more likely to be found in children than in adults. The onset may follow a viral syndrome including measles, mumps, varicella, and infectious mononucleosis, or after pertussis or immunizations. Other disorders associated include the following.

♦ Hysterical Blindness

Most commonly the visual loss is characterized by tunnel vision, in which the visual field loss has distinct sharp margins that do not vary over distances. Complete blindness is less common but is characterized by sudden onset with normal pupillary responses and a normal funduscopic examination.

Arterial Hypotension

Episodes may be accompanied by a temporary loss of vision that may or may not be followed by a loss of consciousness. Lightheadedness and a feeling of weakness occur in most cases.

Increased Intracranial Pressure

Transient visual loss or blurring of vision usually lasts less than 30 seconds. The loss may be precipitated by sudden changes in posture or by excitement. Flashes of light are occasionally associated with the visual loss. Prolonged increased pressure, as with pseudotumor cerebri or hydrocephalus, may lead to optic nerve atrophy and permanent consequences.

Arteriovenous Malformations

The visual loss is unilateral and short-lasting.

Cerebral Embolization

Air may be introduced into the vascular system during cardiac or thoracic surgery or into the dural sinus during neurosurgical procedures. Coma, convulsions, and hemiplegia may occur as well as the visual loss. Fat emboli may enter the pulmonary circulation and reach the brain. Dyspnea, tachypnea, and cerebral signs are present.

Multiple Sclerosis

Occurrence is uncommon in childhood. The onset is usually fairly sudden, often with gait disturbances, paresthesias, and dysesthesias. The course is characterized by remissions and exacerbations.

Cat-Scratch Disease

Acute Meningitis

Encephalitis

Exogenous Drugs or Toxins
Lead Poisoning
Chloramphenicol Toxicity

Acute Disseminated Encephalomyelitis

Similar to multiple sclerosis in sudden onset of neurologic symptoms and signs, including varying combinations of hemiplegia, ataxia, cranial nerve palsies and optic neuritis. Generally, the neurologic symptoms subside and improve, and unlike multiple sclerosis, do not recur. Onset follows viral infections, and, sometimes, immunizations.

Neuromyelitis Optica (Devic Disease)

Visual changes or symptoms of transverse myelitis may occur, as well as various exanthems.

Metabolic Disorders

Sudden cortical blindness has been reported to occur during hypoglycemia.

Systemic Lupus Erythematosus
Cerebral Venous Sinus Thrombosis

Headache, diplopia, nausea, vomiting, blurred vision, and photophobia may be symptoms. Birth control pills may be implicated.

CONGENITAL BLINDNESS

Congenital Malformations

♦ Congenital Optic Atrophy

Signs of this disorder, inherited as an autosomal recessive trait, are evident at birth or shortly thereafter. Nystagmus is generally present.

Retinal Aplasia

Pupillary responses are absent.

Septo-Optic Dysplasia

A congenital optic nerve hypoplasia with hypopituitarism. Hypoglycemia may be a clue in the neonatal period.

Congenital Hydrocephalus
Hydranencephaly

Failure of development and blindness become evident over the first few months of life. Transillumination of the skull is striking.

Porencephalic Cysts

Cysts may involve the visual cortex.

Occipital Encephalocele

Perinatal Anoxia or Hypoxia

Congenital Infections

The TORCH complex of infections may produce blindness present at birth or evidence of visual loss later in life.

♦ CONGENITAL CATARACTS

Cataracts may be extensive enough to interfere with vision (see Chapter 37, Cataracts).

OPTIC ATROPHY

Optic atrophy may be the result of various disorders, both congenital and acquired.

♦ Traumatic Causes

Chronic Subdural Hematoma

In addition to effects on vision, focal or generalized seizures, an enlarged abnormally shaped head, vomiting, developmental delay, and other signs are common.

Increased Intracranial Pressure

Any cause of prolonged increased intracranial pressure may result in optic atrophy and blindness or visual impairment.

Degenerative Disorders

Various neurodegenerative disorders may be associated with optic atrophy, retinitis pigmentosa, and other ophthalmologic signs. A few are listed here (see Harley's text listed at the end of this chapter for a more complete classification).

Tay-Sachs Disease

Symptoms begin in the first few months of life with hyperacusis and irritability. Delayed motor development and decreased visual acuity become apparent by 6 months of age.

Krabbe Disease

The course is similar to that in Tay-Sachs disease, with onset at 4 to 6 months of age, with irritability, failure of motor development, and progressive deterioration. Blindness is usually complete by 1 year of age.

Canavan Disease (Spongy Degeneration of Central Nervous System)

Degeneration of the white matter produces signs and symptoms in the first year of life. Hypotonia, seizures, significant psychomotor retardation, enlarging head size, and decreased visual acuity are prominent features.

Metachromatic Leukodystrophy

Deterioration of psychomotor development follows an initially normal period of development. Optic atrophy occurs late in the course of the disease.

Menkes Kinky Hair Syndrome

This condition is characterized by the early onset of seizures, episodes of hypothermia, significant psychomotor retardation, and striking sparse, short, depigmented hair.

Behr Syndrome

Boys between 3 and 11 years of age are those usually affected; increased extremity tone, hyperreflexia, mild ataxia, and bladder disturbances are found.

GM$_2$ Gangliosidosis

Psychomotor retardation, seizures, and hepatosplenomegaly occur early.

Leber Hereditary Optic Atrophy

This condition usually develops in the second decade but may begin insidiously earlier. The mitochondrial DNA mutation is maternally transmitted and is characterized by progressively increasing central blindness. Early in the course, the eye grounds are normal, but optic atrophy and retinal pigmentary changes develop later. Cardiac dysrhythmias and neurologic findings may be present.

Neuronal Ceroid-Lipofuscinosis

The abrupt onset of seizures resistant to therapy, progressive retardation, and regression to a vegetative state are characteristic features. Optic atrophy occurs later in the course.

Infantile Neuroaxonal Dystrophy

Onset of symptoms in this autosomal-recessive condition is in late infancy, with loss of ability to walk and failure of speech development, and either hypertonia or hypotonia. Late in the course nystagmus and loss of vision occur.

Infantile Optic Atrophy

In this disorder, inherited as an autosomal-dominant trait, progressive visual loss occurs during the school-age years. Central scotomata are most common.

Neoplastic Lesions

♦ Optic Gliomas

Pressure by the tumor on the optic nerve may result in optic atrophy. Visual field cuts and unilateral visual loss are most frequent.

Craniopharyngioma

Visual loss is usually due to compression of the optic chiasm. Visual field defects are the earliest findings.

Other Brain Tumors

Visual defects may occur with other central nervous system tumors depending on their location.

Vascular Lesions

Unilateral blindness may result from compression of the optic nerve by an intracranial aneurysm.

Bony Overgrowth

Osteopetrosis

In this inherited disorder, generalized sclerosis of bone causes decreased size of the cranial nerve foramina, with resulting nerve compression; facial palsy, strabismus, blindness, and deafness may ensue. Hepatosplenomegaly and severe anemia are the result of marrow replacement by bone.

Craniodiaphyseal Dysplasia

Thickening of the cranial bones creates increasing facial distortion. Cranial nerve palsies result from compression by the bony overgrowth.

♦ RETINOPATHY OF PREMATURITY

Varying degrees of retinal scarring and visual loss may be found. Infants at risk should be observed carefully for early signs.

CONGENITAL NYSTAGMUS

Visual acuity may be impaired because of nystagmus (see Chapter 36, Nystagmus).

CHORIORETINITIS

TORCH Complex

Any of the congenital infections may produce chorioretinitis and resultant impaired vision, although toxoplasmosis has been implicated as the most common cause of this lesion.

MACULAR DEGENERATION

Amaurotic Familial Idiocy

Amaurosis means blindness. In the late infantile form (Bielschowsky-Jansky disease) and the juvenile form (Batten-Mayou disease), macular degeneration and loss of vision may occur prior to neurodegeneration with dementia, paralysis, and death.

Familial Degeneration of the Maculae

In this disorder, inherited as an autosomal recessive trait, loss of central vision begins during the second decade. Peripheral vision is maintained for years before total blindness occurs.

GLAUCOMA

A loss of visual acuity may be the result of glaucoma, which may be unilateral or bilateral. (An extensive list of causes may be found in Harley's text, listed at the end of this chapter.) Clinical signs of glaucoma include photophobia, increased tearing, corneal enlargement, and later, clouding of the cornea.

RETINITIS PIGMENTOSA

This condition is characterized by progressive disorganization of the pigment of the retina, usually accompanied by a decrease in the number of retinal vessels and some degree of optic atrophy. Night blindness is often the first symptom of visual loss. A progressive loss of vision may occur over decades. Many heredofamilial disorders feature retinitis pigmentosa, only a few of which are listed here.

Abetalipoproteinemia (Bassen-Kornzweig Syndrome)

Steatorrhea appears early with acanthocytosis of red blood cells. Ataxia and retinitis occur later.

Laurence-Moon-Biedl Syndrome

Prominent features include short stature, obesity, mental retardation, hypogonadism, and polydactyly.

Refsum Disease

Main symptoms include ichthyosis, an unsteady gait, polyneuritis, and deafness.

Usher Syndrome

Retinitis pigmentosa and deafness are the two major signs.

OTHER NEURODEGENERATIVE DISEASES

Schilder Disease

Progressive loss of vision is associated with spastic hemiparesis, seizures, and intellectual deterioration.

Leigh Subacute Necrotizing Encephalomyelopathy

Onset is usually in infancy; the course is rather rapid and includes deterioration of psychomotor development with feeding difficulties, vomiting, seizures, and ataxia.

Progressive Multifocal Leukoencephalopathy

Generalized cerebral and motor function deterioration is associated with major motor seizures. Affected children usually die within 3 to 12 months of onset. A relationship to papovavirus infection has been suggested.

Progressive Infantile Cerebral Cortical Atrophy

Onset is during the first 6 years of life, with deceleration of development, seizures, spasticity, and cerebral blindness.

UVEITIS

Inflammation of the uveal tract (iris, ciliary body, and choroid) may be acute or chronic. In chronic uveitis the symptoms may be subtle and late—predominantly loss of vision—whereas in acute uveitis, pain, photophobia, and increased tearing may be prominent. Some of the important causes are listed subsequently.

Toxoplasmosis

Juvenile Rheumatoid Arthritis

Chronic iridocyclitis is most common in young girls with pauciarticular disease who have positive antinuclear antibody titers.

Sarcoidosis

Ankylosing Spondylitis

Acute inflammation is most common.

Peripheral Uveitis

The pathogenetic mechanism is unknown, but the peripheral form is a common cause of uveitis in children. Onset is usually between 6 and 10 years of age.

PSEUDOBLINDNESS

This is a common cause of "apparent blindness" in children who are severely developmentally delayed.

MISCELLANEOUS CAUSES

Retinoblastoma

Although it may be inherited as an autosomal dominant trait, this condition in most cases appears to be a spontaneous mutation. The tumor may be unilateral or bilateral. The most common presenting signs are a white pupillary reflex and strabismus.

Retinal Detachment

Trauma is the most common cause in children.

Drugs and Toxins

Effects of various drugs and toxins may impair vision. Potential toxins include methanol, steptomycins, quinine, isoniazid, thallium, arsenic, and penicillamine.

Lymphoma

Infiltration of the optic nerve by lymphomatous tissue may mimic optic neuritis.

Mucopolysaccharidoses

Corneal clouding is common in these disorders, most typical of which is Hurler syndrome.

SUGGESTED READING

Duffner PK, Cohen ME. Sudden bilateral blindness in children. *Clin Pediatr* 1978;17:705–712.

Harley RD. *Pediatric ophthamology,* 2nd ed. Philadelphia: WB Saunders, 1983.

Robinson GC, Jan JE. Acquired ocular visual impairment in children: 1960–1989. *Am J Dis Child* 1993;147:325–328.

Taylor D, ed. *Pediatric ophthalmology.* Boston: Blackwell Scientific, 1990.

SECTION V

Nose

41
Epistaxis

Epistaxis, or nose bleed, is a common occurrence in children. In most cases, the episode is brief in duration and related to minor trauma so that medical attention is not sought. Children whose epistaxis is difficult to control or recurrent constitute the bulk of cases brought for evaluation. Even among these groups, trauma is still the most common cause; the injury to the nose may be subtle, such as wiping, picking, or forceful blowing. The tendency to bleed is enhanced by low environmental humidity, allergic rhinitis, or venous congestion. Infections that may cause nose bleeds are usually obvious from systemic symptoms. Bleeding disorders generally have other manifestations of hemostatic problems in addition to the epistaxis, either in the child or in the family.

Ineffective means to control epistaxis are frequently used, such as ice packs placed on the nape of the neck or the bridge of the nose. Surprisingly, few parents realize that "clothespin" constriction of the anterior nares by thumb and finger is effective in most cases. Failure to apply pressure may create a false impression of excessive bleeding.

♦ Most Common Causes of Epistaxis

Trauma–Digital and External	Low Humidity-Dryness
Allergic Rhinitis	Upper Respiratory Infection
Exercise	

● Causes Not to Forget

Thrombocytopenia   von Willebrand Disease

TRAUMA AND IRRITATION

♦ Injury

The most common cause of epistaxis is trauma to the nose, in the form of a direct blow, rubbing, or digital manipulation.

♦ Low Environmental Humidity

This condition is likely to occur during the winter. Chronic dryness may lead to crust formation in the nares. Rubbing or blowing may result in tears of underlying superficial blood vessels.

♦ **Allergic Rhinitis**

Chronic rhinorrhea associated with allergies may cause irritation of superficial blood vessels and result in bleeding.

Foreign Body

A unilateral nasal discharge, especially if bloody, should always suggest this possibility.

Deviated Nasal Septum

A change in normal air flow may produce local irritation to mucous membranes.

Ulcer and Perforation

Chronic digital trauma may result in ulcer formation to the perichondrium. Chronic crusting may enhance bleeding.

♦ **INFECTION**

Rhinorrhea associated with localized or systemic infections may result in epistaxis. In addition, coughing or sneezing may also traumatize congested vessels leading to bleeding. The infections listed here are known to be associated with epistaxis more often than others.

Streptococcosis

Infection of the nasopharynx with Group A β-hemolytic streptococci may produce excoriated nares, generalized lymphadenopathy, and low-grade fever, especially in infants and young children.

Scarlet Fever

Rheumatic Fever

Epistaxis is obviously not a reliable sign.

Infectious Mononucleosis

Pertussis

Epistaxis is most likely to occur during paroxysms of coughing.

Measles

Varicella

Diphtheria

A serosanguineous discharge is an early manifestation.

Other Infections

Epistaxis may be present in malaria, typhoid fever, psittacosis, and syphilis.

BLEEDING DISORDERS

● **Thrombocytopenia**

Epistaxis may be a finding in any of a variety of disorders associated with a decrease in the number of platelets [see Chapter 113, Purpura (Petechiae and Ecchymoses)]. Idiopathic thrombocytopenic purpura is the most common cause; leukemia is the prime concern of parents.

● **von Willebrand Disease**

Recurrent episodes of epistaxis, especially after ingestion of aspirin, may be a presenting sign.

Drugs

Aspirin may predispose to an increased likelihood of bleeding.

Uremia

Children with renal failure have a propensity toward easy bruising and bleeding for multiple reasons, including impaired platelet function.

Coagulation Disturbances

Humoral clotting disorders are less likely to be associated with epistaxis than is thrombocytopenia. There may be evidence of bleeding at other sites.

Factor XI Deficiency

Nosebleeds are common, serious hemorrhages rare.

Hepatic Disease

Depletion of clotting factors is responsible.

TUMORS

Chronic Adenoidal Enlargement

Obstruction of the posterior nasal pharynx may result in chronic rhinorrhea and irritation of the nasal passages. The associated bleeding is usually minimal.

Polyps

Irritation of nasal polyps may lead to bleeding. Allergies and cystic fibrosis are among causes to consider.

Rhabdomyosarcoma

Lymphoma

Juvenile Nasopharyngeal Angiofibroma

This nasopharyngeal tumor occurs most commonly in adolescent boys who present with severe and recurrent nosebleeds and progressive unilateral or bilateral nasal obstruction.

Lymphoepithelioma

This uncommon nasopharyngeal tumor produces unilateral, tender cervical lymphadenopathy, epistaxis, and torticollis.

Midline Reticuloses (Lethal Midline Granulomas)

VASCULAR ABNORMALITIES

Increased Venous Pressure

♦ Exertion

Intense muscular activity with straining may produce vascular congestion, increased pressure, and spontaneous epistaxis.

Superior Vena Cava Syndrome

Obstruction of blood flow from the superior vena cava may greatly increase nasal venous pressure.

Mitral Stenosis

Severe stenosis may produce increased pressure.

Pulmonary Arteriovenous Fistula

Symptoms depend on the size of the arteriovenous shunt. Dyspnea, cyanosis, hemoptysis, epistaxis, and exercise intolerance are common. There may be generalized telangiectasia of the skin and mucous membranes.

Hypertension

Systemic arterial hypertension is an uncommon cause of epistaxis although often considered in the differential diagnosis.

Rendu-Osler-Weber Syndrome (Hereditary Hemorrhagic Telangiectasia)

Epistaxis is the most common presenting sign. The number of cutaneous and mucous membrane telangiectasia increases with age.

Hemangioma

Nasal hemangiomas are uncommon.

Vasculitis

Children with vasculitis frequently have episodes of epistaxis.

MISCELLANEOUS CAUSES

Barometric Changes

Epistaxis may occur especially at high altitudes.

β-Thalassemia

Epistaxis is common in Cooley anemia.

Associated with Menstruation

Adolescent girls occasionally have epistaxis associated with their menstrual periods, but the mechanism is unknown.

Ehlers-Danlos Syndrome

Wegener Granulomatosis

SUGGESTED READING

Katsanis E, Luke K-H, Hsu E, Li M, Lillicrap D. Prevalence and significance of mild bleeding disorders in children with recurrent epistaxis. *J Pediatr* 1988;113:73–76.

McDonald TJ. Nosebleed in children. *Postgrad Med* 1987;81:217–224.

Mulbury PE. Recurrent epistaxis. *Pediatr Rev* 1991;12:213–217.

42

Chronic Rhinitis/Nasal Obstruction

Stuffy or runny nose is a common complaint in children and adults. Chronic rhinitis, a less frequent problem, is defined as inflammation of the nasal mucosa that results in discharge, congestion, and sneezing that occurs for some portion of the day for 2 months or longer. Difficulties resulting from nasal obstruction are more profound in infants who are obligatory nose breathers; however, older children may have significant symptoms as well. Chronic mouth breathers may have complaints of recurrent pharyngitis or snoring; appetite and exercise tolerance may be affected. Chronic cough may accompany chronic rhinitis.

♦ Most Common Causes of Rhinitis/Nasal Obstruction

Recurrent Upper Respiratory Infections   Allergic Rhinitis
Adenoidal Hypertrophy   Sinusitis
Foreign Body   Nasal Septum Deviation
Choanal Stenosis

INFLAMMATORY NASAL OBSTRUCTION

♦ Recurrent Upper Respiratory Infections

May give the impression of persistent rhinitis.

♦ Allergic Rhinitis

The rhinorrhea is usually watery and profuse. It is associated with sneezing; an allergic salute (itchy nose); watery and itchy eyes; and cough during sleep or on arising in the morning due to postnasal drip.

♦ Sinusitis

A chronic mucopurulent nasal discharge should always suggest sinusitis. Headaches and fever may not be present. A persistent "cold" and daytime cough for more than 10 days may reflect involvement of the sinuses.

Infectious Rhinitis

A viral upper respiratory infection may be complicated by bacterial overgrowth and a mucopurulent discharge. **Streptococcosis,** a chronic rhinitis secondary to group

A β-hemolytic streptococci, occurs primarily in young children. It is associated with a prolonged low grade fever, generalized lymphadenopathy, and weight loss. **Congenital syphilis** is a much less common cause of chronic rhinorrhea today, but must not be forgotten as causing "snuffles" in infants.

Adenoiditis

As part of the lymphoid tissue of Waldeyer ring, along with tonsils and pharyngeal lymphoid tissue, the adenoids participate in reactive lymphoid swelling; therefore, agents that cause pharyngitis and tonsillitis can cause adenoiditis as well.

Irritant Rhinitis

Profuse watery or mucoid nasal discharge, with significant congestion, paroxysmal sneezing, and itching may occur from cigarette smoke, pungent odors, or other irritants.

Nonallergic Rhinitis with Eosinophilia (NARES)

Similar in all ways to children with allergic rhinitis, but those affected do not have elevated IgE levels and do not respond to antihistaminics.

Vasomotor Rhinitis

This appears to be a hyperactive cholinergic response. Alternating nasal congestion and, occasionally, watery rhinorrhea may be present. A postnasal drip is a frequent complaint. Triggers include recumbency and temperature and humidity changes.

Atrophic Rhinitis

Atrophic rhinitis is rare in childhood with symptoms of severe nasal obstruction with physiologically widely patent nasal passages. A foul odor may be present. The causes include infection, trauma, nasal surgery, and Wegener granulomatosis. There is also an autosomal dominantly inherited form with onset around puberty.

Retropharyngeal Abscess

This abscess more commonly presents with pharyngitis, dysphagia, meningismus, and stridor. The onset is relatively acute.

ACQUIRED OR IATROGENIC OBSTRUCTION

♦ Adenoidal Hypertrophy

This is a common cause of nasal obstruction. Mouth breathing, noisy respirations when awake, and loud snoring during sleep are prominent features. Severe cases may result in obstructive sleep apnea. Rarely, congestive heart failure secondary to pulmonary hypertension from chronic hypoxia may be the presentation. Enuresis, daytime sleepiness, and decreased attentiveness have also been described in severely affected children.

♦ **Foreign Body**

A unilateral nasal discharge should always suggest this possibility. Bilateral obstructions are not uncommon. A bloody or foul odor to the discharge or even a generalized body odor (bromhidrosis) may be present.

♦ **Septal Deviation**

May be congenital or acquired, after trauma.

Nasal Polyps

A history of progressive nasal obstruction in children with allergic rhinitis, asthma, or chronic purulent nasal discharge may suggest the presence of polyps. Ten percent of children with cystic fibrosis develop polyps. Other causes include Kartagener syndrome, immotile cilia syndrome, recurrent sinusitis, and aspirin intolerance. Woake syndrome is a hereditary disorder with severe recurrent nasal polyposis during childhood, broadening of the base of the nose, tenacious secretions, frontal sinus aplasia, and bronchiectasis.

Rhinitis Medicamentosa

Prolonged use of topical nasal decongestants may cause a rebound phenomenon. Cocaine abuse is a possibility in adolescents. Systemic medications that may cause nasal stuffiness include antihypertensives (e.g., reserpine, hydralazine, guanethidine, and methyldopa), beta blockers (e.g., propranolol, atenolol, nadolol), and antidepressants (e.g., chlordiazepoxide, amitriptyline). Oral contraceptives have also been incriminated.

Trauma

Dislocation of nasal bones and septum may cause an anatomical obstruction. An untreated septal hematoma may result in dissolution of the nasal septal cartilage in as little as 48 hours.

Nasopharyngeal Stenosis

Fusion of the tonsillar pillars and soft palate to the posterior pharyngeal wall by scar tissue may follow tonsilloadenoidectomy.

Hormonal Rhinitis

Pregnancy and hypothyroidism are rare causes.

CONGENITAL OBSTRUCTION

◆ Posterior Choanal Stenosis

If posterior choanal stenosis is severe it may mimic true atresia. Less severe cases present with increased symptoms during feeding. An excessive mucoid discharge may be the only symptom.

Choanal Atresia

Bilateral atresia presents at birth with strenuous but unsuccessful attempts at breathing. Unilateral obstruction presents later with rhinorrhea. Bony obstruction accounts for 90% of the cases. Associated anomalies occur in 50%.

Tornwaldt Cyst

A pharyngeal bursa–diverticulum-like structure is present in 3% of the population. It is a potential space lying in the midline of the posterior wall of the nasopharynx just superior to the adenoidal pad. Symptoms occur when it becomes infected and include a persistent occipital headache accompanied by an annoying postnasal discharge. A lateral soft-tissue radiograph may demonstrate this structure.

Dermoid

A dermoid may occur as a progressively enlarging mass in the midline of the nose. Suspect this possibility whenever a discrete swelling of the nose of a newborn or infant is found. A sinus tract may be present that can extend intracranially.

Encephalocele

An encephalocele is an extrusion of meningeal-lined brain tissue. Sixty percent of anterior encephaloceles are seen externally over the bridge of the nose and another 30% occur intranasally.

Glioma

The presentation of a glioma is similar to that of an encephalocele or dermoid. Most occur intranasally and they are often misdiagnosed as polyps.

Teratoma

A teratoma is a tumor containing derivatives of all three germ cell layers that grows rapidly in early infancy.

NEOPLASMS

Hemangiomas

The tumor tends to grow rapidly during the first 6 months of life. Other cutaneous lesions may or may not be present.

Juvenile Nasopharyngeal Angiofibroma

This is generally seen in adolescent males. Presenting symptoms include recurrent epistaxis, rhinorrhea, and nasal obstruction.

Lymphoma

Hodgkin and non-Hodgkin lymphomas are the most common nasopharyngeal malignancies in childhood.

Rhabdomyosarcoma

Seventy percent occur in children under 12 years of age. The progression is usually silent until eustachian tube obstruction and nasality to the voice occur.

Nasopharyngeal Carcinoma

Nasopharyngeal carcinoma is rare in childhood.

Other Neoplasms

Craniopharyngioma, chordoma, lipoma, and chondroma may occur in this area.

MISCELLANEOUS CAUSES

Fibrous Dysplasia of Facial Bones

This is a cause of slowly progressive obstruction as a result of bony overgrowth. Distortion of the facies and cranial nerve involvement, especially vision, are common.

Cystic Fibrosis

Children with cystic fibrosis tend to have rhinitis with or without polyps.

Sickle Cell Disease

Down Syndrome

Apert and Crouzon Syndromes

Associated with abnormal facial anatomy caused by craniosynostosis.

SUGGESTED READING

Albert D. Nasal obstruction and rhinorrhoea in infants and children. In: Adams DA, Cinnamond MJ, eds. *Paediatric otolaryngology,* 6th ed. Bath, UK: Butterworth/Heinemann, 1997:6/17/1–16.
McIntire SC. Chronic nasal obstruction and rhinorrhea. In: Gartner JC Jr, Zitelli BJ, eds. *Common and chronic symptoms in pediatrics.* St. Louis: Mosby, 1997:201–214.
Simons FER. Chronic rhinitis. *Pediatr Clin North Am* 1984;31:801–819.

SECTION VI

Mouth and Throat

43

Macroglossia

Macroglossia, or enlargement of the tongue, may be caused by tumors, infiltrates, storage products, muscular hypertrophy, or edema; or, the tongue may simply appear enlarged because the mouth is too small to accommodate it. In this chapter, disorders associated with macroglossia are grouped according to age and mode of onset.

MACROGLOSSIA PRESENT AT BIRTH

Beckwith-Wiedemann Syndrome

Clinical presentations are variable but macroglossia and omphalocele or umbilical hernia with neonatal hypoglycemia are key features. Postnatal rapid growth, visceromegaly, and earlobe grooves are found. Abdominal tumors, particularly Wilms' tumors, occur later in a significant number of affected children.

Trisomy 21 Syndrome (Down Syndrome)

The tongue actually may not be enlarged, but the oral cavity is so small that it protrudes.

Hypothyroidism

Athyrotic cretinism is usually associated with an enlarged tongue. Affected infants are lethargic and feed poorly. They may have facial edema; run low temperatures; and tend to have prolonged jaundice. Coarse features become more apparent with age. Tongue enlargement may be noted after a few months of life.

Hemihypertrophy

Congenital hemihypertrophy may include enlargement of one half of the tongue.

Idiopathic Muscular Macroglossia

The tongue may be enlarged without evidence of associated problems or abnormalities.

Robinow Syndrome (Fetal Face Syndrome)

Prominent features include macrocephaly, a large anterior fontanel, frontal boss-ing, hypertelorism, a small upturned nose, short forearms, and a small penis. The small mouth may create an impression of macroglossia.

Generalized Gangliosidosis

The main characteristics are coarse features, prenatal onset of growth deficiency, hypotonia, low nasal bridge, alveolar ridge hypertrophy, and joint contractures.

Duplication 4p Syndrome

Macroglossia is one of many phenotypic abnormalities present in this syndrome.

Simpson-Golabi-Behmel Syndrome

Affected infants are large at birth and continue to be large as adults.

X-linked α-Thalassemia/Mental Retardation Syndrome

Hemangiolymphangioma

MACROGLOSSIA APPEARING AFTER THE NEONATAL PERIOD

Hemangiolymphangioma

The tongue becomes progressively enlarged and protuberant, usually with an irregular or papillary surface. Enlargement may be present at birth.

Hemangioma

Enlargement may become noticeable during the first few months of life as the vascular tumor grows.

Rhabdomyoma

Proliferation of muscle tissue results in enlargement of the tongue. Usually the margins of the tumor are palpable.

Neurofibromatosis

Café au lait spots usually increase in number with age along with cutaneous tumors. Tongue enlargement may be seen in occasional cases.

Fibrous Hamartoma

Mucopolysaccharidoses

In type I (Hurler syndrome), striking features are progressive facial coarseness, deceleration of growth, broad claw hands, hepatosplenomegaly, hernias, kyphosis, alveolar ridge hypertrophy, and macroglossia. In type V (Scheie syndrome), there is a more gradual development of coarse features with a broad mouth, full lips, prognathism, hirsutism, clouding of the corneas, joint limitation, and, occasionally, macroglossia. Intelligence is normal. In type VI (Maroteaux-Lamy syndrome), onset is in the first few years of life, with growth deficiency, coarse facies, large nose, thick lips, prominent sternum, umbilical hernia, cloudy corneas, hepatosplenomegaly, and occasionally, macroglossia.

Pompe Disease (Glycogen Storage Disease, Type II)

This disorder affects skeletal and cardiac muscle. The main features are significant hypotonia, cardiomegaly with early heart failure, and swallowing and respiratory difficulties. Death usually occurs in the first year of life from cardiomyopathy.

Multiple Mucosal Neuroma Syndrome

Gradual coarsening of the facies occurs with age, along with prominent lips, thickened anteverted eyelids, and a nodular tongue. Medullary thyroid carcinoma is common. A Marfanoid body habitus is typical.

Mucolipidosis II

Alveolar ridge hypertrophy gives the impression of macroglossia. Growth deficiency, developmental retardation, and other features similar to those of Hurler syndrome are apparent.

Mannosidosis

In this storage disorder, features include progressively coarsening features, hypotonia, cloudy lenses, and retardation.

Aspartyl-Glucosaminuria

Affected infants appear well at birth but develop diarrhea and recurrent respiratory infections after 4 months of age. Mental retardation is apparent by 1 year of age. Protuberant abdomen and coarse features develop later.

Primary Amyloidosis

Macroglossia develops in about one third of the cases but is usually not apparent until adulthood.

Pachyonychia Congenita

Keratoses of the palms and soles with thickened finger and toenails are striking features. The tongue appears enlarged secondary to a thick white coating.

Sandhoff Disease

This inborn error of metabolism has a clinical presentation mimicking that of Tay-Sachs disease. Macroglossia has been described but is not a prominent feature.

MACROGLOSSIA OF SUDDEN ONSET

Angioneurotic Edema

Infection

Trauma

A hematoma may cause tongue enlargement.

44

Sore Throat

The symptom of sore throat usually means the presence of an infection, either bacterial, mycoplasmal, or, more commonly, viral. Various other factors may produce irritation and soreness of the throat, including postnasal drip associated with allergies, low environmental humidity, smoke, and foreign bodies.

The most common causes of sore throat vary with age and with season of the year. Group A β-hemolytic streptococcus is much more likely to occur in young school-age children, particularly in late winter and early spring; mycoplasma and Epstein-Barr virus infections are more prominent in adolescents. Some causes of sore throat are associated with features that assist in suggesting the diagnosis. Adenovirus infections commonly produce conjunctival inflammation. Herpes simplex and herpangina are associated with ulcerations.

♦ **Most Common Causes of Sore Throat**

Group A Streptococci	Mouth Breathing
Postnasal Drip	Environmental Dryness
Adenovirus	Influenza and Parainfluenza
Epstein-Barr Virus	*Mycoplasma pneumoniae*

INFECTION

Tonsillopharyngitis

♦ **Bacterial Infection**

Primary bacterial tonsillitis is caused by three organisms: group A β-hemolytic streptococci, *Corynebacterium diphtheriae,* and *Neisseria gonorrhoeae.* Gonococcal pharyngitis must be considered in adolescents and young adults with oral or oropharyngeal ulcerations with ragged borders. Diphtheritic pharyngitis may be associated with a grayish membrane, regional adenopathy, and mild fever, but most often its onset is insidious. Tularemia is a much less common cause of primary bacterial tonsillitis.

♦ **Viral Infection**

Most sore throats are caused by acute viral infection, most commonly adenovirus infections, herpes simplex, influenza, coxsackievirus infections, and infectious mononucleosis. Adenovirus infections are commonly associated with conjunctival inflammation. In herpangina, caused by a coxsackievirus, there are tiny vesicles on the anterior tonsillar pillars, whereas in hand-foot-and-mouth disease, shallow ulcers are present in the mouth, and vesicles are found on the hands, feet, and buttocks.

♦ Mycoplasma Infection

Mycoplasma infection as a cause of sore throat may be more common than previously recognized, particularly among adolescents.

Chlamydia pneumoniae

Formerly known as TWAR agent, this organism causes pneumonia in older children and may cause pharyngitis.

Arcanobacterium hemolyticum

An uncommon cause of pharyngitis. May cause a rash that mimics scarlet fever or a drug eruption.

Groups C and G Streptococci

More likely in adolescents or young adults.

Peritonsillar Abscess or Cellulitis

These conditions are usually a result of extension of a tonsillar infection by group A streptococci. The pharyngeal pain is severe, swallowing is difficult, and the uvula is shifted away from the abscess.

Retropharyngeal Abscess

Intense pharyngeal pain and difficulty in swallowing with drooling and hyperextension of the neck are common.

Epiglottitis

Acute epiglottitis is usually caused by *Haemophilus influenzae*, type b. The onset and progression of symptoms is rapid in children and may be preceded by sore throat in adults.

Supraglottitis

Inflammation of the aryepiglottic folds rather than the epiglottis may give the same symptoms as epiglottitis. Group A β-hemolytic streptococci have been implicated.

Laryngotracheobronchitis

Croup is viral in origin; a sore throat may precede the barking cough and stridor.

Laryngitis

Laryngitis is also viral in etiology. Hoarseness is a prominent symptom.

Bacterial Tracheitis

The symptoms are those of croup initially, but they worsen progressively, as a result of tracheal obstruction by mucopurulent secretions. *Staphylococcus aureus* is the usual culprit.

Trench Mouth (Necrotizing Ulcerative Gingivitis)

The tonsils may be involved by this infection, which causes ulcerations, friable and bleeding gums, and the formation of a yellow gray pseudomembrane over the involved tissues.

Oral Moniliasis

Candidal infections, even if extensive, rarely cause pain.

CHRONIC PHARYNGITIS

The sore throat is usually milder than in those associated with the infections as described. There may be a feeling of scratchiness with frequent clearing of the throat. The posterior pharyngeal wall is injected and often has a cobblestone appearance because of lymphoid hypertrophy.

◆ Irritation

Irritation may be caused by dust, smoke, or excessive dryness of the air.

◆ Allergy

A chronic postnasal drip may cause pharyngeal irritation.

Repeated Attacks of Acute Pharyngitis

Lymphonodular Pharyngitis

Nodules of lymphoid tissue are prominent, stimulated by agents such as coxsackie-virus.

TRAUMA

Vocal Abuse

Excessive shouting, singing, or other forms of vocal abuse may result in throat pain as well as hoarseness.

Foreign Body

Sudden onset of throat pain may be caused by the presence of a foreign body. Drooling and difficulty in swallowing are common findings.

Burns

The pharynx may be injured by hot food or drink, or by acids and alkalis.

Smoke

Children may develop pharyngeal irritation from cigarette smoke. Pharyngitis may follow smoke inhalation associated with fires.

♦ PHARYNGEAL DRYING

The mouth and pharynx may become dry and sore from mouth breathing associated with nasal congestion during upper respiratory infections, allergies, or adenoidal hypertrophy. The problem is more common in winter months when the environmental humidity is low.

OTHER CAUSES

Neutropenia

In cyclic neutropenia, or during episodes of neutropenia associated with drug therapy or leukemia, pharyngeal pain may occur with oral ulcerations or membrane formation. While neutropenia is an expected complication of various cancer drugs, neutropenia may occur with other drugs (e.g., propylthiouracil), often heralded by sore throat.

Thyroiditis

A sense of fullness in the throat or true pain may be found in thyroid inflammation. The thyroid gland is enlarged and tender to palpation.

Herpes Zoster

Oropharyngeal lesions may occur, but vesicles are usually present on the face.

Lethal Midline Granuloma

Rare in childhood, this unusual disorder is signified by ulceration of the palate, base of the tongue, or oropharynx with progressive destruction. The lungs and kidneys may also be affected by the vasculitis.

Pharyngeal Carcinoma

This is mainly a disease of middle or old age but has been described in adolescents. The classic triad is pain on swallowing, referred ear pain, and hoarseness.

SUGGESTED READING

Denny FW Jr. Tonsillopharyngitis 1994. *Pediatr Rev* 1994;15:185–190.
McMillan JA, Sandstrom C, Weiner LB, et al. Viral and bacterial organisms associated with acute pharyngitis in a school-aged population. *J Pediatr* 1986;109:747–752.
Putto A. Febrile exudative tonsillitis: viral or streptococcal? *Pediatrics* 1987;80:6–12.

45

Dysphagia

The seemingly simple act of swallowing involves a rather complex array of neuromuscular activities that include sucking or taking food into the mouth and propelling it into the stomach, along with mechanisms that prevent food or liquid from entering the trachea. The process of deglutition may be impaired by various disorders. In addition, one should separate out disorders that cause pain on swallowing (odynophagia), which may be interpreted as difficulty in swallowing.

In this chapter, disorders that may produce dysphagia are divided into two main categories: disorders of the mouth and pharynx and disorders affecting the esophagus.

♦ Most Common Causes of Dysphagia

Prematurity   Gastroesophageal Reflux with Esophagitis
Pharyngitis   Cerebral Palsy
Candidal Esophagitis   Foreign Body

DISORDERS AFFECTING THE MOUTH AND PHARYNX

Mechanical Problems

Cleft Palate

Choanal Atresia and Stenosis

Macroglossia

Macroglossia may be caused by cysts, hemangiomas, or lymphangiomas or may be associated with true muscular enlargement (see Chapter 43, Macroglossia).

Temporomandibular Ankylosis

Lack of movement of the joint may be congenital or associated with inflammatory processes.

Micrognathia

Severe receding chin may interfere with feeding.

Pharyngeal Diverticuli

Congenital Diverticulum

The posterior hypopharynx is the usual site of the diverticulum.

Lateral Pharyngeal Diverticulum

Pulsion Diverticulum

Traumatic Pseudodiverticulum of Pharynx

Foreign Bodies

Tumors of Tongue or Pharynx

Cysts of Larynx or Epiglottis

Infections

♦ **Oral Infection**

Infections of the gums, tongue, tonsils, and buccal mucosa may interfere with swallowing.

Peritonsillar Abscess

The uvula is usually shifted to one side.

Cervical Adenitis

Sinusitis

Epiglottitis

In this life-threatening infection, there are drooling, fever, and a preference to sit upright. An acute onset is typical.

Retropharyngeal Abscess

Children with these abscesses prefer to keep their heads hyperextended.

Guillain-Barré Syndrome

Ascending paralysis associated with this postinfectious syndrome may involve muscles used in swallowing.

Encephalitis and Meningitis

Infants and children with central nervous system infections may lose the ability to coordinate sucking and swallowing.

Botulism

The toxin produces paralysis of muscles involved in swallowing.

Diphtheria

The pseudomembrane or toxin released from nasopharyngeal infection may cause swallowing difficulties.

Tetanus

Muscular spasms may prevent swallowing.

Poliomyelitis

Bulbar paralysis has become uncommon since vaccine development.

Neuromuscular Disorders

♦ Developmental Delay

An effective sucking and swallowing coordination may be delayed in premature infants and in those with severe mental retardation; occasionally, when mild, this may be a normal variation.

♦ Cerebral Palsy

Insults to the central nervous system may produce neuromuscular lesions in many areas, including those necessary for coordination of swallowing.

Hypoxic Brain Damage

Cranial Nerve Palsies

Disorders affecting the fifth, seventh, and ninth through twelfth cranial nerves—either the nucleus or along the course—may interfere with swallowing.

Palatal Paralysis

Paralysis involving the tenth cranial nerve is associated with nasal regurgitation as the infant attempts to feed.

Möbius Syndrome

Facial diplegia occurs along with bulbar palsy. Infants with this uncommon disorder have a striking immobility of the face.

Arnold-Chiari Malformation

Displacement of the brain stem and cerebellum through the foramen magnum usually results in hydrocephalus. Stridor and swallowing difficulties may develop.

Syringomyelia

Depending on the area of the spinal cord or brain stem involved, bulbar symptoms may be present. Loss of pain and of temperature sensation of the extremities or face is often present early.

Cricopharyngeal Incoordination

The disorder is usually present at birth. Muscular spasm prevents effective swallowing. Vomiting, aspiration, and nasal regurgitation are present.

Muscular Problems

Werdnig-Hoffmann Disease

Severe muscle weakness may interfere with effective swallowing.

Myasthenia Gravis

Difficulty in swallowing may be an early sign along with ptosis and strabismus.

Myotonic Dystrophy

In the neonatal period, sucking difficulties may be prominent along with respiratory distress. Muscle weakness occurs later.

Dermatomyositis

Dystonia Musculorum Deformans

Involuntary bizarre posturing may be mistaken for a psychiatric problem.

Miscellaneous Disorders

Prader-Willi Syndrome

Feeding difficulties occur early. Hypotonia, growth retardation, cryptorchidism, and later, obesity are characteristic features.

Juvenile Rheumatoid Arthritis

Involvement of the cricoarytenoid joint usually manifests as stridor, hoarseness, and dyspnea, but swallowing difficulty may ensue.

Angioneurotic Edema

Swelling of soft tissues may interfere with swallowing as well as breathing.

Stevens-Johnson Syndrome

Involvement of the esopharyngeal mucosa and oropharynx with erosive lesions creates swallowing difficulties.

Familial Dysautonomia

Feeding difficulties occur early. Choking and aspiration episodes are common; delayed development, hypotonia, relative pain insensitivity, decreased tearing, absence of fungiform tongue papillae, thermal instability, and emotional lability are other features.

Cerebrohepatorenal Syndrome

Affected infants are also hypotonic and have a characteristic facies with a high forehead.

Sydenham Chorea

There may be feeding difficulties as well as the choreiform movements.

Vitamin Deficiencies

Pellagra

Scurvy

Acrodynia

Mercury poisoning produces a diffuse pink rash, hypotonia, painful extremities, and photophobia and may create feeding difficulties.

Cricopharyngeal Spasm

Trauma to the posterior pharyngeal wall may produce spasm of this muscle group.

Infantile Gaucher Disease

Opisthotonus, bulbar paralysis, stridor, strabismus, and spastic paralysis are prominent features.

DISORDERS AFFECTING THE ESOPHAGUS

Obstruction

♦ **Foreign Body**

This possibility must always be considered in dysphagia of recent onset.

Tracheoesophageal Fistula

Swallowing is normal, but aspiration, choking, and difficulty in handling secretions are noted at birth.

Esophageal Stricture

Stricture may be due to corrosives, reflux esophagitis, or irritation from foreign bodies.

External Compression

Vascular Anomalies

Tracheal compression is usually more severe than esophageal compression. Anomalies include anomalous right subclavian artery, double aortic arch, right aortic arch, and anomalous innominate artery.

Esophageal Duplication

Mediastinal Tumors

Diaphragmatic Hernia

Atopic Thyroid

Thyroiditis

Congenital Esophageal Diverticulum

Esophageal Tumors

Various esophageal tumors have been described including hamartomas, leiomyomas, neuromas, papillomas, and lipomas.

Esophageal Web

Leukemic Infiltrates

Chest pain and dysphagia are usually present.

Psychological Causes: Globus Hystericus

The complaint is usually a lump in the throat with an inability to swallow. Drooling does not occur.

Inflammation

♦ **Candidiasis**

Oral candidal infection is usually present. The immunocompromised host is at risk, as well as patients with hypoparathyroidism and hypoadrenocorticism.

Mediastinitis

Perforation of Esophagus

Herpes Esophagitis

Some immunocompetent patients have been described with this infection without obvious oral involvement.

Crohn Disease

May affect the esophagus resulting in dysphagia.

Corrosives

Acids, alkalis, and, occasionally, medications, may act as corrosives, creating dysphagia.

Altered Motility

◆ Gastroesophageal Reflux

Episodes of vomiting, recurrent aspiration, coughing, wheezing, and failure to thrive may be symptoms. Esophagitis may cause dysphagia.

Achalasia

The esophagus is dilated, and the gastroesophageal junction is narrowed. Difficulty in swallowing and regurgitation after meals are the main complaints.

Esophageal Spasm

Spasm is usually related to stress, eating rapidly, or reflux. There is generally severe substernal pain with intermittent dysphagia and a history of regurgitation.

Chagas Disease

In the chronic phase of trypanosomiasis, heart block and esophageal dilatation may take place.

Miscellaneous Causes

Chronic Pulmonary Disease

Brain Tumors

There may be involvement of cortical motor areas or motor nuclei of the medulla that control sucking and swallowing reflexes.

Collagen Vascular Diseases

Scleroderma

Altered esophageal motility is a relatively common systemic complication.

Dermatomyositis

Sjögren Syndrome

Behçet Disease

Hyperkalemia

With muscle paralysis, dysphagia may occur but is short-lived.

Guillain-Barré Syndrome

Muscular Hypertrophy of the Esophagus

This is a rare disorder of unknown cause, in which the hypertrophy may be localized or diffuse.

Demyelinating Diseases

Epidermolysis Bullosa Congenita

Esophageal or oral lesions may interfere with swallowing.

Lesch-Nyhan Syndrome

Along with choreoathetoid movements and impressive self-mutilation, swallowing difficulties may be present.

Wilson Disease (Hepatolenticular Degeneration)

Coordination of swallowing may be affected. Drooling is a late finding.

Opitz-Frias Syndrome

Difficulty in swallowing with recurrent aspiration may be fatal in infancy. Hypertelorism and hypospadias along with persistent stridor and hoarseness suggest this diagnosis.

Dyskeratosis Congenita

Skin and nail findings are most prominent in this hereditary disorder, but leukoplakia of the mucous membranes including the esophagus leads to dysphagia.

SUGGESTED READING

Derkay CS, Schecter GL. Dysphagia. In: Bluestone CD, Stool SE, Kenna MA, eds. *Pediatric otolaryngology,* 3rd ed. Philadelphia: WB Saunders, 1996:965–973.
Weiss MH. Dysphagia in infants and children. *Otolaryngol Clin North Am* 1988;21:727–735.

46

Increased Salivation and Drooling

Ptyalism, or increased salivation, is a common physiologic sign of teething and is also commonly present in oropharyngeal infections and irritations. The acute onset of excessive salivation with respiratory, gastrointestinal, and central nervous system symptoms suggests the possibility of a poisoning, particularly with organophosphate pesticides.

Drooling, reflecting an inability to contain saliva, occurs in many central nervous system or muscular disorders and needs to be distinguished from increased salivation. Excessive salivation may result in drooling.

PHYSIOLOGIC FACTORS

Teething

Irritation of the gums associated with eruption of teeth causes increased salivation.

Reaction to Foods

Ingestion, sight, or smell of certain foods, particularly spicy or heavily seasoned ones, may increase salivary flow.

Nausea

Any condition causing the sensation of nausea may result in increased salivation, including the morning sickness of pregnancy.

Smoking

Excessive smoking may cause increased salivary flow.

PATHOLOGIC CONDITIONS

Oropharyngeal Lesions

Any oropharyngeal irritation, whether chemical or from infection, can cause increased salivation. In some of these disorders, pain or difficulty in swallowing results in drooling as well. The lesions include gingivostomatitis, aphthous ulcers, dental caries, tonsillar inflammation, peritonsillar and retropharyngeal abscesses, epiglottitis, supraglottitis, and foreign bodies.

Gastroesophageal Reflux

Irritation may stimulate increased salivation.

DRUGS AND CHEMICALS

Various substances may enhance salivation including iodides, histamine, pilocarpine, acetylcholine, methacholine, nicotinic acid, sympathomimetics, mercurial compounds, and organophosphates. Poisoning with organophosphate compounds must always be considered in a child or adult with rather sudden onset of symptoms that include increased sweating, salivation, tearing, coughing, difficulty in breathing, vomiting, diarrhea, weakness, convulsions, coma, and others. The symptoms of acrodynia caused by mercury poisoning include irritability, muscle hypotonia, photophobia, a generalized pink rash, excessive sweating, and painful extremities. Other poisonings causing increased salivation include mushrooms, arsenic, and thallium.

EMOTIONAL STRESS

Pleasurable excitation or, in some individuals, other forms of stress may result in increased salivation.

DROOLING

Central Nervous System and Muscular Disorders

Drooling due to defective swallowing coordination rather than increased salivation is common in neurologic diseases such as cerebral palsy and demyelinating disorders. Children with chorea and encephalitis as well as those with various myopathies and bulbar palsies also drool excessively.

Mental Retardation

Excessive drooling is not uncommon.

Esophageal Obstruction

The appearance of increased salivation is mostly due to inability to swallow secretions. In newborns, esophageal atresia must be a primary consideration in an infant with increased secretions; in later infancy and childhood, an esophageal foreign body is an important possibility. (See Chapter 45, Dysphagia.)

Juvenile Rheumatoid Arthritis

Temporomandibular joint involvement may result in excessive drooling.

Allergies

Children with allergies may drool excessively.

Riley-Day Syndrome (Familial Dysautonomia)

Drooling is a minor symptom compared with dysphagia, recurrent pneumonitis, fevers, postural hypotension, insensitivity to pain, and various other signs. Affected children have increased saliva production as well as drooling.

Rabies

47

Decreased Salivation

A reduction in the production of saliva results in dryness of the mouth (xerostomia). This is a relatively uncommon symptom in childhood and, when present, is most commonly caused by mouth-breathing or mild dehydration secondary to fever or exercise. Drug use and psychogenic disorders must also be considered.

PHYSIOLOGIC CAUSES

Dehydration

The dryness of the mouth may be more severe than would be expected with the degree of clinical dehydration.

Fever

Mouth-Breathing

Mouth-breathing may be a habit but more often is a result of nasopharyngeal obstruction due to adenoidal hypertrophy, allergies, or upper respiratory infection.

Exercise

DRUGS

Xerostomia may be produced by the following: atropine, belladonna, antihistamines, amphetamines, tricyclic antidepressants, opiates, phenothiazines, ergotamine, and phenylbutazone. Dryness of the mouth may be a clue to drug addiction with narcotics or amphetamines in adolescents or young adults.

NEOPLASMS

Primary tumors involving the salivary glands as well as infiltrative neoplasms may disrupt the flow of saliva.

OBSTRUCTION OF SALIVARY DUCTS

A reduction in salivary flow may result from ductal obstruction by stones, tumors, inflammation, or scarring.

PSYCHOGENIC FACTORS

Dryness of the mouth commonly occurs during acute stressful or anxiety provoking situations. Chronic dryness suggests a hysterical trait or depression.

CONGENITAL DISORDERS

Anhidrotic Ectodermal Dysplasia

Sparse hair, an inability to sweat, dryness of the nose, dental abnormalities, and thin, depigmented skin are characteristic of this disorder.

Idiopathic Dry Mouth

This is a distinctly rare disorder in which the mucous membranes of the mouth become glazed, the mouth dry and filled with keratinaceous material.

MISCELLANEOUS CAUSES

Sjögren Syndrome

This condition is characterized by xerostomia and dry eyes (keratoconjunctivitis sicca) with or without manifestations of other autoimmune disorders, most commonly rheumatoid arthritis. The salivary glands may be enlarged.

Salivary Gland Inflammation

The inflammation may be secondary to mumps, sarcoidosis, or tuberculosis.

Central Nervous System Disorders

Multiple sclerosis is a rare cause of dry mouth in the pediatric age group.

Vitamin A Deficiency

Dryness of the eyes with loss of night vision and photophobia is more common than dry mouth.

Hypothyroidism

Uremia

Diabetes Insipidus

Xerostomia is probably secondary to fluid losses.

Progressive Systemic Sclerosis

Botulism

Progressive weakness, ophthalmoplegias, and difficulty in swallowing are more prominent symptoms.

Mikulicz Syndrome

This refers to enlargement of salivary and lacrimal glands due to leukemic infiltration.

Acquired Postganglionic Cholinergic Dysautonomia

This rare disorder of unknown cause is characterized by bilateral internal ophthalmoplegia; lack of tears, saliva, and sweat; atony of the bowel and bladder and normal adrenergic function.

SUGGESTED READING

Deprettere AJ, Van Acker KJ, De Clerk LS, Docx MK, Stevens WJ, Van Bever HP. Diagnosis of Sjögrens syndrome in children. *Am J Dis Child* 1988;142:1185–1187.

48

Hoarseness

Hoarseness is the most important sign of laryngeal disease. The abnormal quality of the voice is usually the result of changes in the mass of the vocal cords or of disorders that interfere with the approximation of the edges of the cords. In infants, the cry may be hoarse because of anatomic abnormalities or cord paralysis. Larnygeal papillomas are an important cause of hoarseness in children between the ages of 1 and 4 years. In the immediate preschool and school-age groups, vocal cord nodules associated with voice misuse are by far the most common cause. Thereafter, larnygitis is most common.

♦ **Most Common Causes of Hoarseness**

   Acute Laryngitis   Laryngotracheitis
   Vocal Cord Nodules

● **Causes Not to Forget**

   Angioedema   Vocal Cord Paralysis
   Laryngeal Papillomas

INFECTIOUS CAUSES

♦ Acute Laryngitis

   Laryngitis is often preceded by or associated with an upper respiratory tract infection. Hoarseness is the chief complaint and fairly sudden in onset. Cough and pain are also common symptoms.

♦ Laryngotracheitis and Laryngotracheobronchitis

   Children with croup commonly have hoarseness and a barking cough before the onset of stridor. Spasmodic croup is usually more acute in onset and is less likely to be preceded by signs of an upper respiratory tract infection.

Postnasal Drip

   Children with acute or chronic postnasal drip caused by upper respiratory infection, sinusitis, or allergies often awaken with a hoarse voice.

Epiglottitis

The voice sounds muffled rather than hoarse. The symptoms of difficulty in swallowing, drooling, and sore throat come on rather quickly with progressive severity.

Laryngeal Diphtheria

The onset of laryngeal signs is usually preceded by a 3- or 4-day period of upper respiratory tract infection, often with a serosanguineous nasal discharge. A posterior pharyngeal membrane may be present.

Tuberculosis

The vocal cords may become distorted by tuberculous nodules.

Tetanus

TRAUMA

♦ Vocal Nodules

Misuse of the voice by excessive shouting or singing is relatively common in children. Tiny hemorrhages in the vocal cords are replaced by fibrous nodules. Hoarseness is the major complaint.

Postintubation Hoarseness

A period of hoarseness and, in young children, stridor commonly follows endotracheal intubation.

Sicca Syndrome

Children with disorders such as cystic fibrosis, ectodermal dysplasia, or collagen-vascular diseases in which mucus and salivary secretions are deficient or abnormal may become hoarse. This symptom is relieved by sips of water. Transient hoarseness may occur in very dry environments or during antihistamine or decongestant drug therapy.

Foreign Body

Hoarseness occurring after a sudden bout of choking suggests this possibility.

Hemorrhage in Vocal Cords

Occurrence is rare in coagulation disorders but has been reported following external or internal trauma, the latter during intubation attempts.

Laryngeal Fracture

Fracture may follow trauma from falls, auto accidents, clothesline injuries, or strangulation attempts. Hoarseness and cough are present immediately after the trauma; dyspnea and dysphagia are common.

Abnormal Arytenoid Cartilage

Displacement of the cartilage may be the result of trauma or may occur congenitally. Hoarseness and stridor are commonly present.

TUMORS

Vocal Cord Polyps

Polyps may develop following prolonged vocal abuse or trauma. The hoarseness may be intermittent.

Hemangioma

These tumors are most likely to appear in the first 2 years of life. Cutaneous hemangiomas may also be present.

● Laryngeal Papillomas

These tumors are seen most frequently in children between 1 and 4 years of age. Hoarseness and loss of voice generally occur first, but difficulty in breathing may develop if the lesions enlarge and obstruct the airway. The papillomas are not malignant but can be life-threatening. This diagnosis must always be considered in young children with persistent hoarseness.

Laryngeal Carcinoma

This lesion is distinctly uncommon in children, but any adult with hoarseness for more than 2 to 3 weeks should undergo laryngoscopic examination.

NEUROLOGIC DISORDERS

● Vocal Cord Paralysis

Stridor, respiratory distress, and feeding difficulties are the common symptoms of bilateral or unilateral cord paralysis in infants; the cry is usually hoarse. In older children, hoarseness tends to be a more prominent symptom. Some causes are:

Central Nervous System Malformation

The Arnold-Chiari malformation may be associated with hoarseness by causing vocal cord paralysis.

Posterior Fossa Tumor

Aberrant Great Vessels

A double aortic arch or abnormally placed subclavian artery may impinge on the recurrent laryngeal nerve.

Left Heart Failure

Hoarseness may be caused by pressure of an enlarged left pulmonary artery or left atrium on the recurrent laryngeal nerve.

Histoplasmosis

Enlarged hilar nodes may entrap the laryngeal nerve and produce hoarseness.

Cardiovocal Syndrome

Left recurrent laryngeal nerve paralysis associated with congenital heart disease. A weak cry and chronic hoarseness are presenting clues.

Bulbar Poliomyelitis

Other signs of pharyngeal dysfunction are also present.

Thiamine Deficiency (Beriberi)

Hyperesthesias and areflexia are early signs, as is hoarseness in infants. Edema and cardiac involvement with tachycardia and cardiomegaly are common.

ALLERGIC REACTION

● **Angioedema**

Hoarseness associated with signs of oropharyngeal edema is a warning of possible impending airway obstruction.

ANATOMIC ABNORMALITIES

Laryngomalacia

Also known as congenital laryngeal stridor, this disorder represents an anomaly of the larynx with laxity of the pharyngeal tissues. The epiglottis, arytenoids, and arytenoepiglottic folds are drawn into the airway during inspiration resulting in partial obstruction. Stridor is the major sign.

Laryngeal Web

Stridor and a weak cry are more common findings in this congenital abnormality.

Subglottic Stenosis

Commonly the sequelae of traumatic or prolonged intubation in the neonatal period.

Laryngeal Cyst

HYSTERICAL

This is an unusual cause in children. The cords are abnormally adducted during speech and coughing. Onset is usually sudden.

MISCELLANEOUS CAUSES

Gastroesophageal Reflux

In severe cases, children may manifest chronic cough and hoarseness.

Hypothyroidism

The voice or cry may take on a hoarse quality in untreated infants.

Hypocalcemia

Infants with tetany secondary to hypocalcemia may have a hoarse cry and stridor.

De Lange Syndrome

The cry of infants with this striking syndrome is growling and coarse. The infants are hirsute, have a distinctive facies, and often have limb reduction defects.

Williams Syndrome

Children with this syndrome have an elflike facies, failure to thrive, and a metallic-sounding voice.

Cricoarytenoid Arthritis

Rarely, a child with juvenile rheumatoid arthritis may have involvement of the cricoarytenoid. Symptoms also include stridor, a feeling of fullness in the throat on swallowing, and referred ear pain.

Gaucher Disease

In the acute or infantile form, the presenting picture is that of pseudobulbar palsy with strabismus, swallowing problems, laryngeal spasm, developmental retardation, and hepatosplenomegaly.

Farber Disease

Hoarseness and stridor may appear at any time in the first few weeks of life. Palpable nodules develop in the skin, painful swellings occur in multiple joints, and hepatomegaly and central nervous system deterioration eventually occur.

Lipoid Proteinosis

Significant hoarseness is a common early symptom that results from lipid deposition in the vocal cords. The tongue and lips become thickened, and papules develop on the skin along with areas of atrophic scarring.

Mucolipidosis II (I-Cell Disease)

Most patients have coarse facial features similar to those seen in Hurler syndrome, along with severe skeletal changes, psychomotor retardation, and frequent respiratory infections.

Amyloidosis

Deposition of amyloid in the vocal cords results in hoarseness.

SUGGESTED READING

Kenna MA. Hoarseness. *Pediatr Rev* 1995;16:69–72.
Waring JP, Lacayo L, Hunter J, Katz E, Suwak B. Chronic cough and hoarseness in patients with severe gastroesophageal reflux disease. Diagnosis and response to therapy. *Dig Dis Sci* 1995;40:1093–1097.

49

Premature Loss of Teeth

The primary (deciduous) or secondary (permanent) teeth may become loose or may be lost for various reasons. Although trauma is the most common cause of tooth loss, this sign may be a prominent clue suggesting the presence of any of several disorders. The loss of one or more primary teeth before age 5 years should suggest the need for evaluation of an underlying cause, while the loss before age 3 years is definitely an indication for additional evaluation (1). Healthy individuals should not lose their permanent teeth. Defects of white blood cells, motility, adhesion, etc., may be the cause of underlying periodontitis, which results in the early loss of teeth.

TRAUMA

During childhood, injury is the most common cause of premature loss or loosening of teeth. Child abuse must always be kept in mind if other suspicious signs and symptoms are present and the explanation of the injury is not consistent with the findings.

ENDOCRINE AND METABOLIC CAUSES

Juvenile Diabetes Mellitus

The loss of teeth is associated with severe oral infections.

Hyperthyroidism

Atrophy of the alveolus with loss of primary teeth may occur.

Hypoparathyroidism

Tetany, hyperreflexia, and seizures are the result of hypocalcemia. The teeth may erupt late but are lost early.

Hypophosphatasia

The clinical picture and radiographic findings are similar to those in rickets. Bone fails to mineralize normally. The early loss of deciduous teeth is an important sign. The serum alkaline phosphatase is low, and increased phosphoethanolamine levels are found in the urine.

Hyperpituitarism

As the mandible grows excessively, the teeth may become separated and loose.

Osteopetrosis

The bones become thick and dense with eventual obliteration of the bone marrow and cranial nerve compression.

Hypophosphatemic Rickets

This inherited abnormality of renal tubular transport is characterized by short stature and bowing of the legs in boys. Loosening of the teeth may be the first clinical indication of the disorder.

HEMATOLOGIC DISORDERS

Leukemia

The gingiva may be swollen and infiltrated with leukemic cells, resulting in a loosening of the teeth. Gingival involvement is more common in acute myelocytic leukemia.

Cyclic Neutropenia

Loosening of the teeth may occur after repeated episodes of oral ulceration associated with the neutropenia, which occurs at about 21-day intervals.

Leukocyte Adhesion Deficiency

Disorders of white cells should be considered as an underlying cause of periodontal disease.

INFECTION AND INFLAMMATION

Periodontitis

Prepubertal periodontitis occurs before age 4 years. It may be localized or generalized. The latter may be associated with otitis media and recurrent infections. In some children white cell defects may be found. Juvenile periodontitis, which occurs in adolescents and young adults, may be inherited.

Osteomyelitis

Mandibular or maxillary osteomyelitis may cause loosening of teeth in the involved area.

Noma (Gangrenous Stomatitis)

This disorder is a rare progressive infection of fusospirochetal origin that occurs in debilitated patients. Gangrenous ulcers develop and spread over the gums and buccal mucosa.

POISONINGS

Acrodynia

This unusual syndrome is the result of mercury poisoning. Affected children are listless, irritable, and hypertonic; they sweat excessively and develop various rashes, often with erythema of the extremities and face. Photophobia and hair loss are common, but loss of teeth occurs only in severe cases.

Arsenic Poisoning

Symptoms of chronic arsenic poisoning include gradual increasing weakness, anorexia, intermittent vomiting, diarrhea or constipation, conjunctival congestion, and stomatitis.

DYSMORPHIC SYNDROMES

Down Syndrome

The early loss of teeth is a result of periodontal disease, which is a common finding. The anterior mandibular region teeth are most commonly affected.

Progeria

A striking disorder, usually evident within the first year, with short stature, alopecia, and other features of aging, including atherosclerosis in the first decade of life.

Werner Syndrome

Another syndrome of early onset of aging. Affected children fail to show an adolescent growth spurt. The skin is thin and atrophic and there is loss of subcutaneous fat.

Coffin-Lowry Syndrome

Early loss of teeth has been described in this syndrome that features mental retardation, coarse features, short stature, and thick, soft hands.

Hajdu-Cheney Syndrome

Early loss of teeth from resorption of the alveolar process is one of the bony abnormalities, which include osteopenia with fractures, acroosteolysis of the digits, and short stature.

Singleton-Merten Syndrome

Affected individuals have skeletal deformities, including ligament ruptures, joint subluxation, short stature, and glaucoma. Early loss of primary and permanent teeth may occur.

MISCELLANEOUS DISORDERS

Langerhans Cell Histiocytosis (Histiocytosis X)

Gingival swelling and tooth disruption is most common in the Hand-Schuller-Christian form of the disease but also occurs in the Letterer-Siwe disease form. The radiologic appearance is referred to as "floating teeth."

Gaucher Disease

In the chronic or adult form, premature loss of teeth is overshadowed by splenomegaly, bone pain, joint swelling, and pathologic fractures.

Familial Dysautonomia

In this rare disorder, findings suggestive of autonomic nervous system dysfunction include abnormal temperature control, absent lacrimation, postural hypotension, indifference to pain, and recurrent pulmonary infection. Grinding of the teeth is responsible for early loss.

Papillon-Lefèvre Syndrome

The principal features of this uncommon disorder are hyperkeratosis of the palms and soles and destruction of the periodontal ligaments with early loss of teeth. The gingivae are red, swollen, and friable.

Pachyonychia Congenita Syndrome

The nails become progressively thickened. The palms and soles often are hyperkeratotic.

Cherubism

Bony structures, especially maxillary, are involved with over expansion leading to displacement of the eyes producing an appearance of upward gaze. The primary and permanent teeth may be exfoliated.

Scurvy

The gums are swollen and fragile, the extremities are painful because of subperiosteal hemorrhage, and petechial hemorrhages occur in the skin.

Acatalasemia

This rare disorder due to lack of catalase in the blood is seen most commonly in Japanese persons. The presenting symptom is painful ulcers around the teeth. Alveolar gangrene and atrophy ensue, with eventual loosening and loss of teeth.

Ehlers-Danlos Syndrome (Type VIII)

This is also known as the periodontal form. There is variable hyperextensibility of the skin, easy bruising, and thin scars.

REFERENCE

1. Hartsfield JK Jr. Premature exfoliation of teeth in childhood and adolescence. *Adv Pediatr* 1994; 41:453–470.

SUGGESTED READING

Shusterman S. Pediatric dental update. *Pediatr Rev* 1994;15:311–318.

50
Delayed Dentition

The first primary (deciduous) teeth usually erupt between 6 and 7 months of age, and by 2 years of age, all 20 deciduous teeth have appeared. Various disorders may interfere with the normal sequence of dental development. Although failure of the dentition to appear by 1 year of age is considered to be a bona fide delay, this finding is a normal variation in a small percentage of children.

Dental eruption reflects bone maturation and provides the opportunity to assess "bone age" clinically. As with delayed bone maturation and growth, the most common causes of delayed appearance of dentition are normal variations, endocrine or metabolic disturbances, and Down syndrome.

♦ **Most Common Causes of Delayed Dentition**

Normal Variation   Down Syndrome
Disorders with Delayed Linear Growth

♦ **NORMAL VARIATION**

The appearance of the first tooth may be delayed until after the first birthday in some children. Check the family history carefully for similar delayed appearance.

ENDOCRINE AND METABOLIC CAUSES

Vitamin D Deficiency and Vitamin D-Resistant Rickets

Signs of florid rickets may not appear until late in the first year of life in deficiency rickets. Frontal bossing, thickening of the wrists and ankles, rachitic rosary (enlargement of the costochondral junctions), and delayed closure of the anterior fontanel may be early signs. The signs in vitamin D-resistant rickets are more subtle, and tibial bowing may be the earliest sign.

Hypothyroidism

In infants with congenital hypothyroidism, delayed eruption of teeth is one of the manifestations of the disorder. Other signs and symptoms predominate, however.

Hypopituitarism

Infants with congenital hypopituitarism have a delayed onset of teething and also retain their primary teeth longer than normal, sometimes throughout life.

Hypoparathyroidism

In primary hypoparathyroidism, delayed eruption of teeth and early loss may occur. Primary features include tetany, hyperreflexia, and convulsions from hypocalcemia. Other signs are diarrhea, dry scaly skin, brittle nails, alopecia, and recurrent candidal infections.

Pseudohypoparathyroidism

Hypocalcemia is also prominent in this disorder. Features of the unusual phenotype include short stature, moon-shaped facies, obesity, mental retardation, and short metacarpals and metatarsals. In pseudopseudohypoparathyroidism the serum calcium and phosphorus levels are normal.

CHROMOSOMAL ABNORMALITY

♦ Down Syndrome

The primary teeth may not appear until after the second birthday, and they are also retained longer than normal.

INHERITED DISORDERS

Achondroplasia

Although inheritance is autosomal dominant, most cases represent spontaneous mutation.

Osteogenesis Imperfecta

Late eruption of dentition is common in this disorder best known for its fragile bones.

Ectodermal Dysplasias

Various types of ectodermal dysplasia have been described. The hair and nails are affected as well as the skin, which tends to be thin and dry. There may be anodontia or hypodontia with abnormally shaped teeth.

Goltz Syndrome (Focal Dermal Hypoplasia Syndrome)

Areas of the skin may appear hypoplastic or sometimes bulging from the presence of lipomatous nodules. Syndactyly, dystrophic nails, strabismus, and dental abnormalities, including late eruption, are common.

Cleidocranial Dysostosis

Features include macrocephaly with a large anterior fontanel, hypoplastic or aplastic clavicles, and delayed eruption of teeth. The inheritance is autosomal dominant.

Treacher Collins Syndrome

Delayed dentition occasionally occurs. The striking facial features of this condition, inherited as an autosomal-dominant trait, include malar hypoplasia, downslanting palpebral fissures, auricular deformities, and a hypoplastic mandible.

Ellis-van Creveld Syndrome (Chondroectodermal Dysplasia)

In this disorder, inherited as an autosomal-recessive trait, small stature, short limbs, polydactyly, cardiac defects, and nail and teeth abnormalities are characteristic features.

Incontinentia Pigmenti

Verrucous or vesicular lesions, often linear, are present in infancy; later, hyperpigmented patches or swirls appear as the initial lesions disappear. Defects of teeth, eyes, nails, hair, and central nervous system are common. It appears to be lethal in utero to males.

Osteopetrosis

In this rare inherited disorder, the development of dense, thick bone obliterates the cranial foramina, with resulting cranial nerve palsies. Pancytopenia results from bone marrow obliteration.

Amelogenesis Imperfecta

This hereditary defect of tooth structure is characterized by thin or absent enamel and brown teeth, which may wear down early in life.

Gardner Syndrome

Delayed eruption of teeth may be the only noticeable sign in the first decade of life. The other features—polyposis of the colon, epidermal and sebaceous cysts, and bony osteomas—do not appear until the second decade. The inheritance is autosomal dominant.

Fibromatosis Gingivae

Overgrowth of the gingiva may cover the dentition giving the appearance of later eruption.

Dubowitz Syndrome

Findings in this unusual disorder are small stature, mental retardation, mild microcephaly, short palpebral fissures, micrognathia, an eczema-like skin disorder, and a lag in eruption of teeth.

Hunter Syndrome (Mucopolysaccharidosis II)

In this X-linked disorder, coarsening of features is more gradual than in Hurler syndrome.

Progeria

This is a most striking and unusual disorder characterized by premature degeneration of body tissues.

ADDITIONAL SYNDROMES ASSOCIATED WITH DELAYED DENTITION

Aarskog

Angelman

Apert

Cockayne

de Lange

Killian/Teschler-Nicola

Maroteaux-Lamy

Miller-Dieker

Pyknodysostosis

INFECTIONS

Congenital Rubella

Congenital Syphilis

OTHER CAUSES

Serious Systemic Illness

Any serious illness may affect development and growth resulting in delayed dentition.

Hemifacial Atrophy

Phenytoin Therapy

SUGGESTED READING

Jones KL. *Smith's recognizable patterns of human malformation*, 5th ed. Philadelphia: WB Saunders, 1997.
Stewart RE, Poole AE. The orofacial structures and their association with congenital abnormalities. *Pediatr Clin North Am* 1982;29:572–573.

SECTION VII

Neck

51
Nuchal Rigidity

A stiff neck in an ill-appearing child with fever usually indicates the presence of meningitis. A lumbar puncture must be performed immediately and the spinal fluid examined for cells, organisms, and protein and sugar content, as well as plated for culture. Nuchal rigidity is not, however, always the result of meningeal irritation secondary to infection; the history and other features of the physical examination may suggest other causes. If the stiff neck is longstanding, a different differential diagnosis is generated. Meningismus is the term given to a sign suggestive of meningitis, such as nuchal rigidity, when meningitis is not present.

The causes of nuchal rigidity have been divided into six categories: infections, vascular abnormalities, neoplasia, bony or muscular problems, metabolic disorders, and intoxications. Torticollis, a twisting of the neck, may also be associated with neck stiffness (see also Chapter 52, Torticollis).

♦ **Most Common Causes of Nuchal Rigidity**

Meningitis	Cervical Adenitis
Trauma	Meningoencephalitis

● **Causes Not to Forget**

Dystonia from Drugs	Myositis
Juvenile Rheumatoid Arthritis	Guillain-Barré Syndrome

INFECTIONS

♦ Meningitis

Meningeal irritation may be the result of bacterial, viral, Rickettsial, mycobacterial, fungal, or protozoal infections. Particularly in the latter three, the infection may be subacute or chronic, whereas in others the onset of symptoms generally are sudden and dramatic. Examination of the cerebrospinal fluid is essential. Special stains or cultures may be required in nonbacterial or nonviral cases.

♦ Cervical Adenitis

Acute adenitis secondary to pharyngitis or associated with other infections may result in nuchal rigidity. The swelling is tender, and the spinal fluid is normal. Posterior cervical adenitis is more likely than anterior to produce this symptom.

♦ **Meningoencephalitis**

The pathogenetic organism may be any of those that cause meningitis. The onset may also be gradual or sudden. Fever, headache, ataxia, altered sensorium, convulsions, and coma are among the possible symptoms.

● **Guillain-Barré Syndrome**

This condition is characterized by acute ascending motor paralysis, often with sensory changes and cranial nerve involvement. Deep tendon reflexes are usually decreased or absent; slight nuchal pain and rigidity are common.

Pneumonia

Nuchal rigidity may be the presenting sign in upper lobe pneumonia prior to auscultatory evidence.

Retropharyngeal Abscess

Other symptoms are prominent including dysphagia, drooling, and muffled voice. The neck is often held hyperextended. Subluxation of C1 and C2 vertebrae may occur.

Epiglottitis

The sudden onset of sore throat, dysphagia, drooling, and muffled voice, with a toxic appearance, is characteristic. Nuchal rigidity with the generalized illness may suggest meningitis, but a lumbar puncture could be catastrophic, a result of airway obstruction.

Acute Cerebellar Ataxia

The onset of ataxia, especially involving the trunk, may be sudden, or signs may develop gradually. This disorder is most frequent in children between 1 and 4 years of age. Nuchal rigidity, if present, is mild.

Cervical Spine Osteomyelitis

Low-grade fever and slowly increasing pain on neck movement may be the only presenting signs.

Other Common Infections

Tonsillitis	Otitis Media
Influenza	Mycoplasma
Pyelonephritis	Mumps
Hepatitis	Shigellosis
Scarlet Fever	Infectious Mononucleosis
Cat-Scratch Disease	Roseola
Typhoid Fever	Herpes Zoster

Lyme Disease

Aseptic meningitis, encephalitis, and a host of other neurologic symptoms and signs may occur.

Brain Abscess

Signs and symptoms depend on the age of the child and the location and size of the lesion. Initially, headache, fever, and seizures may be present. Signs of increased intracranial pressure may be foremost.

Diskitis

These infections usually affect lumbar and thoracic disks, and rarely cause nuchal rigidity.

Malaria
Trichinosis

Periorbital edema, muscle pain, headache, fever, splinter hemorrhages of the nails, and eosinophilia are common signs.

Epidural Abscess

First symptoms are back pain with localized tenderness, and then nuchal rigidity, fever, and headache. Flaccid paralysis with loss of sensation below the level of the lesion then follows.

Less Common Infections
Lymphocytic Choriomeningitis

There is abrupt onset of fever, headache, vomiting, photophobia, and abdominal pain, with cerebrospinal fluid pleocytosis in which the cells are almost all lymphocytes.

Tetanus

Generalized muscle rigidity with muscle spasms occurs. Trismus (clenched jaw) is the classic sign; convulsions may also occur.

Chagas Disease

The findings of intermittent fever, nonpitting edema, lymphadenopathy, hepatosplenomegaly, urticaria, and behavioral problems suggest this disorder, although it is rare in the United States.

Cryptococcosis

India ink stain may be needed to demonstrate the organism.

Leptospirosis

Conjunctivitis, jaundice, albuminuria, and aseptic meningitis suggest this infection.

Dental Abscess

Postinfectious Encephalomyelitis

Poliomyelitis

Poliomyelitis fortunately has become uncommon but was a scourge of the not too distant past. Affected children have rigidity of the back caused by muscle spasm and nuchal rigidity from the aseptic meningitis.

VASCULAR ABNORMALITIES

Subarachnoid Hemorrhage

Meningeal irritation is present with irritability, severe headache, vomiting, loss of consciousness, and possibly coma.

Cerebral Aneurysms

If subarachnoid hemorrhage occurs, nuchal rigidity may develop. Affected children may have recurrent headaches and, rarely, episodes of nuchal rigidity prior to a massive hemorrhage.

Malformation of the Great Cerebral Vein (Vein of Galen)

Usual signs and symptoms occur after a subarachnoid bleed. Children with this anomaly may have cranial nerve palsies, nystagmus, ataxia, vertigo, and personality changes.

Primary Intracranial Venous Thrombosis

Thrombosis can be secondary to local infections, trauma, generalized sepsis, dehydration, and disorders causing a hypercoagulable state. Onset is often precipitous, with seizures, hemiparesis, lethargy and coma, and changing neurologic signs.

NEOPLASMS

Brain Stem Tumors

The triad of findings is characteristic: cranial nerve involvement, especially the seventh, ninth, and tenth nerves; pyramidal tract signs such as abnormal gait and posture and one hand preference; and signs of involvement of cerebellar pathways, such as ataxia, nystagmus, and occasionally, nuchal rigidity.

Meningeal Leukemia

Invasion of the meninges usually occurs when the child is in bone marrow remission. Progressive headache, nausea, vomiting, papilledema, and sixth nerve palsies may be present.

Posterior Fossa Tumors

Nuchal rigidity is more likely when the tumor extends through the foramen magnum into the upper spinal canal. A head tilt is common. Headache and vomiting may be present for long periods before clumsiness, strabismus, and ataxia occur.

Tumors of the Third Ventricle

Pinealomas, in particular, may have ptosis as the first sign. Paralysis of upward gaze is the classic localizing sign. Nuchal rigidity, other signs of increased intracranial pressure, and ataxia also occur.

Osteoid Osteoma

This tumor may occur in cervical vertebrae. Pain is worse at night and may often be relieved by aspirin. Radiographs show a small radiolucent area with surrounding sclerosis.

Eosinophilic Granuloma

This tumor may also occur in cervical vertebrae, giving rise to neck pain and rigidity. A punched out lesion is seen on radiographic examination.

BONY OR MUSCULAR DISORDERS

♦ Subluxations, Dislocations, and Fractures

Rigidity may be a presenting sign in these lesions of the cervical spine. The sudden onset of torticollis, even without a clear history of trauma, should suggest the possibility of these potentially dangerous lesions.

• Myositis and Fibromyositis

A stiff neck may follow exposure to a cold draft or lying in an unusual posture. Neck muscles are tight and tender to palpation.

Vertebral Anomalies

Congenital block vertebrae, such as the Klippel-Feil syndrome may result in some lack of mobility. The condition is not painful, but is evident on radiographs.

Achondroplasia

Forceful flexion of the neck may result in serious spinal cord injury.

Basilar Impression

Invagination of margins of the foramen magnum results in posterior displacement of the odontoid and compression of the spinal cord or brain stem. Other signs may include ataxia, nystagmus, head tilt, and cortical tract signs.

METABOLIC DISORDERS

Infantile Gaucher Disease

This disease is almost always evident during the first 6 months of life. Hyperextension of the neck, strabismus, increased muscle tone, retardation, splenomegaly, laryngeal spasm, and seizures occur.

Maple Syrup Urine Disease

Rigidity and later opisthotonos occur in the first few days of life. Seizures and increased tone may suggest neonatal tetanus. Urine has the characteristic odor.

Kernicterus

Jaundice, irritability, and a shrill cry along with opisthotonos suggest this disorder.

INTOXICATIONS

• Phenothiazines

Dystonic manifestations from idiosyncratic reactions or overdose include nuchal rigidity, torticollis, opisthotonos, trismus, oculogyric crises, cogwheel rigidity, and other frightening signs. The child is usually awake. Intravenous diphenylhydramine promptly relieves the dystonia.

Strychnine

Poisoning results in extreme rigidity of muscles, often intermittently simulating convulsions. Associated pain is intense. The child is awake.

Lead Poisoning

Methanol Poisoning

Hypervitaminosis A

Bone pain, headache, often associated with pseudotumor cerebri, hepatomegaly, and edema are more typical features.

MISCELLANEOUS CAUSES

• Juvenile Rheumatoid Arthritis

Cervical spine involvement rarely may be a presenting sign of this disorder. The presence of fever and leukocytosis may suggest infection. Other joint involvement may occur later.

Black Widow Spider Bite

Muscle spasm, particularly of the back, shoulders, and thighs, is apparent first. Abdominal pain may be exquisite.

Scorpion Sting

Kawasaki Disease

May be the result of an aseptic meningitis associated with this disease.

Paroxysmal Torticollis

Intussusception

REFERENCE

Stein MT, Trauner D. The child with a stiff neck. *Clin Pediatr* 1982;21:559–563.

52

Torticollis

Torticollis literally means "twisted neck." A head tilt is the primary physical sign, although some of the disorders listed below may be associated with neck stiffness as well.

The cause of torticollis may be as innocuous as exposure to a cold draft. A casual approach to the problem is to be condemned, however, because of the possibility of a vertebral subluxation or dislocation. In these conditions, manipulation of the neck or failure to recognize the injury may result in spinal cord compression with all of its serious consequences. For this reason, cervical spine films are suggested as part of the initial evaluation, particularly if pain or muscle spasm is associated with the torticollis. Information helpful in the differential diagnosis includes age of onset, a history of trauma or preceding infection, and associated systemic symptoms and signs.

Early recognition of congenital causes of torticollis is important to prevent facial asymmetry that occurs from the persistent tilting of the head.

♦ **Most Common Causes of Torticollis**

Congenital Muscular	Traumatic
Upper Respiratory Tract Infection	Cervical Adenitis
Klippel-Feil Syndrome	Ocular (Superior Oblique Palsy)
Myositis	

● **Causes Not to Forget**

Paroxysmal of Infancy	Brachial Plexus Palsy
Sandifer Syndrome (GER)	Posterior Fossa Tumor

CONGENITAL CAUSES

♦ **Muscular Origin**

The exact mechanism of production is unknown but may be a stretching of the sternocleidomastoid (SCM) muscle with resultant localized hematoma. Fibrosis of a portion of the SCM muscle develops with resultant shortening. The head is tilted toward the affected side; the chin is rotated to the opposite side. A "tumor" may be felt in the body of the SCM muscle within the first 10 days of life but disappears in 2 to 6 months. There is a higher incidence in breech and difficult forceps deliveries.

◆ Vertebral Anomalies

Failure of segmentation of vertebrae, hemivertebrae, and the Klippel-Feil syndrome may be associated with torticollis. Cervical spine radiographs are diagnostic. In the Klippel-Feil syndrome, there is a reduction in the number of cervical vertebrae as well as fusion; the neck seems to ride on the shoulders. Sprengel deformity (elevation of the scapula) is often found in association with this anomaly. Torticollis may also be associated with the Arnold-Chiari malformation. Anomalies of the odontoid may result in neck injuries with minor trauma. Children with Down syndrome frequently have odontoid hypoplasia and ligamentous laxity leading to atlantoaxial instability.

● Brachial Plexus Palsy

Torticollis may be part of an injury to the brachial plexus at delivery.

Intrauterine Constraint

During late fetal life the head may be fixed in position by the uterus. The head is oblique in shape and the sternocleidomastoid may undergo fibrosis. Most infants respond with postural manipulation for the restricted neck mobility.

TRAUMA

◆ Subluxation

Trauma may be described as minimal or may not be remembered. Subluxation may occur with sudden turning of the neck.

◆ Dislocation

The C1–C2 instability common in various dwarfism syndromes and bone dysplasias may predispose to dislocation.

◆ Fractures

Fracture of the clavicle as well as of vertebral structures may result in torticollis.

◆ Muscle Injury

◆ Ligamentous Injury

INFECTION

◆ Torticollis Following Upper Respiratory Infection

A spontaneous subluxation may occur about 1 week after an upper respiratory infection, thought to be the result of retropharyngeal edema leading to malposition of the atlas on the axis. Children of 6 to 12 years of age are most frequently affected.

♦ **Cervical Adenitis**

Localized irritation of the SCM muscle may cause spasm.

Pharyngitis

Associated tissue swelling may be severe enough to cause instability of the atlas (C1) on the axis (C2).

Retropharyngeal Abscess

Fever, difficulty in swallowing, and drooling are characteristic.

Pneumonia

Characteristically the upper lobe is involved. Cough, tachypnea, and fever are usual findings.

Osteomyelitis

Pain is usually prominent.

Otitis Media

Mastoiditis

Cervical Diskitis

Lemierre Syndrome

Suppurative thrombophlebitis of the internal jugular vein may present with fever, neck pain, sore throat, and torticollis, as well as pulmonary symptoms from emboli.

Tuberculosis

Vertebrae or soft tissues may be affected.

TUMORS

● **Posterior Fossa Tumor**

Headache, nausea, and vomiting are suggestive findings.

Intraspinal Tumor

This tumor is commonly associated with muscle spasm, back pain, and refusal to flex the neck. Muscle weakness, abnormal reflexes, and sensory losses may also occur.

Osteoid Osteoma

Pain at night, relieved by aspirin, is characteristic.

Eosinophilic Granuloma

Erosion of the vertebral structures may cause symptoms.

NEUROGENIC TORTICOLLIS

Myasthenia Gravis

Poliomyelitis

Focal muscle weakness is responsible for the abnormal head posture.

Dystonia Musculorum Deformans

Affected children exhibit prolonged writhing and twisting motions.

Kernicterus

The neonatal history provides the key to diagnosis. Deafness or choreoathetosis may be present.

Huntington Chorea

Affected children have choreiform movements, but onset of symptoms is generally delayed until adulthood. The disorder is inherited as an autosomal dominant trait.

Hepatolenticular Degeneration (Wilson Disease)

Other dystonic movements are present. Inspection of the irises may reveal the Kayser-Fleischer ring.

Neuritis of Spinal Accessory Nerve

The nerve is tender where it enters the neck, at the lateral border of the upper third of the SCM muscle.

Syringomyelia

OCULAR TORTICOLLIS

◆ Superior Oblique Muscle Weakness

Children with fourth cranial nerve palsy may develop torticollis in an effort to prevent diplopia.

Congenital Nystagmus

Refractive Errors

Strabismus

MISCELLANEOUS CAUSES

♦ Myositis or Fibromyositis

This is a fancy name for the common stiff neck following exposure to a cold draft. Neck muscles are tender and painful.

● Reflux Esophagitis

The curious phenomenon of neck torsion without stiffness associated with hiatal hernia is known as Sandifer syndrome.

Juvenile Rheumatoid Arthritis

Cervical spine involvement may result in subluxation of C1 on C2.

Spasmus Nutans

Head nodding, tilt, and nystagmus are the characteristic findings; onset is before 6 months of age.

● Paroxysmal Torticollis

Onset is between 2 and 8 months of age. Episodes last a few hours to 3 days; pallor, vomiting, and agitation may accompany the attacks. A relationship to migraine should be considered.

Drug Induced

Phenothiazines may cause oculogyric crises, dystonia, opisthotonos, or trismus. Unless the overdose was large, the patient is awake and can obey commands. Dystonic reactions may occur with chlorpromazine (Thorazine), droperidol, fluphenazine, haloperidol, metoclopramide (Reglan), prochlorperazine (Compazine), thiethylperazine, thioridazine (Mellaril), thiothixene, trifluoperazine (Stelazine), and trimethobenzamide (Tigan).

Ligamentous Laxity

Laxity of the transverse ligament may be seen in patients on long term oral steroid therapy. Subluxation or dislocation may occur with minimal or no trauma.

Functional Torticollis

This is rare in children.

Polymyositis

Calcification of Intervertebral Disks

In this rare disorder of unknown etiology, the temperature may be mildly increased; there is local tenderness with muscle spasm. Fluffy calcification of the nucleus of the disk is noted on radiographs 1 to 2 weeks after onset.

Fibrodysplasia Ossificans Progressiva

Onset of symptoms of this rare disorder is generally before 10 years of age. Lumpy, hard masses are palpable in the neck.

SUGGESTED READING

Ballock RT, Song KM. The prevalence of nonmuscular causes of torticollis in children. *J Pediatr Orthop* 1996;16:500–504.

Epps HR, Salter RB. Orthopedic conditions of the cervical spine and shoulder. *Pediatr Clin North Am* 1996;43:919–931.

Jones MC. Unilateral epicanthal fold: diagnostic significance. *J Pediatr* 1986;108:702–704.

Lipson EH, Robertson WC. Paroxysmal torticollis of infancy: familial occurrence. *Am J Dis Child* 1978;132:422–423.

Murphy WJ, Gellis SS. Torticollis with hiatus hernia: Sandifer syndrome. *Am J Child* 1977;131:564–565.

SECTION VIII

Chest

53

Chest Pain

The symptom of chest pain in children occurs considerably less frequently than abdominal or limb pain; however, pain in the chest may suggest a more ominous underlying cause to the child or parent than abdominal or limb pain. In a study of 43 children with chest pain, 52% of the children or their parents thought that heart problems were the basis of the symptom, but none of the children actually had cardiac problems (1).

A prospective study of 407 children presenting with chest pain to an emergency department ascribed 21% as idiopathic, musculoskeletal origin 15%, cough 10%, and costochondritis 9% (2). Psychogenic causes were felt to be responsible for 9%, asthma 7%, and trauma 5%. Cardiac findings, almost all mitral valve prolapse, were present in 4% of the children, but they were not necessarily causal. A second report by the same authors of 36% of these children followed over time resulted in a change in their initial diagnosis of chest pain in 34%. Idiopathic pain was assigned to 34%, musculoskeletal pain 11%, asthma 11%, psychogenic 11%, and costochondritis 6% (3).

Although chest pain in adults is a common manifestation of serious underlying problems, in children it infrequently is, as indicated by the studies. Cardiorespiratory causes of chest pain, such as cough, asthma, pneumonia, or heart disease, are more common in young children, while adolescents are more likely to have psychogenic causes of the pain.

In the evaluation of chest pain, the presence or absence of other signs and symptoms should allow clear definition of the etiology of the problem or at least should limit the diagnostic possibilities to a few probable causes.

♦ **Most Common Causes of Chest Pain**

Musculoskeletal: Trauma, Strain   Asthma
Psychogenic   Cough
Costochondritis   Pneumonia
Esophagitis   Sickle Cell Disease

● **Disorders Not to Forget**

Pneumothorax   Myocarditis

CHEST WALL LESIONS

♦ Blunt Injury

The pain may be localized to an area of soft-tissue injury or rib fracture or may be located at costochondral junctions. The history is an important key to diagnosis, as is cutaneous evidence of trauma.

♦ Muscle Strain

A careful history of preceding activities that may have resulted in muscle strain should be obtained. The strain may involve the pectoral, trapezius, latissimus dorsi, serratus anterior and shoulder muscles, and the coracoid process.

♦ Trauma Secondary to Coughing

Protracted or severe coughing as with asthma or bronchitis may produce muscle strain and, occasionally, a rib fracture.

♦ Costochondritis (Tietze Syndrome)

Swelling of one or two costochondral junctions, along with localized pain, is found. The cause is unknown, and the pain and swelling may last for months.

Pubertal Breast Development

Girls and boys may have unilateral tenderness as the nubbin of tissue develops.

Herpes Zoster

Pain in a dermatome distribution may occur days before the appearance of cutaneous vesicles.

Tumors or Infiltrative Processes

Localized swelling or pain in the chest wall without obvious cause mandates a chest film.

Juvenile Rheumatoid Arthritis

Involvement of the costoclavicular joint rarely may be a presenting sign. Pleuritic chest pain is not uncommon.

Slipping Rib Syndrome

This disorder usually is produced by trauma to the costal cartilages of the 8th, 9th, and 10th ribs. The medial fibrous attachments of the ribs are inadequate or ruptured allowing the cartilage tip to slip superiorly and impinge on the intercostal nerve. Pain on palpation is usually present. A hooking maneuver, inserting the fingers under the rib and pulling forward, will reproduce the pain.

Juvenile Ankylosing Spondylitis

Costochondral and costovertebral pain may be present.

Xiphoid Process Syndrome

Pain may be increased by deep breathing.

Cervical Ribs

Symptoms often follow excessive exertion or trauma. Pain often radiates to the arms. Paresthesias are common.

Scalenus Anticus Syndrome

Pain is increased on abduction of the arm.

Costoclavicular Compression Syndrome

Pain is a result of distortion of the thoracic outlet causing compression of the brachial plexus. Paresthesias and signs of vascular compression are often present.

Trichinosis

The combination of muscle pain, periorbital edema, and eosinophilia suggests this diagnosis.

CARDIOVASCULAR DISORDERS

♦ **Sickle Cell Anemia**

Chest pain probably is the result of vascular occlusion.

● **Myocarditis**

A worrisome cause. Shortness of breath may accompany the chest discomfort. The heart sounds may be muffled, tachycardia and a gallop present, as well as fever.

Pericarditis

The pain is usually precordial, dull, increased during inspiration, and sometimes referred to the left shoulder. The pain tends to improve when the child sits up and leans forward. Viruses are responsible for most cases, but collagen vascular diseases, especially systemic lupus erythematosus and juvenile rheumatoid arthritis, are important causes.

Arrhythmias

Chest pain or discomfort may occur during supraventricular tachycardia, ventricular tachycardia, or any arrhythmia affecting coronary artery flow.

Structural Abnormalities

Mitral Valve Prolapse (Barlow Syndrome)

This possibility should be considered in children with an apical, late systolic murmur as well as chest pain. Before blaming mitral valve prolapse as the cause, note that mitral valve prolapse is no more common in children with chest pain than in the general population.

Aortic Stenosis

Severe stenosis may result in decreased coronary artery blood flow and pain.

Pulmonary Stenosis

Severe stenosis may result in chest pain, especially during exercise.

Hypertrophic Cardiomyopathy

Pneumopericardium

A loud, metallic, splashing sound synchronous with the heart sounds may be heard on auscultation. A chest radiograph should confirm the diagnosis.

Rheumatic Fever

Precordial pain may occur during the illness. The Jones criteria must be satisfied to make this diagnosis.

Pulmonary Vascular Obstruction

A pulmonary embolus or infarction produces sudden chest pain and anxiety.

Myocardial Ischemia

This is a distinctly uncommon cause of pain in children unless there is an underlying cardiac defect or coronary artery disease. Consider anomalous coronary arteries, Kawasaki disease sequelae, and longstanding diabetes mellitus.

Chronic Pulmonary Hypertension

Pain may be present on exercise and relieved by rest. The pulmonic component of the second sound is accentuated. Congenital heart disease with increased pulmonary blood flow is the most common cause.

Dissecting Aortic Aneurysm

In children, the initial symptom may be either chest or back pain. This lesion may be associated with the congenital syndromes described subsequently.

Marfan Syndrome

Arachnodactyly, dislocated lenses, pectus carinatum, scoliosis, and other features may be present.

Ehlers-Danlos Syndrome

Manifestations in affected children vary, ranging from hyperextensible joints to cutaneous laxity.

Pericardial Defect

Herniation of the left atrial appendage through the defect produces sharp pain. Recurrent pleural effusions are common. Echocardiography will confirm the diagnosis.

Takayasu Arteritis

The acute phase is characterized by fever, anorexia, weight loss, joint pain, and hypertension.

Pheochromocytoma

Up to 40% of children with this tumor complain of chest or abdominal pain. Hypertension may be paroxysmal or sustained. Tachycardia, palpitations, headache, sweating, and pallor are other findings.

PULMONARY AND PLEURAL DISORDERS

♦ Asthma

The chest pain may be due to muscle strain, pneumothorax or pneumomediastinum, anxiety or hypoxia. Exercise-induced asthma may be a more common cause than recognized in reported reviews of chest pain.

Pleurisy

♦ Pneumonia

Inflammation of the pleural surface of the lung causes a "catching" chest pain during inspiration as the pleural surfaces rub together.

Primary Infection (Bacterial, Viral, or Tuberculous)

The pleural surface may be involved with little parenchymal disease. The pain is increased on inspiration.

Epidemic Pleurodynia (Devil's Grip)

The pain is sharp, stabbing, and accentuated on inspiration. Coxsackie B virus is the usual pathogenic organism.

Familial Mediterranean Fever

Although abdominal pain is more common, any serosal surface may be involved. The pain is sharp, usually lasts a few days, and is recurrent. The family history is important.

Familial Angioneurotic Edema

Chest pain may occur, but more frequent are recurrent episodes of swelling of the extremities and, occasionally, of the tongue and airway structures.

Systemic Lupus Erythematosus

The polyserositis may involve the pleura.

● Pneumothorax

Chest pain may occur with a spontaneous pneumothorax or as a result of a pneumothorax associated with asthma or trauma.

Pneumomediastinum

Crepitus may be noted at the suprasternal notch. Auscultation may reveal a crunching sound, similar to that of walking through snow with a thin film of ice.

Diaphragmatic Irritation

Shoulder pain usually results because the middle and anterior parts of the diaphragm are innervated by the phrenic nerve. A ruptured spleen is the classic cause of left shoulder pain, whereas the right hemidiaphragm may be irritated by a subphrenic abscess, a hepatic abscess, a tumor, or the perihepatitis of the Fitz-Hugh-Curtis syndrome (associated with gonococcal or chlamydial infection).

Tracheitis

Irritation of the trachea may produce a substernal chest pain.

Precordial Catch (Stitch; "Texidor's Twinge")

A sudden, brief catch of pain is common. It occurs in the left lower anterior aspect of the chest, over the heart. It is not associated with exertion. The etiology is unclear.

Cocaine Abuse

The chest pain may be a result of coughing, the development of a pneumomediastinum, or coronary artery spasm.

Interstitial Pneumonitis

Dyspnea on exertion is the first symptom, followed by a dry, nonproductive cough. Anorexia and weight loss ensue. The chest pain may be pleuritic.

Mediastinitis

Mediastinal Tumor

A constant, boring, substernal pain is produced, which may be associated with cough and dysphagia.

Sarcoidosis

Nonspecific chest pain, shortness of breath, a nonproductive cough, and, occasionally, hemoptysis may be the respiratory presentation of symptomatic patients with sarcoidosis. Hilar adenopathy is present in 70% of these cases.

Pulmonary Tumors

ESOPHAGEAL DISORDERS

♦ **Esophagitis**

A much more common cause of chest pain than recognized.

Foreign Body

The pain is usually increased on attempts at swallowing.

Achalasia

Achalasia produces an esophagitis with substernal burning, often worse in the recumbent position.

Ulceration and Strictures

Pain and difficulty in swallowing are primary symptoms.

Esophageal Tear

This may follow pronounced vomiting.

PSYCHOGENIC FACTORS

Hyperventilation

Chest tightness or pain may accompany lightheadedness, headache, acral paresthesias, and carpopedal spasm.

Conversion Reaction

Anxiety and stress may result in the complaint of chest pain, particularly if there is a family member with chest pain related to cardiac disease.

Malingering

Globus Hystericus

The complaint of inability to swallow because of a lump or mass in the throat often has accompanying pain.

NEUROLOGIC DISEASE

Spinal Cord Compression

Pain in the chest may result from impingement on the cord or spinal roots by tumors or abscesses or from compression following vertebral collapse.

EXTRATHORACIC AND REFERRED PAIN

Cholecystitis

Although uncommon in childhood, this inflammation is a notorious mimic of angina in adults.

Pancreatitis

The pain is usually epigastric but may be substernal.

Hiatal Hernia

The substernal pain generally increases in a recumbent position. Esophagitis is common.

Peptic Ulcer

Pancreatic Pseudocyst

Pylorospasm

Pain is usually epigastric but may be over the lower sternum.

Leukemia/Lymphoma

Pain is due to thoracic node involvement.

Nephrolithiasis

Pain may occur in the posterior left lower chest as well as the back, groin, and genitalia.

IDIOPATHIC

REFERENCES

1. Driscoll DJ, Glicklich LB, Gallen WJ. Chest pain in children: a prospective study. *Pediatrics* 1976;57:648–651.
2. Selbst SM, Ruddy RM, Clark BJ, Henretig FM, Santulli T Jr. Pediatric chest pain: a prospective study. *Pediatrics* 1988;82:319–323.
3. Selbst SM, Ruddy R, Clark BJ. Chest pain in children: follow-up of patients previously reported. *Clin Pediatr* 1990;29:374–377.

SUGGESTED READING

Mooney DP, Shorter NA. Slipping rib syndrome in childhood. *J Pediatr Surg* 1997;32:1081–1082.
Mukamel M, Kornreich L, Horev G, Zeharia A, Mimouni M. Tietze's syndrome in children and infants. *J Pediatr* 1997;131:774–775.
Pantell RH, Goodman BW Jr. Adolescent chest pain: a prospective study. *Pediatrics* 1983;77:881–887.
Selbst SM. Chest pain in children. *Pediatr Rev* 1997;18:169–173.
Wiens L, Sabath R, Ewing L, Gowdamarjan R, Portnoy J, Scagliotti D. Chest pain in otherwise healthy children and adolescents is frequently caused by exercise-induced asthma. *Pediatrics* 1992;90:350–353.

54

Gynecomastia

Enlargement of breast tissue in males is common in neonates and adolescents. In both age groups, regression of the enlargement is the rule. In neonates, the gynecomastia invariably disappears, whereas in adolescents the persistence of the swelling, even though for less than 1 to 2 years in 90% of the cases, seems interminable to the young men. Occasionally, the breast enlargement may be so large or last so long that emotional difficulties arise. In some instances, the breast tissue may require surgical removal. Severe gynecomastia, breast tissue more than 4 cm in diameter, may persist into adulthood in up to 4% of adolescent males. Gynecomastia is considered to be a result of an imbalance between circulating estrogens and androgens.

In this chapter, causes of gynecomastia are divided into disorders of either pubertal or prepubertal onset. It is important to ascertain that the enlarged tissue is actually breast parenchyma; a third group of causes of breast enlargement mimicking gynecomastia is, therefore, included.

Braunstein (1) lists the following causes of gynecomastia in patients seeking consultation: idiopathic (25%), acute or persistent due to puberty (25%), drugs (10% to 20%), cirrhosis or malnutrition (8%), primary hypogonadism (8%), testicular tumors (3%), secondary hypogonadism (2%), hyperthyroidism (1.5%), and renal disease (1%).

♦ Most Common Causes of Gynecomastia

Pubertal	Prepubertal	Mimics
Puberty	Transplacental Estrogens	Obesity
Idiopathic	Drugs	
Drugs		
Marijuana		

ONSET DURING OR AFTER PUBERTY

♦ Adolescence (Puberty)

Approximately 70% of boys develop some degree of gynecomastia during adolescence; the peak incidence is between 13 and 15 years of age. The enlargement may be unilateral or bilateral. Generally, the duration of gynecomastia is 1 to 2 years, but in up to 10% it may be as long as 3 to 4 years. Other disorders may cause gynecomastia, but they are uncommon.

♦ Idiopathic

♦ Drugs

Many drugs have been implicated, including digitalis, ketoconazole, metoclopramide, theophylline, sulindac, ergotamine, minoxidil, etretinate, spironolactone, reserpine, phenothiazine, alphamethyldopa, estrogen containing compounds, meprobamate, hydroxyzine, anabolic steroids, androgens, cimetidine, isoniazid, and human chorionic gonadotropin, among others. Smoking marijuana may be associated with breast enlargement. (See reference 2 for additional drug listings.)

Liver Disorders

Gynecomastia may occur in the presence of cirrhosis or liver carcinoma.

Testicular Failure

Failure to produce testicular androgens may be the result of chemotherapy, radiation, cryptorchidism, varicocele, leukemia, and other causes.

Testicular Tumors

Interstitial cell tumors may cause feminization and gynecomastia. Choriocarcinomas of the testes may also cause gynecomastia and are characterized by the presence of large amounts of gonadotropins in the urine. Both kinds of tumors produce unilateral testicular enlargement. Leydig cell tumors secrete increased quantities of estrogens. In Sertoli-cell and sex-cord tumors increased aromatization of estrogen precursors are found.

Klinefelter Syndrome

About one third of boys with this chromosomal abnormality (XXY karyotype) develop gynecomastia during puberty. There is no known phenotypic picture in the preadolescent. Some children may have mental retardation. The small testes are not evident until puberty. Sparse facial hair and a feminine distribution of hair may be present.

Adrenal Tumors

In feminizing adrenal tumors and tumors producing early isosexual maturation with gynecomastia, there are advanced sexual maturation, elevated serum levels of estrogens, and increased urinary 17 ketosteroids. The testes, however, remain small.

Hyperthyroidism

Starvation/Malnutrition

Enlargement primarily appears on recovery.

Renal Disease and Renal Dialysis

Familial Gynecomastia

Reifenstein Syndrome

This condition is characterized by testicular hypoplasia and sclerosis, gynecomastia, and variable degrees of hypospadias.

Kallman Syndrome

Gynecomastia with anosmia, delayed puberty, and testicular atrophy are findings in this rare disorder; transmission is through women who may have anosmia.

Gynecomastia with Hypogonadism and Small Penis

Hyperprolactinemia with galactorrhea is characteristic.

Chromophobe Adenoma of Pituitary

True Hermaphroditism

Gynecomastia in a boy with unilateral cryptorchidism may indicate true hermaphroditism.

Ectopic Production of Human Chorionic Gonadotropin

May be seen in lung, liver, and kidney neoplasms.

Late-Onset Deficiency of Testicular 17-Ketosteroid Reductase

Results in hypogonadism, gynecomastia, and impotence.

Peutz-Jegher Syndrome

A number of males have been described who have developed sex-cord tumors.

PREPUBERTAL ONSET

♦ Neonatal Gynecomastia

Occurrence is common in newborns and is secondary to the transplacental passage of maternal estrogens.

♦ Exogenous Causes

Drugs such as those listed previously may be a cause.

Precocious Puberty

Gynecomastia may occur as part of premature sexual development.

Idiopathic Gynecomastia

This is a rare cause; diagnosis is made by exclusion of other disorders. The condition may be familial and often tends to regress within 1 year.

Liver Disorders

Cirrhosis and carcinomas may cause gynecomastia.

Testicular Tumors

Unilateral testicular enlargement is the primary clue.

Adrenal Tumors

Feminizing tumors accelerate growth and the bone age. Pubic hair may or may not be present. The testes and penis are normal in size for the child's age.

Congenital Adrenal Hyperplasia

Gynecomastia has been described with the 11-β hydroxylase deficiency.

Ectopic Gonadotropin Secreting Tumor

Testicular Feminization Syndrome

Congenital Anorchia

Secondary Testicular Failure

Thyrotoxicosis

Starvation

PSEUDOGYNECOMASTIA

Breast enlargement may not be secondary to hyperplasia of true breast tissue. The following conditions may mimic gynecomastia.

♦ Obesity

Tumors

Lipoma, hemangioma, lymphangioma, neurofibroma, or carcinoma may involve the breast.

Infection

Cellulitis or abscess may cause enlargement.

Fat Necrosis

This condition may ensue following trauma to the breast area.

REFERENCES

1. Braunstein GD. Gynecomastia. *N Engl J Med* 1993;328:490–495.
2. Mahoney CP. Adolescent gynecomastia: differential diagnosis and management. *Pediatr Clin North Am* 1990;37:1389–1404.

SUGGESTED READING

Biro FM, Lucky AW, Huster GA, Morrison JA. Hormonal studies and physical maturation in adolescent gynecomastia. *J Pediatr* 1990;116:450–455.

Rohn RD. Gynecomastia. In: Friedman SB, Fisher M, Schonberg SK, Alderman EM, eds. *Comprehensive adolescent health care*, 2nd ed. St. Louis: Mosby, 1998:1032–1033.

55

Cough

Cough is a common symptom in children. Acute infections, primarily upper respiratory ones, and allergic rhinitis resulting in a postnasal drip are responsible for most coughs. Most causes listed in this chapter produce chronic cough, defined as that lasting more than a few weeks or as recurrent episodes.

Coughing is a reflex that renders an essential protective service: First, it serves to remove substances that may have been accidentally inhaled, and, second, it removes excessive secretions or exudates that may accumulate in the airways. In some cases, cough is produced by extrinsic pressure on airway structures and serves neither of these purposes.

The relative frequency of various causes of chronic coughs differ by age group. In infants, especially neonates, congenital malformations of the airway, pharyngeal incoordination, and gastroesophageal reflux are more common. In preschool and school-aged children asthma, recurrent viral infections, cough variant asthma, environmental irritants, foreign bodies, and sinusitis are most frequent causes. In the prepubertal and adolescent age group, allergic rhinitis, asthma, cough variant asthma, smoking, environmental irritants, and psychogenic coughs are more likely. Pertussis should always be kept in mind. In adults who have had a prolonged cough, for 2 weeks or longer, the prevalence of pertussis was found to be 12.4% to 25% (1).

♦ **Most Common Causes of Chronic Cough**

Infections, Recurrent	Asthma
Cough Variant Asthma	Passive Smoke Exposure
Gastroesophageal Reflux	Allergic Rhinitis/Postnasal Drip
Environmental Irritants	Sinusitis
Pertussis	

● **Disorders Not to Forget**

Cystic Fibrosis	Foreign Body

INFECTION

♦ Upper Respiratory Infection

The common cold is caused by various viruses. Coughing may be produced by pharyngeal irritation, postnasal drip, and other mechanisms.

♦ Bronchitis

Inflammation of the bronchi is most commonly viral in origin, but mycoplasma infection, pertussis, tuberculosis, and secondary bacterial infection may also be causative. In bronchitis, cough is the primary symptom and may initially be dry; later, it becomes loose and productive. Passive smoking may be a cause of chronic bronchitis.

♦ Pneumonia

The majority of pneumonias are also viral in origin. In cases of bacterial origin, the course tends to be more acute and fulminant, sometimes without much cough. Mycoplasma, chlamydia (*Chlamydia trachomatis* in infants; *Chlamydia pnemoniae* in older children), and other organisms may be involved. *Chlamydia trachomatis* pneumonitis, should be considered when an infant between 4 and 18 weeks of age has an afebrile illness with congestion, wheezing, and a distinctive staccato cough. Cytomegalovirus may produce similar symptoms.

♦ Bronchiolitis

Bronchiolitis is generally a disease of young infants primarily caused by viruses, especially respiratory syncytial virus. Tachypnea, wheezing, and cough are typical.

♦ Croup

The croup syndrome has a variety of causes, some of which are infectious. Stridor is a predominant symptom, and the cough is barking in quality.

♦ Sinusitis

Inflammation of the sinus cavities is often associated with a mucoid nasal discharge and postnasal drip, resulting in pooling of secretions in the hypopharynx with cough.

♦ Pertussis

The paroxysmal, repetitive cough of pertussis may last for many weeks. The "whoop" may not be present in young children. Adenovirus and influenza infections also commonly produce prolonged coughs.

Acquired Immunodeficiency Syndrome

Cough may be the result of secondary infections. Of particular concern is *pneumocystis carinii* pneumonia, as well as cytomegalovirus and legionella.

Tuberculosis

Most cases of tuberculosis are asymptomatic. Persistent fever and weight loss may be found. The "classic" bitonal cough and expiratory stridor are rare.

Pleuritis

Localized chest pain accentuated on inspiration is a more common symptom than cough.

Measles

The cough along with coryza, conjunctivitis, and fever followed by the rash completes the typical picture of rubeola. In atypical measles, pulmonary findings are more prominent than is the rash.

Fungal Infection

Histoplasmosis, coccidioidomycosis, and other fungal infections may involve the pulmonary structures, with resultant coughing that is often chronic in nature.

Parasitic Infestation

Cough and wheezing may be prominent during the lung migration phase in visceral larva migrans. In ascariasis, inhalation of the worms as they travel from the esophagus to the hypopharynx may produce coughing.

Psittacosis

Cough generally is not prominent. Fever, malaise, myalgia, and chills are nonspecific symptoms.

Q Fever

This is a rare disease in the United States.

ALLERGY

♦ Rhinitis

Acute or chronic nasal congestion and postnasal drip are common causes of cough. Clinical signs of allergy include allergic "shiners," allergic salute, and Dennies lines (transverse creases on the lower lid).

♦ Asthma

Cough is an integral part of the clinical picture of asthma. Prior to the development of expiratory wheezing, coughing may be the main clue.

◆ Cough Variant Asthma

Cough may be the initial and, occasionally, the only presenting symptom of asthma. Most children who are affected will later have overt asthma. A clinical trial of bronchodilators will be helpful in this diagnosis. In one study of children referred with coughs lasting at least 4 weeks, 39% had this condition (2).

Atelectasis

Recurrent atelectasis commonly develops in asthma due to mucus plugs.

Hypersensitivity Pneumonitis

Various inhalants may trigger recurrent or chronic inflammatory responses with cough and other respiratory symptoms.

Allergic Bronchopulmonary Aspergillosis

This condition may be confused with chronic asthma. A low-grade fever, prolonged wheezing, a peripheral blood eosinophilia, and transient pulmonary infiltrates may be found.

ENVIRONMENTAL IRRITANTS

◆ Dry Air

This is a common cause of coughing that is often overlooked in the differential diagnosis. Dryness of air passages may cause an irritative type cough or result in mucus production and pooling of secretions with a chronic cough, particularly during the winter months when the air in homes lacks proper humidity.

◆ Smoking

The airways may be irritated from tobacco smoke inhaled directly or passively from smoking in the household. Smoke is a common trigger of reactive airways disease.

◆ Fumes

Smoke from tobacco or fireplaces or fumes from chemicals, gases, or paints may trigger coughing following irritation of the airways. Remember glue sniffing.

ASPIRATION

◆ Gastroesophageal Reflux

In infants and young children, recurrent episodes of cough, wheezing or pneumonitis may be associated with aspiration of stomach contents.

- ● **Foreign Body**

  Most foreign bodies are associated with the sudden onset of coughing as they lodge in large airways. Small materials such as seeds or grasses may produce secondary irritation with the clinical picture of asthma or pneumonia. Other findings depend on size, position, and composition of the inhaled body.

Neuromuscular Disorders

Children with various neuromuscular disorders or cricopharyngeal incoordination may experience recurrent episodes of aspiration, particularly during feeding. The cough is wet and often productive.

Hydrocarbons

Ingestion of hydrocarbon containing materials commonly results in aspiration.

Other

Chalasia and achalasia are uncommon causes.

CONGENITAL ANATOMIC DEFECTS

Tracheoesophageal Fistula

In most cases, the onset of symptoms is shortly after birth, with coughing due to aspiration of saliva or feedings.

Tracheomalacia or Bronchomalacia

The lesions may be relatively localized.

Anomalous Blood Vessels

Compression of the trachea or bronchi may produce a cough, often brassy sounding.

Lobar Emphysema

Cough, wheezing, dyspnea, tachypnea, and tachycardia are typical.

Bronchogenic Cyst

These lesions usually are asymptomatic, although in some cases, the cyst may impinge on the bronchi, producing cough.

Pulmonary Sequestration

Recurrent episodes of pulmonary infection, fever, and cough are the usual presenting symptoms.

Tracheal Stenosis

Laryngeal Cleft

Adductor Vocal Cord Paralysis

• **CYSTIC FIBROSIS**

Cystic fibrosis should be included in the differential diagnosis in every child with a chronic cough, particularly when gastrointestinal symptoms are present.

AIRWAY ENCROACHMENT

Mediastinal Tumors

Symptoms occur from airway compression. Stridor or wheezing respiration may be present. A brassy cough may occur if the tumor exerts pressure on the recurrent laryngeal nerve. Lymphomas are best known for this.

Mediastinal Adenopathy

Compression of airway structures by enlarged nodes may occur in various infections and inflammatory disorders.

Pulmonary Tumors

These tumors are rare in childhood. Cough, dyspnea, and signs of obstructive pneumonitis are the most common symptoms.

Hemangiomas

There may also be cutaneous lesions.

Papilloma of Trachea and Bronchi

Dyspnea and stridor are the most common symptoms.

PSYCHOGENIC ORIGIN

Habit Cough (Tics)

There is often a history of school phobia. The cough does not occur during sleep and remains unchanged with exertion, infection, and temperature changes. No systemic symptoms are present. The cough is loud, honking, and very disruptive.

Vocal Cord Dysfunction

Individuals may create adduction of the vocal cords resulting in signs and symptoms of throat tightness, change in voice quality, and airflow obstruction sufficient to cause wheezing, chest tightness, shortness of breath, and cough.

MISCELLANEOUS CAUSES

Exercise Airway Hyperreactivity

This is an important cause of chronic cough that appears not to be mediated through allergic mechanisms. Pulmonary function testing is the most appropriate means of confirming the problem.

Tonsillar Concretions

Whitish balls of dried secretions may accumulate in the tonsillar crypts. They may be dislodged during swallowing and cause episodes of sudden coughing with the production of tiny amounts of this material.

Bronchopulmonary Dysplasia

Infants with this disorder, most commonly prematures who have been mechanically ventilated, commonly have chronic cough.

Auricular Nerve

Stimulation of the auricular branch of the vagus nerve in the external auditory canal by cerumen or a foreign body is an uncommon cause of cough.

Congestive Heart Failure

Other signs and symptoms of failure predominate.

Enlongated Uvula

Rarely, the uvula may drag on the pharyngeal structures, precipitating a cough.

Gilles de la Tourette Syndrome

Cough, with other verbal and motor tics, may support this diagnosis.

Bronchiectasis

This disorder should be considered in the child with chronic cough, persistent atelectasis, and abnormalities on chest roentgenograms despite clinical resolution of infection. It may be associated with measles, pertussis, pneumonia, foreign bodies, cystic fibrosis, and immunodeficiency disorders.

Sarcoidosis

The cough is variable. Bilateral hilar adenopathy is typical on chest roentgenograms.

Pulmonary Emboli

Emboli are uncommon in the pediatric age group. Sudden coughing and dyspnea may occur at the time of embolization.

Interstitial Pneumonitis

The onset of illness is usually insidious. Shortness of breath, tachypnea, and exercise intolerance are typical.

Wegener Granulomatosis

Congenital Immunodeficiency

Children are at risk for recurrent infections.

Immotile Cilia Syndrome

The triad of a productive cough, sinusitis, and otitis has been present in all cases described; in one half, situs inversus was a finding. Infertility is common in affected boys.

Swyer-James Syndrome

This acquired condition follows bronchiolitis obliterans in infancy characterized by repeated bouts of pulmonary infections. A chronic cough may be present and bronchiectasis may occur.

REFERENCES

1. Nennig ME, Shinefield HR, Edwards KM, Black SB, Fireman BH. Prevalence and incidence of adult pertussis in an urban population. *JAMA* 1996;275:1672–1674.
2. Holinger LD. Chronic cough in infants and children. *Laryngoscope* 1986;96:316–322.

SUGGESTED READING

Cloutier MM, Loughlin GM. Chronic cough in children: a manifestation of airway hyperactivity. *Pediatrics* 1981;67:6–12.
Guilbert TW, Taussig LM. "Doctor, he's been coughing for a month. Is it serious?" *Contemp Pediatr* 1998;15:155–172.
Kamei RK. Chronic cough in children. *Pediatr Clin North Am* 1991;38:593–605.
Landwehr LP, Wood RP 2nd, Blager FB, Milgrom H. Vocal cord dysfunction mimicking exercise-induced bronchospasm in adolescents. *Pediatrics* 1996;98:971–974.
Parks DP, Ahrens RC, Humphries CT, Weinberger MM. Chronic cough in childhood: approach to diagnosis and treatment. *J Pediatr* 1989;115:856–862.
Wood RE. Localized tracheomalacia or bronchomalacia in children with intractable cough. *J Pediatr* 1990;116:404–406.
Zitelli BJ. Chronic cough. In: Gartner JC Jr, Zitelli BJ, eds. *Common and chronic symptoms in pediatrics*. St. Louis: Mosby, 1997:189–200.

56

Dyspnea

Normally, breathing is accomplished without a conscious awareness of the effort involved. Dyspnea refers to that condition in which the patient is unpleasantly aware of the work of breathing or in which there is discomfort or difficulty in breathing. Note that children may have an increased rate of breathing (tachypnea) and/or an increased depth of breathing (hyperpnea) without having distress (dyspnea). Dyspnea is both a sign and a symptom: Difficulty in the respiratory effort may be obvious; older children may voice complaints about breathing difficulties. Signs of dyspnea include retractions, use of accessory muscles (e.g., sternocleidomastoid), nasal flaring, and grunting.

The causes of dyspnea are too numerous to list individually. In this chapter, a few important examples are given for each major category; classification is based on the pathophysiologic mechanism involved. The cause of dyspnea does not always reside in the lung. When central nervous system irritation, particularly in meningitis or encephalitis, is the cause, early detection is essential to prevent serious consequences. Metabolic acidosis, with compensatory hyperventilation, may also be mistaken for primary pulmonary disease.

It is also important to try to determine whether the respiratory effort is inspiratory or expiratory: The former suggests disease in the upper or large airways, whereas the latter is indicative of pathologic processes in the smaller airways or lower respiratory tract.

♦ Most Common Causes of Dyspnea

Asthma	Pulmonary Infections
Exercise	Hyperventilation Syndromes
Croup	

INTERFERENCE WITH GAS EXCHANGE

♦ Pulmonary Infections

Gaseous exchange may be impaired in pneumonias of viral, bacterial, fungal, and mycobacterial origin. Air entry may also be compromised. Keep in mind acquired immunodeficiency syndrome with *Pneumocystis carinii* pneumonia.

Aspiration

Gastroesophageal reflux, tracheoesophageal fistula, near drowning, hydrocarbon, and meconium aspiration may result in tissue reactions interfering with gaseous exchange.

Atelectasis

Sickle Cell Disease–Acute Chest Syndrome

Cystic Fibrosis

Pulmonary Edema

Congestive heart failure, allergic pulmonary response, smoke inhalation, and chemical pneumonitis are some of the more common causes.

Neonatal Respiratory Distress Syndrome

Adult Respiratory Distress Syndrome

Pulmonary Fibrosis

Fibrosis resulting in alveolar-capillary block may develop with chronic lung irritation caused by inhalants or oxygen and respirator therapy, or as a consequence of alpha-1-antitrypsin deficiency.

Interstitial Pneumonitis

Various disorders are included under this heading, including lymphocytic interstitial pneumonia associated with humun immunodeficiency virus infection and *Chlamydia trachomatis* pneumonitis in infants.

Idiopathic Pulmonary Hemosiderosis

Recurrent episodes of alveolar hemorrhage may produce attacks of dyspnea, cyanosis, coughing, and hemoptysis.

Sarcoidosis

Pulmonary Lymphangiectasis

May or may not be associated with cardiac disease. The noncardiac associated group may have an early or late onset.

Pulmonary Alveolar Proteinosis

The congenital form is apparent in the newborn period. It is associated with a deficiency of the lung surfactant apoprotein B. The incidence is not known, but it may be responsible for up to 1% of all infant deaths in the first 6 months of life. A sporadic form, rare in children, may be caused by various inciting agents.

INTERFERENCE WITH AIR ENTRY

Bronchial Lumen Compromise

♦ Reactive Airways Disease/Asthma

Bronchiolitis

Foreign Body

There is usually an acute onset of dyspnea, cough, and other pulmonary symptoms.

Upper Airway Obstruction

♦ Croup Syndrome

(See Chapter 59, Stridor.)

Epiglottitis

Adenoidal or Tonsillar Hypertrophy

Compression of Lung

Pneumothorax or Pneumomediastinum

Tumors

If large enough, cysts, teratomas, or other mediastinal growths, including enlarged nodes secondary to malignancies, may compromise pulmonary reserve. Metastatic tumors to lung parenchyma (e.g., Wilms', osteogenic sarcoma) are more common in children than primary lung tumors.

Elevated Diaphragm

The lung may be compressed by elevation the diaphragm caused by abdominal ascites or masses. A diaphragmatic hernia produces the same effect.

Effusions

Lung expansion may be compromised by pleural effusions, empyema, hemothorax, or other fluid collections.

Emphysema

In infants, congenital lobar emphysema may produce early respiratory distress rather than the generalized emphysema seen in adults.

Thoracic Cage Disorders

Flail Chest

Negative pressures cannot be generated to allow air entry.

Body Casts

Thoracic Deformities

Rarely, severe congenital constriction of the thoracic cage occurs, with compromise of pulmonary function. Shwachman and Jeune syndrome are examples.

Extreme Obesity

Painful Breathing

Rib Fracture

Pleurisy

Peritonitis

Kyphoscoliosis

Severe scoliosis may result in respiratory compromise.

CARDIOVASCULAR PROBLEMS

Congenital Heart Disease

Dyspnea is most prominent in disorders with right-to-left shunts that create hypoxic states.

Congestive Heart Failure

Tachycardia, tachypnea, hepatomegaly, and dyspnea are among the earliest signs.

Arrhythmias

Circulation may be compromised as the cardiac pump becomes inefficient. Paroxysmal atrial tachycardia may produce intermittent episodes of dyspnea.

Cardiac Compromise

Pericarditis

Dyspnea and chest pain may be the key symptoms.

Myocarditis

Compromise of circulation may occur with viral myocarditis. Electrocardiogram changes are usually prominent.

Pneumopericardium

Symptoms are consistent with those of a pericardial effusion and pericarditis. A loud, metallic, splashing sound synchronous with the heart sounds may be heard on auscultation. A chest radiograph is diagnostic.

Pulmonary Embolus

Emboli are relatively uncommon in children. The sudden onset of dyspnea, apprehension, cough, and in some cases, chest pain, suggests this diagnosis. Consider a fat embolus in a child with a long bone fracture.

INSUFFICIENT OXYGEN SUPPLY TO TISSUES

◆ Exercise

Exertion is a common nonpathologic cause of dyspnea.

Anemia

High Altitude

Shock

Shock may follow trauma, sepsis, or hemorrhage.

Carbon Monoxide Exposure

Methemoglobinemia

Various drugs and chemicals may alter hemoglobin, decreasing its oxygen carrying capacity.

CENTRAL NERVOUS SYSTEM DISTURBANCES

Acidosis

The respiratory center may be stimulated by changes in pH. In diabetic ketoacidosis, dehydration, inborn errors of metabolism, and salicylate poisoning, hyperpnea may be a primary sign, simulating dyspnea.

Central Nervous System Irritation

Meningitis and Encephalitis

Children with central nervous system irritation from infection are often hyperpneic and appear dyspneic. In some cases, investigation of pulmonary causes of the difficulty has delayed discovery of the primary cause.

Tumors

Hemorrhage

NEUROMUSCULAR PROBLEMS

Guillain-Barré Syndrome

Botulism

Muscular Dystrophy

Werdnig-Hoffmann Disease

Myasthenia Gravis

Hypokalemia

Organophosphate Poisoning

Diaphragmatic Paralysis

Poliomyelitis

PSYCHOGENIC CAUSES

◆ **Hyperventilation Syndrome**

Fright

Pain

Anxiety

MISCELLANEOUS CAUSES

Fever

Hyperthyroidism

SUGGESTED READING

Fan LL, Mullen ALW, Brugman SM, et al. Clinical spectrum of chronic interstitial lung disease in children. *J Pediatr* 1992;121:867–872.

Samaik AP, Lieh-Lai M. Adult respiratory distress syndrome in children. *Pediatr Clin North Am* 1994;41:337–363.

57

Hyperpnea

Hyperpnea is an increase in the depth of respirations. Many of the conditions listed in the classification below feature an increase both in depth (hyperpnea) and in rate (tachypnea) of respiration. More than one pathophysiologic mechanism may be operative in the child with hyperpnea.

Hyperpnea results in increased elimination of carbon dioxide resulting in hypocarbia, which can help compensate for metabolic acidosis and constricts cerebral vessels, which may benefit patients with increased intracranial pressure.

HYPERTHERMIA

Febrile States

Warm Environment

The rate of respirations as well as their depth are increased to assist in heat loss from the body.

METABOLIC ACIDOSIS

Dehydration

Conditions producing dehydration such as severe diarrhea result in decreased renal perfusion and consequent retention of hydrogen ions.

Starvation

Tissue catabolism results in increased hydrogen ion production.

Diabetic Ketoacidosis

This is perhaps the best recognized cause of tissue catabolism leading to metabolic acidosis and hyperpnea.

Inborn Errors of Metabolism

Glycogen Storage Disease Type I

Significant hepatomegaly develops in young children. Recurrent episodes of lactic acidosis may result in death.

Galactosemia

Vomiting, diarrhea, jaundice, and hepatomegaly may occur in the neonatal period.

Ketotic Hyperglycinemia

Methylmalonic Acidemia

Isovaleric Acidemia

A "sweaty sock" odor is characteristic.

Lactic Acidemia

Children with this disorder may have intermittent ataxia, oculomotor nerve palsies, muscle weakness, and progressive motor deterioration.

Cystinosis

Signs of rickets are usually present.

Drugs and Toxins

Various substances may lead to metabolic acidosis.

Salicylates

In acute salicylate intoxication, respiratory alkalosis is transient and metabolic acidosis soon ensues, with hyperpnea. Tachypnea may also be present, the result of brain stem stimulation by salicylate. Hyperpnea is an important clinical sign of toxicity during chronic salicylate therapy.

Respiratory Stimulants

Aminophylline, epinephrine, and nikethamide are examples.

Methanol

Ethylene Glycol

Paraldehyde

The characteristic odor on the breath is readily apparent.

Ammonium Salts

Dinitrophenol

Chronic Renal Failure

Hydrogen ion retention occurs with inadequate renal function.

Renal Tubular Acidosis

In the distal form, the urine remains relatively alkaline despite systemic acidosis.

Intestinal Bicarbonate Loss

May occur during diarrheal disorders.

HYPOXEMIA

Severe Anemia

Shock and Hypotension

Cardiac Failure

Cyanotic Congenital Heart Disease

These disorders tend to produce "painless" hyperpnea in newborns, in contrast with pulmonary disorders.

Chronic Pulmonary Insufficiency of Prematurity

Characteristic pulmonary changes are seen on radiographs. Hyperpnea and retractions resolve slowly.

Pulmonary Edema

NEUROGENIC HYPERPNEA

Hypoglycemia

Encephalitis

Respiratory alkalosis follows stimulation of the respiratory center.

Gram-Negative Sepsis

Increased Intracranial Pressure

(See Chapter 24, Increased Intracranial Pressure and Bulging Fontanel.)

Cerebral Infarction

Acute Salicylate Intoxication

Stimulation of the respiratory center occurs before the metabolic acidosis.

Rett Syndrome

This progressive disorder of females is characterized by autistic behavior, ataxia, stereotypic hand-wringing, dementia, and seizures. Episodes of hyperpnea and apnea may be present.

Oral-Facial-Digital Syndrome, Type VI

A few children with hypoplastic cerebellar vermis have had episodes of hyperpnea. The syndrome features variable oral and facial abnormalities and polydactyly.

Joubert Syndrome

An autosomal recessively inherited disorder that features episodic hyperpnea and apnea in association with partial or complete aplasia of the cerebellar vermis, oculomotor abnormalities, and psychomotor retardation.

MISCELLANEOUS CAUSES

Psychogenic Causes

Anxiety and hysteria are often associated with hyperventilation. Other symptoms include headache, chest tightness, dizziness, and paresthesias of the extremities.

Reflex Hyperventilation

Various stimuli may cause hyperpnea.

Pain

Sudden Cooling of the Skin

Urinary Bladder Distension

Pneumothorax

Pulmonary Vascular Occlusion

For example, a pulmonary embolism may cause occlusion.

=58=
Hemoptysis

The coughing up of blood is frightening for the child, parents, and physician. Children under 6 years of age swallow their sputum, so hemoptysis is a very uncommon complaint in young children.

Massive hemoptysis, defined as bleeding that exceeds 200 to 600 mL per day, may be life-threatening, but in most cases during childhood, hemoptysis does not in itself present a threat to life. In many cases, the origin of the blood is in the nose or oropharynx, and a careful physical examination will disclose the site of bleeding. In young children, one must be careful to differentiate hematemesis from hemoptysis. True hemoptysis of pulmonary origin has various causes, the most common of which are bronchiectasis, cystic fibrosis, an aspirated foreign body, and pulmonary infections.

♦ **Most Common Causes of Hemoptysis**

Cystic Fibrosis   Congenital Heart Disease
Pneumonia   Tracheobronchitis
Bronchiectasis

● **Causes Not to Forget**

Nasal or Oropharyngeal Bleeding   Tuberculosis
Pulmonary Hemosiderosis   Neoplasm

INFECTIONS

♦ **Cystic Fibrosis**

Hemoptysis is rare but may occur in older patients with bronchiectasis. Hemoptysis is a poor prognostic sign because it indicates progressive pulmonary disease. Massive hemoptysis has been reported.

♦ **Pneumonia**

A rusty sputum may occur in bacterial or viral pneumonias, but is a classic sign of pneumococcal pneumonia.

♦ **Bronchiectasis**

A cough, productive of blood tinged sputum, is usually present. Recurrent fever and signs of pneumonia are common. In chronic cases, clubbing of the fingers is found. In addition to cystic fibrosis, causes include damage to the bronchi following lower respiratory tract infection, immunodeficiency disorders, and ciliary dyskinesia, which allow infections and consequent damage to the airways.

Lung Abscess

Pus and sputum are often mixed with the blood.

● **Pulmonary Tuberculosis**

A tuberculin skin test should be performed in all children with hemoptysis. Weight loss, night sweats, intermittent fever, and cough may be present.

♦ **Tracheobronchitis**

This was the most common cause referred to otolaryngologists (1).

Pertussis

Streaks of blood may be seen in the sputum produced after severe coughing episodes.

Influenza

In severe cases a hemorrhagic tracheobronchitis may develop.

Bronchopulmonary Aspergillosis

An underlying pulmonary disorder predisposes to this condition. Fever and a necrotizing pneumonia with cavitation may develop. Hyphae may be found in the sputum.

Coccidioidomycosis

Most cases are asymptomatic, but mild respiratory symptoms develop in a small number with fever, dry cough, malaise, anorexia, and myalgias. Rarely, if the cough is productive, the sputum may be blood tinged.

Blastomycosis

In the pulmonary form, mild respiratory symptoms include a low-grade fever, chest pain, and a nonproductive cough. Progressive disease results in fever, weight loss, night sweats, and hemoptysis.

Hemorrhagic Fevers

This group of disorders, which is found in many parts of the world, is transmitted by arthropods. Some forms are associated with severe prostration, thrombocytopenia, and pneumonitis with hemoptysis.

Paragonimiasis

This infestation is also known as endemic hemoptysis in parts of Africa and Central and South America. A chronic pulmonary infection, caused by a trematode, is associated with cough and hemoptysis.

Stachybotrys atra

Pulmonary hemorrhage, sometimes fatal, has been described with this black fungus toxin when inhaled by infants.

Echinococcosis

TRAUMA

Lung Contusion

Blunt or penetrating injuries of the chest wall may be associated with pulmonary injury and hemoptysis.

Foreign Body

Aspiration of a foreign object may cause hemoptysis following injury to the tracheobronchial tree such as laceration or chronic irritation. Plant fibers are a relatively common culprit.

Endotracheal and Tracheostomy Tubes

Irritation or compression necrosis may erode into blood vessels. Repetitive suctioning may produce hemorrhage.

Smoking Clove Cigarettes

Reaction to inhaled smoke may result in bronchospasm, pulmonary edema, and hemoptysis as well as lesser pulmonary symptoms.

CARDIOVASCULAR CAUSES

♦ Congenital Heart Disease

Hemoptysis tends to occur in infants or in older adolescents, particularly those with pulmonary vascular hypertension and pulmonary venous congestion. The most common congenital heart defects associated with hemoptysis are ventricular septal defect, truncus arteriosus, complex cyanotic heart disease, and transposition of the great arteries (2).

Pulmonary Embolus

Emboli may occur in subacute bacterial endocarditis or in peripheral venous thrombosis. Symptoms depend on the size of the embolus, the number of emboli, and the severity of the lesions. Dyspnea, pallor, cyanosis, and chest pain with a shocklike picture may be present.

Multiple Pulmonary Telangiectasis

This condition may be part of hereditary hemorrhagic telangiectasia (Rendu-Osler-Weber syndrome). The family history is important because the disorder is transmitted as an autosomal dominant trait.

Pulmonary Arteriovenous Malformations

The size of the malformation determines prerupture symptoms, which may include finger clubbing, polycythemia, and cyanosis. The lesion may be associated with the Rendu-Osler-Weber syndrome.

Mitral Stenosis

Hemoptysis may occur during paroxysmal dyspnea or pulmonary edema. Occasionally, the bleeding may be brisk when a bronchial or pleurohilar vein ruptures.

Endomyocardial Fibrosis

Hemoptysis is a late finding during left-sided heart failure.

Necrotic Pulmonary Arterial Lesions

Children with systemic lupus erythematosus and periarteritis nodosa may develop hemoptysis secondary to pulmonary vascular lesions.

TUMORS

Laryngotracheal Papilloma

These recalcitrant lesions are usually the result of exposure to human papilloma virus at the time of vaginal delivery.

● **Bronchial Adenoma**

Bronchogenic Cysts

Enterogenic Cysts

Duplications of the bowel may be present in the thoracic cavity. Symptoms depend on the size and position of the cyst and include recurrent pulmonary infections, chest pain, and hemoptysis.

Mediastinal Teratoma

The gastric mucosa of the teratoma may produce secretions that ulcerate into the lung parenchyma.

Bronchogenic Carcinoma

Occurrence in childhood is rare.

Metastatic Tumors

Bronchial Submucosal Gland Tumors

The two most common types are carcinoid tumors and adenoid cystic carcinomas. Cough is the most common presenting symptom, often with hemoptysis. Wheezing may confound the diagnosis.

Plasma Cell Granuloma of Lung

Additional findings may include clubbing, cough, chest pain, and weight loss.

Bronchial Carcinoid Syndrome

Endometriosis

VASCULITIS

Henoch-Schönlein Purpura

Systemic Lupus Erythematosus

A pulmonary hemosiderosis picture may appear long before other features occur.

Wegener Granulomatosis

Necrotizing granulomas of the upper and lower respiratory tract may result in hemoptysis. Evidence of renal vasculitis is usually present.

Polyarteritis Nodosa

Rheumatoid Arthritis

Behçet Syndrome

Antiphospholipid Syndrome

Immunoglobulin A Nephropathy

MISCELLANEOUS DISORDERS

Sickle Cell Anemia

Pulmonary intravascular sickling resulting in infarction has been described.

Hemorrhagic Disorders

Mild, undetected hemophilia may present with hemoptysis.

Pulmonary Hemorrhage

Premature infants who have suffered hypoxic insults are most commonly affected.

• Pulmonary Hemosiderosis

A number of types of pulmonary hemosiderosis have been described, characterized by recurrent pulmonary symptoms including cough, dyspnea, wheezing, and hemoptysis, as well as changes seen on radiographs and iron-deficiency anemia.

Idiopathic Primary Pulmonary Hemosiderosis

Primary Pulmonary Hemosiderosis with Hypersensitivity to Cow Milk

Affected children usually have high titers of precipitins to cow milk proteins. Chronic rhinitis, recurrent otitis media, and gastrointestinal symptoms are also present.

Primary Pulmonary Hemosiderosis with Glomerulonephritis (Goodpasture Syndrome)

Drugs and Toxins

Cocaine

Aspirin

Propylthiouracil

Diphenylhydantoin

Inhalation of Resins

Sarcoidosis

Patients with symptomatic respiratory presentations may occasionally have hemoptysis.

Pulmonary Sequestration

Ehlers-Danlos Syndrome

Bronchial Artery Aneurysm

Swyer-James Syndrome

Unilateral hyperlucent lung acquired following bronchiolitis obliterans in infancy. Repeated bouts of pulmonary infection occur and may be followed by bronchiectasis.

• BLEEDING WITHOUT PULMONARY INVOLVEMENT

The child must be examined carefully for evidence of upper airway disorders associated with bleeding that may be mistaken for hemoptysis.

Epistaxis

Oral or Nasopharyngeal Trauma

Acute Tonsillitis

Gingivitis

Munchausen Syndrome by Proxy

Hematemesis

REFERENCES

1. Fabian MC, Smitheringale A. Hemoptysis in children: the Hospital for Sick Children experience. *J Otolaryngol* 1996;25:44–45.
2. Coss-Bu JA, Sachdeva RC, Bricker JT, Harrison GM, Jefferson LS. Hemoptysis: a 10-year retrospective study. *Pediatrics* 1997;100:E7.

SUGGESTED READING

Etzel RA, Montaña E, Sorenson WG, Kullman GJ, Allan TM, Dearborn DG. Acute pulmonary hemorrhage in infants associated with exposure to *Stachybotrys atra* and other fungi. *Arch Pediatr Adolesc Med* 1998;152:757–762.
Pianosi P, Al-Sadoon H. Hemoptysis in children. *Pediatr Rev* 1996;17:344–348.
Sherman JM. When you see red. *Contemp Pediatr* 1997;14:79–90.

59

Stridor

Stridor is defined as a crowing sound heard usually during inspiration. The sound may be high pitched or low pitched and may also be present during expiration. Generally, stridor is indicative of obstruction somewhere along the respiratory tract, from the pharynx down to the major bronchi. This symptom demands immediate attention and thorough evaluation to uncover the precise cause.

It is important to determine whether the cause of the stridor is an acute or a chronic disorder. The following clues may be helpful in evaluating this sign. The presence of a weak cry, hoarseness, or aphonia strongly suggests a laryngeal problem. Obstructive lesions above the laryngeal glottis usually produce inspiratory crowing, whereas expiratory stridor is the result of lesions below this area. Biphasic stridor, inspiratory and expiratory, is usually the result of obstructive lesions in the glottis or subglottis, but lesions extending into the midtrachea may also produce biphasic stridor. If the child prefers to hold the neck in a hyperextended position, extrinsic pressure on the airway should be suspected.

In the classification that follows, the causes of stridor are divided into acute and chronic disorders. Associated signs and symptoms that may aid in the differential diagnosis are included.

♦ **Most Common Causes of Stridor**

Neonates	**Acute**	**Chronic**
Laryngomalacia	Viral Croup	Laryngomalacia
Vocal Cord Paralysis	Spasmodic Croup	Subglottic Stenosis
Vascular Ring	Psychogenic	

● **Causes Not to Forget**

Laryngeal Webs	Foreign Body	Gastroesophageal Reflux
Hypocalcemic Tetany	Retropharyngeal Abscess	Vascular Ring
	Angioedema	
	Severe Asthma	
	Diphtheria	

ACUTE CAUSES OF STRIDOR

◆ Laryngotracheitis (Viral Croup)

Viral croup is the most common cause of acute stridor. There is usually a history of a preceding upper respiratory infection followed by the development, usually at night, of inspiratory stridor and a cough that sounds like a seal's bark. Hoarseness may be prominent. The term *laryngotracheobronchitis* should be reserved for cases in which the lower respiratory tract is involved, evidenced by both stridor and wheezing.

◆ Spasmodic Croup

Episodes of inspiratory stridor, not preceded by an upper respiratory infection, may occur without fever. Affected children are generally older than those in whom acute laryngotracheitis is found. The episodes may be recurrent.

◆ Psychogenic

May cause difficulties in diagnosis. On laryngoscopy, paradoxical closure of the vocal cords on inspiration is found.

● Severe Asthma

With significantly prolonged expiratory phase, the inspiratory phase may be foreshortened to a stridulous gasp.

● Foreign Body Aspiration

Inspiratory stridor occurs if the foreign body is lodged in the subglottic area or above; both expiratory and inspiratory stridor are usually present if the obstruction is lower. A sudden choking episode followed by stridor and dyspnea suggests a foreign body.

● Angioedema

Acute swelling of the upper airway may cause alarming dyspnea and stridor; fever is uncommon. Swelling of the face, tongue, or pharynx may be present as well.

Esophageal Foreign Body

Stridor may occur if the foreign body is lodged in the cervical esophagus. Drooling, dysphagia, and anorexia without signs of infection may be prominent.

Epiglottitis

Epiglottitis usually does not cause stridor. Onset of the infection is sudden, with fever, difficulty in swallowing, drooling, a muffled voice, and preference to sit upright. The child appears acutely ill. The incidence has fallen dramatically with the introduction of *Haemophilus influenzae* type b vaccine.

Supraglottitis

The aryepiglottic folds rather than the epiglottis are inflamed. Group A, β-hemolytic streptococcus may be the cause. Symptoms are similar to epiglottitis.

Ingestion of Corrosives

Stridor results from swelling of oral and pharyngeal structures. Drooling, mouth ulcers, and a history of ingestion are most important clues.

Trauma

Falls, auto accidents, clothesline injuries, and violent blows may result in laryngeal fracture. Hoarseness and cough are presenting symptoms. Crepitation of the neck may be present, as well as dyspnea and dysphagia.

Peritonsillar Abscess

Stridor is a late sign as edema of the hypopharynx develops. Early signs are sore throat, dysphagia, drooling, and difficulty in opening the mouth. The uvula is shifted from the midline.

Bacterial Tracheitis

Acute serious upper airway obstructive illness may be the result of this infection, usually due to *Streptococcus aureus*. Initial signs are indistinguishable from croup, but instead of improving over days, children develop high fever and toxicity. Copious, thick, purulent tracheal secretions are present and may be life-threatening. It is critical to differentiate this infection from laryngotracheitis.

• Retropharyngeal Abscess

Stridor develops as the pharyngeal wall becomes edematous, the abscess exerts a mass effect, and the inflammation creates a "stiff" airway. Drooling and dysphagia are present. Affected children hold the neck hyperextended.

• Hypocalcemic Tetany

This is a rare cause of stridor due to the greatly reduced incidence of rickets. Other signs include carpopedal spasm, tremors, irritability, twitchings, and convulsions.

• Diphtheria

Stridor may be produced as the faucial membrane forms or drops into the glottic area. Fever, hoarseness or aphonia, a serous or serosanguineous nasal discharge, and cervical adenopathy may be prominent.

Laryngeal Candidiasis

Laryngeal Aplasia

In a newborn with significant inspiratory effort, cyanosis, and chest retractions, laryngeal aplasia or severe stenosis should be considered. Aplasia is not consistent with life unless a tracheostomy is performed immediately.

CHRONIC CAUSES OF STRIDOR

♦ Congenital Laryngeal Stridor

This disorder, also called laryngomalacia, is thought to be caused by a relative immaturity of the laryngeal framework. On inspiration the loose tissues collapse inward, producing stridor that is more significant in the supine position. The stridor is more sonorous or stertorous in quality; the cry, however, is normal. The condition usually resolves with growth by 1 year of age. Direct laryngoscopy should be performed to confirm the diagnosis.

♦ Subglottic Stenosis

Stridor is present from birth, but pronounced respiratory difficulty does not usually occur until an upper respiratory infection results in swelling or increased mucus production.

Floppy Epiglottis (Omega-Shaped Epiglottis)

The epiglottis may fall back into the airway, causing partial obstruction, like laryngomalacia. Stridor is more severe in the supine position.

• Gastroesophageal Reflux

The onset of stridor may be anywhere from 7 days to 3 months of age. Some infants have no history of recurrent vomiting or spitting.

♦ Hypertrophied Tonsils

Tonsillar tissue may be so large that the supraglottic airway becomes obstructed. Stridor is especially noticeable during sleep. Pulmonary hypertension and congestive heart failure may follow.

• Vascular Ring/Aberrant Vessels

In vascular ring anomalies such as a double aortic arch, anomalous innominate artery, or abnormally placed subclavian artery, regurgitation of food with cyanotic attacks and inspiratory or expiratory stridor may be the presenting signs. The infant may prefer to keep the neck hyperextended. An aberrant left pulmonary artery and aneurysmal dilation of the pulmonary arteries associated with absent pulmonary valve can produce dyspnea, stridor, and wheezing.

Hemangiomas

Subglottic lesions gradually enlarge during the first few months of life. The stenosis produces a musical stridor similar to that of viral croup.

♦ Laryngeal Paralysis

The paralysis may be present at birth or develop later. The voice may take on a higher pitch with hoarseness and dyspnea in bilateral vocal cord paralysis, which usually signifies a brain stem injury or central nervous system malformation. Unilateral paralysis may follow recurrent laryngeal nerve entrapment by mediastinal tumor, aberrant great vessels, or aortic arch, or damage during cardiac surgery. Onset of paralysis may be sudden in the Arnold-Chiari deformity. The cry is generally weak. Intubation may injure the vocal cords.

● Laryngeal Web

A weak cry and stridor are evident. Direct laryngoscopy reveals failure of separation of the anterior portions of the vocal cords.

Micrognathia

In severe defects, as in the Pierre Robin syndrome, the tongue may fall back over the supraglottic aperture, producing stridor.

Abnormal Arytenoid Function

The arytenoid cartilage may be displaced congenitally or secondary to trauma. Hoarseness and stridor are present.

Laryngeal Papillomatosis

These lesions should be considered in any child who develops hoarseness and breathing difficulty without evidence of infection. Stridor may occasionally be present. The human papillomavirus is usually picked up from the mother during passage through the birth canal.

Chronic Laryngeal Stenosis

Stenosis is a frequent occurrence after tracheostomy due to granuloma formation or cartilaginous overgrowth; it may also develop after infections, trauma, burns, or radiation.

Tracheal Stenosis

A congenitally small tracheal cartilaginous ring or absent cartilage may be associated with obstruction. If the defect is extrathoracic, the stridor is inspiratory; if intrathoracic, both inspiratory and expiratory crowing are present.

External Compression

Cystic masses, including lingual cysts, tonsillar teratomas, nasopharyngeal angio-fibromas, and cystic hygromas, may obstruct the supraglottic area.

Acquired Subglottic Cysts

Low-birth weight infants may develop these cysts.

Aberrant Thyroid Tissue

A lingual thyroid or thyroglossal duct cyst may cause partial obstruction.

Mediastinal Cyst or Teratoma

Thoracic pain, a choking sensation, dyspnea, and stridor may be present.

Bronchial or Esophageal Cysts

Symptoms are suggestive of bronchial stenosis: cough, wheeze, progressive dyspnea, stridor, and cyanosis.

Internal Laryngocele

The voice is muffled, and stridor is present. The mucosal pocket lies between the true and false cords.

Macroglossia

The tongue may be enlarged enough to obstruct the hypopharynx.

Farber Disease

Hoarseness and stridor may appear at any time during the first few weeks of life. Palpable nodules develop in the skin, along with painful swelling of multiple joints. Hepatomegaly and central nervous system deterioration eventually occur.

Coccidioidomycosis

One case of subglottic infection has been reported.

Rheumatoid Arthritis

Involvement of the cricoarytenoid joint produces stridor and dyspnea.

Opitz-Frias Syndrome

Affected infants have feeding difficulties, often with recurrent aspiration, hypertelorism, and hypospadias. Stridor and a hoarse voice are often lifelong findings.

Marshall-Smith Syndrome

A sporadic disorder with poor growth, advanced bone age, prominent eyes, low nasal bridge, and upturned nose.

Laryngotracheoesophageal Cleft

Partial clefts are the most common form of this rare anomaly. Respiratory distress, feeding difficulty, and recurrent aspiration inevitably develop.

SUGGESTED READING

Geist R, Tallett SE. Diagnosis and management of psychogenic stridor caused by conversion disorder. *Pediatrics* 1990;86:315–317.

Mancuso RF. Stridor in neonates. *Pediatr Clin North Am* 1996;43:1339–1357.

Nielson DW, Heldt GP, Tooley WH. Stridor and gastroesophageal reflux in infants. *Pediatrics* 1990;85:1034–1039.

Smith RJH, Catlin FI. Congenital anomalies of the larynx. *Am J Dis Child* 1984;138:35–39.

60

Wheezing

The old adage "All that wheezes is not asthma" is perhaps overworked; yet many physicians have been fooled by the apparent asthmatic child in whom elevated sweat chloride levels are later demonstrated or by the child who is subsequently found to have an airway foreign body. Sometimes expiratory noises cannot be distinguished from inspiratory ones, and at times both may be present. What may sound like wheezing may really be stridor, snoring, sighing, or just noisy breathing.

Wheezing is a musical sound caused by partial obstruction of the airway and is most often expiratory. Stridor is a coarser sound produced on inspiration. The following list of causes of wheezing has been divided into three primary categories: The first group represents the conditions that should be considered in the primary differential diagnosis; the second group represents much less likely causes of wheezing. In the third group are disorders in which wheezing is rarely found, or in which the respiratory noise may be mistaken for wheezing.

♦ **Most Common Causes of Wheezing by Age Group**

Infants	Preschool–Early Grades	Adolescents
Bronchiolitis	Asthma	Asthma
Gastroesophageal Reflux	Bronchitis	Vocal Cord Dysfunction
Asthma	Gastroesophageal Reflux	Bronchitis
Bronchopulmonary Dysplasia		

● **Causes Not to Forget**

Vascular Ring/Aberrant Vessel	Cystic Fibrosis	Cystic Fibrosis
	Foreign Body	"Cardiac" Asthma

COMMON CAUSES OF WHEEZING

♦ **Asthma/Reactive Airways Disease**

Overall, asthma is the most common cause of wheezing in children. Repeated attacks of labored breathing, a tight cough, air trapping manifested by an increased anteroposterior diameter of the chest, and a "garden of sounds" heard on auscultation of the lungs (crackles, snaps, pops, rhonchi, whistles, etc.) are characteristic. The family history is frequently positive for atopy. Attacks can be precipitated by exposure to various allergens, infection, exercise, ingestants, and, sometimes, emotions.

♦ Bronchiolitis

Wheezing is a hallmark of this viral infection of the lower airway, usually caused by respiratory syncytial virus. Adenovirus and influenza virus are other common causes. Fever may or may not be present; tachypnea and retractions are common. Bronchiolitis is most frequent in infants between 1 and 6 months of age and unusual in those older than 18 months.

♦ Bronchitis

Infections (viral, bacterial, protozoal, or mycotic) that affect lower airways may be associated with wheezing. There may also be a diffuse pneumonitis, but notably, classic lobar pneumonia does not cause wheezing. Diffuse chest film changes, a clinical picture consistent with nonbacterial infection, and failure to respond completely to bronchodilators are findings that help in differentiation from asthma. The more common viruses involved include adenovirus, parainfluenza, and influenza viruses. Lower respiratory infections with wheezing in school-aged children in the fall are frequently related to *Mycoplasma pneumoniae*. In infants 3 weeks to 3 months of age, *Chlamydia trachomatis* may be the culprit.

Aspiration
♦ Gastroesophageal Reflux

Especially during infancy, reflux with aspiration into the lungs may produce recurrent episodes of wheezing mimicking asthma. There may not be a history of vomiting. Incidence is greater in the developmentally disabled. Hiatal hernia or, rarely, esophageal stenosis may be demonstrated.

● Foreign Body

There is usually a sudden onset of respiratory symptoms with cough, stridor, or wheezing. Symptoms depend on the type of foreign body, its size, where it is trapped, and the size of the patient. Signs may be unilateral on auscultation. Secondary infection may occur. Stridor is usually more prominent than wheezing. An esophageal foreign body may compress the trachea, producing a wheeze.

Pharyngeal Incoordination

Children with familial dysautonomia, bulbar palsy, and cleft palate may be predisposed to aspiration.

♦ Vocal Cord Dysfunction

By adducting the vocal cords, a wheezing sound may be generated on expiration, mimicking asthma. Care must be taken not to confuse this psychogenic problem with reactive airways disease. Direct laryngoscopy may be necessary in difficult cases, to confirm that the cords are adducted during expiration rather than relaxing.

● **Cystic Fibrosis**

This is not a common cause of wheezing, but one that should not be missed. Affected children may have associated wheezing and they sometimes have asthma. Other signs and symptoms of cystic fibrosis should be sought: chronic cough, repeated respiratory infections, persistent pulmonary changes on radiograph films, steatorrhea, clubbing of the nails, and failure to thrive. A sweat test provides a definitive diagnosis.

♦ **Bronchopulmonary Dysplasia**

This condition is a sequelae of respiratory distress syndrome in neonates.

● **Vascular Ring**

This defect usually causes early onset of respiratory problems: brassy cough, dyspnea, stridor (much more common than wheeze), and repeated infections. Symptoms are often worse after feeding, and there may be some difficulty in swallowing. The neck may be held hyperextended. Double aortic arch and aberrant subclavian arteries are the most common anomalies.

● **Aberrant Vessels**

In addition to vascular rings other vessels may impinge on the airway. An aberrant left pulmonary artery, absent pulmonary valve with aneurysmal dilation of the pulmonary arteries, and an aberrant innominate can also produce similar signs.

LESS COMMON CAUSES OF WHEEZING

Human Immunodeficiency Virus Infection

Pulmonary infections may lead to wheezing.

● **"Cardiac Asthma"**

Bronchial compression from cardiac enlargement may cause wheezing along with other symptoms. Congestive heart failure as a cause is usually obvious, with hepatomegaly, cardiomegaly, tachycardia, and tachypnea.

Congenital Obstructions

Tracheal or Bronchial Stenosis

Stridor is more common with tracheal stenosis; wheezing, with bronchial stenosis. Repeated lower respiratory infections are common.

Bronchomalacia

Bronchi may collapse on expiration, causing obstructive symptoms of cough, wheezing, and dyspnea with recurrent infections.

Tracheobronchomegaly

This disorder may be associated with cutis laxa. Redundancy of structures may result in recurrent infections and obstructive symptoms.

Lobar Emphysema

Tachypnea is a presenting sign in early infancy. Uncommonly, a wheeze is heard over the affected lobe.

Sequestration

Recurrent infection, sometimes with hemoptysis, is a common manifestation.

Alpha$_1$-Antitrypsin Deficiency

Adults are much more likely than children to present with respiratory symptoms; infants and children generally manifest signs of liver disease.

Visceral Larva Migrans

Toxocara larvae may pass through the lung, producing an asthmalike picture. Affected children may have hepatomegaly, anorexia, and anemia; eosinophilia is usually pronounced.

Hypersensitivity Pneumonitis

Causes are numerous; it is more prevalent in adults. Drugs (including aspirin), organic dust particles, chemicals, and fungi (*Aspergillus* and *Candida*) have been implicated.

Tumors

Tracheal and Bronchial Tumors

Symptoms depend on tumor location as well as its size. Cough, wheezing, and recurrent infection are prominent. Hemangiomas on neck and chest may be a clue but are not reliable indicators of respiratory tract hemangiomas. External compression of the airway by cysts, hilar adenopathy, lymphomas, and other mediastinal masses may produce dyspnea, chest pain, cough, and stridor as well as wheezing.

Carcinoid Tumors

These are very unusual in children. Wheezing, diarrhea, and sudden flushes of the skin may be present.

Miscellaneous Causes

Tracheoesophageal Fistula

The H-type fistula is an uncommon cause of recurrent pneumonia or wheezing.

Pulmonary Vasculitis

Collagen vascular diseases, especially systemic lupus erythematosus, may involve the pulmonary system. Pneumonitis, pleurisy, cough, hemoptysis, dyspnea, and, sometimes, wheezing may be found.

Pulmonary Hemosiderosis

Episodes of cough, wheezing, dyspnea, and hemoptysis are recurrent. Anemia develops. Various types have been described: idiopathic, secondary to cow milk, associated with myocarditis, and associated with glomerulonephritis (Goodpasture).

Immune Deficiency States

Affected children may have wheezing as a symptom in recurrent pulmonary infections.

Fibrous Mediastinitis

Involvement of the tracheobronchial tree may result in wheezing. There may be esophageal obstruction as well.

Ciliary Dyskinesis

The triad of cough, sinusitis, and otitis media have been present in all cases.

Anomalous Left Coronary Artery

Infants may present with wheezing, primarily from congestive heart failure. The danger is administration of beta-adrenergic drugs in this situation, which may cause arrhythmias and death.

CONDITIONS WITH RESPIRATORY NOISES MIMICKING WHEEZING

Other respiratory noises or symptoms may be mistaken for wheezing. Most discussions of the differential diagnosis of asthma or causes of wheezing include the disorders listed here. There should be no difficulty in distinguishing the associated dyspnea or stridor from wheezing.

Infections

Laryngotracheobronchitis

Inspiratory stridor is the key feature. Rarely, wheezing may be a finding when the lower airways are involved.

Other Causes of Croup Syndrome

Upper airway obstruction, as in spasmodic croup, epiglottitis, diphtheria, and retropharyngeal abscess, produces stridor rather than wheezing.

Pertussis

The repetitive cough should not be confused with wheezing.

Upper Airway Obstruction

Stridor or noisy respirations are produced. Causes include enlarged tonsils and adenoids, choanal stenosis or atresia, polyps, laryngeal papillomas, vocal cord paralysis, tetany, lingual thyroid, and allergic edema.

Congenital Malformations of Lungs

Dyspnea, tachypnea, and cyanosis are symptoms.

Hypoplasia

Cysts

Arteriovenous Malformation

Miscellaneous Causes

Neck Injury

Compression of the trachea produces stridor rather than wheezing.

Hysteria

Apparent respiratory difficulty in the hyperventilation syndrome should not be confused with wheezing.

Salicylate Intoxication

Deep, rapid respirations rather than an increased expiratory phase of respiration are found in salicylate toxicity. Salicylate hypersensitivity may cause true wheezing.

SUGGESTED READING

Kemper KJ. Chronic asthma: an update. *Pediatr Rev* 1996;17:111–117.
McFadden ER Jr, Gilbert IA. Exercise-induced asthma. *N Engl J Med* 1994;330:1362–1367.
Morgan WJ, Martinez FD. Risk factors for developing wheezing and asthma in childhood. *Pediatr Clin North Am* 1992;39:1185–1203.

61

Hypertension

Hypertension can be said to be a physical sign that has come of age. Over the last two decades considerable advances have been made in uncovering the pathogenesis and etiology of hypertension as well as improving the treatment of elevated blood pressure. As with so many other diseases that have become a focus of attention, hypertension has been found to be much more frequent after routine measurement became commonplace.

There have been so many good reviews published on this subject, some of which are listed at the end of this chapter, that no attempt is made here to cover the many important considerations in obtaining and interpreting blood pressure readings. A few general points do require emphasis, however. The blood pressure must be obtained accurately. The appropriate size of blood pressure cuff must be used. The width of the rubber inflatable bladder should be approximately 40% of the arm circumference midway between the olecranon and the acromion. This should result in a cuff that encircles 80% to 100% of the circumference of the extremity and covers two thirds of the length of the upper arm; a narrow cuff results in an elevated reading. If the pressure is taken in the sitting position, the arm should be supported at the level of the heart. Fear, agitation, apprehension, and other emotional factors, in addition to heat and exercise, may cause elevations in blood pressure. The importance of repeating measurements over time (if the elevations are not severe) cannot be overstated. If possible, a series of home readings should be attempted.

Rames and colleagues (1) found that 13.4% of school children 5 to 18 years of age had a blood pressure reading in excess of the 95th percentile on standard charts for age, or greater than 140/90 mm Hg, on the initial examination. On repeated screening, however, less than 1% of all children had a sustained high level. In addition, more than one half of these children had relative weights of 120% or more of the expected norm for height and body build. The association of obesity with high blood pressure in children is more prevalent than previously recognized. The implications for future health need additional clarification, however.

The younger the child and the more severe the hypertension, the more likely a cause for the pressure elevation will be found. The majority of children with secondary hypertension (hypertension secondary to a defined condition) have a renal or renovascular cause. Generally, in office practice, the incidence of demonstrable causes of secondary hypertension, particularly renal, is not as high as that reported in studies of cases seen in referral centers. Essential hypertension was considered rare in the

1960s; by the late 1970s, however, essential hypertension was recognized to cause over one half of blood pressure elevations in teenagers.

The following classification of causes of hypertension groups disorders by the organ system involved. Where possible, associated signs and symptoms are included to offer diagnostic clues. Most frequently, the elevation is "silent." Routine measurement of blood pressure is critical. Signs and symptoms that may be associated with hypertension are protean: headache, dizziness, nausea or vomiting, visual disturbances, facial nerve palsy, irritability, seizures, convulsions, personality changes, changes in conscious state, polyuria, polydipsia, weight loss, and so forth.

♦ Most Common Causes of Hypertension by Age Group

Newborn	**Infants, Children and Adolescents**
Renal Artery Thrombosis	Essential (Primary)
Renal Artery Stenosis	Renal Parenchymal Disease
Congenital Renal Malformations	Renal Vascular Disease
Coarctation of the Aorta	Coarctation of the Aorta
Aortic Thrombosis	

Pseudohypertension
Small Cuff Size	Apprehension

MISCELLANEOUS COMMON CAUSES

♦ Pseudohypertension

Inappropriate Cuff Size

In the past, this has been the most frequent cause of elevated blood pressure. The measurement must be repeated with use of the appropriate cuff.

Apprehension

The effects of the procedure and the milieu in which the pressure is obtained should not be underestimated. Repeated measurements over time (especially at home) are most helpful.

Obesity

Hypertension in obese children may be due in part to cuff size inaccuracy; however, do not ignore signs and symptoms of other disorders. Weight reduction is the key to therapy; lower readings following desired weight loss confirm the diagnosis.

♦ Essential Hypertension

This form is asymptomatic, with no abnormal findings on physical examination. Often one or both parents also have essential hypertension. It is most commonly identified in teenagers, especially those who are obese.

Immobilization

Hypertension is a relatively common accompaniment of immobilization following orthopedic or surgical procedures. Children in body casts or cervical traction are particularly prone to develop hypertension.

Orthopedic Manipulation

Leg lengthening procedures brought this cause to attention.

RENAL CAUSES

♦ Pyelonephritis

Renal parenchymal disease, especially pyelonephritis, acute as well as chronic, is the most common renal cause. Chronic pyelonephritis may be surprisingly asymptomatic.

♦ Unilateral Renal Parenchymal Disease

In addition to pyelonephritis, parenchymal disease may result from obstructive uropathy, congenital defects, infarction, or trauma.

♦ Reflux Nephropathy
♦ Renal Artery Abnormalities

Stenosis, aneurysms, arteritis, fistula, fibromuscular dysplasia, and thrombosis may all cause hypertension. Auscultation of the flanks may disclose bruits. If occlusion is severe, the onset is more abrupt. Headache, polyuria, polydipsia, and growth failure may be nonspecific symptoms. Café au lait spots of neurofibromatosis may be a clue. These abnormalities are second only to parenchymal disease as a cause of renal related hypertension.

♦ Acute Glomerulonephritis

This is a relatively common cause of hypertension of acute onset. Evidence of preceding streptococcal infection should be sought. Symptoms may be nonspecific such as malaise, headache, and anorexia, but edema, hematuria, and oliguria are common. Seizures and congestive heart failure may occur abruptly.

Other Nephritides

A host of other causes of glomerulonephritis must be considered. The presence of protein and cellular elements in the urine suggests this group of disorders; renal biopsy is usually required for differentiation. (See Chapter 78, Hematuria.)

Henoch-Schönlein Syndrome (Henoch-Schönlein Purpura)

A purpuric rash is characteristic. Abdominal pain, periarticular swelling, and soft-tissue swelling are also common. The renal disease is caused by IgA deposits and generally lags behind other findings.

Renal Trauma

Acute injury may have caused notable hematuria, gross or occult.

Hydronephrosis

The acute onset of hydronephrosis from obstruction may be associated with vomiting. A flank mass may be palpable.

Familial Nephritis

Recurrent episodes of hematuria, especially with intercurrent infections, are common; deafness may be a finding, especially in males. Renal failure occurs in family members in the third and fourth decades.

Hemolytic Uremic Syndrome

Persistent diarrhea, often bloody, and severe pallor draw attention to the hemolytic anemia and thrombocytopenia. Acute renal failure may follow. Burr cells from the associated microangiopathy are seen on the peripheral blood smear.

Renal Vein Thrombosis

Fever, hematuria, oliguria, and a flank mass are often present.

Renal Stones

There may be a history of renal colic with intermittent flank pain and hematuria. If stones obstruct the ureter, vomiting follows.

Nephrotic Syndrome

Edema, proteinuria, hypoalbuminemia, and hypercholesterolemia are present. The cause is most frequently idiopathic, with multiple names such as nil disease, minimal change disease, and childhood nephrosis.

Hypoplastic Kidney

There may be unilateral involvement of the entire kidney, or the defect may be segmental (Ask-Upmark), perhaps associated with vesicoureteric reflux.

Wilms' Tumor

The usual presenting sign is an abdominal mass that has been discovered by the parents. Abdominal pain and hematuria may also be present. Two thirds of affected children are under 3 years of age.

Neuroblastoma

Symptoms vary. Associated hypertension has been reported in from 10% to 50% of cases.

Acute Renal Failure

Polycystic Disease

The infantile form results in renal failure in the first or second decade. The kidneys are palpable early as abdominal masses. Hypertension is present in infancy and may be difficult to control. The liver is cystic also and leads to portal hypertension and varices in late childhood. Inheritance pattern is autosomal recessive. In the adult form, hypertension begins in the second or third decade or later; renal insufficiency is prominent. Inheritance pattern is autosomal dominant.

Renal Tuberculosis

The classic finding is "sterile pyuria."

Radiation Nephritis

Retroperitoneal Fibrosis

Renin Secreting Tumors

These lesions are a rare cause of severe hypertension. Symptoms may include polyuria, polydipsia, and enuresis. Hypokalemic alkalosis is usually present.

Liddle Syndrome

This is another cause of hypokalemic alkalosis with hypertension. Polyuria and polydipsia with an inability to concentrate urine are present. Inheritance pattern is probably autosomal dominant.

ENDOCRINE CAUSES

Hyperthyroidism

Systolic pressure is elevated. Weight loss, irritability, tremor, tachycardia, sweating, and exophthalmos are strongly suggestive.

Adrenogenital Syndrome

Hypertension does not occur with 21-hydroxylase deficiency, which accounts for 95% of cases of adrenogenital syndrome.

17-Hydroxylase Deficiency Syndrome

This rare deficiency results in hypogonadism with lack of secondary sex characteristics. Affected boys display pseudohermaphroditism; girls have amenorrhea.

11-β-Hydroxylase Deficiency

This defect results in rapid virilization with rapid somatic growth.

Cushing Syndrome

Obesity, moon facies, buffalo hump, arrested linear growth, acne, hirsutism, striae, malar flush, and elevated blood pressure are characteristic.

Pheochromocytoma

This tumor may produce episodic elevations in blood pressure with flushing, sweating, tachycardia, and headache. There may be a family history, or the lesion may be associated with neurofibromatosis or Sipple syndrome (multiple endocrinopathy).

Primary Aldosteronism

The picture may include periodic muscular weakness, paresthesias, tetany, growth failure, polyuria, and polydipsia. Serum sodium levels are high, serum potassium low, and serum bicarbonate high.

Primary Hyperparathyroidism

This is an unusual cause of hypertension. Symptoms are primarily those of hypercalcemia: muscle weakness, anorexia, nausea, vomiting, constipation, polyuria, polydipsia, weight loss, and fever. Calcium deposits in the kidney may result in renal damage and hypertension.

Diabetes Mellitus

Chronic nephropathy in childhood is unlikely unless the diabetes has been present for 10 or more years.

CARDIOVASCULAR CAUSES

♦ Coarctation of Aorta

Diminished or absent femoral pulses with hypertensive upper extremity pressures are characteristic.

Patent Ductus Arteriosus

Increased systolic pressure, wide pulse pressure, and a machinery-type murmur are findings.

Arteriovenous Fistula

Systolic pressure is increased; cardiac rate may also be increased.

Polycythemia

Anemia

In severe cases, systolic pressure may be elevated.

Subacute and Acute Bacterial Endocarditis

Aortic Insufficiency

Leukemia

Williams Syndrome

Hypertension is common in this syndrome that features short stature, mental retardation, an outgoing personality, characteristic facies, and supravalvular aortic stenosis.

Pseudoxanthoma Elasticum

Yellowish papules on the neck, in the axillae, and around the umbilicus and groin become more apparent with age. There may be angioid streaks in the retina with hemorrhages. Systemic vascular disease usually occurs later in life.

Takayasu Disease (Pulseless Disease)

Unequal pulses develop or are lost; large vessels are affected. The etiology is unknown.

NEUROLOGIC CAUSES

Increased Intracranial Pressure

Cerebral edema resulting from trauma, vascular accidents, pseudotumor cerebri, or infection (meningitis, encephalitis, abscesses) may cause systemic hypertension, presumably as a homeostatic mechanism designed to preserve cerebral perfusion. (See Chapter 24, Increased Intracranial Pressure and Bulging Fontanel.)

Guillain-Barré Syndrome (Acute Febrile Polyneuritis)

Progressive ascending paralysis is characteristic. Hypertension may be a sign of impending respiratory failure.

Familial Dysautonomia

Absent lacrimation and fungiform papillae on the tongue, diminished response to pain, recurrent episodes of vomiting, emotional lability, and paroxysmal hypertension are common.

Poliomyelitis

DRUG-INDUCED HYPERTENSION

Sympathomimetics

In particular, nose or eye drops and cough preparations have been implicated. Phenylephrine, ephedrine, isoproterenol, epinephrine, amphetamines, methylphenidate, and phenylpropanolamine are examples.

Corticosteroids

Oral Contraceptives

Anabolic Steroids

Abuse of these drugs by teens is more common than recognized.

Cocaine

Methysergide

Phencyclidine

Licorice

Licorice may contain glycyrrhizinic acid a mineralocorticoid-like substance that causes sodium retention, potassium wasting, and hypertension.

Reserpine Overdose

MISCELLANEOUS CAUSES

Acute Pain

Pain may cause the release of catecholamines and resultant hypertension.

Hypernatremia

Acute sodium overload, which may be iatrogenic rather than hypernatremic dehydration, is implicated.

Burns

Collagen Vascular Diseases

Systemic Lupus Erythematosus

Scleroderma

Dermatomyositis

Periarteritis

Heavy Metal Poisoning

Lead and mercury poisoning may cause hypertension.

Hypercalcemia

Hypercalcemia may be idiopathic or secondary to metastatic disease, sarcoidosis, or subcutaneous fat necrosis.

Stevens-Johnson Syndrome

This is a severe bullous form of erythema multiforme with mucous membrane involvement.

Sickle Cell Anemia

Malignancies

Rhabdomyosarcoma is an example.

Tuberous Sclerosis

Hypopigmented macules, café au lait spots, facial papules, and seizures are common. Inheritance pattern is autosomal dominant.

Acute Intermittent Porphyria

Fabry Disease (Angiokeratoma Corporis Diffusum)

Minute reddish blue or black lesions (angiokeratomas) are noted over the lower abdomen and scrotum late in the first decade of life. Paresthesias of extremities, recurrent fever, and proteinuria are other findings.

Amyloidosis

Neurofibromatosis

The hypertension is not always renovascular in origin.

Chronic Hypoxia

Includes sleep-apnea-associated hypertension.

Malignant Hyperthermia

The hypertension is associated with tachycardia, tachypnea, and stiff muscles. Fever develops and later a shocklike picture supervenes.

REFERENCE

1. Rames LK, Clarke WR, Connor WE, et al. Normal blood pressures and the evaluation in childhood: the Muscatine study. *Pediatrics* 1978;61:245–251.

SUGGESTED READING

Daniels SR. The diagnosis of hypertension in children: an update. *Pediatr Rev* 1997;18:131–135.

Hanna JD, Chan JCM, Gill JR Jr. Hypertension and the kidney. *J Pediatr* 1991;118:327–340.

Hohn A. Hypertension. In: Finberg L, ed. *Saunders manual of pediatric practice.* Philadelphia: WB Saunders, 1998:587–590.

National High Blood Pressure Education Program Working Group on Hypertension Control in Children and Adolescents. Update on the 1987 Task Force report on high blood pressure in children and adolescents: a working group report from the National High Blood Pressure Education Program. *Pediatrics* 1996;98:649–658.

Rocchini AP (editor). Childhood hypertension. *Pediatr Clin North Am* 1993;40:1–212.

Sinaiko AR. Hypertension in children. *N Engl J Med* 1996;335:1968–1973.

62

Syncope

Syncope or fainting refers to the sudden and transient loss of consciousness, usually as a result of decreased cerebral perfusion and anoxia. Syncopal episodes are usually of short duration; however, if they last for over 20 seconds, a few clonic twitches may occur that may falsely suggest epilepsy. By adulthood, as many as 15% of children will have had a syncopal episode (1).

Vasovagal syncope is responsible for the great majority of syncopal episodes, and, as such, is generally benign. The history is extremely important in helping direct attention to syncopal episodes that necessitate additional investigation. Individuals with vasovagal (neurocardiogenic) syncope have recurrent episodes of near syncope usually associated with nausea, diaphoresis, pallor, and blurred vision. Tilt table testing has been shown to offer the most diagnostic support for the probability of vasovagal syncope in individuals with a consistent history (2). If syncope occurs during exercise, the underlying cause may be a potentially fatal one; investigation for underlying pathology, particularly cardiac, is mandatory. Similarly, if there is a family history of syncope, sudden death, myocardial disease, or arrhythmias, investigation should be undertaken.

♦ Most Common Causes of Syncope (1)

Vasovagal (75% or Greater)	Hysterical Fainting
Migraine	Arrhythmia
Seizure	Breath Holding

VASOVAGAL (VASODEPRESSOR; NEUROCARDIOGENIC) SYNCOPE

The most common cause of sudden fainting is termed vasovagal syncope. A familial history of syncope can often be obtained. Occurrence is most common in adolescence. Episodes may be provoked by factors such as pain, sudden emotional upset, hunger, fatigue, prolonged standing, heat, or the loss of or sight of blood. Most cases are not associated with an identifiable factor, however. A prodrome of lightheadedness, dizziness, cold sweat, and pallor is common. Vasovagal syncope has been described in the following.

♦ **Postural Hypotension**

Assuming a standing position suddenly after recumbency may be associated with lightheadedness or syncope.

Cough

Prolonged coughing episodes may raise intrathoracic pressure, decrease venous return to the heart, and lower cardiac output, resulting in syncope.

♦ **Migraine**

Basilar artery migraine may cause a loss of consciousness and, possibly, syncope.

Pregnancy

Micturition

This unusual form of syncope occurs during urination.

Swallowing

An unusual cause in children related to increased vagal tone with second-degree heart block.

Esophageal Foreign Body

The mechanism may be transient hypoxia, exaggerated vagal response, or vasovagal syncope.

Paracentesis

Syncope may occur after the sudden removal of fluid from the pleural space, peritoneal cavity, or bladder.

Hair Grooming

Has been described as a precipitant of vasovagal syncope.

♦ **HYSTERICAL FAINTING**

Fainting may be an attention getting device. The situation tends to be dramatic, often is repeated, and has no prodrome; usually the child shows little concern for the episode. The period of unresponsiveness is generally much longer in duration than with vasovagal syncope.

CARDIOVASCULAR CAUSES

Cardiovascular causes account for a small percentage of actual syncopal episodes.

Structural Cardiac Disease

Syncopal episodes may occur with a number of cardiac disorders, particularly after exercise.

Severe Aortic Stenosis

Hypertrophic Cardiomyopathy (IHSS)

Severe Pulmonic Stenosis

Tetralogy of Fallot

Truncus Arteriosus

Transposition of the Great Vessels

♦ **Arrhythmias**

Paroxysmal Atrial Tachycardia/Supraventricular Tachycardia

Ventricular Tachycardia

Stokes-Adams Syncope

Complete atrioventricular block causes loss of consciousness.

Familial Paroxysmal Ventricular Fibrillation

Mitral Valve Prolapse

Usually, children or adults with prolapse of a mitral leaflet are asymptomatic. In some, arrhythmias may occur, or precordial chest pain may be a presenting symptom. The presence of an apical late systolic murmur or a mid-systolic click suggests this disorder. Prolapse may coexist with Marfan syndrome, the straight back syndrome, idiopathic hypertrophic subaortic stenosis, or ostium secundum defect of the atrial septum. Note, however, that the incidence of syncope in individuals with mitral valve prolapse is no higher than in the general population.

Cardioauditory Syndrome (Jervell and Lange-Nielsen)

Fainting attacks may begin in infancy or childhood, usually precipitated by emotions or physical exertion. The attacks may be mild, severe, or even fatal and are probably secondary to ventricular fibrillation. The electrocardiogram is useful in demonstrating large T waves and a prolonged QT interval. Perceptive, profound, and symmetric deafness is part of this disorder inherited as an autosomal-recessive trait and is congenital or very early in onset.

Long QT Syndrome Without Deafness (Romano-Ward Syndrome)

Syncopal episodes commonly begin in early childhood and may be mild and transient or severe, leading to several minutes of unconsciousness or even sudden death. As many as one half of those affected by this autosomal-dominant disorder die before adolescence. Attacks are most commonly precipitated by violent emotions or physical exercise.

Long QT Associated with Drugs

Various drugs may result in complications of a long QT interval, including cisapride, quinidine, procainamide, terfenadine, when used in combination with erythromycin or ketoconazole, and astemizole.

Sinus Node Dysfunction

Dysfunction may occur with or without structural heart disease. Irregular cardiac rhythms or abnormally slow heart rates are clues. Other symptoms include chest pain with exercise, palpitations, and dizzy spells.

Emery-Dreifuss Muscular Dystrophy

Initial features include toe walking, partial flexion of the elbows, and inability to fully flex the neck and spine. A distinct pattern of contractures in the absence of major weakness is the earliest clue to diagnosis. In early adulthood, atrial conduction abnormalities occur with exertional chest pain and recurrent syncope. If rhythm disturbances are untreated, the disorder proves fatal by mid-adulthood. There is an X-linked inheritance.

Bradycardia in Highly Trained Athletes

Heart block may develop in athletes during intense training.

Primary Pulmonary Hypertension

The onset may be insidious. Symptoms include chest pain, shortness of breath, and fatigue.

Cardiomyopathy

May be idiopathic, familial, associated with myocarditis, or caused by coronary artery anomalies.

Carotid Sinus Syncope

Attacks appear to be related to a hyperactive carotid sinus reflex with slowing of the heart and hypotension.

Large Pulmonary Embolus
Left Atrial Myxoma

A pedunculated myxoma may suddenly block left atrial outflow. A changing murmur may be a clue. This lesion may occur in tuberous sclerosis.

Anomalous Coronary Arteries

Although most cases present in infancy, anomalies of the origin of the coronary artery may lead to cardiac ischemia at any age.

♦ BREATH HOLDING

Some young children may have recurrent episodes of breath holding and sometimes syncope. The breath holding occurs during crying precipitated by injury or a deliberate attention-getting device during anger or frustration. During the syncopal episode there may be a few muscular twitches that may be mistaken for seizures by the parents. Two types of breath holding spells have been described: (a) a cyanotic spell following crying, and (b) a pallid one with the sudden onset of pallor and collapse without prior crying.

HYPERVENTILATION

Prolonged deep breathing, either intentional or unrecognized during emotional stress, may lead to lightheadedness, generalized weakness, carpopedal spasm, and chest tightness. Occasionally, if the $PaCO_2$ is reduced far enough, syncope may occur. A dangerous form of intentional hyperventilation has been reported in swimmers prior to races, who may subsequently become unconscious while underwater and drown.

♦ EPILEPSY

Convulsive episodes, particularly akinetic or drop seizures, may mimic syncopal episodes; there is no postictal phase, and they are not associated with jerking movements. Affected older children do not report lightheadedness or other symptoms prior to the collapse.

METABOLIC CAUSES

Hypoxia

Hypocalcemia

Hyponatremia

Hypokalemia

Hypoglycemia

An extremely rare cause in children.

MISCELLANEOUS CAUSES

Drugs

Some antihypertensive agents may cause postural hypotension and fainting. Antihistamines often cause dizziness and sometimes syncope.

Hypovolemia

May be the result of blood loss or dehydration.

Severe Anemia

Iron deficiency anemia seems to be more prone to cause syncope than other causes.

Arnold-Chiari Malformation

Has been described in a small percentage of individuals who present after infancy with evidence of this malformation.

Cerebellar or Brain Stem Tumors

Syncopal episodes may occur in children with these tumors after coughing or straining.

Adrenal Insufficiency

Weakness, lightheadedness, and fainting may occur in adrenocortical insufficiency, most commonly after the withdrawal of oral steroids.

Anterior Mediastinal Tumors

Stridor, orthopnea, cough, and edema of the head and neck should suggest this possibility.

Familial Dysautonomia

Other features are more prominent including recurrent aspiration, temperature elevation, lack of tears, and reduced sensitivity to pain.

Acquired Postganglionic Cholinergic Dysautonomia

This is a rare disorder of unknown cause characterized by strabismus, lack of tears, saliva, and sweat, and atony of the bowel and bladder. Orthostatic hypotension may lead to syncope.

REFERENCES

1. McHarg ML, Shinnar S, Rascoff H, Walsh CA. Syncope in childhood. *Pediatr Cardiol* 1997;18:367–371.
2. Strieper MJ, Auld DO, Hulse E, Campbell RM. Evaluation of recurrent pediatric syncope: role of tilt table testing. *Pediatrics* 1994;93:660–662.

SUGGESTED READING

Braden DS, Gaymes CH. The diagnosis and management of syncope in children and adolescents. *Pediatr Ann* 1997;26:422–426.
Driscoll DJ, Jacobsen SJ, Porter CJ, Wollan PC. Syncope in children and adolescents. *J Am Coll Cardiol* 1997;29:1039–1045.
Hannon DW, Knilans TK. Syncope in children and adolescents. *Curr Probl Pediatr* 1993;23:358–384.
Kanter RJ. Syncope and sudden death. In: Garson A Jr, Bricker JT, Fisher DJ, Neish SR, eds. *The Science and Practice of Pediatric Cardiology*, 2nd ed. Baltimore: Williams & Wilkins, 1998:2169–2199.
Ruckman RN. Cardiac causes of syncope. *Pediatr Rev* 1987;9:101–108.

SECTION IX

Abdomen

63
Abdominal Distension

A distended or protuberant abdomen may result from a variety of disorders. The diagnostic possibilities may be rapidly narrowed by information supplied by the history and a careful physical examination.

If abdominal enlargement occurs suddenly and is associated with vomiting and pain, intestinal obstruction or peritonitis must be considered. An abdominal mass or visceromegaly is easily distinguishable from other less well-defined causes. The presence of ascites opens another list of diagnostic possibilities.

In the past, the most common abdominal masses in children, which often result in abdominal enlargement, were renal in origin. In newborns about one half were due to hydronephrosis and one third to cystic lesions. In children under 1 year of age, about 40% were due to hydronephrosis and 40% due to tumors, while in children over age 1 year tumors accounted for 70% of renal masses (1). It is not known what effect prenatal ultrasound has had in these statistics.

◆ Most Common Causes of Abdominal Distension

Posture	Aerophagia
Constipation	Intestinal Obstruction
Ileus	Abdominal Mass
Pregnancy	

GENERAL CONSIDERATIONS

◆ Posture

An excessive lordosis from poor posture or the normal curve in toddlers may make the abdomen appear protuberant.

◆ Aerophagia (Air Swallowing)

The excessive swallowing of air may result from improper feeding techniques, with pacifiers, from gum chewing, and during times of excitement or stress. The abdomen tends to be tympanitic; excessive gas passage, from both above and below, is a helpful clue.

◆ Chronic Constipation

A careful history of elimination patterns is helpful. If the stool is hard, left lower quadrant masses may be palpable. A rectal examination reveals a distended rectal vault filled with stool. An abdominal radiograph may reveal massive fecal retention not apparent on palpation.

Excessive Feeding

This is most commonly seen in infants, but older children may voluntarily ingest large enough quantities of food or drink to distend the abdomen.

Malnutrition

Wasted extremities contrast with the potbellied appearance in kwashiorkor.

Muscle Weakness

Disorders causing muscle weakness may be associated with an increased lumbar lordosis and consequent abdominal protuberance.

Chilaiditi Syndrome

This is a rarely discussed entity in recent times; it refers to the presence of pain in the right upper quadrant associated with excessive air swallowing.

♦ INTESTINAL OBSTRUCTION

In most instances obstruction produces an acute onset of symptoms. Vomiting, pain, and failure to pass stools along with the abdominal distension should direct attention to this group of disorders.

Neonatal Disorders

Duodenal Atresia

Vomiting develops shortly after the first feeding or prior to it as a result of amniotic fluid ingestion. The vomitus may be bile tinged; the epigastric area is distended.

Gastrointestinal Atresia or Stenosis

The time of onset of symptoms depends on the level of obstruction, but in most, symptoms begin in the first day or two. Meconium may be passed despite obstructive lesions.

Imperforate Anus

Tracheoesophageal Fistula

Generally, coughing and regurgitation of saliva are more common than the abdominal distension that may occur with some types.

Meconium Ileus

Up to 25% of children with cystic fibrosis have been reported to present in the neonatal period with obstructive symptoms secondary to meconium ileus.

Meconium Peritonitis

Most frequently the peritonitis is the result of an intestinal atresia or meconium ileus. Generally, affected infants appear quite ill, with a hugely dilated abdomen, flank and genital edema, and distended abdominal wall veins.

Necrotizing Enterocolitis

Infants particularly at risk are those who may have had a neonatal insult. Early signs are vomiting, lethargy, temperature instability, apnea, and abdominal distension.

Hirschsprung Disease (Congenital Megacolon)

Vomiting, distension, and constipation are the usual presenting signs, but symptoms may not appear until later.

Gastric Perforation

Vomiting, refusal to feed, respiratory distress, and cyanosis are followed quickly by abdominal distension.

Enteric Duplication
Disorders with Later Onset
Incarcerated Hernia

Inguinal hernia incarceration is most common.

Intussusception

This disorder is usually characterized by episodic crampy abdominal pain; distension occurs later. "Currant jelly" stools provide evidence of vascular compromise. Intussusception generally occurs in children between 6 months and 3 years of age.

Malrotation With Volvulus

The sudden onset of vomiting followed by the rapid development of abdominal distension, particularly in the first months of life, should suggest this possibility. Shock follows rapidly.

Bezoar

Hair, vegetable matter, or casein from formulas may agglutinate to form an obstructive mass. Distension may not be as evident as is the epigastric mass.

Intestinal Tumors

These are relatively rare causes of obstruction in children.

♦ ABDOMINAL MASSES

(See also Chapter 68, Abdominal Masses, for a more complete listing.)

Visceromegaly

(See Chapter 66, Hepatomegaly, and Chapter 67, Splenomegaly.)

Neoplasia
Wilms' Tumor

Generally, parents note abdominal enlargement during bathing of the child.

Neuroblastoma

In young infants, hepatic metastases may produce the enlargement.

Hepatic Tumors

Hepatomas, hemangiomas, or abscesses may be large enough to distend the abdomen.

Lymphoma

Particularly American Burkitt lymphoma, a rapidly growing abdominal tumor in young children.

Ovarian Tumors

There may be abdominal pain as well due to torsion of the ovarian pedicle.

Pancreatic Cyst

Fullness in the left upper quadrant and epigastrium may be present, sometimes associated with ascites. There may be a history of abdominal trauma.

Gallbladder Disease
Choledochal Cyst

The triad of abdominal pain, mass in the right upper quadrant, and jaundice is often present.

Hydrops

Acute swelling of the gallbladder is usually associated with abdominal pain, jaundice, and swelling of the right upper quadrant in an acutely ill child.

Genitourinary Disorders

Hydronephrosis

Bladder Distension

Polycystic Kidneys

In the infantile form, abdominal enlargement may be the only presenting sign.

♦ Pregnancy

In the postpubertal girl with lower abdominal distension, pregnancy must always be considered.

Hydrometrocolpos

An imperforate hymen or vaginal atresia may result in massive distension of the uterus due to retained secretions. The McKusick-Kaufman syndrome features polydactyly and other congenital abnormalities as well as hydrometrocolpos.

Storage Diseases

Hepatic and splenic enlargement may produce abdominal distension. (See Chapter 66, Hepatomegaly, and Chapter 67, Splenomegaly.)

Tay-Sachs Disease

Gaucher Disease

Glycogen Storage Diseases

Mucopolysaccharidoses

Peritoneal, Mesenteric, or Omental Cysts

Usually, progressive abdominal enlargement is the only symptom.

Amyloidosis

Primary or secondary amyloidosis may be associated with significant hepatic enlargement.

Anterior Meningocele

ASCITES

Flank fullness, generalized dullness to percussion, and demonstration of a fluid wave indicate the presence of ascitic fluid. (See Chapter 64, Ascites, for diagnostic possibilities.)

INFECTION AND INFLAMMATION

Crohn Disease

Distension may be part of the clinical presentation along with weight loss, recurrent or persistent fevers, anorexia, and intermittent diarrhea.

Ulcerative Colitis

Diarrhea and abdominal pain are the most common presenting symptoms. Abdominal distension may also occur, but it is most pronounced during the complication of toxic megacolon in which there are stasis and significant bowel dilatation.

Peritonitis

Bacterial Peritonitis

Abdominal pain is usually intense. Bowel sounds are decreased or absent. The peritonitis may be primary (e.g., nephrotic syndrome, liver disease), or secondary (e.g., ruptured viscus).

Bile Peritonitis

The leakage of bile produces a sudden, severe illness with distension, abdominal pain, fever, and shock.

Tuberculous Peritonitis

Onset may be insidious without much pain or tenderness.

Abdominal Abscess

Botulism

Symptoms may begin several hours or days after toxin ingestion. Nausea, vomiting, blurred vision, diplopia, and abdominal fullness are followed by weakness and dysphagia. In infants, the most common age group to develop botulism, constipation and ptosis are the earliest signs.

Malaria

Splenic and hepatic enlargement may result in abdominal distension.

Amebiasis

A large hepatic abscess may produce distension of the right upper quadrant. General abdominal distension may also be part of the picture, as well as diarrhea, abdominal pain, and growth failure.

Congenital Cytomegalovirus Infection

ENDOCRINE AND METABOLIC DISORDERS

Hypothyroidism

The abdomen is often protuberant with an umbilical hernia.

Rickets

A potbelly appearance may be part of the picture of developing rickets, along with poor muscle tone, lordosis, and difficulty in walking.

MALABSORPTION/MALNUTRITION

Celiac Disease

The symptoms of full blown gluten enteropathy include failure to thrive, chronic diarrhea, muscle wasting, irritability, and anorexia, along with the abdominal distension.

Cystic Fibrosis

Abdominal distension may be present in the child with steatorrhea and failure to thrive or as part of the meconium ileus equivalent with recurrent abdominal pain and intermittent obstruction from fecal impactions.

Congenital Lymphangiectasia

Chylous ascites may be present.

Kwashiorkor

Protein insufficiency may lead to the characteristic potbellied appearance and orangish hair color. Protein-calorie malnutrition (marasmus) generally does not result in abdominal distension.

Abetalipoproteinemia

Growth failure during the first few months of life is followed by the development of steatorrhea and abdominal distension during the first year. Ataxia and weakness develop later.

MISCELLANEOUS CAUSES

♦ Ileus

A silent abdomen may result from various causes.

Hypokalemia

This condition may produce an ileus with vomiting and abdominal distension.

Carbohydrate Intolerance

Abdominal bloating may be noticeable along with crampy abdominal pain and loose bowel movements.

Irritable Bowel Syndrome

Abdominal distension has been described in adults. Air swallowing does not appear to be responsible.

Postviral Gastroparesis

Abdominal distension, vomiting, abdominal pain, and early satiety may be symptoms and signs of gastroparesis following an acute viral illness. Rotavirus may be a common culprit.

Toxic Megacolon

Underlying causes include Hirschsprung disease, ulcerative colitis, and *Clostridium difficile* infection.

Necrotizing Enterocolitis

Although primarily seen in low-birth weight infants, older infants and children may be affected. Bloody stools and pneumatosis intestinalis are usually present.

Intestinal Pseudo-Obstruction

Clinical manifestations include periodic vomiting, abdominal distension, constipation, urinary retention, and weight loss. The condition may be idiopathic or associated with a host of conditions including scleroderma, amyloidosis, various endocrinopathies, narcotic or laxative abuse, electrolyte disturbance, and vasoactive secreting tumors.

β-Thalassemia

During the second half of the first year of life, pallor, irritability, anorexia, fever, and an enlarging abdomen due to hepatosplenomegaly become part of the picture.

Absence of Abdominal Wall Musculature

The prune-belly (Eagle-Barrett) syndrome is associated with renal abnormalities. The classic triad is absent abdominal musculature, undescended testes, and dilated ureters.

Pneumoperitoneum

Perforation of the bowel or stomach may result in the accumulation of free abdominal air. Peritonitis usually accompanies or quickly follows this emergent condition.

Beckwith-Wiedemann Syndrome

Macroglossia, visceromegaly, and omphalocele or umbilical hernia should suggest this syndrome.

Drug-Induced Ileus

Peripheral neuropathy causing drugs such as vincristine, may lead to ileus, constipation, and abdominal distension.

Scurvy

Distension is a late manifestation of vitamin C deficiency.

Beriberi

Thiamine deficiency is usually manifested by a peripheral neuritis, encephalopathy, and cardiac failure.

Chloramphenicol Toxicity

The "gray baby syndrome" may occur in infants treated with chloramphenicol. Toxic accumulations result in a shocklike picture with abdominal distension.

REFERENCE

1. Vane DW. Left upper quadrant masses in children. *Pediatr Rev* 1992;13:25–31.

SUGGESTED READING

Sigurdsson L, Flores A, Putnam PE, Hyman PE, DiLorenzo C. Postviral gastroparesis: presentation, treatment, and outcome. *J Pediatr* 1997;130:751–754.

=64=
Ascites

Ascites is the intraperitoneal collection of fluid. In general, there are three underlying mechanisms for the production of this fluid: (a) a reduction in the oncotic pressure of the plasma; (b) an obstruction to venous or lymphatic drainage; and (c) irritation of the peritoneum by infection, trauma, or neoplasia. In diseases that are associated with ascites, combinations of these mechanisms may often be operative.

In this chapter, disorders that may be associated with the production of ascitic fluid have been divided into four groups, among which there may be some overlap. It seems especially worthwhile to separate the neonatal period from other age groups, particularly for enumeration of diseases that may produce a hydropslike picture. The other three groups reflect an attempt to categorize disorders associated with ascites by their mode of onset and associated symptoms; sudden onset in an ill-appearing child; subacute onset, with other symptoms; and insidious onset.

♦ **Most Common Causes**

Cirrhosis of the Liver
Congestive Heart Failure

Nephrotic Syndrome
Protein-Losing Enteropathy

Neonate: Urine: Perforation/Obstruction

Hydrops Fetalis

● **Causes Not to Forget**

Hepatic Vein Thrombosis

Turner Syndrome

NEONATAL PERIOD

Genitourinary Causes

♦ Urinary Tract Obstruction with Perforation

Urine is the most commonly found ascitic fluid in the neonate. In some cases the actual leakage site may be difficult to locate; posterior urethral valves, unilateral ureteral stenosis, and urethral atresia must be considered as possible causes of obstruction.

Hydrometrocolpos

The clinical picture may falsely suggest ascites when the uterus is grossly distended with retained secretions. These secretions may spill into the peritoneal cavity, producing ascites.

Ruptured Perinephric Cyst

Congenital Nephrosis

Nephrosis is usually not present at birth, but edema and ascites may be noticeable in the neonatal period.

Renal Vein Thrombosis

Ascites is a late finding. Flank mass, oliguria, and hematuria occur first.

Peritonitis

Meconium Peritonitis

Most infants with prenatal perforation of the bowel are acutely ill, with tachypnea, grunting, and cyanosis. The abdominal wall is distended with prominent superficial veins. In some infants, mild-to-moderate distension and hydroceles may be the only presenting signs. Bowel perforation occurring suddenly after birth causes acute illness. Air as well as fluid may be identified on abdominal radiographs.

Bile Peritonitis

Newborns are rarely affected; they may not be as acutely ill as older children with peritoneal irritation from bile. Fluctuating jaundice and acholic stools, inguinal hernias, and abdominal distension are diagnostic clues.

Acute Bacterial Peritonitis

Affected infants are acutely ill. Underlying causes include acute appendicitis, perforation of a hollow viscus, gangrenous bowel, trauma, and septicemia.

Chylous Ascites

The etiology usually cannot be determined. Generally, these infants do not appear ill. The ascitic fluid is milky due to a high fat content. The onset is insidious and may be associated with pleural effusions and lymphedema of the extremities.

◆ Disorders That May Produce a Hydropslike Picture

For an expanded list refer to the article by van Maldergem et al. (1).

Erythroblastosis Fetalis

Infants with severe isoimmune disease, most commonly a result of Rh incompatibility, may present with ascites and anasarca. ABO incompatibility is a rare cause.

Congestive Heart Failure

In utero causes include premature closure of the foramen ovale and supraventricular tachycardia.

Circulatory Abnormalities

Arteriovenous malformations, hemangioendothelioma, umbilical or chorionic vein thrombosis, twin-to-twin transfusions, and fetal-maternal hemorrhage may be causes.

Fetal Infections

Cytomegalovirus, toxoplasmosis, congenital hepatitis, congenital syphilis, leptospirosis, and Chagas disease have all been implicated. Parvovirus B19 is the most frequent.

Neoplasia

Placental chorioangioma, choriocarcinoma in situ, and fetal neuroblastomatosis may be causes.

Miscellaneous Causes

● **Turner Syndrome**

The most common cause of fetal hydrops.

α-Thalassemia (Bart's Hemoglobin)

Maternal Diabetes

Infantile Polycystic Kidney

Achondroplasia

Achondrogenesis Type III

Pulmonary Lymphangiectasia

Ruptured Ovarian Cyst

Cystic Adenomatoid Malformation of the Lung

Lysosomal Storage Diseases

Congenital ascites may be a presenting sign of these disorders, which include infantile sialidosis, Salla disease, GM_1 gangliosidosis, and Gaucher disease.

SUDDEN ONSET IN AN ILL-APPEARING CHILD

Acute Bacterial Peritonitis

Severe, sudden onset of abdominal pain with fever and distension is characteristic. Some ascitic fluid or exudate may form. Children with nephrotic syndrome are particularly predisposed to bacterial peritonitis.

- **Hepatic Vein Occlusion (Budd-Chiari Syndrome)**

  There is usually an abrupt onset of abdominal enlargement. Abdominal pain, hepatomegaly, and, less commonly, splenomegaly and jaundice may be present. This syndrome may be secondary to a number of underlying disorders including hepatoma, hypernephroma, leukemia, sickle cell disease, inflammatory bowel disease, and allergic vasculitis.

Fulminant Hepatic Failure

Bile Peritonitis

  Escape of bile into the peritoneal cavity results in a sudden, severe illness with abdominal distension, tenderness, fever, and shock.

Bowel Perforation or Infarction

Acute Hemorrhagic Pancreatitis

  Clues include a bluish discoloration around the umbilicus (Cullen sign) or in the flanks. There may be a hemorrhagic pleural effusion.

Acute Glomerulonephritis

  Ascites is uncommon and usually overshadowed by other signs and symptoms.

SUBACUTE ONSET WITH OTHER SYMPTOMS

Ascites develops during the course of some diseases that have other more prominent signs and symptoms.

- ◆ **Cirrhosis**

  A large variety of disease processes may cause cirrhosis, the leading cause of ascites after the neonatal period. Although the first manifestations of cirrhosis may be those of portal hypertension (splenomegaly and esophageal varices, with hematemesis and ascites), there are often other clues in the past history or on physical examination that may suggest a specific cause. The development of ascites may be insidious or acute.

Obstructive Biliary Diseases

Biliary Atresia

  In the neonate, the initial picture is that of obstructive jaundice, followed by liver and spleen enlargement. Growth failure and, later, ascites become evident.

Choledochal Cyst

  Early signs are the triad of abdominal pain, jaundice, and a mass in the right upper quadrant.

Cystic Fibrosis

Biliary cirrhosis may occur late in the course.

Ascending Cholangitis

Stones and tumors are rare causes of obstruction of the biliary tree that may produce cirrhosis if longstanding.

Infection and Inflammation

Hepatitis

A, B, and other forms have been implicated.

Rubella; Coxsackievirus Infection; Cytomegalovirus Infection; Herpes Simplex

Toxoplasmosis

Syphilis

Neonatal Hepatitis

A catchall group of diseases, not caused by the previous diseases.

Mycobacterium Avium-Intracellulare

A few cases have been described associated with acquired immunodeficiency syndrome.

Chronic Active Hepatitis

Persistent jaundice, of 4 weeks duration or longer, or relapsing episodes may be clues. Other symptoms include arthritis, fever, erythema nodosum, lethargy, and hepatosplenomegaly.

Ulcerative Colitis and Regional Enteritis

Vascular Causes

Constrictive Pericarditis

Signs of heart disease may or may not be present. Hepatomegaly and dyspnea on exertion precede the ascites. The liver may be tender to palpation.

Cardiac Failure

Ascites is present only in children with chronic right heart failure, as in pulmonic stenosis, tricuspid atresia, and pulmonary hypertension.

Hereditary Hemorrhagic Telangiectasia

Cutaneous telangiectasia may suggest liver involvement. Cirrhosis develops as a result of hepatic cell fibrosis that follows shunting of blood.

Genetic and Metabolic Disorders

Some of the more common causes are listed here.

Cystic Fibrosis

Wilson Disease (Hepatolenticular Degeneration)

There may be neurologic, hematologic, or gastrointestinal signs. Cirrhosis with ascites or hematemesis may be the initial symptom.

Alpha$_1$-Antitrypsin Deficiency

Affected children may present in the neonatal period with jaundice or later in life with cirrhotic manifestations.

Galactosemia

Vomiting, jaundice, hepatosplenomegaly, failure to thrive, and corneal clouding may precede the signs associated with cirrhosis.

Glycogen Storage Disease, Type IV

Hepatomegaly and poor muscle tone precede signs of cirrhosis.

Tyrosinemia

Infants with the acute form present in the first 6 months of life with vomiting, diarrhea, hepatosplenomegaly, edema, ascites, and failure to thrive. Jaundice is present in one half of the cases. In the chronic form, cirrhosis may be a later presenting sign.

GM$_1$ Gangliosidosis

Congenital ascites and hepatosplenomegaly may be the initial clues.

Drugs

Hepatotoxic Drugs

Methotrexate and similar preparations may result in ascites.

Hypervitaminosis A

Although uncommon, ascites has been described along with headache (increased intracranial pressure), bone pain, and scaly dermatitis.

Veno-Occlusive Disease

Cirrhosis, splenomegaly, and ascites may occur following ingestion of toxins such as "bush tea" in the Caribbean islands.

Renal Disorders

♦ Nephrotic Syndrome

Edema, proteinuria, hypoproteinemia, and hypercholesterolemia constitute the syndrome, all stemming from the massive proteinuria. Ascites may be a prominent finding.

Chronic Renal Failure

Malignancy

Lymphoma

Leukemia

Hodgkin Disease

Granulosa Cell Tumor of Ovary

Ascites occasionally is part of the symptom complex in young girls, as well as early breast development, advanced height for age, pubic hair, and intermittent vaginal bleeding.

Mesenteric Fibromatosis

Systemic Lupus Erythematosus

Serosal involvement may uncommonly result in ascites.

Kwashiorkor

Hypersensitivity Peritonitis

Abdominal distension and pain, nausea, vomiting, diarrhea, and weight loss appear gradually. Hypersensitivity angiitis probably represents an allergic reaction.

Chronic Granulomatous Disease

Ascites may occur as a result of hepatic granulomatosis.

Cystic Mesathelioma of Peritoneum

May be benign or malignant.

INSIDIOUS ONSET

♦ Nephrotic Syndrome

♦ Protein-Losing Enteropathies

Various disorders may be causative. Abdominal symptoms, such as diarrhea and cramping, may be chronic. Ménétrier disease (hypertrophic gastropathy) frequently mimics nephrotic syndrome.

Pancreatitis

Abdominal pain is the most constant symptom, but it may be mild and ascitic fluid formation gradual. Inapparent or intentional abdominal trauma (as in a battered child) may result in chronic pancreatic fluid leakage.

Chylous Ascites

Affected children rarely have symptoms other than abdominal swelling. This form is usually the result of an injury to, obstruction of, or anomaly of the thoracic duct. Child abuse must always be considered.

Portal Vein Obstruction

Intraperitoneal Tumors

These tumors may cause occlusion of inferior vena cava or hepatic veins, or they may seed the peritoneal cavity or metastasize to the liver, resulting in fluid formation.

Tuberculous Peritonitis

Presentation may be vague, with low-grade fever and few localizing symptoms.

MIMICS OF ASCITES

Omental or Mesenteric Cysts

Celiac Disease

Severe Megacolon

REFERENCE

1. Van Maldergem L, Jauniaux E, Fourneau C, Gillerot Y. Genetic causes of hydrops fetalis. *Pediatrics* 1992;89:81–86.

SUGGESTED READING

Cochran WJ. Ascites. In: Oski FA, Deangelis CD, Feigin RD, McMillan JA, Warshu JB, eds. *Principles and practice of pediatrics*, 2nd ed. Philadelphia: JB Lippincott, 1994:1902–1907.
McGillivray BC, Hall JG. Nonimmune hydrops fetalis. *Pediatr Rev* 1987;9:197–202.

65

Abdominal Pain

Abdominal pain is a common pediatric problem with such a variety of causes that a listing of all the diagnostic possibilities would read like the index of a pediatrics textbook. In the classification that follows, abdominal pain has been divided into two general categories, recurrent and acute. However, there may be a great deal of overlap between these two groups: Separate instances of recurrent pain may appear to be acute; conversely, disorders with acute presentations often may become recurrent.

For both recurrent and acute abdominal pain, common causes, less common ones, and then unusual causes are listed. An additional category of trauma-induced causes has been included for acute abdominal pain.

The history is important in the evaluation of this symptom and should include information about the site of the pain, its pattern of radiation, duration and events surrounding onset of pain, and systemic symptoms, as well as past medical history, social history, and familial history. The physical examination obviously is also critically important, there are extra-abdominal causes of abdominal pain as well.

♦ **Most Common Causes of Abdominal Pain**

Recurrent	**Acute**
Chronic, Nonspecific	Gastroenteritis
Constipation	Mesenteric Adenitis
Carbohydrate Malabsorption	Appendicitis
Functional	Dietary Indiscretion
	Bacterial Enterocolitis
	Trauma

● **Abdominal Pains Not to Forget**

Pneumonia	Pharyngitis (Streptococcal)
Pyelonephritis	Diabetic Ketoacidosis
Volvulus	Incarcerated Hernia

RECURRENT ABDOMINAL PAIN

Common Causes

♦ **Chronic Nonspecific Abdominal Pain of Childhood**

Up to 10% of all children, particularly those between 5 and 12 years of age, may have chronic "bellyaches." This disorder, despite its undetermined pathogenetic mechanism, is so common that whole books have been written about it (1). Characteristics of the pain may vary, but generally, the pain is poorly localized— most children vaguely refer to the periumbical area; in fact, according to Apley, the further the pain is from the umbilicus, the more likely an organic cause for the pain. The episodes are generally less than an hour's duration and frequently only minutes long. The children prefer to lie down and may look pale; on cessation of the pain they are up and about as if nothing had happened. Appetite and growth are unaffected. A familial history of abdominal pain may be elicited.

♦ Constipation

Chronic stool withholding may be associated with vague, recurrent abdominal pain resulting from colonic spasm or dilatation of the proximal intestine. The etiology of constipation may be varied. History of elimination habits and rectal examination lead to the diagnosis.

♦ Carbohydrate Malabsorption

Liebman (2) found lactose intolerance in about one third of children with chronic nonspecific abdominal pain. Bloating and cramping after lactose ingestion is common in populations at high risk (e.g., blacks, Asians, and Native Americans). Other carbohydrates may be important causes as well including sucrose, sorbital from sugarless gums, etc., and fructose from fruit drinks.

♦ Functional Pain

The subjective complaint of pain in a child has special meaning: It may represent a wish to avoid school or a cry for attention or help, as in abuse or molestation. It is also a common familial somatic response to stress, among other causes. The difficult but important task for the physician is to uncover, if possible, the situational forces being experienced by the child.

Irritable Colon

The crampy episodes of abdominal pain may be especially increased at times of stress. There may be a family history of the disorder. Stools are usually pelletlike and frequent but occasionally may be loose.

Dysmenorrhea

This poorly understood disorder is common in adolescents and young adults. The discomfort does not begin until regular ovulation is established and seems to be related to endometrial prostaglandin release.

Mittelschmerz

Ovulatory pain midway through the menstrual cycle often occurs only on one side, especially the right. Affected girls usually have some abdominal tenderness; guarding and even an increased white blood cell count may be present.

Allergic-Tension Fatigue Syndrome

Abdominal pain may be a primary complaint in this poorly understood complex of symptoms attributed to food allergy. Headaches, irritability, lethargy, and leg pains may accompany the pain. Elimination diets should be tried in suspected cases (3).

Less Common Disorders

Air Swallowing (Aerophagia)

This may be a more common cause of crampy abdominal pain than has been considered. The child may have increased belching and flatulence as well. Excessive gum chewing may be one cause. Pain in the right upper quadrant associated with air swallowing, called Chilaiditi syndrome in the past, is thought to be caused by interposition of the colon between the liver and the diaphragm.

Migraine

Controversy exists whether recurrent pains are a manifestation of a migraine variant or precede the classic picture. Cyclic vomiting is sometimes present.

Gastritis

Antral nodular gastritis has been found to be associated with *Helicobacter pylori*.

Peptic Ulcer

This may perhaps be more common than has been recognized. Only one half of children with a peptic ulcer manifest the classic picture of burning epigastric pain increased on fasting and relieved by foods or antacids. Vomiting and gastrointestinal blood loss are prominent symptoms.

Inflammatory Bowel Disease

Regional enteritis and ulcerative colitis may have few symptoms early in their development. Diarrhea, blood loss, weight loss, unexplained fever, anemia, growth failure, and a host of other symptoms may occur during the course of the illness.

Sickle Cell Anemia

Abdominal crises may be seen along with other vaso-occlusive syndromes. The pain is severe. Fever is often present.

Urinary Tract Disorders

Chronic pyelonephritis, hydronephrosis, ureteroceles, and other urinary tract disorders may be associated with recurrent abdominal pain.

Hiatus Hernia

Epigastric or substernal discomfort is common. Associated reflux of gastric contents into the distal esophagus may also result in "heartburn" symptoms that may increase during recumbency. Torsion spasms of neck (Sandifer syndrome) is another clue to the presence of a hiatus hernia.

Esophagitis

Chronic reflux may result in abdominal as well as chest pain.

Drug Therapy

The diagnosis is usually obvious, especially with aspirin, but effects of antibiotics, anticonvulsants, and bronchodilators should also be considered.

Parasites

Most children harboring intestinal parasites have no symptoms, although these organisms are frequently suggested as a cause of abdominal pain. *Giardia lamblia* infection should be considered, even without altered bowel patterns. Ascariasis, infestation by the large roundworm, rarely causes symptoms. Large numbers of parasites may cause some cramping, but other symptoms such as lethargy, flatulence, bloating, diarrhea, and anorexia usually accompany the cramps. When eosinophilia occurs in association with peptic ulcer symptoms, strongyloidiasis should be suspected.

Masses and Tumors

Vague symptoms or recurrent pain may be seen with any intra-abdominal mass or tumor, including splenomegaly, hepatomegaly, ovarian cysts, teratomas, bezoars, Wilms' tumor, and neuroblastomas. Careful palpation of the abdomen for a mass is mandatory in every child with this symptom.

Collagen Vascular Diseases

Abdominal pain is common in the systemic form of juvenile rheumatoid arthritis and systemic lupus erythematosus.

Uncommon and Unusual Causes

● Malrotation With or Without Volvulus

Partial small bowel obstruction may cause intermittent symptoms of abdominal pain. Likewise, volvulus may be intermittent but is a catastrophe waiting to happen.

Heavy Metal Poisoning

Abdominal pain may be an early sign of lead, arsenic, or mercury poisoning.

Diskitis

Abdominal pain may be a presenting symptom of inflammation of an intervertebral disk space. Back pain or decreased movement becomes apparent over time.

Endometriosis

Recurrent Pancreatitis

This condition may be hereditary as well as associated with cystic fibrosis, hyperparathyroidism, and hyperlipoproteinemia. Pancreatic calcifications on plain films of the abdomen are a later finding. Pain is generally intense.

Arrhythmias

Particularly, paroxysmal supraventricular tachycardia may cause pain.

Brain Tumor

Signs and symptoms of increased intracranial pressure predominate.

Hyperthyroidism

Irritability, weight loss, heat intolerance, and tachycardia are usually present.

Addison Disease

Anorexia, weight loss, lethargy, and muscular weakness are common symptoms.

Meconium Ileus Equivalent

As many as 10% of children with cystic fibrosis may develop severe constipation and abdominal pain.

Hematocolpos

A bulging imperforate hymen may be seen on pelvic examination. A lower abdominal mass is usually palpable.

Linea Alba Hernia

In some cases, pain may not be localized to the palpable nodule, which is most often near the umbilicus.

Mesenteric Cysts

Coarctation of the Aorta

Hypertension with weak femoral pulses is characteristic.

Porphyria

Moderate or severe pain, often colicky, is characteristic. Constipation is usually significant. Onset before puberty is rare.

Duplication of Bowel

Affected children usually present with symptoms of obstruction but may have ectopic gastric mucosa resulting in ulceration.

Tuberculosis of Spine

Choledochal Cyst

A mass in the right upper quadrant, jaundice, and abdominal pain suggest this lesion.

Abdominal Epilepsy

Even greater controversy abounds here than with migraine. Some researchers feel these episodes are migrainous; others have described children whose pain ceased during anticonvulsant therapy.

Superior Mesenteric Artery Syndrome

This syndrome may be seen in teenagers who have recently lost weight or have been in body casts. Vomiting, nausea, bloating, and early satiety on eating are common. The mechanism is compression of the intestine in the "nutcracker" formed by the aorta and the superior mesenteric artery, without the cushion effect of peritoneal fat.

Abdominal Angina

Colicky abdominal pain occurs after meals; weight loss usually follows. A bruit is frequently heard over the epigastrium.

Hyperlipoproteinemia

Familial, type I, is characterized by eruptive xanthomatosis, lipemia retinalis, recurrent abdominal pain, pancreatitis, and hepatosplenomegaly. Type IV may be associated with pancreatitis when serum triglyceride levels are very high.

Transient Protein-Losing Enteropathy

This disorder is ushered in by the onset of anorexia, emesis, or abdominal pain followed by generalized edema.

Spinal Cord Tumors

Leg weakness or pain, back pain, and bowel or bladder problems are much more common.

Slipping Rib Syndrome

Pain is often localized to the upper quadrants. Palpation of the chest wall over the costal cartilages 8 to 10 will often localize the pain.

Familial Mediterranean Fever

This disease is characterized by febrile attacks of peritonitis, pleuritis, or synovitis, usually brief in duration. Inheritance pattern is autosomal recessive.

Hereditary Angioedema

Recurrent attacks of abdominal pain are often accompanied by swelling of the extremities and occasionally life-threatening laryngeal edema.

Wegener Granulomatosis

Recurrent abdominal pain may be seen in this rare disorder primarily characterized by renal vasculitis and upper and lower respiratory tract necrotizing granulomas.

Familial Dysautonomia

ACUTE ABDOMINAL PAIN

Any cause of recurrent abdominal pain may produce acute symptoms. Of those listed, the most severe acute pain is caused by sickle cell disease and pancreatitis, though the presentation of any given child depends on the pain threshold and associations from previous episodes.

Common Causes

♦ **Gastroenteritis**

Viral origin is most common. Diarrhea is usually a more prominent symptom than in appendicitis. There is no rebound tenderness; bowel sounds are hyperactive. Pain tends to be diffuse.

♦ **Bacterial Gastroenteritis/Enterocolitis**

Infection by *Shigella, Yersinia, Campylobacter,* and occasionally *Salmonella* organisms may produce abdominal pain.

♦ **Acute Appendicitis**

The variations in appendiceal position may result in "atypical" pictures. Fever, anorexia, and vomiting are helpful clues.

◆ Mesenteric Adenitis

Enlargement of lymph nodes in the terminal ileum, is most often caused by a viral infection. When associated with *Yersinia* or streptococcal pharyngitis the pain may mimic acute appendicitis, but it is less localized.

◆ Dietary Indiscretion

The amount and type of food or fluid intake prior to onset of the pain should be ascertained.

Food Poisoning

Vomiting and diarrhea are frequent accompaniments. Other family members may be ill.

● Pharyngitis

Especially when streptococcal, pharyngitis may be associated with abdominal pain and vomiting, simulating an acute intestinal process.

● Pneumonia

Children with pneumonia of the lower lobe may present with abdominal pain. Careful auscultation of the chest and timing of respiratory rate are required.

● Acute Pyelonephritis

Presenting symptoms may be gastrointestinal—vomiting, abdominal pain, and diarrhea—with none of the classic urinary tract signs.

Less Frequent Causes

Pelvic Inflammatory Disease

Pain is most frequent during the menstrual period. Pain in the right upper quadrant may result from gonorrheal or chlamydial perihepatitis (Fitz-Hugh-Curtis syndrome).

Acute Pancreatitis

Pain is initially epigastric. As symptoms progress, vomiting of bile may occur.

Electrolyte Disturbances

Ileus and pain are associated with hypokalemia.

● Hernias

Pain is severe if the hernia is strangulated or incarcerated.

- **Diabetic Ketoacidosis**

    Abdominal pain is an often overlooked presentation of diabetic ketoacidosis (DKA). Polyuria persists even though the child may appear dehydrated. Respirations are heavy and deep. A test useful in differentiating DKA as a cause of abdominal pain from other causes (e.g., appendicitis) precipitating DKA, is the serum bicarbonate level. If DKA is the cause, the bicarbonate is less than 10 mEq per dL, and the pain recedes when the bicarbonate exceeds 10 mEq per dL.

Hepatitis

    In both infectious and serum hepatitis, vomiting and anorexia are common. Pain is usually not well localized.

Infectious Mononucleosis

Henoch-Schönlein Syndrome (Henoch-Schönlein Purpura)

    Hemorrhagic rash, especially on the lower extremities, is the most consistent finding. Arthritis, nephritis, and areas of skin edema are common. Abdominal pain is associated with submucosal and subserosal bleeding in the intestinal wall; intussusception is a complication in approximately 3% of cases.

Intussusception

    The sudden onset of acute severe recurring episodes of pain may be accompanied by vomiting; there may be an unusual degree of lethargy. Dark blood-tinged mucousy ("currant jelly") stools occur later.

Peritonitis

    A rigid, tender abdomen with rebound tenderness is typical, with diminished or absent bowel sounds. Affected children appear acutely ill.

Obstruction Secondary to Adhesions

    There is usually a prior history of surgery or peritonitis. Bowel sounds are high-pitched, with rushes; vomiting is common.

- **Volvulus**

    There may be a history of intermittent pain prior to midgut volvulus. Shock may quickly ensue.

Cholecystitis; Cholelithiasis; Acute Hydrops of Gallbladder

    Gallstones may be a finding in disorders with hemolysis. A hydropic gallbladder is often palpable.

Herpes Zoster

Acute abdominal pain may precede the appearance of the vesicles over the abdominal wall.

Acute Glomerulonephritis

Hypoglycemia

Meckel Diverticulum

Profuse, painless rectal bleeding is a more common presentation than pain. Pain symptoms may mimic appendicitis. Perforation may lead to peritonitis. Diverticulum may be the lead site of intussusception.

Leukemia, Lymphoma

Cat-Scratch Disease

Children may have hepatosplenomegaly with abdominal pain as a significant finding or chief complaint.

Dietl Syndrome (Crisis)

Intermittent obstruction of the uteropelvic junction, particularly following the ingestion of large amounts of fluid. Symptoms include crampy upper abdominal pain, nausea, and vomiting.

Iliac Adenitis

There may be a history of lower extremity injury or infection days to weeks before onset of abdominal pain. Hip pain may also be present.

Myocarditis

Acute Rheumatic Fever

In one series, 5% of children presented with abdominal pain of such severity that appendectomy was performed.

Abdominal Abscesses

Abscesses may be perinephric, psoas, subdiaphragmatic, and so forth.

Uncommon and Unusual Causes

Mesenteric Artery Occlusion

Abdominal distension, nausea, and vomiting develop, followed rapidly by shock.

Testicular Torsion or Neoplasm

Pain is usually scrotal or lower abdominal, allowing separation from other abdominal processes.

Nephrotic Syndrome

Ménétrier Syndrome

Hypertrophic gastropathy, may be associated with abdominal pain as well as protein-losing enteropathy.

Ascites

Renal Colic

Stone formation may occur because of urinary infection or obstruction, with immobilization, or in genetic and metabolic defects. Gross hematuria is present as well as the colicky abdominal or flank pain.

Hemolytic Crisis

Children with hereditary spherocytosis may present with acute abdominal pain and anemia associated with infections. The spleen is usually palpable.

Pericarditis

Epigastric as well as chest pain may be present

Hypertensive Crisis

Abdominal pain and vomiting may be primary symptoms.

Serositis

Connective tissue disorders, especially systemic lupus erythematosus, may be associated with episodes of serositis and chest or abdominal pain.

Vasculitis

Vasculitis from numerous causes may be associated with abdominal pain. Periarteritis nodosa and mucocutaneous lymph node syndrome are best known in children.

Spinal Cord Tumors

Erythromycin-Induced Cholestasis

The estolate ester may induce cholestasis, particularly in children over age 12 years. The abdominal pain may be acute or the picture may resemble one of obstructive jaundice.

Paroxysmal Cold Hemoglobinuria

Most commonly seen after viral infections. After cold exposure the child experiences back or abdominal pain, followed by chills, fever, and hemoglobinuria.

Eosinophilic Gastroenteritis

Nausea, vomiting, and diarrhea with recurrent abdominal pain and peripheral blood eosinophilia are found in this unusual disorder.

Black Widow Spider Bite

Trauma Induced

♦ Abdominal Wall Muscle Bruise or Strain

This is by far the most common of the traumatic causes of acute pain. Tenderness is superficial. There may be a history of a blow to the abdomen or of new or excessive exercise activity such as sit-ups.

Splenic Rupture or Hematoma

Left shoulder pain may be an early clue.

Liver Laceration or Hematoma

Injury is usually the result of blunt trauma and should be suspected if the hematocrit continues to drop following abdominal trauma.

Pancreatic Pseudocyst

Symptoms of pain, fever, and vomiting, with a palpable epigastric mass, usually begin some time after trauma. Serum amylase levels are usually elevated. Ascites and pleural effusions may be present.

Perforated Viscus

Signs of peritonitis develop. Free air may be seen on upright films of the abdomen.

Intraperitoneal Blood

The presence of blood in the peritoneum from any cause produces abdominal pain.

REFERENCES

1. Apley J. *The child with abdominal pains,* 2nd ed. Oxford: Blackwell Scientific Publications, 1975.
2. Liebman WM. Recurrent abdominal pain in children: lactose and sucrose intolerance, a prospective study. *Pediatrics* 1979;64:43–45.
3. Crook WG. Food allergy—the great masquerader. *Pediatr Clin North Am* 1975;22:227–238.

SUGGESTED READING

Boyle JT. Recurrent abdominal pain: an update. *Pediatr Rev* 1997;9:310–320.
Bugenstein RH, Phibbs CM. Abdominal pain in children caused by linea alba hernias. *Pediatrics* 1975;56:1073–1074.

Chong SKF, Lou Q, Asnicar MA, et al. *Heliobacter pylori* infection in recurrent abdominal pain in childhood: comparison of diagnostic tests and therapy. *Pediatrics* 1995;96:211–215.

Hoffenberg EJ, Rothenberg SS, Bensard D, Sondheimer JM, Sokol RJ. Outcome after exploratory laparotomy for unexplained abdominal pain of childhood. *Arch Pediatr Adolesc Med* 1997;151:993–998.

Hyams JS. A simple explanation for chronic abdominal distress. *Contemp Pediatr* 1991;8:88–104.

Hyams JS, Hyman PE. Recurrent abdominal pain and the biopsychosocial model of medical practice. *J Pediatr* 1998;133:473–478.

Silverberg M. Chronic abdominal pain in adolescents. *Pediatr Ann* 1991;20:179–185.

Walker LS, Guite JW, Duke M, Barnard JA, Greene JW. Recurrent abdominal pain: a potential precursor of irritable bowel syndrome in adolescents and young adults. *J Pediatr* 1998;132:1010–1015.

66

Hepatomegaly

Hepatomegaly, or the presence of an enlarged liver, is a relatively common finding in the pediatric age group. Diseases that may be associated with hepatomegaly are numerous; pathophysiologic mechanisms of enlargement include vascular congestion, hyperplasia of Kupffer cells, cholestasis, cellular infiltrates, storage products, inflammation, fatty infiltration, and intrinsic tumors. Because the liver can be a site of extramedullary hematopoiesis and is part of the reticulo-endothelial system, enlargement often represents a secondary process rather than one primarily focused on the liver.

The amount of extension of the liver below the right costal margin at the midclavicular line must not be used as the sole criterion for enlargement. The diagnosis of hepatomegaly is best based on liver span measurements. A discussion of the technique of measurement and graphs of the normal range for children can be found in the article by Walker and Mathis (1).

In this chapter, causes of hepatomegaly have been divided into groups by age of onset and by the presence or absence of systemic signs or illness. The largest group contains disorders that may appear at any age.

♦ **Most Common Causes of Hepatomegaly**

Reactive (Associated with Viral Infections)   Viral Hepatitis
Drug and Toxins (Especially Acetaminophen)   Iron Deficiency Anemia
Sickle Cell Disease   Hemolytic Anemias
Congestive Heart Failure

● **Causes Not to Forget**

Acetaminophen Toxicity   Storage Disorders
Peroxisomal Disorders   Cystic Disease
Hemangiomas   Pseudomegaly-displaced down

APPEARANCE IN NEONATAL PERIOD

♦ Intrauterine and Neonatal Hepatitis

A diffuse array of infections, congenital and acquired, may be associated with hepatomegaly. Fulminant intrauterine infections may be recognized during the first few days of life. Jaundice is common. Microcephaly, petechiae, and splenomegaly may also be present. Infections that should be considered include cytomegalovirus, rubella, toxoplasmosis, herpes simplex, syphilis, parvovirus, and varicella. Bacterial sepsis and acquired viral infections, including enterovirus infections, may also be causes.

Maternal Diabetes

Infants are generally large for gestational age and appear plethoric, hypotonic, and lethargic.

Isoimmunization Disorders

Infants with erythroblastosis fetalis, most commonly as a result of Rh or ABO sensitization, may have significant hepatomegaly, because of extramedullary hematopoiesis, and in severe cases, congestive heart failure.

Congestive Heart Failure

Cardiac failure, especially right-sided, produces significant hepatomegaly.

Hemolytic Anemias

Children with disorders associated with hemolytic anemia such as congenital spherocytosis, may have liver enlargement.

Biliary Atresia

In extrahepatic atresia, infants appear normal at birth. Jaundice appears after the first week of life. Intrahepatic atresia must also be considered in any unexplained obstructive jaundice. The liver becomes slightly enlarged and smooth.

Inspissated Bile Syndrome

This syndrome usually follows a moderately severe hemolytic disease. Persistent low-grade hyperbilirubinemia and hepatomegaly are found. Stools are pale to dark yellow in color.

• Hemangioma of Liver

The development of congestive heart failure of obscure origin in a child with hepatomegaly may be the presenting sign. Occasionally, cutaneous hemangiomata may be found.

Neonatal Lupus Erythematosus

Infants with neonatal lupus may have cholestatic hepatitis as well as hematologic abnormalities including thrombocytopenia, neutropenia, and hemolytic anemia. Rashes generally appear at 6 weeks of age. Most mothers are asymptomatic.

Metastatic Neuroblastoma

Cutaneous as well as hepatic tumor involvement may be present.

Hemorrhage into the Liver

Birth trauma may result in bleeding into the liver with hepatic enlargement and anemia.

Galactosemia

Affected infants appear normal at birth but then develop vomiting, diarrhea, hepatosplenomegaly, and jaundice. They often die of early fulminant sepsis, usually with *Escherichia coli*. Failure to thrive and cataracts are often present in survivors.

Disorders of the Urea Cycle

Citrullinemia, argininosuccinicaciduria, or argininemia should be considered in infants with vomiting, lethargy, coma, and seizures. Earliest signs appear in the first 2 months of life. Hypoglycemia, hypoproteinemia, and a hemorrhagic diathesis are attributed to acute hepatic necrosis.

Methylmalonic Acidemia

Infants with the vitamin B_{12}-responsive form present with early nursing difficulties, vomiting, episodes of metabolic acidosis during infections or following increased protein intake, failure to thrive, and microcephaly or macrocephaly.

Beckwith-Wiedemann Syndrome

Macroglossia, omphalocele or umbilical hernia, and postnatal gigantism are suggestive findings. Neonates may have severe hypoglycemia.

• Zellweger Syndrome

Hypotonia with a high forehead, flat and narrow facies, redundant skin folds of the neck, and hepatomegaly are characteristic findings.

Alpha$_1$-Antitrypsin Deficiency

Signs of cholestatic disease such as jaundice and hepatosplenomegaly may occasionally be present in the neonate. More commonly, the deficiency produces an anicteric hepatitis that progresses to cirrhosis.

Achondrogenesis

Affected infants usually die shortly after birth. Very small stature is obvious.

♦ **Infantile Sialidosis**

This is a rare, primary neuraminidase deficiency characterized by dwarfism, failure to thrive, congenital ascites, pericardial effusions, skeletal abnormalities, and early death.

APPEARANCE IN INFANCY WITH PROMINENT SYSTEMIC FINDINGS

♦ **Sickle Cell Disease**

Splenomegaly is common during infancy. Hepatomegaly is present in almost all affected infants and children and becomes more severe during crises.

Neuroblastoma

Liver enlargement occurs with hepatic metastases. The primary tumor may also be mistaken for liver enlargement.

β-Thalassemia

First symptoms usually begin after 6 months of age. Hepatosplenomegaly is striking; pallor, irritability, fever, anorexia, and frontal bossing are other findings.

Klippel-Trenaunay-Weber Syndrome

There is hypertrophy of one or more limbs, with hemangiomas, varicosities, and arteriovenous fistulae.

Histiocytosis X (Letterer-Siwe Disease)

Onset of symptoms is generally in infancy, with scaly, crusted skin lesions, enlargement of liver and spleen, lymphadenopathy, fever, anemia, thrombocytopenia, and leukopenia.

Mucopolysaccharidoses

● **Mucopolysaccharidosis I (Hurler Syndrome)**

Coarse features gradually appear; macrocephaly, claw hands, hirsutism, hepatosplenomegaly, and mental deterioration become prominent.

Mucopolysaccharidosis II (Hunter Syndrome)

Features are less coarse than in Hurler syndrome, but stiff joints, dwarfism, and hepatosplenomegaly occur.

Mucopolysaccharidosis III (Sanfilippo Syndrome)

Onset is between 1 and 3 years of age. Splenomegaly is minimal, but mental retardation is severe. Features are coarse.

Mucopolysaccharidosis VI (Maroteaux-Lamy Syndrome)

Affected children have coarse features as well as stiff joints, cloudy corneas, and hepatosplenomegaly.

Glycogen Storage Diseases

● **Type I (von Gierke Disease)**

The abdomen is protuberant; the enlarged, firm, smooth liver may extend to the iliac crest. Splenomegaly and cardiomegaly are absent. Profound hypoglycemia and acidosis may be present in early infancy. Short stature and a doll-like facies are other features.

Type II (Pompe Disease)

Cardiac and skeletal muscle are involved. Signs including profound hypotonia with decreased reflexes develop in the first few weeks of life. Cardiac failure is common and probably the cause of hepatomegaly.

Type III (Forbes Disease)

Hepatomegaly and failure to thrive may be the only symptoms. Fasting hypoglycemia and hyperlipidemia may be present.

Type IV (Andersen Disease)

Infants present at approximately 1 year of age with enlarged nodular liver and splenomegaly. Cirrhosis develops, and death eventually occurs as a result of portal hypertension.

Type V (Hers Disease)

An enlarged liver and growth retardation may be prominent.

Hereditary Fructose Intolerance

Affected infants are normal at birth. Clinical manifestations appear after dietary introduction of fructose and sucrose. Vomiting and diarrhea occur early; hepatomegaly develops after continued ingestion of fructose; bleeding, jaundice, and renal tubular acidosis may follow.

Generalized Gangliosidosis (Type I)

Accumulation of the ganglioside GM_1 results in hepatosplenomegaly and an appearance resembling that of Hurler syndrome. Foam cells are present in the bone marrow.

Fucosidosis

Moderate hepatosplenomegaly, dementia, spasticity, and cardiomyopathy are characteristic.

- **Gaucher Disease**

    The malignant infantile form can develop at any time in the first few months of life. Feeding problems, vomiting, hepatosplenomegaly, muscular hypertonia, and developmental deterioration are characteristic. Cough and respiratory difficulty are common. Splenomegaly is more prominent than hepatomegaly.

    Niemann-Pick Disease

    The infantile form is characterized by hepatosplenomegaly and developmental retardation. A cherry-red retinal spot develops early in the course.

    Farber Disease

    Hoarseness and stridor may appear in the first few weeks of life. Painful nodules develop in the skin and subcutaneous tissues, particularly over joints. Hepatomegaly and central nervous system deterioration occur later.

    Wolman Disease

    Failure to thrive with vomiting and diarrhea may be present from birth; massive hepatosplenomegaly occurs. A key finding is enlarged, calcified adrenal glands on abdominal radiographs.

    Crigler-Najjar Syndrome

    This disorder is characterized by a severe, persistent hyperbilirubinemia with the unconjugated form, often with early kernicterus.

    Mannosidosis

    Coarse facies, opacities of lens, and psychomotor retardation are present.

    Familial Intrahepatic Cholestasis

    Jaundice, pruritus, and abdominal distension with hepatosplenomegaly are found. Some types are familial with phenotypic characteristics.

    Albers-Schönberg Syndrome

    Severe osteopetrosis. The bones are thick, dense and fragile. Macrocephaly, frontal bossing, pancytopenia, and cranial nerve palsies occur.

    Mucolipidosis I

    Myoclonus, mental retardation, cherry red spots of the retina, skeletal dysplasia, small stature, coarse features, and hepatosplenomegaly are findings.

Mucolipidosis II (I-Cell Disease)

Alveolar ridge hypertrophy with limited joint mobility is found. Liver enlargement is minimal.

Aase Syndrome

Triphalangeal thumb and hypoplastic anemia are the major features.

Systemic Carnitine Deficiency

This disorder is characterized by acute episodes of encephalopathy associated with hepatic dysfunction and progressive muscle weakness. Symptoms may mimic Reye syndrome.

Familial Erythrophagocytic Lymphohistiocytosis

This is a rapidly fatal illness with fever, pancytopenia, central nervous system involvement, and hepatosplenomegaly.

Lysinuric Protein Intolerance

This rare autosomal recessive disorder also features splenomegaly, muscle weakness, and osteoporosis.

Multiple Sulfatase Deficiency

An autosomal recessive disorder characterized by an initial period of normal development followed by the onset of motor and mental difficulties during the first or second year. In later stages, most patients have coarse facial features, ichthyosis, hepatosplenomegaly, and skeletal abnormalities. Appearance may be confused with mucopolysaccharidoses.

APPEARANCE IN FIRST DECADE WITHOUT APPARENT CHRONIC ILLNESS

♦ Iron Deficiency Anemia

Hepatomegaly may occur in iron deficiency anemia, especially in young children.

Acquired Immune Deficiency Syndrome

Other common features include generalized lymphadenopathy, recurrent opportunistic infections, splenomegaly, and failure to thrive, but hepatomegaly may be an early finding and become an apparent chronic illness.

Chronic Hepatitis

Infants with chronic viral hepatitis B may have hepatomegaly without other overt signs of illness. Liver enzymes are elevated.

Hepatoblastoma

Asymptomatic abdominal enlargement is the most frequent sign. This tumor is most likely to appear before 3 years of age; as it progresses, other symptoms such as poor appetite, failure to gain weight, and pallor are common.

Wilms' Tumor

When right sided, the tumor may distort the liver and give the sense of enlargement or it may be mistaken for hepatomegaly.

Congenital Lipodystrophy

There is a striking absence of subcutaneous fat. Hepatomegaly eventually develops.

Type I Hyperlipoproteinemia

Hepatosplenomegaly develops early in the first decade. Episodes of abdominal pain may occur; xanthomata can occur early. Serum chylomicrons and cholesterol levels are increased.

Homocystinuria

Arachnodactyly, subluxation of lenses, malar flush, and mental retardation with minimal hepatomegaly may be found. Vascular thromboses frequently occur, especially as these children age.

Moore-Federmann Syndrome

Hepatomegaly may be found in this familial syndrome characterized by short stature that becomes evident during childhood.

APPEARANCE IN FIRST DECADE WITH APPARENT ILLNESS

● Pseudohepatomegaly

The liver may seem enlarged if displaced downward by the diaphragm. Asthma is the most common cause of air trapping and displacement of the liver.

◆ Hemolytic Anemias

Various types of hemolytic anemia, such as congenital spherocytosis, may be associated with hepatomegaly.

Metastatic Tumors

Chronic Granulomatous Disease

Recurrent infections, suppurative lymphadenopathy, dermatitis, osteomyelitis, chronic enteritis, and malabsorption are prominent symptoms.

Visceral Larva Migrans (Toxocariasis)

This infestation should be considered in any child with recurrent fever, cough, and wheezing in the presence of hepatomegaly, especially if a significant eosinophilia is found.

Hand-Schuller-Christian Disease

The classic triad of exophthalmos, diabetes insipidus, and punched-out lesions of the skull seen on radiographs suggests this form of histiocytosis. Letterer-Siwe disease has a rash, usually petechial, in addition to hepatosplenomegaly.

Chédiak-Higashi Syndrome

Affected children usually have problems with recurrent infections. Partial albinism, variable hepatosplenomegaly, neutropenia, anemia, and thrombocytopenia are found. Large cytoplasmic inclusions are seen in the white blood cells.

APPEARANCE AT ANY AGE–RELATIVELY ASYMPTOMATIC

♦ Reactive Hepatomegaly

Slight liver enlargement may frequently be associated with a mild, self-limited illness, often viral, with some gastrointestinal involvement.

Cirrhosis

Several disorders producing cirrhosis are associated with liver enlargement early in the course (see Chapter 64, Ascites). Many of these disorders may be silent in their progression.

Obesity

Hyperalimentation/Lipid Infusion

Cholestasis is the cause of enlargement.

Hepatic Tumors

Most tumors produce asymmetric liver enlargement.

Hepatocarcinoma

This tumor is uncommon before 3 years of age. There may be some abdominal discomfort as the tumor enlarges. Hemihypertrophy, macroglossia, and absence of a kidney have been described in some cases.

- **Hemangioendotheliomas and Cavernous Hemangiomas**

    Associated cutaneous lesions are common.

Hamartomas

Solitary Cysts

Inflammatory Bowel Disease

Although there may have been symptoms of inflammatory bowel disease, hepato-megaly may be insidious during an asymptomatic period.

- **Polycystic Disease of the Liver**

    This disease is often discovered incidentally. The hepatic enlargement is asymp-tomatic.

Ascariasis

Hepatomegaly may occur during the extraintestinal migration of the worm. If the child is symptomatic, colicky abdominal pain is the most common complaint.

Hemochromatosis

Hepatomegaly, increased skin pigmentation, and diabetes mellitus are the clas-sic features.

Tangier Disease

Striking, enlarged orangish-yellow tonsils may be the initial clue. The liver is occasionally enlarged.

Echinococcosis (Hydatid Disease)

Liver enlargement is localized, distinct, smooth, and round.

Amyloidosis

In primary amyloidosis many organs are involved. Hepatic function is rarely disturbed. Secondary amyloidosis is occasionally seen in children with chronic ill-nesses, but again the liver involvement is usually asymptomatic.

Rendu-Osler-Weber Syndrome (Hereditary Hemorrhagic Telangiectasia)

Cutaneous telangiectatic lesions suggest this possibility.

Mulibrey Nanism

The early onset of growth failure, a triangular facies, prominent forehead, and hepatomegaly with pericardial constriction characterize this disorder.

APPEARANCE AT ANY AGE–GENERALLY APPEARING ILL

♦ Hepatitis

Several viruses may cause hepatitis. Mononucleosis affects the liver in most cases. A granulomatous hepatitis may be seen in tuberculosis and sarcoidosis.

♦ Drugs and Toxins

Hepatocellular injury or cholestasis may occur during treatment with a number of drugs or on exposure to toxic materials. Phenobarbital, hydantoins, sulfonamides, tetracyclines, and corticosteroids are commonly used drugs that may produce hepatomegaly. Beware of acetaminophen toxicity from unsuspecting, unsupervised administration by care givers. Anabolic steroids may be responsible. Insulin administration in a child with diabetes who has been without insulin for awhile may cause sufficient new glycogen deposition to produce hepatomegaly.

♦ Congestive Heart Failure

Liver enlargement is more common in right heart failure.

Sepsis

Hepatomegaly may occur during acute viral and bacterial infections.

Starvation

Malaria

Rocky Mountain Spotted Fever

Histoplasmosis

Tuberculosis

The declining incidence of this disease may catch us off guard in considering this diagnosis.

Leukemia and Lymphoma

Generally, children with these diseases manifest other signs and symptoms.

Cystic Fibrosis

Signs of pulmonary and pancreatic involvement are the usual presenting symptoms. Abdominal distension, ascites, or esophageal varices with bleeding may be the first sign of the cirrhosis.

Constrictive Pericarditis

This disorder may be chronic, with an insidious onset of fatigue, dyspnea, abdominal swelling, and hepatosplenomegaly.

Diabetes Mellitus

Hepatomegaly may be an acute phenomenon during ketoacidosis or may be chronic with poor disease control.

Chronic Active Hepatitis

Persistent or relapsing jaundice is the earliest finding. Hepatosplenomegaly is present in most children. Arthritis, arthralgias, fever, erythema nodosum, or colitis may be present.

Babesiosis

This protozoal illness has been reported with increasing frequency in the United States. Fever, chills, hepatomegaly, and signs of hemolysis may be present.

Juvenile Rheumatoid Arthritis

Hepatomegaly may be a finding in the systemic form.

Systemic Lupus Erythematosus

Brucellosis

Brucellosis is often associated with a remittent type of fever; fatigability and vague muscle pains may be the only symptoms.

Liver Abscess

Incidence is greater in children receiving anti-inflammatory or antineoplastic drugs. Pain in the right upper quadrant is an early symptom, with tenderness over the liver. Weight loss, anorexia, fever, and jaundice may be present.

Parasitic Disorders

Amebiasis

This is most commonly seen in the tropics or subtropics. Hepatic involvement is characterized by high fever, profuse sweating, hepatic tenderness, and occasionally, right shoulder pain.

Schistosomiasis

Fever, urticaria, malaise, weight loss, and anorexia with eosinophilia are the most prominent symptoms.

Liver Flukes

Fever, dyspnea, and hepatomegaly with eosinophilia are common. Pain in the upper quadrant, urticaria, and jaundice may also be found.

Leptospirosis

Symptomatic disease is characterized by an abrupt onset of fever, myalgia, headache, and vomiting. The associated vasculitis may affect any organ system.

Alpha₁-Antitrypsin Deficiency

The first symptoms may be those of an acute hepatitis or an anicteric hepatitis progressing to cirrhosis. Chronic lung disease occurs in some older children.

Wilson Disease

The presentation of this inherited disorder is varied. Children may present with an acute hepatitis, asymptomatic cirrhosis with portal hypertension and bleeding from varices, acute hemolysis, renal disturbances, or neurologic symptoms.

Budd-Chiari Syndrome

This syndrome must be considered in children with the abrupt onset of ascites in the absence of known liver disease. Splenomegaly is generally present.

Veno-Occlusive Disease

This disorder occurs in certain endemic areas such as Jamaica and India. Ascites, hepatomegaly, and jaundice develop rapidly, usually after exposure to a toxin.

Hyperlipoproteinemia

Onset of symptoms in types IV and V is after the first decade. Xanthomata and premature arteriosclerotic heart disease in family members are clues.

Infantile Pyknocytosis

Hepatosplenomegaly with pallor and jaundice is found, as well as characteristic burr cells on peripheral blood smear.

Hypervitaminosis A

Leg and forearm pain, anorexia, and irritability are other symptoms.

Primary Sclerosing Cholangitis

This rare disorder is occasionally associated with ulcerative colitis. Progressive liver failure, cholestatic jaundice, weight loss, and steatorrhea are other features.

Generalized Histiocytic Proliferation Syndromes

Several of these syndromes show erythrophagocytosis and have been reported under various names (e.g., virus-associated hemophagocytic syndrome). Clinical findings are similar and include organomegaly and pyrexia. One group is precipitated by viral infections, usually in immunosuppressed patients.

♦ Reye Syndrome

Vomiting follows a prodromal illness such as in influenza B or chickenpox. Delirium and coma may follow.

REFERENCE

1. Walker WA, Mathis RK. Hepatomegaly: an approach to differential diagnosis. *Pediatr Clin North Am* 1975;22:929–942.

SUGGESTED READING

Gartner JC Jr. Hepatosplenomegaly. In: Gartner JC Jr, Zitelli BJ, eds. *Common & chronic symptoms in pediatrics.* St. Louis: Mosby, 1997:355–364.

67

Splenomegaly

The spleen serves two primary functions: (a) filtration of particulate matter and formed elements from the blood, and (b) assistance in protection from infection by means of the production of humoral factors needed for opsonization. During the first 5 or 6 fetal months, it also serves as a site of blood formation.

Although it has been stated that the spleen is not palpable until enlargement to 3 or 4 times its normal size occurs, this is not always the case. As outlined under the section on **Normal Variants**, as many as 1% of all children, and a higher percentage of children under 1 year of age, have palpable but normal spleens. Whereas the normal palpable spleen is soft and just barely felt, the pathologically enlarged spleen is usually more easily palpated; it often has an abnormal surface or consistency; and it is generally associated with other signs and symptoms.

♦ **Most Common Causes of Splenomegaly**

Malaria (Worldwide)	Viral Infections (Various)
Infectious Mononucleosis	Bacterial Infections
Sickle Cell Anemia	Acquired Immunodeficiency Syndrome
Portal Hypertension	Hereditary Spherocytosis
Pseudosplenomegaly	
(Low Diaphragm)	

● **Causes Not to Forget**

Leukemia	Gaucher Disease
Thalassemia	Hemolytic Anemias

♦ **NORMAL VARIANTS**

The spleen is usually palpable in most premature infants and in as many as 30% of term infants. By 1 year of age, 10% of healthy infants still have a palpable spleen, and even after 10 years of age approximately 1% of children and adolescents have palpable spleens. In older infants and children the spleen tip is just barely palpable in the left mid-clavicular line and is soft; it can often only be palpated on deep inspiration. Most of these children have visceroptosis of the spleen, that is, the spleen hangs in a slightly lower position than normal. A wandering spleen, the result of elongated mesenteric connections, may appear in unusual places and may be mistaken for another organ or mass.

INFECTION

The most common cause of splenomegaly overall is infection. In most cases the enlargement subsides over a few weeks.

Acute Infections

♦ Malaria

Worldwide, malaria may be the most common cause of splenomegaly.

♦ Viral

A number of viral infections may cause splenic enlargement, particularly infectious mononucleosis and cytomegalovirus infection.

♦ Bacterial

Many bacterial infections are accompanied by splenic enlargement: severe pneumonia, septicemia, bacterial endocarditis, typhoid fever, brucellosis, tularemia, plague, and others. A splenic abscess must also be considered. Usually the splenomegaly is only one part of a systemic illness.

Rickettsial

Rocky Mountain spotted fever and typhus are examples.

Protozoal

Malaria should be considered; a travel history is mandatory. Trypanosomiasis may also be a cause. Babesiosis seems to be increasing in the United States. Fever, chills, signs of hemolysis, and hepatosplenomegaly may be present. The peripheral blood smear should be examined for parasitized erythrocytes.

Spirochetal Infection

Leptospirosis may be associated with splenomegaly.

Chronic Infections

♦ Bacterial

Subacute bacterial endocarditis, brucellosis, and staphylococcal infection involving ventriculoatrial shunts are examples.

♦ Viral

Splenomegaly may especially accompany congenital infections such as rubella, herpes, and cytomegalovirus infection.

Protozoal

Toxoplasmosis, malaria, schistosomiasis, and visceral larva migrans may cause splenic enlargement.

Fungal

Histoplasmosis and coccidioidomycosis are examples.

Mycobacterial

Splenomegaly may be a finding in tuberculosis, especially miliary tuberculosis.

Spirochetal

Don't forget syphilis.

Altered Host Defense

♦ Acquired Immune Deficiency Syndrome

More prominent features include recurrent opportunistic infections, hepatomegaly, generalized lymphadenopathy, and failure to thrive.

Chronic Granulomatous Disease

This disorder is characterized by recurrent infections, significant adenopathy, and furunculosis with onset at an early age. Hepatic and splenic enlargement may signify abscesses.

Immunodeficiency Disorders

The spleen may be greatly increased in size, especially after repeated infections.

Chediak-Higashi Syndrome

Features include recurrent infections, partial albinism, variable degrees of hepatosplenomegaly, neutropenia, anemia, and thrombocytopenia.

Familial Lipochrome Histiocytosis

This rare disorder is similar to chronic granulomatous disease. Splenomegaly, pulmonary infiltration, and arthritis, with increased susceptibility to bacterial infections, are prominent features.

HEMATOLOGIC DISORDERS

Iron Deficiency

If splenomegaly is present, it is mild.

Hemolytic Disorders

Altered red blood cell properties, either surface immunoglobulins or loss of deformability, may result in their trapping and removal by the spleen, with consequent splenic enlargement.

◆ Sickle Cell Anemia

As the child ages the spleen usually shrinks due to repeated infarction. Acute, life-threatening enlargement of the spleen is seen in sequestration crises, most commonly occurring during the second 6 months of life and less frequently after age 2 years.

◆ Hereditary Spherocytosis

Jaundice may be present in infancy. Later, affected children present with pallor and splenomegaly, occasionally with aplastic crises. Spleen size increases with age.

Isoimmunization Disorders

Rh and ABO incompatibilities in infants are the best known of these disorders.

Autoimmune Hemolytic Anemia
● Thalassemia Major

Hepatosplenomegaly and pallor are prominent in affected children over 6 months of age.

Other Red Cell Disorders

Hemoglobin C disease, SC disease, elliptocytosis, stomatocytosis, pyruvate kinase deficiency, glucose-6-phosphate dehydrogenase deficiency, and other enzyme disorders may be associated with splenomegaly.

Congenital Erythropoietic Porphyria

Prominent features include cutaneous lesions (vesicles, bullae, and scarring) on sun exposure, red urine, hypertrichosis, and splenomegaly.

Extramedullary Hematopoiesis

Osteopetrosis and myelofibrosis may be associated with splenomegaly as fetal sites of blood formation again become active.

Idiopathic Myelofibrosis

Fibrosis of the bone marrow usually begins before 3 years of age. Anemia, thrombocytopenia, leukoerythroblastosis, splenomegaly, and, occasionally, hepatomegaly are found.

STORAGE DISEASES

Lipid Storage Diseases

• Gaucher Disease

Splenic enlargement occurs in acute and chronic forms. In early-onset types progressive developmental deterioration is generally seen; in the chronic or adult form, onset is insidious, with splenomegaly followed by hepatomegaly, patchy brown or yellow skin discoloration, and bony lesions. This disorder should be considered in anyone with splenomegaly and an unexplained mild anemia.

Niemann-Pick Disease

Various types have been described, with onset ranging from 6 months to 5 years of age. Hepatosplenomegaly and progressive mental deterioration are common. Cherry-red spots are commonly found on funduscopic examination, and foam cells abound in the bone marrow.

Gangliosidoses

An increasing number of forms of this storage disorder are being described. Coarse features, often resembling those seen in Hurler syndrome, are characteristic of the forms involving gangliosides GM_1 and GM_3. Progressive deterioration is common.

Mucolipidodoses

Affected children also have coarse features like those of Hurler syndrome, progressive deterioration, and progressive hepatosplenomegaly. Mucolipidoses I and II, mannosidosis, and fucosidosis may all be associated with splenomegaly.

Metachromatic Leukodystrophy

Mild visceromegaly may be present with the progressive neurologic deterioration.

Wolman Disease

Failure to thrive and diarrhea are present from birth. Calcified adrenal glands seen on abdominal radiographs are pathognomonic.

Lactosyl Ceramidosis

Onset of symptoms is by 1 year of age, with failure to thrive, mental deterioration, and hepatosplenomegaly.

Cholesterol Ester Storage Disease

Hepatomegaly is a constant feature; splenomegaly occurs less frequently. Affected children may have advanced atherosclerosis. Hyperlipemia is usually present.

Analphalipoproteinemia (Tangier Disease)

A red-orange coloration of the tonsils is characteristic; splenomegaly is common. A peripheral neuropathy is the most serious complication.

Hyperchylomicronemia (Type 1 Hyperlipoproteinemia)

The spleen and liver are occasionally enlarged; hyperlipemia is typical. Attacks of abdominal pain and crops of eruptive xanthomata are found.

Mucopolysaccharidoses

The syndromes of Hurler, Hunter, Sanfilippo, and Maroteaux-Lamy may be associated with splenomegaly. Dysmorphogenic features of these disorders overshadow the splenomegaly. (See Chapter 66, Hepatomegaly.)

Glycogen Storage Disease

In type IV (Andersen disease), the liver is enlarged and nodular with early onset of cirrhosis. Splenomegaly may be a later finding.

Other Storage Diseases

Amyloidosis

Proteinuria with hepatosplenomegaly in a child with a chronic inflammatory disease suggests this diagnosis.

Sea Blue Histiocyte Disease

Reticuloendothelial cells contain large blue cytoplasmic granules. Splenomegaly is common. The clinical course may be mild, with purpura caused by thrombocytopenia, or may be characterized by progressive hepatic cirrhosis.

VASCULAR CONGESTION

◆ Portal Hypertension with Congestive Splenomegaly
Cirrhosis

This is the most common cause of portal hypertension. Various infectious and hereditary disorders may be responsible (see Chapter 66, Hepatomegaly).

Hepatitis

Both infectious and serum types have been implicated.

Chronic Active Hepatitis
Biliary Atresia

Cystic Fibrosis

Wilson Disease

Galactosemia

Alpha$_1$-Antitrypsin Deficiency

Cystinosis

Hemosiderosis

Tyrosinosis

Fructose Intolerance

♦ **Extrahepatic Lesions**

Cavernous Transformation of Portal Vein

This lesion may be a sequela of umbilical vein catheterization in the neonatal period.

Splenic Vein Thrombosis

Splenic Artery Aneurysm

Congenital Portal Vein Stenosis or Atresia

Chronic Congestive Heart Failure

Constrictive Pericarditis

Hepatomegaly appears before splenomegaly.

Splenic Trauma

A splenic hematoma may follow abdominal injury.

TUMORS AND INFILTRATIONS

● **Leukemia**

Over one half of children with acute lymphocytic leukemia will have splenomegaly sometime during their disease.

Lymphomas

Splenomegaly may be an isolated finding in some cases of both Hodgkin disease and other forms of lymphoma.

Metastatic Disease

Neuroblastoma is most common.

Cysts

Cysts may be congenital or follow trauma. An asymptomatic smooth mass is typical.

Splenic Hemangioma

Cutaneous hemangiomas are sometimes present.

Splenic Hamartoma

This rare disorder is characterized by failure to thrive, recurrent infections, and pancytopenia.

Histiocytosis-X

Both Letterer-Siwe disease and Hand-Schuller-Christian disease may be associated with splenomegaly. Other signs and symptoms predominate.

Generalized Histiocytic Proliferation Syndromes

Several of these disorders show erythrophagocytosis and have been reported under various names (e.g., virus associated hematophagocytic syndrome). Clinical findings are similar and include organomegaly and pyrexia.

MISCELLANEOUS CAUSES

♦ Pseudosplenomegaly

The spleen may seem large because of downward displacement by the diaphragm.

Serum Sickness
Connective Tissue Disorders
Juvenile Rheumatoid Arthritis
Systemic Lupus Erythematosus
Beckwith-Wiedemann Syndrome

Splenomegaly may be part of the generalized visceromegaly.

Hemihypertrophy

Splenic enlargement may be found if the left side of the body is hypertrophied.

Situs Inversus

The "splenomegaly" is the normal transposed liver.

Sarcoidosis

Hyperparathyroidism

In neonatal disease, early symptoms include failure to thrive, constipation, hepatosplenomegaly, anemia, seizures, polyuria, polydipsia, and hypotonia.

Cockayne Syndrome

Hepatosplenomegaly has been reported in affected children who have short stature, pinched facies, microcephaly, and progressive deterioration.

Gingival Fibromatosis and Digital Anomalies

Absent or dysplastic nails, clubbed digits, gingival overgrowth, and soft, bulky nose and ear cartilage are prominent signs. One half of cases have hepatosplenomegaly.

Hyperdibasic Aminoaciduria

Splenomegaly is occasionally found in affected children, whose protein intolerance causes failure to thrive, diarrhea, vomiting, and aversion to protein-rich foods.

Miller-Dieker Syndrome (Lissencephaly)

This disorder is characterized by severe failure to thrive, microcephaly, high and narrow forehead, prominent occiput, anteverted nares, and micrognathia. Cyanotic attacks are frequent in the neonatal period.

Infantile Pyknocytosis

Pallor, jaundice, hepatosplenomegaly, and the presence of burr cells on the peripheral smear are characteristic findings.

Dyskeratosis Congenita

This rare genetic disorder is characterized by atrophy and a reticular pigmentation of the skin, dystrophic nails, and leukoplakia. There is a significant risk of development of aplastic anemia.

Lysinuric Protein Intolerance

This rare autosomal recessive disorder also features hepatomegaly, muscle weakness, and osteoporosis.

SUGGESTED READING

Gartner JC Jr. Hepatosplenomegaly. In: Gartner JC Jr, Zitelli BJ, eds. *Common & chronic symptoms in pediatrics.* St. Louis: Mosby, 1997:355–364.

= 68 =

Abdominal Masses

In differential diagnosis of abdominal masses in childhood, the age group of the affected child should be considered: In newborn infants over one half of all abdominal masses are renal in origin, and of these, most are caused by multicystic kidney disease or congenital hydronephrosis. In older infants and children, most abdominal masses are due to enlargement of the liver and spleen, often from diseases such as leukemia or lymphoma or as a result of portal hypertension. However, retroperitoneal tumors, especially Wilms tumors and neuroblastomas, make up a sizeable percentage of masses found in children over 1 year of age.

In this chapter, masses that are the result of hepatomegaly (see Chapter 66) or splenomegaly (see Chapter 67) are not included. Abdominal masses from other causes generally lie in the area of the organ of origin, which aids in the selection of diagnostic studies. Before extensive laboratory investigations are undertaken, it is important to rule out the presence of large amounts of stool in the large intestine or of urine in the bladder as the cause of the distension.

♦ **Most Common Causes**

Neonate
Renal: Hydronephrosis
Multicystic-Polycystic
Bladder Distension
Mesoblastic Nephroma

Infancy–Adolescence
Feces
Intrauterine Pregnancy
Bladder Distension
Wilms' Tumor
Neuroblastoma

GENITOURINARY DISORDERS

Renal Disease

♦ **Hydronephrosis**

♦ **Polycystic or Multicystic Kidney Disease**

Solitary Cysts

Renal Vein Thrombosis

This lesion is more likely to occur in newborn infants, especially in those of diabetic mothers, or rarely, during severe dehydration. Hematuria is common.

Ectopic or Horseshoe Kidney

Ureterocele

Perinephric Abscess

◆ **Bladder Distension**

The mass is globular and located in the midline, usually below the umbilicus. In the newborn, obstruction of urine outflow—for instance, as a consequence of posterior urethral valves—should be considered. In older infants and children, causes of bladder distension include anticholinergic drugs, spinal cord tumors, spinal cord abnormalities, and bladder irritation from inflammatory conditions in the pelvis or infection within the bladder. Urethral irritation may also cause urinary retention.

Urachal Cyst

The cyst may be palpated as a midline swelling below the umbilicus attached to the abdominal wall.

Bladder Diverticulum

Uterine Enlargement

◆ **Pregnancy**

Pregnancy must always be considered in adolescents with midline, lower abdominal masses.

Hydrometrocolpos

In early infancy, a suprapubic mass and vomiting as a result of hydronephrosis from obstruction of the ureters may be signs. Adolescents with an imperforate hymen may have uterine distension from retained secretions and menses.

Ovarian Disorders

Ovarian Cyst

Occasionally, the ovary may twist on its pedicle, producing symptoms similar to those of acute appendicitis.

Ovarian Tumors

These tumors are uncommon in childhood.

NEOPLASIA

◆ **Wilms' Tumor**

The mass is often discovered by parents while bathing the child. In over 60% of the cases, the tumor is found before 5 years of age. The mass may extend to the midline and into the iliac fossa, or it may simulate splenomegaly or hepatomegaly.

♦ **Neuroblastoma**

About one half of these tumors arise in the abdomen. The mass frequently crosses in the midline. The tumor may produce excessive catecholamines, resulting in tachycardia, diarrhea, hypertension, skin flushing, and perspiration. Almost 50% occur within the first 2 years of life.

Lymphoma

Enlargement of the liver and spleen is generally found, but abdominal lymph nodes are frequently enlarged as well.

Teratoma

An abdominal mass, high in the retroperitoneal region, usually becomes evident in the first 2 years of life. Radiographs of the tumor often reveal spotty calcifications.

Retroperitoneal Lymphangioma

This tumor is palpable as an ill-defined cystic mass.

♦ **Congenital Mesoblastic Nephroma**

This embryonic tumor is usually present at birth.

Embryonal Rhabdomyosarcoma

The origins may be bladder, prostate, or retroperitoneal.

INTESTINAL DISORDERS

♦ **Fecal Material**

Masses of stool are frequently palpable in the left lower quadrant or on the entire left side, corresponding to the course of the descending colon. Generally, the masses are mobile, multiple, and disappear after a cleansing enema.

Intussusception

Other symptoms such as pain and vomiting, may be much more prominent than the mass, which is palpable in the right lower or upper quadrant.

Regional Enteritis

Palpable masses may be caused occasionally by mesenteric node inflammation or by fistula or abscess formation, in inflammatory bowel disease.

Intestinal Duplication

In addition to the mass, abdominal pain, vomiting, or gastrointestinal hemorrhage may be present.

Incarcerated Hernia

Malrotation with Volvulus

The sudden onset of abdominal pain and vomiting heralds this catastrophic event.

Bezoar

In premature infants fed milk with a high casein content, lactobezoars may form. Hair ingestion may also result in gastric masses.

Intestinal Tumors

Leiomyosarcomas and other solid tumors are uncommon. Peritoneal, mesenteric, or omental cysts may occur.

Pyloric Stenosis

Projectile vomiting in a hungry young infant is usually the first clue. The mass is the stomach, if fluid or air filled. The pyloric tumor (the olive) is rather small and deep.

BILIARY DISORDERS

Choledochal Cyst

Symptoms include a mass in the right upper quadrant with jaundice or pain.

Hydrops of the Gallbladder

Infants with acute hydrops of the gallbladder present with poorly localized, continuous abdominal pain, and a mass in the right upper quadrant.

Distended Gallbladder

Distension occurs occasionally in cystic fibrosis.

MISCELLANEOUS CAUSES

Abscesses

Abdominal abscesses are generally associated with fever, abdominal discomfort, anorexia, and, frequently, vomiting and diarrhea. They are generally not palpable.

Pancreatic Cyst

Blunt injury to the abdomen may be the cause. The mass is palpable in the epigastrium and left upper quadrant. Ascites may accompany the cyst.

Anterior Meningocele

Adrenal Hemorrhage

Aortic Aneurysm

The occurrence of aortic aneurysm is rare in children. The mass is pulsatile.

SUGGESTED READING

Brodeur AE, Brodeur GM. Abdominal masses in children: neuroblastoma, Wilms tumor, and other considerations. *Pediatr Rev* 1991;12:196–206.
Schwartz MZ, Shaul DB. Abdominal masses in the newborn. *Pediatr Rev* 1989;11:172–179.
Vane DW. Left upper quadrant masses in children. *Pediatr Rev* 1992;13:25–31.

SECTION X

Gastrointestinal System

69

Vomiting

Vomiting is such a common symptom in childhood that it is difficult to present a nice, neat, clear classification of possible causes. Fortunately, in most cases, vomiting is merely part of a relatively benign gastrointestinal infection; the problem ceases in a day or two. Vomiting is a worrisome symptom when it persists; develops in the neonatal period; is associated with abdominal distension or severe abdominal pain; is projectile (see Chapter 70, Projectile Vomiting/Cyclic Vomiting); when the vomitus contains blood or bile; or when there are other significant systemic signs and symptoms or other warning signals.

The acute onset of vomiting suggests different disorders from those associated with chronic or recurrent vomiting; however, there may be some overlap between these groups. The various other clues obtained from the history and physical examination should quickly narrow the diagnostic possibilities to a few likely causes.

It is important to ascertain that the symptom complaint is vomiting and not regurgitation or spitting up. This differentiation is particularly important in infancy: Is the infant bringing up stomach contents forcefully, or is there a nondramatic flow of small amounts of fluids or food from the mouth? Is the vomiting preceded by a cough or choking that in turn precipitates the vomiting? In this latter case, disorders involving areas other than the gastrointestinal tract should be considered.

The classification of causes of vomiting begins with some general possibilities and then groups disorders by the organ system involved.

♦ **Most Common Causes of Vomiting**

Infants
Overfeeding
Gastroesophageal Reflux
Gastroenteritis
Pylorospasm
Systemic Infection

Children and Adolescents
Gastroesophageal Reflux
Gastroenteritis
Cough
Peptic Ulcer
Systemic Infection
Medications/Ingestions

● **Causes Not to Forget (All Ages)**

Intestinal Obstruction (e.g., Volvulus)
Central Nervous System Infection
Congenital Adrenal Hyperplasia
Diabetic Ketoacidosis
Appendicitis
Amino and Organic Acidurias

Pyelonephritis
Brain Tumor
Pregnancy
Pancreatitis
Migraine

GENERAL CONSIDERATIONS

Poor Feeding Technique

♦ Overfeeding

This is usually seen in infants but may occur in youngsters who consume excessive amounts of food or drink.

Improper Formula Preparation

The formula may contain excessive amounts of protein or solutes, or mistaken ingredients that may cause vomiting.

Excessive Air Swallowing

The nipple opening may be too small. A propped bottle may also cause excessive air swallowing with consequent vomiting.

Inappropriate Handling After Feeding

Bouncing the infant on the knee after feeding may bring up what just went down.

Psychogenic Vomiting

Vomiting may be self-induced or may be caused by anxiety or stress, or it may be brought on by sights, smells, or occasionally sounds.

The Active Child

Spitting up and occasional vomiting may be found in the infant who is constantly moving, or the child who engages in excessive activity after eating.

♦ Coughing

Coughing episodes may trigger vomiting. Pertussis is a classic example. The chief complaint may be vomiting rather than coughing!

Postnasal Drip

Excessive mucus production may cause pharyngeal gagging with vomiting; the presence of large amounts of mucus in the stomach may induce vomiting in some children. Allergic rhinitis and sinusitis are examples.

Emotional Deprivation

Vomiting may be a nonspecific symptom of the altered maternal-infant relationship.

Cyclic Vomiting

See Chapter 70, Projectile Vomiting/Cyclic Vomiting.

Immobilization

Occasionally, young children or infants who are immobilized by casts may vomit for unexplained reasons.

GASTROINTESTINAL DISORDERS

Pharyngeal and Esophageal Disorders

♦ Gastroesophageal Reflux

Recurrent coughing spells, choking, wheezing episodes, and pneumonia may be prominent features.

Hiatus Hernia

Recurrent episodes of vomiting begin at an early age. Affected children may develop failure to thrive, anemia secondary to blood loss from esophagitis, and torsion spasms of the neck (Sandifer syndrome).

Chalasia

Chalasia is a common cause of regurgitation in neonates. The lower esophageal sphincter fails to close fully, allowing reflux of gastric contents. Rarely, the condition may persist, giving rise to recurrent episodes of regurgitation, often with pneumonitis and esophagitis.

Achalasia

The occurrence of achalasia is uncommon in childhood; usually older children are affected. The lower esophagus fails to relax with swallowing.

Tracheoesophageal Fistula

Choking and coughing may be associated with vomiting.

Esophageal Stenosis or Web

Infants with congenital lesions present with early onset of vomiting and dysphagia.

Esophageal Tumors
Esophageal Duplication

Compression by the duplication causes stenosis. Dyspnea owing to tracheal compression may be present.

Cricopharyngeal Incoordination

The inability to swallow liquids and secretions results in recurrent aspiration, choking, and occasionally vomiting.

Congenital Short Esophagus

Gastric Disorders

♦ **Pylorospasm**

♦ **Peptic Ulcer**

Vomiting, intestinal blood loss, and abdominal pain are more common after 6 years of age; the abdominal pain is uncommon under 6 years and is often atypical after age 6.

Gastritis

Irritation of the gastric mucosa may result from aspirin and other drugs or toxic ingestants including corrosives and alcohol.

Postviral Gastroparesis

Abdominal distension, vomiting, abdominal pain, and early satiety may be symptoms and signs of gastroparesis following an acute viral illness. Rotavirus may be a common culprit.

Pyloric Stenosis

Gastric Bezoars

Bezoars may be composed of hair, vegetable fibers, or, in small infants, coagulated milk protein.

Gastric Mucosal Diaphragm or Antral Web

The egress of contents from the stomach may be blocked.

Pyloric Atresia

Gastric Volvulus

Onset may be acute, with epigastric pain and vomiting, or the condition may be chronic, with recurrent postprandial discomfort, vomiting, belching, and upper gastrointestinal bleeding.

Gastric Tumors

Large tumors or those close to the pylorus may cause obstruction.

Gastric Duplication

Generally is associated with blood loss from irritation of the gastric mucosa.

Microgastria

A congenital small stomach results in an inability to take normal-sized feedings.

Chronic Granulomatous Disease (CGD)

Gastric outlet obstruction resulting from granulomatous inflammation of the antral wall may be the first manifestation of CGD. Blood in the stool, anorexia, and poor weight gain are other features.

Intestinal Disorders

• Obstruction

A host of congenital or acquired obstructive lesions may result in vomiting. Whether the distension is epigastric or abdominal depends on the site of the obstruction. Bilious vomitus indicates obstruction unless proven otherwise.

Malrotation

• Volvulus

Intestinal Atresia or Stenosis

Incarcerated Hernias

Intussusception

Episodic crampy abdominal pain with vomiting should suggest this disorder. Lethargy is often a prominent feature.

Hirschsprung Disease

Adhesions

Following previous surgery or injury.

Paralytic Ileus

A number of conditions including infections (e.g., pneumonia), hypokalemia, perforation, pancreatitis, diabetic ketoacidosis, medications, and others may produce an ileus with resultant vomiting.

Meconium Ileus or Equivalent Syndrome

A meconium plug may occur in small or sick infants. In older children, thick secretions may cause an obstructive picture.

Congenital Adhesions or Bands

Duodenal Web

Intestinal Duplication

Imperforate Anus

Foreign Body

Superior Mesenteric Artery Syndrome

Duodenal compression is most likely to be seen in children in body casts or during prolonged recumbency and is associated with rapid weight loss. The duodenum is compressed between the aorta and the superior mesenteric artery as a result of loss of mesenteric fat.

Tumors

Mesenteric Cysts

Vomiting occurs if the cyst becomes infected or filled with blood.

Duodenal or Intestinal Hematomas

If there is no clear history of a traumatic episode, child abuse should be considered.

Omental Infarction

Increasing abdominal pain and nausea, sometimes with vomiting, may be seen. Abdominal tenderness is usually diffuse.

Intestinal Pseudo-Obstruction

Clinical manifestations include periodic vomiting, abdominal distension, and constipation. Causes include scleroderma, amyloidosis, various endocrinopathies, narcotic or laxative abuse, electrolyte disturbances, and vasoactive intestinal peptide secreting tumor, as well as an idiopathic primary form.

Inflammation and Irritation

• Appendicitis

Anorexia and vomiting are often early manifestations.

Food Poisoning

Abdominal pain, vomiting, and diarrhea develop within the first 12 hours following ingestion of the contaminated food. Enterotoxins are responsible.

Regional Enteritis

Crohn disease uncommonly causes vomiting unless there are complications or unless inflammation involves the stomach or duodenum, resulting in symptoms of obstruction.

Peritonitis

Ulcerative Colitis

Diarrhea, rectal bleeding, and weight loss are the most frequent symptoms. Vomiting may occur later, particularly with toxic dilatation of the colon.

Necrotizing Enterocolitis

Ileocecal Inflammation in Leukemia (Typhlitis)

Right lower quadrant pain, abdominal distension, diarrhea, and vomiting in a child with leukemia should alert the physician to this diagnosis.

♦ Infection

Almost any systemic infection may result in vomiting. A few intestinal infections and infestations are listed.

♦ Gastroenteritis

Viral infections affecting the gastrointestinal tract, such as those caused by the rotavirus group, commonly produce vomiting and diarrhea.

Shigellosis

Onset of symptoms may be abrupt, with fever, abdominal pain, anorexia, and vomiting. Diarrhea, crampy abdominal pain, tenesmus, and occasionally meningismus may follow.

Toxogenic *Escherichia coli*

Vomiting may be an early manifestation before onset of diarrhea or may accompany it.

Yersinia enterocolitica

This disease may begin as an upper respiratory tract infection and progress to a prolonged illness with vomiting, diarrhea, fever, and abdominal pain.

Cholera

Vomiting may be severe. Profuse, watery diarrhea without fecal characteristics is the primary symptom.

Giardiasis

Symptomatic infestations usually result in diarrhea and abdominal distension. Uncommonly the infestation may mimic peptic ulcer disease, with epigastric pain and vomiting.

Strongyloidiasis

Upper gastrointestinal involvement may be associated with abdominal pain and vomiting. Migration of the larvae to the lung results in cough, dyspnea, and pneumonia.

Hookworm

Amebiasis

Ascariasis

Other Intestinal Disorders

Gastrointestinal Allergy

Abdominal pain, diarrhea, and occasionally vomiting may be related to the ingestion of certain foods.

Lactose Intolerance

Familial forms may be associated with prominent vomiting. Acquired forms are generally characterized by diarrhea.

Gluten Enteropathy (Celiac Disease)

Diarrhea and growth failure are the most common symptoms, but vomiting and abdominal pain may be prominent.

Ménétrier Disease

Vomiting may be part of this disorder characterized by a protein losing enteropathy.

EXTRAINTESTINAL ABDOMINAL DISORDERS

Hepatitis

Nausea and vomiting may appear early. Lethargy, right upper quadrant tenderness, and jaundice strongly suggest hepatitis.

• Pancreatitis

Children with the hereditary form have episodes of recurrent abdominal pain progressing to nausea and vomiting lasting 4 to 6 days. In acute pancreatitis, epigastric abdominal pain predominates.

Acute Cholecystitis

This is an uncommon cause of vomiting in children. Abdominal pain is right sided, with tenderness to palpation. Nausea and vomiting are found in most cases.

Cholelithiasis

Intermittent colicky pain is characteristic. There may be vomiting and fatty food intolerance.

Testicular or Ovarian Torsion

Choledochal Cyst

Typical symptoms are abdominal pain, jaundice, and a right upper quadrant mass. Vomiting, fever, and alcoholic stools are occasionally present.

Liver Abscess

Hepatoma

GENITOURINARY TRACT DISORDERS

● **Pregnancy**

"Morning sickness" may be the cause in the sexually active adolescent.

● **Pyelonephritis**

Symptoms of fever, chills, and abdominal and back pain with vomiting may falsely suggest an acute gastroenteritis.

Hydronephrosis

Urinary Tract Obstruction

Any acute obstruction of the urinary tract with proximal distension may cause vomiting. Dietl's crisis refers to episodes of acute abdominal pain and vomiting following ingestion of large quantities of liquids and is the result of ureteropelvic junction obstruction.

Renal Stones

Hydrometrocolpos

Uterine distension from retained products may produce vomiting that may be projectile in young infants.

METABOLIC AND ENDOCRINE DISORDERS

● **Diabetic Ketoacidosis**

Abdominal pain and vomiting may be prominent as an initial presentation of diabetes or in the known diabetic whose disease is poorly controlled.

● **Amino Acid and Organic Acid Disorders**

Many of the inborn errors of amino acid and organic acid metabolism or transport may be associated with vomiting, particularly after feedings are begun in the neonatal period. Ketoacidosis, changes in sensorium, seizures, and abnormal odors should suggest the possibility of any of the following: phenylketonuria, methylmalonic acidemia, maple syrup urine disease, hypervalinemia; hyperlysinemia; ketotic hyperglycinemia (propionic acidemia), butyric or hexanoic acidemia, isovaleric acidemia, or the urea cycle disorders: argininosuccinic aciduria, citrullinemia, ornithine transcarbamylase deficiency, and carbamyl phosphate synthetase deficiency.

Fatty Oxidation Defects

Uremia

Hypercalcemia

Renal Tubular Acidosis

- **Congenital Adrenal Hyperplasia (Adrenogenital Syndrome)**

Vomiting progressing to shock in the first few weeks of life in an infant with ambiguous genitalia demands investigation for this disorder.

Corticosteroid Withdrawl

Diabetes Insipidus

Galactosemia

Onset of vomiting, diarrhea, and jaundice coincides with the introduction of milk to the diet.

Fructose Intolerance

Consider this possibility in infants who begin vomiting after introduction of fruits into the diet.

Fructose 1,6-Deficiency

Lysosomal Acid Phosphate Deficiency

Gangliosidoses

Wolman Disease

Niemann-Pick Disease

Glycogen Storage Disease, Type I

Hypoparathyroidism

Vomiting may be the result of increased intracranial pressure associated with the hypocalcemia. Seizures, cataracts, tetany, headaches, and mucocutaneous candidiasis may be findings.

DISORDERS OF THE CENTRAL NERVOUS SYSTEM

Any of the large number of diseases causing central nervous system irritation or increased intracranial pressure may produce vomiting.

- **Migraine**

    Vomiting is a common symptom, especially early in the onset of the attack. In young infants who cannot report the symptom of headache, recurrent vomiting attacks may be the primary symptom. A history of motion sickness is found in up to one half of the children.

- **Infections**

    Meningitis, encephalitis, or brain abscess may be a cause. Some infections may be subacute; in tuberculous meningoencephalitis, for example, presenting symptoms may suggest a gastroenteritis.

    Trauma

    Vomiting frequently follows head injury. Collections of blood (acute or chronic) may also be associated with vomiting: subdural hematoma, subarachnoid hemorrhage, or epidural hematoma.

- **Brain Tumors**

    Morning vomiting and headache should suggest the presence of central nervous system tumors. Other signs include cranial nerve palsies, ataxia, increasing head size, and a bulging fontanel.

    Hydrocephalus

    Other Causes of Increased Intracranial Pressure

    Lead poisoning and pseudotumor cerebri may be causes. (See Chapter 24, Increased Intracranial Pressure and Bulging Fontanel.)

    Epilepsy

    Episodes of vomiting may accompany convulsive attacks.

OTHER SYSTEMIC DISORDERS

◆ **Parenteral Infections**

    Any systemic infection may cause vomiting. The neonate with septicemia may have bile-stained vomitus, suggesting obstruction.

    Streptococcoccus

    Acute Group A β-hemolytic streptococcal infections may produce symptoms of fever and vomiting, particularly in young children.

◆ **Medications**

    Always check to see if the child has been taking prescription or nonprescription drugs.

♦ Toxic Ingestions

Must always be considered in children. Organophosphate exposure produces a classic presentation that includes vomiting.

Emetic Ingestion

May be voluntary, as in adolescents with bulimia, or involuntary, as in Munchausen syndrome by proxy.

Vestibular Injury or Inflammation

Middle ear disorders associated with vertigo may stimulate intense vomiting on movement.

Familial Dysautonomia

Affected children may have recurrent aspiration, postural hypotension, absent lacrimation, absent deep tendon reflexes, and episodic fevers, among other signs and symptoms.

Acrodermatitis Enteropathica

Other symptoms such as a malabsorptive diarrhea, skin lesions, alopecia, and irritability overshadow the occasional vomiting.

Black Widow Spider Bite

Reye Syndrome

Recurrent vomiting ushers in the encephalopathy.

SUGGESTED READING

Forbes D. Differential diagnosis of cyclic vomiting syndrome. *J Pediatr Gastroenterol* 1995;21(Suppl. 1): 11–14.

Glassman M, Spivak W, Mininberg D, et al. Chronic idiopathic pseudoobstruction: a common misdiagnosed disease of infants and children. *Pediatrics* 1989;83:603–608.

Li BUK. Cyclic vomiting: new understanding of an old disorder. *Contemp Pediatr* 1996;13:48–62.

Orenstein SR. Gastroesophageal reflux. *Pediatr Rev* 1992;13:174–182.

Ramos AG, Tuchman DN. Persistent vomiting. *Pediatr Rev* 1994;15:24–31.

Sigurdsson L, Flores A, Putnam PE, Hyman PE, DiLorenzo C. Postviral gastroparesis: presentation, treatment, and outcome. *J Pediatr* 1997;130:751–754.

Zitelli BJ. Persistent vomiting. In: Gartner JC Jr, Zitelli BJ, eds. *Common & chronic symptoms in pediatrics.* St. Louis: Mosby, 1997:275–289.

70

Projectile Vomiting/Cyclic Vomiting

Forceful or projectile vomiting in an infant usually brings immediately to mind the diagnosis of pyloric stenosis. However, a knowledge of other possible causes is important, particularly in cases where other findings make this diagnosis unlikely; for example, the child may be beyond the usual age for presentation, or the symptoms may be abrupt in onset.

In this chapter are listed some disorders that may be associated with projectile vomiting; many of the others cited in Chapter 69, Vomiting, whatever the cause, may also produce occasional projectile episodes. However, the disorders listed here are somewhat more notorious.

Cyclic vomiting syndrome must be separated from chronic vomiting. Children with cyclic vomiting have frequent episodes of vomiting during an "attack," but they have vomiting-free intervals between. Children with chronic vomiting tend to have fewer episodes of emesis but on a daily basis and not separated by long symptom-free intervals. One definition separates the two on these two quantitative criteria: Cyclic vomiting has a peak intensity of at least four emeses per hour and frequency of no more than nine episodes per month (1). The differentiation is helpful in considering diagnoses; cyclic vomiting tends to have non-gastrointestinal causes, whereas chronic vomiting is much more likely to have gastrointestinal disorders responsible.

PROJECTILE VOMITING

Gastrointestinal Disorders

Pyloric Stenosis

Vomiting usually begins within the first few weeks of life and becomes progressively more severe and projectile. Visible gastric peristalsis may be noted. Affected infants feed avidly, even after vomiting.

Hiatal Hernia

In severe cases in which symptoms begin in the first few weeks of life, the vomiting may be projectile, mimicking pyloric stenosis.

Peptic Ulcer

Channel or antral ulcers may produce colicky symptoms with episodes of forceful vomiting.

Pylorospasm

Some researchers have questioned the existence of this disorder; perhaps it represents one end of the spectrum of which pyloric muscle hypertrophy is the other. Most cases respond nicely to conservative treatment.

Pyloric Atresia

Signs are obvious at the first feeding.

Gastric Volvulus

Onset may be acute, with epigastric pain and vomiting, or the disorder may be chronic, with recurrent postprandial discomfort, vomiting, belching, and upper gastrointestinal tract bleeding.

Duodenal Obstruction

Atresia, stenosis, or webs commonly produce projectile vomiting. The epigastrium may appear distended, and the vomitus usually contains bile.

Gastric Mucosal Diaphragm

Folds of mucosa may intermittently block the egress of stomach contents.

Infection

Sepsis

Systemic infections, particularly in neonates, may be associated with projectile vomiting. The vomitus may be bile stained. Affected infants appear sick, and the onset is acute.

Pyelonephritis

Unsuspected pyelonephritis is a notorious mimic of pyloric stenosis, especially in young infants.

Genitourinary Tract Disorders

Urinary Tract Obstruction

Significant dilatation of any part of the urinary tract from obstruction, such as renal stones, ureteral kinking, or tumor, may result in forceful emesis.

Hydrometrocolpos

Children with imperforate hymen or vaginal atresia resulting in uterine distension from retained secretions may present with projectile vomiting along with a lower abdominal mass.

Central Nervous System Disorders

Vomiting may occur in several central nervous system disorders, although projectile vomiting is infrequent. Infection, irritation, and increased intracranial pressure must be considered. Usually, changes in sensorium and other central nervous system signs indicate a central lesion.

Meningitis and Encephalitis

Acute Intracranial Hemorrhage

Intraventricular, epidural, or subarachnoid bleeding should be considered, especially if associated with headache and changes in sensorium.

Hydrocephalus

Sudden blockage of cerebrospinal fluid flow is a much more likely cause than gradual ventricular enlargement.

Brain Tumors

Sudden obstruction of cerebrospinal fluid flow is most likely to produce projectile vomiting.

Lead Encephalopathy

Other Disorders

Congenital Adrenal Hyperplasia (Adrenogenital Syndrome)

Hypoadrenalism in young infants may be associated with forceful vomiting. Virilization and ambiguous genitalia are important clues.

Hypercalcemia

Associated symptoms include anorexia, constipation, polydipsia, and polyuria, along with nausea and vomiting.

Wolman Disease

In this rare disorder of cholesterol storage, diarrhea, weight loss, and hepatosplenomegaly occur in the first few weeks of life. Calcifications in enlarged adrenal glands are characteristic on abdominal radiographs. Forceful vomiting occasionally occurs.

Phenylketonuria

Vomiting (sometimes projectile) and irritability may be seen in the first few months of life.

CYCLIC VOMITING SYNDROME

Migraine and Abdominal Migraine

This is the most common cause of cyclic vomiting, perhaps accounting for almost 50% of cases (1). The diagnostic criteria include: a familial history of migraine, recurrent identical attacks, no abdominal symptoms between attacks, and attacks lasting several hours (2).

Chronic Sinusitis

Surprisingly, this was the second most common cause found in one study (1).

Metabolic/Endocrinologic Disorders

Addison Disease

Regional Enteritis

Acute Intermittent Porphyria

Ornithine Transcarbamylase Deficiency

Partial defects of a number of amino or organic acidurias may cause cyclic episodes of vomiting.

Propionic Aciduria

Methyl Malonic Acidemia

Isovaleric Acidemia (Chronic Intermittent Form)

Disorders of Fatty Oxidation

Medium chain acyl-CoA dehydrogenase deficiency.

Hereditary Fructose Intolerance

Gastrointestinal Disorders

Malrotation with Intermittent Volvulus

Although most children with malrotation and volvulus are diagnosed in the first year of life, the clinical presentation may occur at any age.

Peptic Ulcer Disease

More likely to cause chronic vomiting.

Pancreatitis

Pancreatic Pseudocyst

Chronic Idiopathic Pseudo-Obstruction

Intestinal Duplication/Cyst

Superior Mesenteric Artery Syndrome

Urinary Tract Disorders

Intermittent Ureteropelvic Junction Obstruction

Dietl's crisis refers to the onset of vomiting secondary to ureteropelvic junction obstruction following the ingestion of large amounts of fluids. Increased urine production kinks the ureteropelvic junction resulting in obstruction and renal pelvic distension.

Renal Stones

◆ **Other**

Psychogenic

Munchausen Syndrome by Proxy

Recurrent vomiting may be the result of ipecac administered by a parent or caregiver.

Familial Dysautonomia

Idiopathic

Unfortunately, this is still a relatively common cause, i.e., we do not know.

REFERENCES

1. Li BUK. Cyclic vomiting: new understanding of an old disorder. *Contemp Pediatr* 1996;13:48–62.
2. Lundberg PO. Abdominal migraine—diagnosis and therapy. *Headache* 1975;15:122–125.

SUGGESTED READING

Fleisher DR, Matar M. The cyclic vomiting syndrome: a report of 71 cases and literature review. *J Pediatr Gastroent Nutr* 1993;17:361–369.
Forbes D. Differential diagnosis of cyclic vomiting syndrome. *J Pediatr Gastroenterol Nutr* 1995; 21(Suppl. 1):S11–S14.
Pfau BT, Li BUK, Murray RD, Heitlinger LA, McClung HJ, Hayes JR. Differentiating cyclic from chronic vomiting patterns in children: quantitative criteria and diagnostic implications. *Pediatrics* 1996;97:364–368.

71

Diarrhea

Diarrhea denotes the passage of an increased number of stools of variable nonsolid consistency. The passage of an excessive amount of fluid with the stool is the primary manifestation of diarrhea. The complaint of diarrhea is more frequent than the identification of a pathologic process, particularly in infants; for example, breast fed infants commonly have a loose bowel movement with each feeding (gastrocolic reflex). There are four basic pathophysiologic mechanisms that may produce this fluid loss: secretory, cytotoxic, osmotic, and dysenteric. More than one of these malfunctions may be present at the same time. (For discussion of these mechanisms, see the **Suggested Reading** list at the end of this chapter.)

Fortunately, most of the common causes of diarrhea either are not life threatening or are disorders that can be managed fairly easily. Of the many possible causes, only a few are commonly seen: dietary indiscretions, viral and bacterial infections, extraintestinal infections, carbohydrate intolerance, and the irritable bowel syndrome.

Causes of diarrhea have been divided into those seen in the newborn infant, in the well appearing child, and finally, in the ill appearing child. The more common disorders are listed first; the less common ones follow.

♦ **Most Common Causes of Diarrhea**

Acute	**Chronic**
Viral (Rotavirus and Others)	Nonspecific Diarrhea of Childhood
Bacterial	Overfeeding
Extraintestinal Infections	Carbohydrate Malabsorption
Antibiotic Induced	Milk Protein Allergy

● **Causes Not to Forget**

Cystic Fibrosis	Celiac Disease
Encopresis (Around Impaction)	Acquired Immunodeficiency Syndrome
Inflammatory Bowel Disease	Intestinal Parasites

DIARRHEA IN THE NEWBORN

♦ **Overfeeding**

Excessive caloric or fluid intake may result in loose stools.

♦ **Viral Infections**

Rotavirus and other viral infections are not common, but may occur in nursery outbreaks.

Drug Withdrawl Syndrome

Infants manifesting withdrawl are irritable and have frequent small watery bowel movements.

Extraintestinal Infections

Diarrhea may occur with systemic infections.

Bacterial Infections

Escherichia coli and *Salmonella* infections are most common, but other organisms may also be responsible.

Cow Milk Allergy

This is a rare cause of diarrhea in the newborn.

Necrotizing Enterocolitis

Abdominal distension, lethargy, temperature irregularities, and vomiting are findings.

Congenital Lactase Deficiency

Occurrence is rare. Stools are frothy and contain sugar.

Glucose or Galactose Malabsorption

Familial Chloride Diarrhea

Profuse watery diarrhea may begin even *in utero*. The stools resemble urine. Abdominal distension and ileus develop as part of hypokalemic-hypochloremic alkalosis.

Enterokinase Deficiency

Intermittent diarrhea may be present from birth. Vomiting, irritability, and failure to thrive become prominent features.

Hypoadrenalism

The adrenogenital syndrome is the most likely cause of this problem.

Maternal Ulcerative Colitis

Infants born to affected mothers may have transient diarrhea for the first few days of life.

Congenital Villous Atrophy

A rare disorder that results in chronic, life-threatening diarrhea beginning in the newborn period. Intestinal biopsy is required to make the diagnosis.

DIARRHEA IN A WELL APPEARING CHILD

♦ **Normal Variation**

Parents, particularly of breast-fed infants, may need reassurance that a loose bowel movement with each feeding is normal.

♦ **Overfeeding**

Excessive food or liquid intake may result in frequent loose stools.

♦ **Irritable Colon Syndrome or Chronic Nonspecific Diarrhea of Childhood**

These two disorders may be related. Chronic nonspecific diarrhea, seen in healthy thriving children from 6 months to 3 years of age, is characterized by frequent loose stools, most prevalent in the morning, and more frequent after ingestion of cold liquids. In the irritable colon syndrome, seen in older children, the stools are frequent and small, often passed with gas and sometimes preceded by mild cramping. This is the most common cause of chronic diarrhea in young children.

♦ **Milk (or Soy) Protein Allergy**

A true allergic reaction to cow milk or soy protein may cause diarrhea and mild abdominal cramps. A protein losing gastroenteropathy may result in significant generalized edema and significant anemia. Heiner syndrome, caused by severe milk allergy, is characterized by bloody diarrhea and shock after ingestion of small amounts of cow milk protein.

Inadequate Dietary Fat

The deficiency may result in frequent stools.

Other Dietary Causes

A careful history may reveal excessive intake of a number of foodstuffs that may result in diarrhea. Dietetic candies and gums, a source of sorbitol, if eaten in excess may result in diarrhea. Apple and other juices may provide excess fructose, which can provide an excessive osmotic load. Fruit juice excess is commonly associated with chronic nonspecific diarrhea of childhood. Always ask what the child eats each day.

♦ **Antibiotics**

Diarrhea may be associated with or follow a course of antibiotics. Causes include the vehicle for the antibiotic, a change in bacterial flora, and overgrowth of *Clostridium difficile;* other mechanisms, as yet unidentified, may also be involved.

Medications

Ingestion of various medications, such as decongestants and theophylline preparations, may be associated with the passage of frequent loose stools.

● **Constipation with Leakage**

Children with fecal impactions may present with the complaint of diarrhea due to leakage of loose stool around the bolus of hard stool.

Laxative Abuse

This may be inflicted by caregivers or may be part of a scheme to lose weight in adolescents with eating disorders.

Allergic Tension Fatigue Syndrome

Some children, particularly those with an atopic background, may manifest a host of signs and symptoms including headache, abdominal pain, lethargy, irritability, and diarrhea secondary to intolerance of various foods, particularly milk, chocolate, nuts, and eggs.

♦ **Carbohydrate Intolerance**

The defect may be primary or follow gastrointestinal infections. Lactose intolerance is most common. The stools are frothy, smell like vinegar, and contain reducing substances.

● **Parasites**

Children with infestation by any of a variety of parasites may not appear ill. *Giardia* and *Cryptosporidium* as well as amebiasis, and ascariasis are possibilities.

Familial Polyposis

Although diarrhea is not a common manifestation, its presence may lead to a rectal examination and discovery of the diagnosis.

Well Water

The high mineral content of some well water may result in diarrhea. Bacterial contamination is another mechanism.

DIARRHEA IN AN ILL APPEARING CHILD

Infectious Gastroenteritis

◆ Viral

A host of viruses have been found to cause diarrhea. Rotavirus is the most important cause of vomiting and diarrhea in the United States during the winter months, particularly in children 6 months to 2 years of age. Adults and older children have diarrhea with severe abdominal cramps but no vomiting. Other causes of viral gastroenteritis include Norwalk virus, calicivirus, coronavirus, and the enteric adenoviruses.

◆ Bacterial

Salmonella, shigella, and *E coli* are the best known bacterial causes of diarrhea, but *Campylobacter jejuni* and *Yersinia enterocolitica* are being recognized with increasing frequency. Intermittent relapses with a chronic diarrheal picture are not uncommon. *C difficile* toxin must be considered in children who had previously been treated with antibiotics.

• Parasitic Infestation

Giardia infection is the most common cause of parasitic diarrhea. *Cryptosporidium* is being recognized with increased frequency, particularly in daycare settings and in immune compromised individuals. Other parasitic infestations that may cause chronic diarrhea with weight loss and abdominal distension include amebiasis, strongyloidiasis, and hookworm infestation.

Fungal

Candida and *Histoplasma* are among the fungal pathogens.

◆ Extraintestinal Infections

Many extraintestinal infections may be associated with diarrhea, especially in younger children. Otitis media, urinary tract infections, sepsis, and pneumonias are the most frequently recognized. This is sometimes referred to as parenteral diarrhea.

◆ Carbohydrate Malabsorption

Watery, frothy stools that smell like vinegar and contain sugar should suggest this possibility. Lactose absorption is most frequently affected; congenital, acquired, and developmental lactose intolerances are well recognized. Sucrose, isomaltose, and glucose or galactose malabsorptions may be found.

• Inflammatory Bowel Disease

Ulcerative colitis is characterized by abdominal cramps, tenesmus, and the passage of stools containing mucus and blood. In Crohn disease, the presentation may be more subtle with abdominal pain, fever of unknown origin, and weight loss or failure of development.

- **Cystic Fibrosis**

  Failure to thrive, recurrent pneumonias, and steatorrhea are the most frequent manifestations.

- **Celiac Disease**

  This disorder is now being recognized more frequently in the United States. An accurate diagnosis is critical, because of the harsh dietary restrictions. Diarrhea generally begins after the introduction of wheat containing foods but is not present in one third of affected children.

Maternal Deprivation Syndrome

Children with growth and developmental retardation secondary to psychosocial factors may present with chronic diarrheal stools.

Anatomic Abnormalities of the Bowel

Hirschsprung Disease (Congenital Megacolon)

Diarrheal leakage may occur. The development of an enterocolitis in this disorder is particularly dangerous.

Short Bowel Syndrome

Blind or Stagnant Loop

Diarrhea, steatorrhea, abdominal distension, weight loss, and intermittent episodes suggestive of intestinal obstruction may be present.

Malrotation and Partial Small Bowel Obstructions

The initial symptom may be diarrhea.

Enteric Fistulas

Intestinal Lymphangiectasia

This disorder should be suspected in a child with edema, hypoproteinemia, steatorrhea, and loose stools.

Intestinal Pseudo-Obstruction

Constipation and abdominal distension may be prime signs, but affected children may also have recurrent diarrhea.

Immune Deficiency

Diarrhea with failure to thrive, recurrent infections, and chronic cough should suggest any of several immune deficiency diseases, generally those with reduced cellular immunity or deficient IgA.

- **Acquired Immunodeficiency Syndrome**

  IgA Deficiency

  Hypogammaglobulinemias or Agammaglobulinemias

  Combined Immunodeficiency

  Wiskott-Aldrich Syndrome

  Ataxia Telangiectasia

Endocrine Causes

Hyperthyroidism

Hypoparathyroidism

Diarrhea is unusual but may be associated with hypocalcemia. Seizures, tetany, and muscular cramps dominate the clinical picture.

Adrenal Insufficiency

Weakness, lethargy, vomiting, anorexia, and diarrhea are characteristic. Serum sodium levels are low; serum potassium levels are high.

Tumors

Neuroblastoma; Ganglioneuroma; Ganglioneuroblastoma

Carcinoid Tumors

These tumors are rare in children; findings may include episodes of cutaneous flushing, wheezing, and diarrhea.

Vasoactive Intestinal Peptide-Secreting Tumors

Findings include failure to thrive, abdominal distension, hypertension, sweating episodes, metabolic acidosis, and low serum potassium levels. Diarrhea may be intermittent at first but then becomes unremitting.

Intestinal Lymphosarcoma

Abdominal pain, malaise, anemia, and diarrhea are the primary features.

Pancreatic Disorders

Exocrine Pancreatic Insufficiency

Malabsorption, failure to thrive, cyclic neutropenia, anemia, and metaphyseal dysostosis are found in the Shwachman-Diamond syndrome.

Chronic Pancreatitis

Hepatic Disturbances

Hepatitis

Children with acute hepatitis may have diarrhea or constipation.

Chronic Hepatitis

Cirrhosis

Bile Acid Deficiency

Steatorrhea develops along with anorexia and vomiting.

Biliary Atresia

Progressively deepening jaundice, failure to thrive, malnutrition, and abdominal distension in the first months of life are prominent findings.

Protein Calorie Malnutrition

Metabolic Disorders, Inherited

Galactosemia

Jaundice, failure to thrive, cataracts, hepatomegaly, vomiting, and diarrhea are important findings. The urine should be checked for the presence of reducing substances.

Tyrosinemia

Failure to thrive, vomiting, diarrhea, abdominal enlargement, edema, ascites, and hepatosplenomegaly are the leading symptoms.

Methionine Malabsorption

This defect is characterized by diarrhea, convulsions, retardation, and a sweet odor to the urine.

Familial Protein Intolerance

Vomiting and diarrhea begin between 3 and 13 months of age.

Wolman Disease

Chronic diarrhea develops in the first few weeks of life. Hepatosplenomegaly and significant failure to thrive are found. Areas of calcification in the adrenal glands are seen on abdominal roentgenograms.

Abetalipoproteinemia

Ataxia, retinitis pigmentosa, and steatorrhea with acanthocytes on peripheral smear are clues.

Selective Malabsorption of Vitamin B$_{12}$

Gaucher Disease

Niemann-Pick Disease

Vascular Disorders

Mesenteric Artery Insufficiency

Early Portal Hypertension

Intestinal Ischemia

Miscellaneous Disorders

Clostridium difficile Toxin

A chronic watery diarrhea with poor weight gain may be caused by this toxin. Prior antibiotic therapy may or may not have preceded its onset. Oral vancomycin usually proves helpful.

Acrodermatitis Enteropathica

Perioral and perianal psoriatic-like plaques and vesicobullous lesions of the extremities with diarrhea, irritability, and alopecia should suggest this disorder. Dramatic improvement follows zinc therapy.

Zollinger-Ellison Syndrome

This disorder is associated with multiple gastric and peptic ulcers.

Scleroderma

Skin changes usually precede the intestinal manifestations.

Folic Acid Deficiency

Neurofibromatosis

Café au lait macules and, after puberty, neurofibromas are present.

Familial Dysautonomia (Riley-Day Syndrome)

Recurrent vomiting, aspiration, absent lacrimation, absent filiform papillae on the tongue, emotional lability, and postural hypotension are associated findings.

Whipple Disease

This disorder, usually seen in adults, causes foul-smelling diarrhea with fever. An infectious pathogenesis is presumed.

Toxic Diarrhea

Diarrhea may be secondary to chemotherapy or irradiation.

SUGGESTED READING

Cohen MB, Balistreri WF. Diagnosing and treating diarrhea. *Contemp Pediatr* 1989;6:89–114.
DeWitt TG. Acute diarrhea in children. *Pediatr Rev* 1989;11:6–12.
Gartner JC Jr. Chronic diarrhea. In: Gartner JC Jr, Zitelli BJ, eds. *Common & chronic symptoms in pediatrics.* St. Louis: Mosby, 1997:247–258.
Judd RH. Chronic nonspecific diarrhea. *Pediatr Rev* 1996;11:379–384.
Kenney RT. Parasitic causes of diarrhea. *Pediatr Ann* 1994;23:414–422.
Murphy MS, Walker WA. Celiac disease. *Pediatr Rev* 1991;12:325–330.
Northrup RS, Flanigan TP. Gastroenteritis. *Pediatr Rev* 1994;15:461–472.

72

Constipation and Fecal Retention

Although the old adage "one man's constipation may be another man's diarrhea" is a bit of an exaggeration, it serves to remind us that there are wide variations in normal elimination habits. In infancy, changes in stool type or frequency are common. In some families, excessive attention to elimination details may cause normal patterns to be perceived as abnormal.

Generally, constipation refers to a state in which the stools are hard and difficult to pass (obstipation), but also infrequent, less than three times per week. Infants have relatively weak abdominal musculature and are at a mechanical disadvantage attempting to stool in a supine position; they commonly increase their intraabdominal pressure by a Valsalva maneuver, which causes them to become "red in the face," convincing the parents that they are constipated.

The causes of constipation range from chronic stool-holding, in which huge fecal impactions may be found, to "spastic colon," in which scybalous (rabbit pellet-like) stools are characteristic; from dietary causes to metabolic disorders; and from neurogenic problems to psychogenic ones.

In 95% of neonates, meconium is passed within the first 24 hours of life; failure to do so requires careful evaluation and is considered separately in the following classification of causes of constipation. A careful history including diet and a description of the stools should not be neglected in any age group, nor should a familial history of elimination patterns. A rectal examination should be performed. Keep in mind that the great majority, well over 90% in most studies, of children with constipation have chronic idiopathic constipation, sometimes referred to as functional constipation.

♦ **Most Common Causes**

Chronic Idiopathic   Painful Defecation
Dietary Causes

● **Causes Not to Forget**

Infantile Botulism   Lead Poisoning
Meconium Ileus Equivalent   Hypokalemia
Spinal Dysraphism   Hirschsprung Disease

DELAYED PASSAGE OF MECONIUM

Intestinal Obstruction

Infants with atresias, webs, volvulus, or other causes of obstruction may present with failure to pass stools as well as abdominal distension and vomiting. The passage of meconium does not rule out a high or low obstruction.

Hirschsprung Disease (Congenital Megacolon)

This disorder accounts for 20% to 25% of the cases of neonatal intestinal obstruction. Abdominal distension is followed by decreased appetite; the finding of bile-stained vomitus is common. Digital examination or saline enema may induce stool passage and relief of symptoms and signs. Occasionally, the disorder may not be diagnosed until later in life. The stools passed are never normal.

Meconium Ileus

Symptoms usually begin on the second day of life with abdominal distension and vomiting. Most affected infants have cystic fibrosis.

Meconium Plug

Plugs may block the intestines, especially in premature infants. Hirschsprung disease must always be considered.

Functional Ileus

Sepsis, respiratory distress syndrome, pneumonia, and electrolyte imbalance may be responsible for the ileus.

Small Left Colon Syndrome

Clinical presentation is typical of bowel obstruction. Barium enema demonstrates the significantly decreased caliber of the left colon. Maternal diabetes is common.

Drugs Administered to Mother

Magnesium sulfate, opiates, and ganglionic blocking agents given to the mother prior to delivery may cause delayed passage of meconium in the neonate.

Hypothyroidism

Prolonged jaundice, lethargy, and low body temperature are additional suggestive signs.

PHYSIOLOGIC CAUSES

♦ Dietary

Breastfeeding

Breast-fed infants initially have frequent stools, often with every feeding; however, many at around 6 weeks of age begin to have prolonged periods, often many days, without the passage of stool.

Cow Milk

The casein curd, often difficult to digest, is one of the reasons why unaltered cow milk often leads to constipation. Although this effect is most commonly seen in young infants, a high intake of milk or other dairy products (e.g., cheese) at any age may result in constipation.

Low Dietary Roughage

A diet low in vegetable fiber or other bulk results in hard, difficult to pass stools. This is a common condition in children whose diet consists largely of milk, sugared cereal, and snack foods.

Deficient Fluid Intake

Any condition or illness that results in a reduced fluid intake or excessive fluid losses (e.g., fever) may result in a decreased fecal bulk with less frequent elimination.

Febrile States

Hot Weather

Insufficient Intravenous Fluids

In hospitalized children.

Immobility

Constipation may be a problem in children confined to bed, especially after surgery or following the application of casts, especially body casts.

Anorexia Nervosa

Starvation

VOLUNTARY WITHHOLDING

♦ Chronic Idiopathic Constipation

A great deal has been written about the common problem of the "stool hoarder." The problem generally begins after 2 1/2 to 3 years of age. Parental concern may not begin until the child begins soiling the underwear because of spillage around a huge fecal impaction distending the rectum. A rectal examination and a careful history for possible precipitating events are essential. Any of a number of causes may result in painful defecation and subsequent withholding, creating an ever increasing problem.

♦ **Painful Defecation**

    Anal Fissure

    Perianal Dermatitis or Irritation

    Perianal Streptococcal Cellulitis

    Sexual Abuse

    Hemorrhoids

Intentional Withholding

This may occur during travel or at school, with a change in environment, or during periods of family stress or upheaval.

Improper Toilet Training

Constipation may be the result of the parents failing to set standards for toilet training or as a result of excessive compulsion regarding training.

Emotional Disturbance

Severe Mental Retardation

Depression

INTESTINAL DISORDERS

● **Hirschsprung Disease (Congenital Megacolon)**

Uncommonly, the onset of symptoms is delayed until after the newborn period. The condition may have been obscured by repeated digital examinations or enemas with relief of obstructive symptoms. Stools are infrequent and ribbon-like rather than the huge masses seen with the acquired form. Generally, the rectal ampulla is empty on digital examination.

● **Meconium Ileus Equivalent**

A significant number of older children with cystic fibrosis may develop constipation to the degree of obstruction. This phenomenon may be due to the accumulation of intestinal luminal mucus that adheres to the intestinal wall and to which food adheres.

Anal or Rectal Stenosis

Stenosis is most commonly acquired rather than congenital, especially after imperforate anus repair or with neoplasms or pelvic abscesses.

Malrotation

Anteriorally Placed Anus

This may represent an aborted imperforated anus.

Dolichocolon

An abnormally long colon is often a familial trait. Increased extraction of water creates hard, compacted stools. Affected children require a high-bulk diet.

Appendicitis

Constipation is a minor feature, overshadowed by the abdominal pain.

Celiac Disease

Although diarrhea is more common, a small number of affected children may have fecal impactions and vomiting, mimicking obstruction.

NEUROGENIC DISORDERS

Intestinal Pseudo-Obstruction

This uncommon disorder, of various causes, with progressively severe motility problems leads to abdominal distension and failure to pass stools. The primary form is familial and presents in infancy. The acquired forms may be associated with scleroderma, amyloidosis, various endocrinopathies, narcotic or laxative abuse, electrolyte disturbance, and vasoactive secreting tumors.

Cerebral Palsy

Children with the athetoid variety and those who are severely spastic are most likely to have constipation.

Myelomeningocele

Spinal Cord Injury

Sacral Agenesis

Diastematomyelia

The spinal cord may become tethered by bony spicules. There may be cutaneous abnormalities over the spine, as well as gait and urinary disturbances.

● **Spinal Dysraphism**

Fibrous bands, lipomas, septa or dermal sinuses may cause traction or pressure lesions. Look for cutaneous clues over the spine. The onset of symptoms may occur later in childhood or even adolescence.

Neurofibromatosis

Constipation or obstipation is an unexplained common association. Colonic neuro-fibromas may produce obstruction or an acquired megacolon.

Muscular Weakness

Various causes include spinal muscular atrophy (Werdnig-Hoffman disease), the myotonias, prune-belly syndrome, and muscular dystrophies. Lack of muscle power to create intra-abdominal pressure makes evacuation difficult.

Guillain-Barré Syndrome

The ascending weakness overshadows the constipation.

Neuronal Dysplasia

Is associated with increased numbers of ganglion cells in the lower colon, in contrast to aglanglionic disease. Problems may appear throughout childhood with variable degrees of constipation or as pseudo-obstruction. This disorder is associated with neurofibromatosis and multiple endocrine neoplasia type IIb.

Familial Dysautonomia

Acquired Postganglionic Cholinergic Dysautonomia

Associated findings include bilateral internal ophthalmoplegia, impaired secretion of tears and saliva, and absence of sweating as well as gastrointestinal atony.

ENDOCRINE AND METABOLIC DISORDERS

- ### Hypokalemia

Reduced peristalsis or ileus may occur.

Hypercalcemia or Hypocalcemia

Children immobilized with casts, traction, and so forth, may develop hypercalce-mia with its attendant problems, including constipation.

Hypothyroidism

Other features of hypothyroidism are generally more prominent than constipation.

Diabetes Mellitus

Constipation may be related to lack of adequate bowel water early in the disease, and after many years to a neuropathy.

Pheochromocytoma

Affected children occasionally have severe constipation. More typical features include hypertension, headache, tachycardia, palpitations, nausea, and vomiting.

Conditions Associated with Polyuria

Polyuria results in deficient stool water. Diabetes insipidus and renal tubular acidosis may be causes.

Acute Intermittent Porphyria

Abdominal pain, vomiting, and constipation may be the initial manifestations.

Amyloidosis

Lipid Storage Disorders

Constipation may be a minor feature of some of these disorders.

MISCELLANEOUS DISORDERS

• Infant Botulism

Facial and ocular palsies, a poor suck, and hypotonia should suggest this possibility. Constipation may be an early complaint.

• Lead Poisoning

When plumbism was more common, constipation was a relatively common presenting complaint.

Drugs

Antihistamines, opiates, and phenothiazines may be constipating. Methylphenidate, phenytoin, calcium channel blockers, vincristine, and aluminum antacids may also cause constipation.

Viral Hepatitis

Diarrhea and constipation occur with equal frequency.

Salmonellosis

In the systemic form, fever for 1 to 3 weeks, rose spots, anorexia, splenomegaly, constipation, and leukopenia may be presenting signs.

Lupus Erythematosus

Dermatomyositis

Scleroderma

Intestinal involvement may result in decreased intestinal motility.

Graft Versus Host Disease

Tetanus

Chagas Disease

SUGGESTED READING

Abi-Hanna A, Lake AM. Constipation and encopresis in childhood. *Pediatr Rev* 1998;19:23–30.
Loening-Baucke V. Constipation in early childhood: patient characteristics, treatment, and longterm follow up. *Gut* 1993;34:1400–1404.
McClung HJ, Boyne L, Heitlinger L. Constipation and dietary fiber intake in children. *Pediatrics* 1995;96:999–1000.
Urbach AH. Constipation. In: Gartner JC Jr, Zitelli BJ, eds. *Common & chronic symptoms in pediatrics.* St. Louis: Mosby, 1997:233–246.

73

Fecal Incontinence and Encopresis

Most children achieve full bowel control and acquire regular bowel habits during the fourth year of life. Occasionally, episodes of fecal incontinence occur; most parents recognize these as "accidents." When episodes of incontinence become frequent or regular, medical evaluation is required.

Encopresis refers to the voluntary or involuntary evacuation of feces into the underwear or in places that are not socially acceptable depositories. The most common cause of encopresis is a large fecal impaction, which in most cases develops from withholding stool after a series of painful defecations. A careful history will usually differentiate chronic constipation with characteristic overflow incontinence from those with a voluntary, anatomic, or neurologic cause.

INVOLUNTARY CAUSES

♦ Chronic Constipation with Encopresis

This is by far the most common cause of fecal soiling. As the fecal impaction enlarges the anal sphincter becomes chronically stretched and unable to prevent spillage of stool. Two types of incontinence, which may coexist, have been reported: One is the rubbing of the hard fecal impaction as it extends through the anal sphincter onto the underwear, giving a linear caking of stool. The more common form is the frequent passage of small amounts of liquid stool around the bolus of impacted stool, causing soiling of the underwear. Abdominal and rectal examination will disclose the cause of the soiling. The causes of chronic constipation producing the encopresis are numerous (see Chapter 72, Constipation and Fecal Retention).

♦ Diarrheal Conditions

During acute or chronic diarrheal diseases the child may not be able to voluntarily control the peristaltic rushes of liquid stool by using the external anal sphincter. Although this is more likely to occur in young children, older children and adults with these diseases may occasionally lose control because of fatigue, inaccessibility of toilets, or general illness.

Seizures

Fecal incontinence may occur during a convulsive episode.

VOLUNTARY CAUSES

Failure to Achieve Control

The child may never have been toilet trained for various reasons, such as family disinterest or resistance by the child to the training approach. The severely mentally retarded child may never achieve control.

Regressive Behavior

Previously toilet trained young children may resume soiling at the time of stressful situations, such as birth of a sibling, illnesses, separations, death in the family, or moves.

Emotional Disturbances

The soiling may occasionally be a manifestation of severe psychologic problems.

ANATOMIC CAUSES

Anorectal Anomalies

Anatomic abnormalities such as perineal fistulas may result in soiling.

Regional Enteritis (Crohn Disease)

Must be considered in the older child.

Scarring of the Anus

Control of defecation may be lost following anorectal surgery, particularly for imperforate anus or Hirschsprung disease, or from anorectal trauma.

Sexual Abuse

Fecal incontinence may be the result of damage to the rectum, but may also have psychogenic reasons.

NEUROGENIC CAUSES

Myelomeningocele

Fecal incontinence is very common in children with myelomenigoceles. The incontinence may be overflow associated with constipation, or associated with diarrheal stools.

Muscular Dystrophies

Incontinence may occur associated with constipation or inability to hold back the urge to defecate.

Diastematomyelia

Low back pain, progressive weakness of the lower extremities, and bladder and bowel incontinence may be present. Cutaneous changes over the spinal column may be a clue.

Spinal Cord Tumors

Lipomas, teratomas, neurofibromas, gliomas, arteriovenous malformations, and other tumors may be associated with encopresis along with back pain, weakness of the lower extremities, and reflex or sensory changes. Cutaneous clues may be present over the spinal column.

Spinal Dysraphism

Fibrous bands, lipomas, septa or dermal sinuses may cause traction or pressure lesions. Look for cutaneous clues over the spine. The onset of symptoms may occur later in childhood or even adolescence. Fecal incontinence may be a presentation.

Sacral Agenesis

Spinal Cord Injuries

Syringomyelia

Transverse Myelitis

A sudden onset of paralysis of the lower extremities occurs.

Epidural Abscess

Severe back pain over the infected area and lower extremity weakness are the more prominent symptoms.

Guillain-Barré Syndrome (Infectious Polyneuritis)

Constipation is common; incontinence is rare.

Poliomyelitis

SUGGESTED READING

Benning MA, Buller HA, Heymans HS, Tytgat GN, Taminiau JA. Is encopresis always the result of constipation? *Arch Dis Child* 1994;71:186–193.
Loening-Baucke V. Encopresis and soiling. *Pediatr Clin North Am* 1996;43:279–298.
Nolan T, Oberklaid F. New concepts in the management of encopresis. *Pediatr Rev* 1993;14:447–451.

74

Hematemesis

Hematemesis, or the vomiting of bright red blood or coffee ground material, quickens the pulse of all who see it; if significant blood loss occurs, the child may have tachycardia as well. The vomiting of blood, rather than finding blood in the stool only, implies that the site of the bleeding is proximal to the ligament of Treitz. Hematemesis is so often a sign of a serious underlying disorder that it must be considered a medical emergency.

In the following classification of possible causes, hematemesis in neonates has been separated from that occurring in older infants and children. Swallowed blood, during parturition in the newborn or from epistaxis thereafter, must always be included in the differential diagnosis. The other causes are grouped by anatomic site or by hematologic origin.

In the past, as many as one third to one half of cases of hematemesis in children were unexplained; however, newer technology such as fiberoptic endoscopy may significantly lower this percentage. Unfortunately, hematemesis often occurs suddenly without warning in previously asymptomatic children. A careful history and physical examination may uncover subtle clues that may help in sorting out possible causes.

♦ **Most Common Causes of Hematemesis**

Swallowed Blood (Maternal)   Swallowed Blood (Epistaxis)
Gastritis   Esophagitis
Duodenal Ulcer   Esophageal Varices

● **Causes Not to Forget**

Maternal Breast Fissure   Milk Protein Intolerance
Munchausen by Proxy

NEONATAL CAUSES

♦ **Swallowed Maternal Blood**

The newborn may swallow maternal blood during the birth process. Almost always hematemesis of this variety occurs within the first 12 to 24 hours after birth. The

Apt test, using the fact that fetal hemoglobin resists alkali denaturization, is helpful in documenting the presence of maternal blood.

- **Swallowed Blood by Breast-Fed Infants**

  Always check the breasts of breast-feeding mothers whose infants vomit blood, in search of a nipple fissure.

  ### Hemorrhagic Gastritis

  This disorder may occur in the sick neonate following a stressful delivery or a neonatal complication such as sepsis or meningitis.

  ### Peptic Ulcer

  Neonatal events may be stressful enough to result in ulcer formation or perforation.

  ### Hemorrhagic Disease of the Newborn

  Otherwise healthy appearing infants may vomit significant amounts of blood in the first few days of life. A bleeding site is not usually found; instead, there may be significant oozing from multiple foci. There may be evidence of bleeding from other areas of the body (umbilicus, penis if circumcision has been done, or puncture sites) or petechiae and purpura. Vitamin K deficiency is less common now, but maternal aspirin ingestion during the few days prior to delivery or use of anticonvulsants or anticoagulants by the mother should be considered.

  ### Spontaneous Rupture of Esophagus

  Occurrence is uncommon in infants, but this disorder should be suspected in the infant who appears well initially and then develops respiratory distress (secondary to the development of a tension pneumothorax), increased with feeding, and sometimes associated hematemesis.

♦ SWALLOWED BLOOD

The site of bleeding may be in the upper respiratory tract, particularly with epistaxis or following dental extractions, tonsillectomy, and oral or pharyngeal lacerations. In breast-fed infants be sure to check the mother's breast for fissures!

ESOPHAGEAL DISORDERS

♦ Chalasia/Gastroesophageal Reflux

If these conditions are associated with blood mixed in with the vomitus, the amount is generally small. Reflux of stomach acids into the esophagus may result in erosions. Early symptoms may be vomiting after meals, irritability, poor appetite, recurrent coughing episodes, or pneumonitis.

◆ Hiatal Hernia

Vomiting or excessive regurgitation after feedings may begin shortly after birth. Some infants have dysphagia, poor weight gain, and recurrent aspiration pneumonitis. The amount of blood in the vomitus is quite small.

◆ Esophageal Varices

Massive hematemesis is the most frequent presentation. The two most common underlying conditions are portal vein thrombosis and hepatic cirrhosis. It is essential to obtain a careful neonatal history to uncover possible causes of longstanding portal vein thrombosis such as omphalitis, neonatal sepsis, diarrhea with shock, exchange transfusions, and umbilical vein catheterization. Hepatic cirrhosis may result from a host of disorders (see Chapter 64, Ascites) including obstructive biliary disease, infections and inflammatory disorders, cardiovascular problems, genetic and metabolic disorders, and drugs. Some inherited causes of cirrhosis that may produce hematemesis and are worthy of consideration are cystic fibrosis, Wilson disease, alpha$_1$-antitrypsin deficiency, galactosemia, Gaucher disease, porphyria, and Rendu-Osler-Weber syndrome (hereditary hemorrhagic telangiectasia). Other less frequent presenting signs of portal hypertension include splenomegaly, prominent veins of collateral circulation over the abdominal wall, hepatomegaly, clubbing, and ascites.

Foreign Bodies

Ingested foreign bodies may cause lacerations along the alimentary tract with resultant bleeding.

Mallory-Weiss Syndrome

Excessive retching may cause a tear in the esophagus.

Corrosive Agents

Acid and alkali substances may produce significant bleeding as they erode through the mucosa.

Congenital Microgastria

In this rare disorder the stomach is small, resulting in reflux and esophagitis.

Esophageal Tumors

GASTRODUODENAL LESIONS

◆ Peptic Ulcer

Symptoms may vary with the age of the child. Children under 3 years of age may have a poor appetite, vomiting, crying after meals, and abdominal distension; those 3 to 6 years of age often have vomiting related to eating, periumbilical pain, and pain that may awaken them at night. Children older than 6 years of age may complain of a burning or gnawing epigastric pain, most frequent after fasting or at night, that may occasionally be relieved by food or milk. In the Zollinger-Ellison syndrome, gastric hypersecretion results in multiple duodenal or jejunal ulcers.

Stress Ulcers

These ulcers occur during times of other serious illness, such as central nervous system disease or burns.

◆ Gastritis

Irritation of the stomach may follow ingestion of corrosives, nonsteroidal anti-inflammatory agents, aspirin, iron, acetaminophen, aminophylline, boric acid, fluoride, heavy metals, phenol, or bacterial food poisoning.

Helicobacter pylori Gastritis

This bacterium has become the leading cause of secondary gastritis in older children.

Gastric Outlet Obstruction

Small amounts of blood may appear in the vomitus in pyloric stenosis, antral ulcers, or pyloric webs.

Duplications

Esophageal or gastric duplications may become ulcerated and bleed. Abdominal pain or, occasionally, a palpable mass may be present.

Tumors

Leiomyomas, leiomyosarcomas, and lymphomas may erode vessels and cause hematemesis.

Infections

Hemorrhagic Fevers

In various parts of the world, the bites of ticks and mites may produce disorders characterized by fever, chills, muscle aches, headache, bleeding diatheses, hematemesis, and shock.

Mycotic Infections

Debilitated patients are predisposed. Progressive sinusitis, cellulitis, and pneumonitis are common findings.

Malaria

Drugs

(Also see Gastritis.)

Theophylline

Caffeine Intoxication

Pseudoxanthoma Elasticum

This rare disorder has skin changes resembling a plucked chicken in areas such as the neck and axillae. Alterations in elastic tissue of the gastrointestinal vessels may lead to bleeding.

HEMATOLOGIC DISORDERS

Thrombocytopenia

Disseminated Intravascular Coagulation

Aplastic Anemia

Leukemia

von Willebrand Disease

MISCELLANEOUS DISORDERS

● **Milk Protein Intolerance**

Occult blood loss is more common, but hematemesis may occur.

● **Munchausen Syndrome by Proxy**

Blood may be placed in vomitus or around the mouth by a caregiver.

Henoch-Schönlein Purpura

This disorder rarely causes hematemesis.

Pulmonary Bleeding

Hematemesis may occur in disorders that produce hemoptysis if the blood is not swallowed. Idiopathic pulmonary hemosiderosis should be considered.

Blunt Trauma to the Abdomen

Particularly, duodenal injuries may cause hematemesis.

Rendu-Osler-Weber Syndrome

Hereditary hemorrhagic telangiectasia is an autosomal dominant disorder associated with mucocutaneous telangiectasia.

Scurvy

The clinical presentation may mimic that of a peptic ulcer. There may be other signs of hemorrhage into the skin and periosteitis that may manifest as tender extremities.

SUGGESTED READING

Ament ME. Diagnosis and management of upper gastrointestinal tract bleeding in the pediatric patient. *Pediatr Rev* 1990;12:107–116.

Gryboski JD. Peptic ulcer disease in children. *Pediatr Rev* 1990;12:15–21.

Mezoff AG, Preud'Homme DL. How serious is that GI bleed? *Contemp Pediatr* 1994;11:60–92.

75

Melena and Hematochezia

Hematemesis is generally associated with lesions located above the ligament of Treitz. Melena, the passage of black, tarry stools due to the presence of blood altered by intestinal juices, and hematochezia, the passage of gross blood in the stool, may indicate upper and lower gastrointestinal bleeding. In fact, melena rather than hematemesis may be a presenting sign of upper tract bleeding. Melena denotes bleeding proximal to the ileocecal valve. Hematochezia most frequently reflects a colonic source of bleeding, but may also be caused by bleeding from the upper tract if the transit time of gastrointestinal contents is so short that blood has not changed color.

The amount of blood passed, age of the child, associated symptoms and condition of the child, and location of the blood in the stool are important diagnostic considerations. In the past, gastrointestinal bleeding went unexplained in as many as one half the cases; at present, with more sophisticated tools such as fiberoptic endoscopy, a definitive diagnosis should be possible more often.

The predominant causes of gastrointestinal bleeding vary with age. Some disorders listed in Chapter 74, Gastrointestinal Bleeding: Hematemesis, are repeated here in order to include the most common causes of bleeding in three age groups. Any disorder causing hematemesis, however, may also produce melena.

◆ Most Common Causes of Gastrointestinal Bleeding (1)

Neonate	Infants	Children
Anal Fissure	Anal Fissure	Polyps
Swallowed Maternal Blood	Infectious Diarrheas	Anal Fissure
	Milk Protein Intolerance	Infectious Diarrheas
Infectious Diarrheas	Meckel Diverticulum	Swallowed Blood
Hirschsprung Disease	Intussusception	(Epistaxis)
Necrotizing Enterocolitis	Gastrointestinal Duplication	Inflammatory Bowel Disease
Volvulus		
Stress Ulcer	Peptic Ulcer	Peptic Ulcer
		Meckel Diverticulum
		Gastritis

● **Disorders Not to Forget**

Esophageal Varices   Hemolytic-Uremic Syndrome
Foreign Bodies   Coagulopathies
Esophagitis

NEONATAL PERIOD

♦ **Swallowed Maternal Blood**

The Apt test, which makes use of the resistance of fetal hemoglobin to alkali denaturization, may be helpful in separating out maternal from newborn blood.

♦ **Swallowed Blood from Maternal Breast Fissure**

♦ **Gastroenteritis**

Irritation or invasion of the gastrointestinal tract may occur during viral and bacterial infections. Generally, small amounts of blood are passed.

Hemorrhagic Gastritis

Peptic Ulcer

♦ **Stress Ulcer**

Sepsis

May cause a stress ulcer, or result in intravascular coagulation.

Milk Intolerance

Cow and soy milk protein intolerance may result in gastrointestinal bleeding, sometimes manifested as hematochezia.

♦ **Necrotizing Enterocolitis**

Occurrence is most common on the third to fifth day of life in premature infants. Vomiting, abdominal distension, temperature instability, lethargy, and apnea are other symptoms. Diarrhea and, later, red to "currant jelly" stools may follow.

Hirschsprung Disease

Enterocolitis developing in an infant with this disorder is a medical emergency.

Hematologic Problems

Thrombocytopenia

Disemminated Intravascular Coagulation

Hypoprothrombinemia

Afibrinogenemia

Trauma to Rectum

An anal fissure or more severe internal injuries may result from improper use of a rectal thermometer.

Severe Congenital Heart Disease

Ischemia of the bowel may occur resulting in oozing of blood from intestinal mucosal surfaces.

♦ Malrotation with Midgut Volvulus

Intermittent episodes of bile-stained vomiting generally precede the onset of shock that occurs when the bowel twists on itself.

Acute Ulcerative Colitis

This disorder is rare in neonates. Signs include irritability and blood and mucus in the stool.

Intestinal Obstruction

Peritonitis

Hypoglycemia

INFANCY

♦ Anal Fissure

Fissure is the leading cause in this age group. Blood generally is present on the outside of the stool and is bright red. Constipation often leads to fissure formation.

♦ Enterocolitis and Infectious Diarrheas

The amounts of blood passed are generally small. Fever and diarrhea are often present. Viruses and bacteria (especially *Salmonella,* shigella, *Campylobacter,* and *Escherichia coli*) are the most common causes.

● Esophagitis

(See Chapter 74, Hematemesis.)

♦ Peptic Ulcer

♦ Milk Allergy

The passage of small amounts of occult blood is common. Occasionally, the allergy may be characterized by more active bleeding and a shocklike picture.

♦ Intussusception

Intussusception must be suspected in the young child with episodic, crampy abdominal pain lasting 5 to 10 minutes during each attack. Vomiting, pallor, and lethargy are usually present. The passage of "currant jelly" stools is a later finding.

♦ Meckel Diverticulum

This lesion is characterized by the painless passage of large amounts of bright to dark red blood in a previously well child. Symptoms begin in the first 2 years of life in one half of the cases and, occasionally, may mimic those of appendicitis.

Volvulus

• Esophageal Varices

Gangrenous Bowel

Interference with the blood supply of the bowel, particularly with venous congestion, will eventually lead to the passage of blood.

♦ Duplication of Bowel

This anomaly is particularly likely to be associated with bleeding if ectopic gastric mucosa is present in the duplication. A mass may be palpated on careful abdominal examination.

Hemorrhagic Colitis

Enterohemorrhagic *E coli* 0157:H7 is an important cause. Bright red, grossly bloody stools follow fever, severe abdominal cramps, diarrhea, and emesis.

Hemangiomata of Bowel

Occasionally, cutaneous hemangiomas may be clues.

Acute Intestinal Ischemia

Clinical features include hematochezia, abdominal distension, and pneumatosis intestinalis. Stenosis of the superior mesenteric artery is a rare cause. Hypotension and necrotizing enterocolitis are other causes.

von Willebrand Disease

Occasionally, bleeding may occur with this disorder. It may be precipitated by the use of salicylates.

Drugs

Infants treated with steroids, nonsteroidal anti-inflammatory drugs, and others may have gastrointestinal bleeding.

CHILDHOOD

◆ Juvenile Polyps

The passage of blood, mixed in with the stool or on the outside, is painless; 75% of polyps are within 25 cm of the rectum.

◆ Anal Fissures

◆ Peptic Ulcers

◆ Enterocolitis and Infectious Diarrheas

The amounts of blood passed are generally small. Fever and diarrhea are often present. Viruses and bacteria (especially *Salmonella,* shigella, *Campylobacter,* and *E coli*) are the most common causes.

● Hemorrhagic Colitis

Escherichia coli serotype 0157:H7 may play a significant role in this disorder as well as in hemolytic uremic syndrome. Severe abdominal cramps, watery diarrhea followed by bright red, grossly bloody stools and enuresis are common.

◆ Inflammatory Bowel Disease

Ulcerative Colitis

Most frequent symptoms include loose stools, weight loss, rectal bleeding, abdominal pain, growth failure, tenesmus, arthritis, and uveitis. Onset may be insidious or acute.

Regional Enteritis (Crohn Disease)

Diarrhea, abdominal pain, weight loss, anemia, fever, rectal bleeding, growth failure, and arthritis are the primary symptoms.

Drugs

Steroids, nonsteroidal anti-inflammatory agents, and other drugs may cause gastrointestinal bleeding.

● Esophageal Varices

Henoch-Schönlein Purpura

Rash, abdominal pain, arthralgia, periarticular swelling, and nephritis should suggest this disorder.

♦ **Meckel Diverticulum**

Blood Dyscrasias

  Thrombocytopenia

  Leukemia

  von Willebrand Disease

Immunocompromised Patients

Children whose immune system is compromised by chemotherapy are susceptible to infections with cytomegalovirus, herpes, and *Candida,* which may cause esophagitis and other mucosal damage leading to melena or hematemesis.

Intestinal Duplication

Hemorrhoids

● **Intestinal Foreign Bodies**

Lymphosarcoma

MISCELLANEOUS CAUSES

● **Hemolytic-Uremic Syndrome**

The clinical picture develops after an episode of diarrhea. Affected children present with pallor, edema, and symptoms resembling those of an acute glomerulonephritis. Thrombocytopenia is present along with the hemolytic anemia and acute renal failure.

Hemangiomas and Telangiectasias

These disorders are associated usually with painless bleeding. Gastrointestinal hemangiomas may be associated with cutaneous lesions. The Rendu-Osler-Weber syndrome (hereditary hemorrhagic telangiectasia) is an autosomal dominant disorder associated with mucocutaneous telangiectasia. Cavernous hemangiomas may extend throughout the intestinal submucosa and are commonly associated with cutaneous lesions as well.

Munchausen Syndrome by Proxy

Blood may be placed in the stool as an attention getting action.

Polyposis

Other types of intestinal polyposis may rarely produce gastrointestinal bleeding.

Familial Polyposis

Inheritance pattern is autosomal dominant, with a high incidence of intestinal carcinoma. Diarrhea is a common early symptom. Polyps may number in the hundreds.

Peutz-Jeghers Syndrome

Polyps are in the upper intestine; melanotic patches occur on the oral mucosa.

Intestinal Parasitism

Blood loss is either occult or small in amount. Diarrhea, abdominal cramps, and weight loss may be present. In the United States, amebiasis, hookworm, and whipworm infestations are the most frequent parasitic causes of blood in the stool.

Nodular Lymphoid Hyperplasia

This disorder is often preceded by an infectious diarrheal disease. Small, sessile, polypoid lesions are found in the colon and rectum. The bleeding is painless and in small amounts.

Cryptitis

Inflammation may be caused by constipation or diarrhea. Symptoms include pain on defecation, rectal burning, and tenesmus.

Diverticulitis

This disorder, rare in children, may produce a clinical picture of a "left-sided appendicitis."

Uremia

Blunt Injury to the Bowel

Injury to the bowel wall may result in hematomas with associated bleeding into the intestinal lumen.

Necrotizing Enterocolitis

Older infants and children may also develop this condition. Sudden abdominal distension and pneumatosis intestinalis are other features.

Pseudoxanthoma Elasticum

The alteration of elastic tissue in gastrointestinal vessels may lead to bleeding. Skin changes, which are usually not recognizable until the second decade, present as yellowish papules resembling a plucked chicken on the neck, below the clavicles, in the axillae, perineum, and thighs.

Chronic Granulomatous Disease

Gastric outlet obstruction, resulting from granulomatous inflammation of the antral wall, may be the first clinical manifestation. Vomiting, anorexia, and poor weight gain are other features.

Solitary Rectal Ulcer Syndrome

An unusual disorder in children. Characterized by recurrent rectal bleeding, mucous discharge, tenesmus, and pain located in the perineum or sacral area.

Scorpion Bite

Scurvy

MIMICS

It is important to ascertain that the black tarry or bright red stool color is due to blood.

Black Stools

Bismuth

Pepto-Bismol is a commonly used over the counter preparation.

Iron

Charcoal

Licorice

Spinach

Grape Juice

Red Stools

Food Coloring Additives

Kool-aid, jello, and a host of other foods may contain the additive.

Red Beets

Tomatoes

REFERENCE

1. Mezoff AG, Preud'Homme DL. How serious is that GI bleed? *Contemp Pediatr* 1994;11:60–92.

SUGGESTED READING

Ament ME. Diagnosis and management of upper gastrointestinal tract bleeding in the pediatric patient. *Pediatr Rev* 1990;12:107–116.
Berezin S, Schwarz SM, Glassman M, Davidian M, Newman LJ. Gastrointestinal milk intolerance of infancy. *Am J Dis Child* 1989;143:361–362.
De la Rubia L, Ruiz Villaespesa A, Cebrero M, Garcia de Frias E. Solitary rectal ulcer syndrome in a child. *J Pediatr* 1993;122:733–736.
Milov DE, Andres JM. Sorting out the causes of rectal bleeding. *Contemp Pediatr* 1988;5:80–104.
Silber G. Lower gastrointestinal bleeding. *Pediatr Rev* 1990;12:85–93.

SECTION XI

Genitourinary Tract

76
Dysuria

Painful urination is most frequently attributed to infection. Urethral or perineal irritation, however, may be an even more common cause. The perineum should be closely inspected, the urinary stream observed if possible, and urine obtained for microscopic examination and culture.

♦ Most Common Causes of Dysuria

Cystitis   Urethritis (Infectious or Irritant)
Perineal Irritation

INFECTIOUS CAUSES

♦ Urinary Tract Infection

Bladder infections, usually bacterial in origin, are a common cause of dysuria. Urinary frequency, lower abdominal pain, and enuresis may also be present.

♦ Urethritis

Pain on urination and a urethral discharge suggest gonococcal or chlamydial urethritis.

Herpes Simplex

Herpetic lesions in the periurethral area will cause pain on urination.

Varicella

Young girls with varicella may have periurethral lesions that are painful on urination. In some cases urinary retention may occur.

Hemorrhagic Cystitis

Onset is usually sudden, with frequency and dysuria. Suprapubic pain, enuresis, and fever are less common. Most cases are thought to be of viral origin, particularly adenovirus.

Prostatitis

This uncommon disorder may affect adolescent boys. Fever and chills may be associated with low back pain and testicular aching. On rectal examination the prostate is enlarged, boggy, and tender. Gonorrheal organisms are the most common pathogen, but others have been described.

Vaginitis

In adolescent girls, dysuria in most cases is secondary to a gynecologic infection.

Renal Tuberculosis

This is a rare cause of dysuria. Most cases are asymptomatic and are discovered during the evaluation of sterile pyuria.

IRRITATION

♦ Trauma

Trauma to the perineum may cause urethral irritation and dysuria. The injury may occur after a fall against a bicycle frame or a direct kick to the perineum, or it may follow sexual abuse. Chronic irritation, for instance from a bicycle seat, may be responsible. Masturbation may cause urethral irritation and transient dysuria. Occasionally, the urethra may be irritated by insertion of a foreign body.

♦ Primary Irritant Dermatitis

This condition occurs primarily in infants and young children in diapers. Prolonged contact of the skin with urine or leaching out of detergents from diapers may cause local irritation and pain on urination. Other irritants include perfumes, deodorants, and chemicals found in some soaps, feminine hygiene deodorants, and spermicides.

♦ Meatal Ulceration

Infant boys may develop meatal ulcers from contact with diapers.

♦ Bubble Bath

Any strong detergent used in bath water may cause a chemical urethritis.

♦ Shampoo

Urethritis may be caused by shampoo used to wash the child's hair while the child is sitting in the tub.

♦ Diarrhea

Severe diarrhea may produce local irritation of the perivaginal and periurethral area.

Pinworms

Pinworm infestation is more likely to be a cause in young girls. The pinworms may migrate out of the anus at night and enter the urethra, occasionally causing irritation. Night crying in young girls should suggest the possibility of pinworms, which may be seen on inspection of the hymenal ring and anus.

Meatal Stenosis

True stenosis is a debated cause of dysuria in boys. Splaying of the urinary stream may cause a burning sensation. The meatal opening is a pinhole rather than a slit.

Urethral Stricture

Stricture formation may follow trauma or irritation. The quality of the urinary stream should be checked.

Urethral Diverticulum

Post voiding meatal bleeding and dysuria may be associated with a distal urethral diverticulum associated with the valve of Guerin (lacuna majora).

Urinary Calculi

Pain on urination may occur during passage of a stone. Hematuria is almost always present.

Idiopathic Hypercalicuria

Although occult hematuria is a more common finding, dysuria has been described with hypercalicuria without calculi.

MISCELLANEOUS CAUSES

Bladder Outlet Obstruction

Symptoms include dysuria, urinary hesitancy, and sometimes dribbling.

Bladder Diverticulum

Dysuria, lower abdominal pain, urinary frequency, and difficulty in initiating urination are possible symptoms.

Appendicitis

If the inflamed appendix or a peri-appendiceal abscess lies low in the iliac fossa, urination may be frequent and painful. Any pelvic abscess may produce similar symptoms.

Labial Adhesions

Drugs

Various drugs may cause cystitis with resulting dysuria. Amitriptyline hydrochloride, isoniazid, imipramine, cyclophosphamide, heparin, dicumarol, sulfonamides, and antihistaminics may be associated with dysuria.

Urethral Prolapse

This disorder has primarily been described in young, black females. A purplish, mulberry like mass, usually bloody, is found an perineal inspection.

Acute Nephritis

Acute glomerulonephritis is rarely associated with dysuria.

Reiter Disease

Occurrence is uncommon in children. The classic triad of symptoms is arthritis, urethritis, and conjunctivitis.

Wilms' Tumor

Rarely, this tumor may be associated with dysuria and hematuria.

SUGGESTED READING

Fleisher GR. Pain-dysuria. In: Fleisher GR, Ludwig S, eds. *Textbook of pediatric emergency medicine.* Baltimore: Williams & Wilkins, 1993:366–368.
Heldrich FJ. Dysuria. In: Hoekleman RA, Friedman SB, Nelson NM, Seidel HM, Weitzman ML, eds. *Primary pediatric care.* St. Louis: Mosby, 1997:929–931.

77

Pyuria

Pyuria, the presence of white blood cells in the urine, is frequently equated with a urinary tract infection, either bacterial or nonbacterial. One definition of pyuria is the presence of 5 or more white blood cells per high powered field of urine; the specimen for examination must be 5 mL carefully collected by the clean catch method and then centrifuged at 3000 rpm for 3 minutes. An enhanced method of urinalysis has been recommended that uses a hemocytometer in which to count white blood cells (1). The urine is obtained by catheterization. Normal specimens contain fewer than 10 white blood cells per mm^3.

A variety of disorders may cause white blood cells to be shed in the urine, with fever probably the most common cause. If one is to make a diagnosis of a bacterial cause of pyuria, a positive culture must be obtained. Leukocytes from sources other than the urinary tract, such as found in vaginal leukorrhea or balanitis, must not be mistaken for those from the urinary tract.

INFECTION

Urinary Tract Infection

♦ Pyelonephritis

Although pyuria cannot be equated with infection, urinary tract infection must be the diagnosis of exclusion. Pyelonephritis is likely to produce systemic signs such as fever and chills; gastrointestinal symptoms and back pain are common.

♦ Cystitis

Bladder infections may be bacterial or viral. Dysuria and frequency are common complaints.

♦ Urethritis

Urethral discharge is typical. Nonspecific urethritis is probably most commonly caused by *Chlamydia* infection.

Renal Abscess

Tuberculosis

Renal tuberculosis must be considered in cases of sterile pyuria.

Blastomycosis

Disseminated blastomycosis, though rare, may involve the urinary tract.

Systemic Infection

Gastroenteritis

Pyuria may occur in viral infections of the gastrointestinal tract.

Other Systemic Infections

Pyuria may be found in other systemic infections, particularly those associated with high fever.

NEPHROPATHIES

Glomerulonephritis

(See Chapter 78, Hematuria.)

Acute Glomerulonephritis

Hematuria and proteinuria are more prominent, but the number of white blood cells may be increased significantly.

Chronic Glomerulonephritis

Lupus Nephritis

Hereditary Disorders

Alport Syndrome

Affected children most commonly present with gross hematuria, especially with intercurrent upper respiratory infections. Striking pyuria may be found. Deafness may occur in late childhood or adolescence.

Nail-Patella Syndrome (Arthro-Onychodysplasia)

In this disorder, inherited as an autosomal dominant trait, small or atrophic patellae, nail dysplasia, elbow deformities, and the presence of iliac horns are features. The nephropathy may be benign or progressive, leading to chronic renal insufficiency.

Renal Tubular Acidosis

Permanent distal renal tubular acidosis may have a low level proteinuria and pyuria. The urinary pH is 6.0 to 6.5 with a low blood pH and hyperchloremia. Growth retardation may be the only abnormality. Nephrocalcinosis is almost constant.

Polycystic Kidney Disease

In the infantile form, inherited as an autosomal recessive trait, early onset with abdominal masses is characteristic.

IRRITATION

Chemical Irritation

Urethritis and cystitis may be caused by irritation from strong detergents such as bubble bath.

Masturbation

Irritation of the urethra may produce pyuria.

Instrumentation

Calculi

Stones may be formed in or cause irritation to various parts of the urinary tract. Hematuria is commonly associated with the pyuria.

Primary Hyperoxaluria Type 1

Pyuria may be an early sign of renal damage secondary to the accumulation of oxalate crystals in the kidney.

OTHER CAUSES

♦ Fever

Pyuria commonly occurs in febrile states.

Dehydration

Kawasaki Disease

Pyuria from urethritis is commonly associated with this disorder.

Toxic Shock Syndrome

Renal Vein Thrombosis

Hematuria is more prominent than pyuria.

Urethral Stricture

Only boys are affected. The severity of the stricture usually dictates symptoms such as poor urinary stream, dribbling of urine, and occasionally dysuria.

Urinary Tract Tumor

Bladder tumors are rare but may cause pyuria.

Lymphoma

Renal involvement may occur, resulting in pyuria and proteinuria, sometimes with palpable kidneys, hypertension, and azotemia.

Bladder Diverticuli

Renal Papillary Necrosis

Intramuscular Iron Injection

Oral Polio Vaccine

Sarcoidosis

The kidneys are rarely affected. The extent of renal involvement may be correlated with the degree of hypercalcemia. Cough, weight loss, and chest pain are the most common symptoms.

REFERENCE

1. Hoberman A, Wald ER. UTI in young children: new light on old questions. *Contemp Pediatr* 1997;14:140–144, 148, 150–152, 154–156.

78

Hematuria

Hematuria, the presence of blood in the urine, may be gross or microscopic; it may also be symptomatic or asymptomatic. During the course of the responsible disorder the nature of the hematuria may change. In addition, hematuria may also be intermittent.

A number of studies of hematuria in children have found prevalence rates of less than 0.5% for both sexes combined. Ingelfinger and colleagues (1) reported gross hematuria in 1.3 per 1000 pediatric emergency room patients. Vehaskari and colleagues (2) screened an unselected population of over 8,000 school children and found that in 1.1%, two or more urine specimens revealed microscopic hematuria, defined as 6 or more red blood cells (RBC) per 0.9 mm^2 of fresh uncentrifuged midstream urine. Other studies of hematuria in children have used different criteria, such as more than 3 RBC per high powered field (HPF) of urine centrifuged at 2,500 rpm for 5 minutes, with the supernatant poured off leaving 0.2 mL. The use of urine dipsticks may disclose as few as 3 RBC per HPF.

There are a few rules of thumb that can aid in the differentiation of renal from extrarenal causes of hematuria (Table 78-1). Hematuria without proteinuria does not rule out a renal cause, but a combination of persistent proteinuria and hematuria must be considered presumptive evidence of renal parenchymal disease. The microscopic appearance of the red cells should be examined; if the majority of the cells are dysmorphic the source of bleeding is the renal parenchyma.

Be sure that what appears to be hematuria, is truly red blood cells and that the source is the urine. Menstrual blood mixed with urine is a common source of confusion. If the hematuria seems to be the result of trauma, keep in mind that underlying structural disorders may be the cause. In asymptomatic children with hematuria check the urine of other family members and check the hearing of at least the child. Finally, a child with recurrent episodes of gross hematuria during viral infections should suggest IgA nephropathy.

♦ **Most Common Causes of Hematuria**

Gross Hematuria

Cystitis	Irritation of Perineum
Urethritis	IgA Nephropathy
Meatal Ulceration	Trauma
Urolithiasis	

TABLE 78-1. *Differentiating renal from extrarenal causes of hematuria*

	Renal causes	Extrarenal causes
Three-tube test	Number of RBCs similar in each tube	Increased RBCs in tube I or III
Color	Brown and smokey	Pink or red
RBC casts	May be present	Absent
Clots	Generally absent	May be present
Pain	Not usually present	May be present
Edema	May be present	Not usually present
Hypertension	May be present	Not usually present

Microscopic Hematuria

Trauma   IgA Nephropathy
Benign Familial Hematuria   Hypercalciuria
Drugs   Coagulopathy

• Causes Not to Forget

Alport Syndrome   Sickle Cell Trait and Disease
Factitious   Exercise

IMMUNOLOGIC INJURY

Acute Glomerulonephritis (Poststreptococcal)

This disorder may follow pharyngeal or skin infection. Streptococcal serum antibody titers are usually elevated. Various signs and symptoms include fever, headache, malaise, abdominal pain, periorbital edema, and convulsions.

Chronic Glomerulonephritis

Several types have been described; the clinical picture in one may resemble that in another, so that differentiation is difficult.

Focal Segmental Glomerulosclerosis

Membranous Glomerulopathy

Causes include systemic lupus erythematosus, hepatitis B, and syphilis.

Membranoproliferative

Mesangial Proliferative

◆ IgA Nephropathy (Berger)

Henoch-Schönlein Purpura

The presence of petechial or purpuric lesions, primarily involving the lower extremities, should suggest this diagnosis. Abdominal pain and arthralgia with periarticular swelling are common features. Renal histology is indistinguishable from IgA nephropathy.

Collagen-Vascular Diseases

Systemic Lupus Erythematosus

Renal involvement occurs eventually in most patients with lupus.

Polyarteritis Nodosa

The most common clinical features include fever, signs of cardiac failure, abdominal complaints, and a diffuse maculopapular rash.

Subacute Bacterial Endocarditis

The nephritis may be the result of septic emboli or immune complexes. There may be subtle changes in heart sounds or evidence of microembolic phenomena in the skin.

Goodpasture Syndrome

The combination of hemoptysis, anemia, and renal disease suggests this disorder.

Wegener Granulomatosis

Renal vasculitis is responsible for the glomerulopathy. Necrotizing granulomas occur in the upper and lower respiratory tract.

Nephrotic Syndrome

Hematuria is uncommon in NIL disease but is more common in a secondary nephrotic syndrome, caused by one of the chronic glomerulonephritides.

"Shunt" Nephritis (Ventriculojugular Shunt Infection)

Immune complexes against bacteria infecting the shunt, usually staphylococcus, may develop. Anemia, splenomegaly, and arthritis may also be present.

INFECTIOUS DISEASES

Pyelonephritis (Acute or Chronic)

Hematuria is frequently present during active infections.

Nephritis Associated with Infection

Bacterial Infections

Staphylococcal, pneumococcal, brucellar, and meningococcal infections may be associated with hematuria.

Viral Infections

Hepatitis B, mumps, echovirus and coxsackievirus infections, rubeola, and varicella-zoster are examples.

Other Infections

Syphilis, malaria, toxoplasmosis, leptospirosis, and Rickettsial infection have been implicated.

♦ Hemorrhagic Cystitis

The origin is probably viral. Signs of lower urinary tract infection are common. Adenovirus is the most common virus responsible.

Urethroprostatitis

The prostate is tender on rectal examination.

♦ *Chlamydia*

A urethritis produced by this common, sexually transmitted pathogen may present with dysuria and hematuria. Small clots in the urine are common.

♦ *Neisseria Gonorrhoeae*

Macroscopic hematuria, with a purulent urethral discharge and dysuria, may result from the toxic action of this bacterium on the urethral epithelium.

Renal Tuberculosis

This is an uncommon cause but should be considered when sterile pyuria is a finding.

Schistosomiasis

Epidemic Nephropathy

This unusual disorder, endemic in northern Scandinavia, is caused by a serotype of hantaviruses. The main symptoms are fever, abdominal pain, and renal tenderness with oliguria followed by polyuria.

FAMILIAL AND CONGENITAL URINARY TRACT DISORDERS

• Chronic Hereditary Nephritis

Various types have been described, some benign and some progressive and fatal. Alport syndrome, inherited as a sex linked dominant trait, is associated with deafness in 30% to 40% of cases; cataracts are a finding in 10%. Affected men die younger than women of renal failure, but usually do not until the fourth or fifth decade. In cases of unexplained hematuria, urine of family members should be examined.

♦ Benign Familial Hematuria

Microscopic hematuria, almost always a finding, may become gross with intercurrent systemic infection; proteinuria is unusual. The inheritance pattern is autosomal dominant. Family members should be checked. Thin basement membrane disease is the proposed new name for this familial disorder.

Polycystic Disease of the Kidney

Infantile Form

Early death is common. The kidneys are usually easily palpable; liver cysts are common. Inheritance pattern is autosomal recessive.

Adult Form

Onset of symptoms including hypertension may be delayed, even to beyond the fourth decade; 10% die in the first decade of cerebral aneurysms. Inheritance pattern is autosomal dominant.

Congenital Urinary Tract Abnormalities

Structural aberrations may lead to hematuria. Posterior urethral valves may go unnoticed. Hematuria may occur after trauma in disorders such as hydronephrosis. Urethral diverticuli may cause dysuria as well as hematuria.

Nail-Patella Syndrome

Dystrophic nails and absent or hypoplastic patellae are the prominent external signs of this disorder inherited as an autosomal dominant trait. The onset of nephritis is late.

BLEEDING OR VASCULAR DISORDERS

♦ Coagulation Disorders

Coagulation Factor Deficiencies

Platelet Deficiencies

von Willebrand Disease

Vitamin K Deficiency

● Hemoglobinopathies

Sickle Cell Disease or Trait

Hematuria is more common in sickle cell trait.

Sickle Cell Hemoglobin C Disease (SC Disease)

Sickle Cell Thalassemia Disease

Hemoglobin C Disease

Vascular Abnormalities

Hemangiomas

Occasionally, cutaneous hemangiomas may also be present.

Hereditary Hemorrhagic Telangiectasia (Rendu-Osler-Weber Syndrome)

Telltale purplish telangiectasia are found on the skin, particularly the mucous membranes. Inheritance pattern is autosomal dominant.

Renal Vein Thrombosis

This is more likely to occur in dehydrated infants or infants of diabetic mothers. Diminished urine output with an enlarging flank mass strongly suggests this diagnosis.

Varices of the Renal Pelvis or Ureter

Loin Pain Hematuria Syndrome

This disorder, characterized by episodes of severe flank pain and hematuria, is associated with the use of contraceptives. Tortuous intraglomerular arterioles are found.

Nutcracker Syndrome

A rare vascular abnormality with compression of the left renal vein between the aorta and the superior mesenteric artery. This situation may result in venous hypertension and the formation of ureteral and renal pelvic venous varicosities.

NEOPLASTIC DISEASE

Renal Neoplasms

Children with Wilms' tumors rarely have hematuria, whereas children with renal cell carcinoma commonly do. The hematuria is usually painless.

Leukemia

Bladder Tumors

Papillomas or, less commonly, rhabdomyosarcomas.

URINARY TRACT TRAUMA

♦ Direct Trauma

Football, lacrosse, or any contact sport (including many noncontact varieties), as well as accidents, battering, and the like, may cause urinary tract injury and hematuria. Keep in mind that there may be an underlying structural disorder of the urinary tract. In banana seat hematuria in bicycle riders, the trauma is to the prostatic urethra.

◆ Meatal Ulceration or Perineal Excoriations

These lesions are most prevalent in infant boys in diapers.

◆ Urolithiasis

Colicky flank pain is characteristic if a stone becomes lodged in a ureter. Bladder stones may otherwise be asymptomatic. The presence of stones may indicate pyelonephritis, hypercalciuria, structural abnormalities, or cystinuria.

Indirect Trauma

Hematuria may follow episodes of shock or anoxia.

Acute Tubular Necrosis

Cortical and Medullary Necrosis

Renal Infarction

Foreign Bodies

Urethral foreign bodies are more common in girls than boys.

Masturbation

Masturbation may cause microscopic hematuria; sperm are usually present on microscopic examination.

Prolapsed Urethra

Inspection reveals a purplish periurethral mass in a young girl.

◆ DRUG-INDUCED INJURY

Several drugs must be monitored for their nephrotoxic effects. Hematuria may be related to large doses or long-term therapy with methicillin and other penicillins, cephalosporins, sulfonamides, furosemide, mercurial diuretics, and nonsteroidal analgesics.

MISCELLANEOUS CAUSES

● Exercise

The heavier the exercise, the more likely is the tendency for hematuria. Almost 20% of marathon runners will have microscopic hematuria that clears within 48 hours of the race.

♦ **Hypercalciuria**

The site and mechanism of injury are not clear. Children with unexplained hematuria should be evaluated for hypercalciuria. Children with juvenile rheumatoid arthritis seem more prone to this problem, and it may be part of a number of other systemic diseases.

Appendicitis

Microscopic hematuria may be present in almost one third of cases.

Hydronephrosis

Acquired structural anomalies of the urinary tract may also be associated with hematuria.

Hemolytic-Uremic Syndrome

This occurs most commonly in young infants, usually following an acute gastroenteritis; pallor and oliguria are presenting features. Thrombocytopenia and a hemolytic anemia with bizarre-shaped red blood cells on peripheral smear are characteristic.

Allergy

Rarely, allergic reactions result in the passage of blood in the urine.

Polyps

Congestive Heart Failure

Scurvy

Uric Acid Crystals

Cystinuria

Oxalosis (Primary Hyperoxaluria)

Sarcoidosis

Idiopathic Hematospermia

Emotional Factors: Autoerythrocyte Sensitization

This is a bizarre disorder characterized by spontaneous bleeding, especially in the skin, seen primarily in young women with psychological problems.

RECURRENT MONOSYMPTOMATIC (ESSENTIAL, BENIGN, IDIOPATHIC) HEMATURIA

Hematuria may be recurrent, especially associated with upper respiratory infections. The etiology is unknown.

MIMICS OF HEMATURIA

♦ Menstruation

In any postmenarchal girl in whom urinalysis shows hematuria, menstruation is the most likely cause of the spurious presence of heme in the urine.

♦ Perineal Irritation

May leave traces of blood on diapers of underpants suggesting hematuria.

Urate Crystals

Urate crystals may precipitate in an acid urine, giving the appearance of a pink sediment.

Hemoglobinuria

This may occur with blood dyscrasias, severe infections, burns, or transfusion reactions.

Myoglobinuria

Occurrence is most likely in the postinfluenzal syndrome and during malignant hyperthermia. The urine is brownish; the dipstick is positive, but there are no red blood cells seen on microscopic examination.

Porphyrinuria

Children with congenital erythrocytic porphyria pass a bright red urine.

"Beeturia"

Certain people after ingesting red beets will excrete the coloring in the urine. In children, this usually indicates iron deficiency.

● Factitious

On occasion, the patient or a caregiver, may introduce blood into the urine.

Biliuria

Povidone Iodine (Betadine)

Results of a dipstick test may be positive for blood if this agent is present in the urine.

Drugs

Phenytoin, phenothiazines, and pyridium are examples.

Food Dye

Red Diaper Syndrome

Serratia marcescens in the stool may impart a reddish color to diapers after hours of incubation in the diaper pail.

REFERENCES

1. Ingelfinger JR, Davis AE, Grupe WE. Frequency and etiology of gross hematuria in a general practice setting. *Pediatrics* 1977;59:557–561.
2. Vehaskari VM, Rapola J, Koskimies O, et al. Microscopic hematuria in school children: epidemiology and clinicopathologic evaluation. *J Pediatr* 1979;95:676–684.

SUGGESTED READING

Abarbanel J, Benet AE, Lask D, Kimche D. Sports hematuria. *J Urol* 1990;143:887–890.
Fitzwater DS, Wyatt RJ. Hematuria. *Pediatr Rev* 1994;15:102–108.
Garcia CD, Miller LA, Stapleton FB. Natural history of hematuria associated with hypercalciuria in children. *Am J Dis Child* 1991;145:1204–1207.
Kalia A, Travis LB. Hematuria, leukocyturia, and cylindruria. In: Edelmann CM Jr, ed. *Pediatric kidney disease,* 2nd ed. Boston: Little, Brown & Co., 1992:553–563.
Lieu TA, Grasmeder HM 3rd, Kaplan BS. An approach to the evaluation and treatment of microscopic hematuria. *Pediatr Clin North Am* 1991;38:579–592.
Ruley EJ. Hematuria. In: Hoekleman RA, Friedman SB, Nelson NM, Seidel HM, Weitzman ML, eds. *Primary pediatric care.* St. Louis: Mosby, 1997:996–999.
Yadin O. Hematuria in children. *Pediatr Ann* 1994;23:474–485.

79

Changes in Urine Color

The color of the urine may range from pale yellow or almost colorless to amber, depending on the amount of liquid ingested and the types of foods eaten. Various dyes in foods and drink and certain drugs and diseases may also cause discoloration of the urine. Interesting urine colors may result when children suck on magic markers!

This chapter highlights only a few of the causes of discolored urine. A more complete listing can be found in the **Suggested Readings**.

RED URINE

Heme

Hematuria

Hemoglobinuria

Intravascular hemolysis occurring in various disorders may result in the passage of a pink to red-wine urine. The plasma also takes on a pinkish color.

Myoglobinuria

This occurs during muscular necrosis, such as after trauma, ischemia, intense exercise, and ingestion of drugs such as alcohol or barbiturates, and in inflammatory and degenerative diseases of muscle. Characteristic symptoms include muscle weakness, tenderness, and edema. The urine is more brownish, than reddish.

Urate Crystals

This cause is most prevalent in newborns, but a pinkish (brick-dust) sediment of urate crystals may also appear in urine specimens refrigerated for later urinalysis.

Food Pigments

Beets

About 10% of the population will have "beeturia" normally following the ingestion of red beets, but the incidence is greatly increased in children with iron deficiency.

Blackberries

Anthocyanine

This is a pigment found in berries.

Dyes

Pyridium
Aniline: These dyes are used in candies.
Rhodamine B: This dye is used to color foods and drinks.
Phenolphthalein
Congo red

Drugs

Pyrvinium pamoate	Phenothiazines
Methyldopa (Aldomet)	Aminopyrine
Phenytoin sodium	Ibuprofen
Sulfasalazine	Senna
Adriamycin	Chloroquine

Deferoxamine (Desferal)

Urine discoloration ("vin rose") occurs when serum iron levels are elevated.

Porphyrins

The passage of a pink to red urine may be the first sign of congenital erythropoietic porphyria in the neonatal period. Photosensitivity and hirsutism occur later. In all probability the "werewolves" of old probably were afflicted with this malady. Children with other forms of porphyria are less likely to pass red or pink urine.

Other Causes

Serratia Marcescens

This is a nonpathogenic chromobacterium that produces a red pigment when grown aerobically, particularly on wet diapers (red diaper syndrome).

Biliuria

A reddish yellow color may be present.

GREEN URINE

Food Color

Excessive ingestion of Clorets, containing chlorophyll, has been reported to produce a green urine.

Biliverdin

Biliverdin may be passed in the urine in disorders producing chronic obstructive jaundice.

Drugs

Amitryptyline Hydrochloride (Elavil)   Adriamycin
Methocarbamol (Robaxin)   Indomethacin

Pseudomonas Infection

Other Causes

Phenol   Resorcinol
Tetrahydronaphthalene   Methylene Blue
Riboflavin   Carotene Excessive Ingestion

BLUE URINE

Methylene Blue

Triamterene (Dyrenium)

Doan's Kidney Pills

Blue Diaper Syndrome

A bluish discoloration of the diaper may be caused by the dye indigotin, an oxidative product of indican, produced in a defect in tryptophan absorption.

DARK BROWN OR BLACK URINE

Globins (Hemoglobin, Myoglobin)

Decomposition of hemoglobin to acid hematin results in a Coca-Cola or tea-colored urine.

Drugs

Metronidazole (Flagyl)

Nitrofurans (Nitrofurantoin [Furadantin] and Others)

Methocarbamol (Robaxin)

Quinine

Phenacetin

Dyes

Aniline dyes, used to color candies, may produce a dark urine.

Other Causes

Nitrates

Naphthol

Phenols

Rhubarb

Alkaptonuria

Homogentisic acid produces a dark color of the urine only after the specimen stands for hours.

Cascara

Chlorinated Hydrocarbons

Carotene

Ingestion of foods containing large amounts produces discoloration.

Vitamin B Complex

Melanoma

Widely disseminated melanoma may result in excretion of a dark urine.

YELLOW URINE

Bile Pigments

Riboflavin

Picric Acid (Trinitrophenol)

ORANGE URINE

Rifampin

Pyridium

Sulfisoxazole Phenazopyridine (Azogantrisin)

MILKY WHITE URINE

Pus

Phosphate Crystals

Chyle

PURPLE URINE

Phenolphthalein

SUGGESTED READING

Baker MD, Baldassano RN. Povidone iodine as a cause of factitious hematuria and abnormal urine coloration in the pediatric emergency department. *Pediatr Emerg Care* 1989;5:240–241.

Cone TE Jr. Some syndromes, diseases and conditions associated with abnormal coloration of the urine or diaper. *Pediatrics* 1968;41:654–658.

Shirkey HC. Drugs that discolor the urine and feces. In: Shirkey HC, ed. *Pediatric therapy.* St. Louis: CV Mosby, 1980:163–166.

80

Enuresis

Enuresis, the involuntary passage of urine, is a common symptom in children. It is, of course, normal in young children. Noctural enuresis refers to the involuntary passage of urine during sleep, while diurnal enuresis refers to the involuntary or intentional passage of urine into clothing while awake by a child old enough to maintain bladder control. By $3\frac{1}{2}$ years of age, approximately 75% of children are dry by day and night. At 5 years of age, 10% to 15% of children still wet the bed at night; in 5%, nocturnal enuresis remains a problem at age 10; and at 15 years of age, 1% of children may still be enuretic. Affected boys outnumber girls. There is a strong hereditary background: 32% of fathers and 20% of mothers have a history of enuresis. About two thirds of monozygotic twins are concordant for enuresis; dizygotic twins are likely to be discordant.

Each child with enuresis must be evaluated with consideration of the many possible causes, about which a great deal has been written (see the **Suggested Reading** list for a few examples). A careful history must be obtained and a thorough physical examination, including observation of the urinary stream, must be performed. The approach to enuresis may vary with the specialist seeing the child. To the urologist, obstructive disorders of the urinary tract seem the most likely explanation; the psychiatrist may favor an emotional origin. The pediatrician generally subscribes to the theory of developmental delay of bladder control.

It is useful to distinguish primary from secondary enuresis. Primary enuretics are those who never have achieved a period of consistent dryness; secondary enuretics are those who relapse after a period of dryness generally of 6 months or longer. Children with congenital abnormalities resulting in enuresis or those with maturational delay in bladder control are more likely to have primary rather than secondary enuresis.

Despite the long list of possible causes, developmental or maturational delay is responsible for most cases of primary enuresis. Many organic abnormalities have been suggested as possible causes, but most reports of valves, strictures, contractures, and the like are anecdotal or come from studies that lack appropriate controls. A history of poor urinary stream, dribbling, daytime incontinence, or urinary tract infection suggests the need for additional evaluation.

♦ **Most Common Causes of Enuresis**

Nocturnal: Primary

Maturational/Developmental Delay

Nocturnal: Secondary

Urinary Tract Infection
Polydipsia/Polyuria Associated

Diurnal

Micturition Deferral   Unstable Bladder (Urge Syndrome)
Urinary Tract Infection   Stress Incontinence

● **Causes Not to Forget**

Constipation   Obesity (Trapping of Urine)
Spinal Dysraphism   Obstructive Sleep Apnea

♦ DEVELOPMENTAL DELAY

Most pediatricians subscribe to this theory, which is supported by hereditary data, the demonstration of small functional bladder capacity, urinary frequency and urgency, and the fact that most children eventually attain control with maturation. Despite urinary frequency, the 24-hour output of urine is not increased and the urinary stream and neurologic examination are normal. Although most children in this group have primary enuresis, one fourth to one third have a dry period of several months or more before relapsing; from 10% to 25% also have encopresis.

PSYCHOGENIC ENURESIS

Toilet Training

Some cases are felt to be related to pressures experienced by the child around the time of toilet training—either premature training, excessive parental rigidity, associated punishment, or excessive leniency.

♦ Emotional Stress

Bladder control may never be attained or may be lost because of various stressful conditions: illness, separation from parents, birth of a sibling, death of a family member, or fear of abandonment.

Psychological Disturbances

These are an uncommon cause, but may be a factor in severe cases.

ORGANIC ABNORMALITIES

Obstructive Lesions

● **Chronic Constipation**

Children with known or unsuspected constipation may have enuresis as well as encopresis. Resolution of the constipation may control the enuresis. Constipation is also associated with an increased incidence of urinary tract infection.

Labial Fusion

Urine is trapped behind the fused labia minora, which leaks out while the child is playing.

Significant Phimosis

Urethral Valves

A poor urinary stream and dribbling may be findings.

Ectopic Ureters

In girls, dribbling or constant wetting may occur because of vaginal placement of the ureter.

Diverticulum of Anterior Urethra

May be associated with dysuria and hematuria.

Urethral Stricture

Meatal Stenosis

There may be no relationship to enuresis, because meatotomy usually does not solve the problem.

Bladder Diverticuli

Prostatic Tumor or Abscess

Hydrocolpos or Hematocolpos

Examination may reveal absence of hymenal patency or the presence of a perineal bulge.

Neurogenic Disorders

♦ Unstable Bladder

Characterized by involuntary, uninhibited detrusor muscle contraction in a child who should have achieved volitional control. Symptoms include frequent urination, urgency, daytime incontinence, and nocturnal enuresis. It is often associated with attention deficit hyperactivity disorder, as is most frequent in girls. Squatting is used as an attempt to control the bladder detrusor contraction.

Occult Neuropathic Bladder

Clinical manifestations include diurnal wetting, encopresis, urinary tract infections, trabeculated bladder, vesicourethral reflux, upper tract deterioration, and "emotional imbalance" (1). The etiology is uncertain, but perhaps this disorder represents one end of a spectrum of developmental delay.

- ### Spinal Dysraphism

  Fibrous bands, lipomas, septa, or dermal sinuses may cause traction or pressure lesions on the spinal cord with resultant loss of bladder control. Look for discolorations, hair, or lumps over the vertebral column.

Spinal Cord Tumors

Various types of tumors include gliomas, neurofibromas, teratomas, lipomas, and arteriovenous malformations. Back pain, encopresis, lower extremity weakness, reflex or sensory changes, bony abnormalities of spinal column, or cutaneous abnormalities may be findings.

Diastematomyelia

There may be cutaneous abnormalities over the spinal column. Low back pain or progressive weakness of legs may be present.

Seizures

Incontinence may be a sign of nocturnal seizures, but this is unusual.

Myelomeningocele

Sacral Agenesis

Spinal Cord Injuries

Infections

- ### Urinary Tract Infections

  Cystitis, urethritis, or trigonitis may be associated with enuresis, but infection may not be the primary cause.

Osteomyelitis of Vertebral Body

Compression of the spinal cord by the infection is the cause.

Spinal Epidural Abscess

Exquisite pain over the infected area is the predominant symptom.

- ## Disorders Associated with Polyuria and Polydipsia

  The possibilities are numerous (see Chapter 18, Polydipsia). Diabetes mellitus or insipidus, sickle cell anemia, and renal disorders are included in this group, as well as psychogenic water drinking.

MISCELLANEOUS CAUSES

◆ Micturition Deferral

This is the most common cause of diurnal enuresis among preschool age children, who do not choose to interrupt play.

Allergies

Some authors believe various allergies, particularly hidden food allergies, are responsible for some cases. Elimination diets, particularly of milk, chocolate, or eggs, may be tried.

● Obesity

In extremely obese girls, urine may be trapped in the vagina during micturition. Subsequently, they may have wetting upon standing.

Global Retardation

● Obstructive Sleep Apnea

Children who develop hypoxemia as a result of intermittent upper airway obstruction while sleeping may have enuresis. Snoring with obstructive type breathing patterns may be the clue.

Giggle Micturition

Giggle micturition is an unusual form of incontinence with complete emptying of the bladder brought on by giggling or hearty laughter. The loss of urine is sudden, involuntary, and uncontrollable.

Hypercalciuria

Some have ascribed this condition as a cause in some children.

Complete Heart Block

A child has been described who developed nocturnal enuresis associated with progressive bradycardia during sleep.

REFERENCE

1. Hinman F. Urinary tract damage in children who wet. *Pediatrics* 1974;54:142–150.

SUGGESTED READING

Foxman B, Valdez RB, Brook RH. Childhood enuresis: prevalence, perceived impact, and prescribed treatments. *Pediatrics* 1986;77:482–487.

O'Regan S, Yazbeck S, Hamberger B, Schick E. Constipation: a commonly unrecognized cause of enuresis. *Am J Dis Child* 1986;140:260–261.

Robson WLM. Diurnal enuresis. *Pediatr Rev* 1997;18:407–412.

Schmitt BD. Nocturnal enuresis. *Pediatr Rev* 1997;18:183–190.

Tietjen DN, Husmann DA. Nocturnal enuresis: a guide to evaluation and treatment. *Mayo Clin Proc* 1996;71:857–862.

81

Precocious Puberty

Precocious puberty refers to the appearance of signs and symptoms of sexual maturity earlier than expected. In the United States, pubertal development in girls before 8 years of age or in boys before 9 years of age is generally considered to be abnormal. A recent study in pediatricians' offices in the United States revealed that girls show earlier sexual development than a generation ago, when previous norms were established (1). Moreover, racial differences were detected, with African-American girls developing faster than white girls (1). In this chapter, true isosexual precocity is considered separately from incomplete forms.

Sexual precocity is more common in girls than boys, and in most cases it is idiopathic. In girls between 6 and 8 years of age, early sexual development is rarely associated with central nervous system lesions, whereas in boys a central nervous system lesion is more likely. The ability to measure serum gonadotrophins and gonadal steroids has helped immensely in assessing the causes of sexual precocity. Two major categories of sexual precocity, central and peripheral, are defined by dependence on gonadotrophins: Central precocious puberty is gonadotrophin releasing factor (GnRH) dependent, while peripheral is GnRH independent. The peripheral forms occur with elevated levels of gonadal steroids independent of hypothalamic-pituitary activation. A physical finding in the peripheral forms in boys is the lack of testicular enlargement compared with true precocious puberty of the central type. The **Suggested Reading** list at the end of this chapter gives a few sources for review of the laboratory methods required for precise definition of the causes of precocity.

Particular attention should be paid to premature thelarche (breast development) and premature adrenarche (pubic hair), which are briefly discussed here. Differentiation of incomplete forms of precocity from true isosexual precocious puberty is mandatory.

◆ **Most Common Causes of Precocious Puberty**

Females	**Males**
Idiopathic	Central Nervous System Hamartoma
Exogenous Hormones	Anabolic Steroids
	Congenital Adrenal Hyperplasia

● **Disorders Not to Forget**

Neurofibromatosis   McCune-Albright Syndrome

TRUE ISOSEXUAL PRECOCIOUS PUBERTY

♦ Idiopathic Precocity (Constitutional)

Cryptogenic or idiopathic precocious puberty is by far the most common cause in girls, accounting for as many as 80% of the cases. Girls close in age to the established norms may need no additional evaluation; the earlier the development, the greater is the need for making this a "diagnosis of exclusion." In boys, however, only 20% of the cases are idiopathic and the rest are secondary to underlying central nervous system, adrenal, or other causes. The first sign of pubertal development may be breast development or labial enlargement in the girl, pubic hair in either sex, testicular or phallic enlargement in the boy, and a growth spurt in both sexes. The true incidence of idiopathic precocious puberty is unknown, however, because occult lesions may be found at routine autopsy in these children years later. Occult hypothalamic hamartomas may be responsible for many of these cases.

Familial Trait

Premature activation of the hypothalamic-pituitary axis with subsequent stimulation of the gonads occurs in boys but is apparently uncommon in girls.

Disorders of the Central Nervous System

A number of types of central nervous system lesions may disrupt the inhibitory neural paths that influence the hypothalamic-pituitary axis and result in precocious puberty.

♦ Hamartoma of the Tuber Cinereum

With the use of magnetic resonance imaging technology, this lesion has become the most common cause of precocious puberty in males, particularly those with onset under age 4 years. The hamartomas are not true neoplasms but a congenital malformation of ectopic GnRH neurosecretory cells.

Tumors

A number of tumors may stimulate the hypothalamic-pituitary-gonadal axis. Neurologic and ophthalmologic signs and symptoms are important clues, but some tumors may be completely asymptomatic. The following tumors may trigger precocious puberty: gliomas, astrocytomas, ependymomas, pinealomas, suprasellar cysts, and craniopharyngiomas. Pineal tumors producing sexual precocity have been described only in boys. Craniopharyngiomas more frequently are associated with pubertal delay.

Infections

Precocious puberty may follow central nervous system insults such as encephalitis, tuberculous meningitis, and brain abscesses.

Irradiation

Depending on the total dose, the pathways that inhibit GnRH pulse generator may be affected. In high doses of irradiation growth hormone production may be knocked out, but precocious pubertal signs present.

Head Trauma

Hydrocephalus

Various causes of hydrocephalus have been associated with precocious puberty, including congenital syphilis and toxoplasmosis.

Cerebral Malformations

Empty sella, septo-optic dysplasia, microcephaly, Arnold-Chiari malformation, and other disorders may be associated with precocious puberty.

Diffuse Cerebral Atrophy

Tuberous Sclerosis

Hypopigmented macules, ash leaf patches, facial papules (adenoma sebaceum), and seizures are prominent signs of this disorder inherited as an autosomal dominant trait.

Sarcoid and Tuberculous Granulomas

Adrenal Causes

The testes remain small in adrenal causes of precocious puberty.

Tumors

The feminizing effects of adrenal tumors are difficult to differentiate from hypothalamic (idiopathic) precocious puberty. Urinary 17-ketosteroids are increased in both but not suppressed by dexamethasone in adrenal tumors. Adrenal tumors can cause either virilization or feminization of either sex.

♦ Congenital Adrenal Hyperplasia (Adrenogenital Syndrome)

The virilization of genitalia in boys may not be noticeable at birth but appears later. Affected girls undergo virilization *in utero* and, therefore, have ambiguous genitalia at birth.

Corticosteroid-Treated Congenital Virilizing Adrenal Hyperplasia

In a number of infant girls who were somewhat virilized and advanced in general development but not treated with glucocorticoids until after infancy, onset of thelarche and menarche was reported to occur early.

Ovarian and Testicular Causes
Ovarian Tumors

These are a rare cause of true isosexual precocity. The tumors generally are responsible for incomplete precocity as a result of estrogen production, with breast enlargement, some nipple development, and vaginal mucosa changes. Ovarian cysts are most common, followed by granuloma or theca cell tumors. Most of these tumors are palpable on bimanual examination. Urinary estrogen levels are greatly increased. Less frequent causes are choriocarcinomas, teratomas, and arrhenoblastomas.

Familial Leydig-Cell Hyperplasia (Testotoxicosis)

This is an autosomal dominant or sporadic disorder with autonomous Leydig cell function. The onset is 2 to 3 years, and features the rapid progression of pubertal development with increased muscle mass, virilization, pubic hair, and penile enlargement. The testes are slightly enlarged, but not to the degree expected for the pubertal development.

Testicular Tumors

In idiopathic sexual precocity both testes are enlarged. Unilateral enlargement suggests a Leydig cell tumor. Virilizing adrenal hyperplasia is usually associated with small testes, but adrenal rests of aberrant tissue may cause bilateral enlargement in some of these cases.

Peutz-Jegher Syndrome

The presence of ovarian tumors has been described in several patients. Some males have had Sertoli cell tumors. Brown macules on the lips and oral mucosa and intestinal polyposis are the clues.

Miscellaneous Causes
• Polyostotic Fibrous Dysplasia (McCune-Albright Syndrome)

This syndrome, often associated with precocious puberty, features bony lesions, often causing bending or bowing of limbs, abnormal gait, or pathologic fractures, and large patches of skin pigmentation with an irregular border. In girls, the first sign of precocious puberty may be menarche. In boys, the development of precocious puberty rarely begins before 8 years of age.

Hypothyroidism

Severe congenital hypothyroidism may be associated with sexual precocity and galactorrhea in girls. The clinical signs of hypothyroidism are usually obvious.

Russell-Silver Syndrome

Low birth weight, short stature, a triangular face, and a large appearing head are characteristic. Asymmetry and the early onset of puberty have been reported.

♦ **Exogenous Hormones**

Estrogens in contraceptive pills, foods, medications, and even hand creams contaminated by estrogens, have been implicated. Increased pigmentation of the areolae and external genitalia is a common finding. Anabolic steroids are of particular concern in young athletes.

Gonadotropin Producing Tumors

Hepatoblastoma

This tumor is seen only in boys with precocious puberty. Physical findings include an enlarged liver that is sometimes nodular, phallic and muscular enlargement, and advanced skeletal growth, with little or no testicular enlargement.

Chorioepitheliomas

These rare but highly malignant tumors produce large amounts of gonadotropic substances.

Teratoma

Reported tumors have been presacral in location, and some have produced increased chorionic gonadotropins.

● **Neurofibromatosis (von Recklinghausen Disease)**

Hypothalamic gliomas associated with neurofibromatosis type 1 may cause precocious puberty. The presence of 6 or more smooth edged café au lait spots greater than 1 cm in diameter is an important skin clue.

PREMATURE THELARCHE

This benign disorder usually occurs before 4 years of age and may be unilateral or bilateral. It is not accompanied by other signs of puberty. There is no growth spurt, and no enlargement of the uterus or labia. The bone age is not advanced, urinary 17-ketosteroid excretion is not increased, gonadotropins are low or absent, and the vaginal smear shows no estrogen effect. The breast enlargement is nonprogressive and may regress. The onset of puberty is not advanced. Premature thelarche must be differentiated from true precocious puberty, ovarian cysts, and ovarian tumors, which are associated with other estrogen effects. The hypothesized cause is an increased sensitivity of breast tissue to stimulation by relatively low concentrations of estradiol.

PREMATURE ADRENARCHE (PUBARCHE)

Pubarche and adrenarche are terms frequently used interchangeably to describe early onset of the development of pubic hair. Pubarche is a more general term; adrenarche denotes the source of stimulation. Early pubic hair predominantly occurs in girls and is occasionally associated with mental deficiency or preceding cerebral damage. It is defined as the appearance of pubic or axillary hair without other signs of virilization or feminization before the age of 8 years. There is no pubertal type of growth spurt or rapid skeletal maturation or phallic enlargement. The bone age and height age are slightly advanced, and urinary 17-ketosteroid levels are slightly high. Pregnanetriol and gonadotropic hormones are not found in the urine. This disorder must be differentiated from true precocious puberty or if clitoral enlargement is present, from congenital adrenal hyperplasia, adrenal carcinoma, or a virilizing ovarian tumor.

ISOLATED MENSES

These may occur with no other signs of sexual development. Usually found in females from 1 to 9 years of age. Most affected girls have a limited number of menses. Height velocity and bone age are normal. The condition appears to be benign. Plasma estradiol concentrations may be significantly elevated above the prepubertal normal range. A transient functional ovarian cyst may be responsible.

INCOMPLETE SEXUAL PRECOCITY

Feminizing Disorders

Ovarian Cysts

Ovarian cysts may enlarge and produce enough estrogen to induce signs of feminization, usually breast enlargement, nipple development, and vaginal mucosal effects.

Granulosa or Theca Cell Tumors

These rare tumors produce estrogen. The majority are palpable on bimanual examination.

Rare Sources of Estrogen

Gonadoblastomas, lipoid tumors, cystadenomas, and ovarian carcinomas are examples.

Exogenous Estrogens

Disorders with Virilization

Both ovarian and adrenal disorders may promote incomplete sexual precocity with virilization.

Ovarian Tumors

Arrhenoblastoma, lipoid tumors, cystadenomas, ovarian carcinomas, and gonadoblastomas are examples.

Adrenal Carcinoma

Signs of glucocorticoid excess may also be present with growth failure, obesity, moon facies, and other cushingoid features. Urinary excretion of 17-ketosteroids and pregnanetriol is not suppressed by dexamethasone.

Congenital Adrenal Hyperplasia (Adrenogenital Syndrome)

REFERENCE

1. Herman-Giddens ME, Slora EJ, Wasserman RC, et al. Secondary sexual characteristics and menses in young girls seen in office practice: a study from the Pediatric Research in Office Settings network. *Pediatrics* 1997;99:505–512.

SUGGESTED READING

Habiby R, Silverman B, Listernick R, Charrow J. Precocious puberty in children with neurofibromatosis type 1. *J Pediatr* 1995;126:364–367.

Kappy MS, Ganong CS. Advances in the treatment of precocious puberty. *Adv Pediatr* 1994;41:223–261.

Merke DP, Cutler GB Jr. Evaluation and management of precocious puberty. *Arch Dis Child* 1996;75:269–271.

Pescovitz OH. Precocious puberty. *Pediatr Rev* 1990;11:229–237.

Styne DM. New aspects in the diagnosis and treatment of pubertal disorders. *Pediatr Clin North Am* 1997;44:505–529.

82

Pubertal Delay

Puberty is considered to be delayed when there are no signs of sexual development at 12 to 13 years of age or no menses in girls by age 15, or testicular length smaller than 2.5 cm in boys by age 14 years. An abnormality in pubertal development should also be considered if more than 5 years has elapsed between the onset of breast development and the occurrence of menarche in girls or between the start of enlargement of testes in boys and the completion of genital growth.

Delayed puberty, a more common concern in boys than in girls, is usually a result of constitutional delay; a family history of a similar delay is especially helpful in making this diagnosis. The wide variation in normal pubertal development calls for prolonged observation rather than initiating extensive and expensive laboratory evaluations, unless other clues to a different process are present. In girls with pubertal delay, a demonstrable cause such as X chromosomal abnormalities is likely to be found. Chronic systemic diseases also frequently result in a delay of sexual development.

One way of approaching pubertal delay is to divide the causes into two major categories: hypergonadotropic and hypogonadotropic hypogonadism. In hypogonadotropic hypogonadism there is decreased secretion of the pituitary hormones, luteinizing (LH) and follicle-stimulating (FSH), as a result of a disorder in the hypothalamic-pituitary axis. In hypergonadotrophic hypogonadism the primary disorder is in the gonadal tissues. Measurement of these hormones will help direct the laboratory evaluation of possible causes. Eugonadotropic pubertal delay is primarily found in females with primary amenorrhea.

◆ Most Common Causes of Pubertal Delay

Constitutional (As much as 90%)   Chronic Disease
Turner Syndrome

● Causes Not to Forget

Klinefelter Syndrome   Kallman Syndrome

◆ CONSTITUTIONAL DELAY

Constitutional or physiologic delay of sexual development is the most common cause of pubertal delay in boys. The diagnosis is based on progressive growth from early childhood at the low normal rate of 5 cm (2 inches) per year. A history of similar delay in other family members, particularly fathers, is helpful. The hypothalamus and pituitary fail to stimulate gonadal development.

HYPERGONADOTROPIC HYPOGONADISM

Gonadal Dysgenesis

♦ Turner Syndrome and X Chromosomal Abnormalities

These are the most common causes of hypogonadism and delayed adolescence in girls; probably mosaics are more common than the 45X karyotype. There is a great variation in the phenotypic picture such as webbed neck, shield chest, high arched palate, cubitus valgus, and multiple nevi. Girls with an XO karyotype are rarely taller than 63 inches.

● Klinefelter Syndrome (XXY Karyotype)

Diagnosis is rarely possible before puberty because there is no characteristic phenotype. This disorder should be suspected in boys with pubertal delay who are tall with euchnoid proportions and have gynecomastia and small, atrophic testes (less than 2 cm in length).

Mixed Gonadal Dysgenesis (45X/46XY Karyotype)

Affected children usually present at puberty with an unmasculinized Turner syndrome phenotype or some sexual ambiguity.

Noonan Syndrome

Characteristic features are short stature, web neck, low hairline, leading to the characterization as "male Turner" syndrome. Additional findings include hypertelorism, scoliosis, and pulmonary stenosis. Cryptorchidism is common.

Swyer Syndrome

The phenotype is female with a 46XY karyotype. Streak gonads are present. The disorder is inherited as an X-linked recessive trait.

Defects in Steroidogenesis

Congenital Adrenal Hyperplasia (Adrenogenital Syndrome)

Deficiency of 17-α-hydroxylase in the genetic male or female is associated with gonadal failure and hypertension. 17-ketosteroid reductase deficiency in the genetic male may be a cause. Less common forms, e.g., desmolase deficiency and 17,20-lyase deficiency, cause hypogonadism in phenotypic females.

Prepubertal Castration

Congenital Anorchia

The testes are absent.

Testicular Atrophy

This may occur *in utero* or following testicular torsion or hemorrhage before puberty. Mumps orchitis may be responsible.

Autoimmune Oophoritis

This condition may be associated with other endocrinopathies such as Hashimoto thyroiditis, Addison disease, diabetes mellitus, and hypoparathyroidism.

Ovarian Trauma

Cytotoxic Drugs

The gonads may be damaged by cytotoxic agents used in the treatment of neoplasia, blood disorders, or collagen vascular diseases.

Irradiation of the Gonads

Ovarian Failure

May develop in course of other disorders such as ataxia-telangiectasia, myotonic dystrophy, and galactosemia. Infection of the ovary is another cause of failure.

Resistance to Gonadotropin Action (Savage Syndrome)

A rare cause of pubertal delay.

Reifenstein Syndrome

Testicular hypoplasia and sclerosis with gynecomastia at adolescence and a variable degree of hypospadias are features.

HYPOGONADOTROPIC HYPOGONADISM

Pituitary Defects

Pituitary Dysgenesis

Other features of panhypopituitarism are present long before pubertal delay becomes a concern. Isolated defects of LH, FSH, or both may occur.

Pituitary Tumors

Autoimmune Hypophysitis

Hypothalamic Defects

Congenital Anomalies

- #### Kallmann Syndrome

   This disorder represents a familial metabolic defect of gonadotropin releasing factor. Key features include a decreased or absent sense of smell in about 80%

of cases, and, in some cases, a complaint of inability to taste. There is a familial history of infertility. It is four times as common in males than females. Abnormalities of facial fusion may be present.

Septo-Optic-Dysplasia

Midline malformations may be associated with hypothalamic pituitary deficiencies. The septum pellucidum may be absent, and optic dysplasia may be present. Vision is often impaired. Nystagmus is present on physical examination.

Encephalocele

Hypothalamic structures may be involved.

Congenital Hydrocephalus

Isolated Deficiency of Gonadotropic Releasing Factor (GnRH)

Hypothalamic Tumors

Craniopharyngioma

Usual features include growth failure, symptoms of increased intracranial pressure, and visual disturbances.

Gliomas of the Optic Chiasm

Histiocytosis-X

Diabetes insipidus and growth failure are more notable than eventual sexual infantilism.

Other Tumors

Hypothalamic Trauma

Injuries to the hypothalamus may occur as a result of blunt trauma to the head, hemorrhage, or infection.

Irradiation

Syndromes with Hypogonadism

Prader-Willi Syndrome

Short stature, hypotonia, hypogonadism, and obesity are the characteristic features.

Laurence-Moon-Biedl Syndrome

This disorder, inherited as an autosomal recessive trait, is characterized by short stature, polydactyly, obesity, mental retardation, and retinitis pigmentosa.

Pseudopseudohypoparathyroidism

Obesity, mental retardation, delayed puberty, short hands, and round facies are present.

Other Endocrinopathies

Hypothyroidism

This is an uncommon cause of delayed puberty. Growth failure with a delayed bone age are common.

Addison Disease

Cushing Syndrome

Hyperprolactinemia

May result in functional hypogonadotropism. Galactorrhea is present in about one half of those affected. Approximately one third of hyperprolactinemic women have a pituitary adenoma.

♦ Chronic Disease

Any chronic disease may potentially be associated with a delay in pubertal development as a result of functional gonadotrophin deficiency.

Chronic Malnutrition

One speculation is that the onset of puberty is triggered by the attainment of a critical body weight.

Anorexia Nervosa

Celiac Disease

Inflammatory Bowel Disease

Chronic Pulmonary Disorders

Chronic Renal Failure

Neoplasia

Collagen Vascular Disorders

Hemoglobinopathies

Sickle Cell Disease

Psychiatric (Severe Emotional Stress)

FAILURE TO REACH MENARCHE

Androgen Insensitivity (Testicular Feminization)

The karyotype is 46XY, but the testes fail to respond. The phenotype is female with good breast development but little or no axillary or pubic hair. The vagina is short. Inguinal hernias may contain testes. The usual presenting complaint is failure to reach menarche.

Gonadal Dysgenesis and Variants

Hyperprolactinemia

Polycystic Ovary Disease

Anatomic Defects

Imperforate Hymen

Transverse Vaginal Septum

Congenital Absence of Uterus

Renal, skeletal, and cardiac anomalies may also be present.

SUGGESTED READING

Kulin HE, Müller J. The biological aspects of puberty. *Pediatr Rev* 1996;17:75–86.
Schwartz ID, Root AW. Puberty in girls: normal or delayed. *Contemp Pediatr* 1989;6:83–104.

83
Amenorrhea

Amenorrhea may reflect an underlying pathologic process, but it is also a normal state for the first 10 to 16 years of life. Some adolescents who visit pediatricians with concern over the failure to reach menarche simply have a physiologic delay in beginning menstruation, which may be familial. Attention to details of secondary sexual development is important in determining whether this delay is physiologic. Other adolescents may have experienced menarche but have not had another period for 4 to 6 months; here again the cause may be physiologic, anovulatory menstrual cycles.

Amenorrhea may be primary or secondary. Failure to achieve menarche by age 16 years is classified as primary amenorrhea. In the evaluation of primary amenorrhea, it is important to distinguish patients with full development of secondary sexual characteristics from those with a prepubertal appearance: Girls who fail to show any development of secondary sexual characteristics by 14 years of age require investigation for delayed puberty (see Chapter 82, Pubertal Delay), whereas adolescents who have attained full secondary sexual development without the onset of menstruation within a year or so should have a careful examination for anatomic causes of menstrual failure.

Secondary amenorrhea, defined as absence of menses for longer than 3 months following menarche, is a far more common complaint than primary amenorrhea. Irregular menstrual periods are common for the first few years after menarche because of anovulatory cycles. Psychogenic interference with hypothalamic function is also a common cause of missed periods. Various stresses, depression, and dietary misadventures may result in secondary amenorrhea. Naturally of great concern to the parents is the fear that pregnancy is the cause. Signs of androgen excess should be looked for, particularly hirsutism and acne, to narrow the diagnostic possibilities.

In this chapter, pathologic conditions that should be considered in the differential diagnosis have been divided into those causing primary and secondary amenorrhea.

♦ **Most Common Causes of Amenorrhea**

Primary	Secondary
Physiologic	Pregnancy
Chronic Illness	Stress/Exercise
Pregnancy	Systemic Disease
Turner Syndrome	Hormonal Contraceptives
	Anorexia Nervosa
	Hyperandrogenic Chronic Anovulation

PRIMARY AMENORRHEA

♦ **Physiologic Causes**

Delayed Menarche

Menarche may occur normally between 10 and 16 years of age, but failure to show any signs of pubertal development by 14 years of age requires investigation (see Chapter 82, Pubertal Delay). Anatomic causes should be suspected in the adolescent who has attained full breast and pubic hair development without menarche within the next year (see the following text). Examination for signs of normal pubertal development is often helpful in determining whether the delay in menarche is physiologic. A family history of similar delays in the mother, aunts, or siblings is obviously valuable.

Pregnancy

Pregnancy is an uncommon cause of primary amenorrhea, but must also be considered in the sexually active adolescent.

Anatomic Causes

If the secondary sexual development is complete, anatomic causes of failure to menstruate must be considered first.

Imperforate Hymen

The typical complaint is lower abdominal pain, sometimes at monthly intervals, in a 14- or 15-year-old girl. There also may be urinary difficulties. A bluish bulge may be seen when the labia are separated (hydrometrocolpos).

Vaginal Atresia

In the Mayer-Rokitansky-Kuster-Hauser syndrome the uterus varies from normal to streak, to completely absent. Ovarian function is normal. Other anomalies, especially renal and skeletal, are frequently present.

Asherman Syndrome

Ablation of the uterine lining secondary to trauma or infection.

Congenital Atresia of Cervix

Absent Uterus

Chromosomal Abnormalities

♦ **Turner Syndrome**

The classic phenotype, with short stature, webbed neck, shield chest, increased carrying angle of the arms, short fourth and fifth metacarpals, increased nevi, aortic stenosis or coarctation of the aorta, and a history of lymphedema at birth, is difficult to miss. Most cases are not so well defined. Short stature in an adolescent with deficient sexual development indicates the need for chromosomal studies.

Turner Syndrome Variants

The clinical picture may range from that of Turner syndrome, to some degree of masculinization, to a normal female appearance.

Mosaics

X Chromosomal Abnormalities

Balanced X Autosomal Translocations

Gonadal Problems

Pure Gonadal Dysgenesis

Secondary sexual maturation is delayed or absent. Affected girls may be tall. On laparoscopy only gonadal streaks are found.

Resistant Ovaries Syndrome

Although lutenizing hormone (LH) and follicle stimulating hormone (FSH) levels are increased, the ovarian follicles fail to respond. Ovarian biopsy is required to distinguish this disorder from pure gonadal dysgenesis.

Androgen Insensitivity (Testicular Feminization)

Affected children are phenotypic "females" with an XY karyotype. They have excellent breast development but infantile nipples, absent pubic and axillary hair, a short, blind vagina, and an absent or rudimentary uterus. There is often a positive familial history on the maternal side.

Incomplete Testicular Feminization

Here there is also an XY karyotype, but hirsutism, clitoral enlargement, and absence of breast development are features.

True Hermaphroditism

Most affected children have some virilization, usually incomplete, and are raised as boys. Breasts develop at puberty.

Ovarian Tumors

Granulosa cell tumors secrete estrogens at a high level that is constant. Androgen producing tumors are associated with virilization.

Polycystic Ovaries

The amenorrhea is usually secondary.

Ovarian Failure

This disorder may follow radiation treatment for an abdominal malignancy in infancy or childhood or the use of chemotherapy.

Hypothalamic-Pituitary Causes

Congenital Disorders

Panhypopituitarism

Sexual infantilism, as well as growth deficiency and evidence of other endocrine deficiencies, usually suggests this disorder before delayed menarche becomes a concern.

Kallman Syndrome

A genetic disorder with failure of secretion of normal amounts of gonadotrophin releasing factor. Anosmia is a common accompanying symptom.

Laurence-Moon-Biedl Syndrome

Features include obesity, mental deficiency, polydactyly or syndactyly, retinal pigmentation, and hypogonadism with genital hypoplasia.

Prader-Willi Syndrome

Hypotonia, obesity, short stature, retardation, and small hands and feet are characteristic features.

Hypogonadotropic Hypogonadism

These disorders produce sexual infantilism with normal or increased height; plasma levels of LH are low. It may occur alone or be associated with the disorders previously mentioned.

Olfactogenital Syndrome

In this form of hypogonadotropic hypogonadism, the sense of smell is decreased or absent.

Acquired Disorders

Suprasellar or Infrasellar Tumors

Craniopharyngiomas, gliomas, and other tumors are rare causes of primary amenorrhea. Visual field defects, symptoms of diabetes insipidus, lethargy, and rarely obesity may be additional features. A prolactinoma may be responsible.

Trauma

Damage may have been done to the hypothalmic-pituitary axis.

Neurosarcoidosis

A rare cause of amenorrhea. Generally, other signs and symptoms of sarcoidosis are present.

Psychogenic Amenorrhea

Stress

Reactions to stress of various types may involve primary but more commonly secondary amenorrhea. Depression over family conflicts, moves, school, and so forth may delay the onset of menses.

Anorexia Nervosa

Obesity

For unexplained reasons, significant obesity may be associated with amenorrhea.

Endocrine Disorders

Congenital Adrenal Hyperplasia (Adrenogenital Syndrome)

Affected children may have a partial defect in adrenal steroid synthesis and may develop clitoromegaly and subsequent virilization at genital puberty.

Hypothyroidism

This condition is more likely to produce menstrual irregularities rather than amenorrhea.

Hyperthyroidism

Hyperthyroidism resulting from toxic goiter is more often associated with amenorrhea than with menstrual irregularities.

Diabetes Mellitus

Longstanding, untreated diabetes mellitus with growth failure is now rare.

Cushing Syndrome

Truncal obesity, hypertension, and a falling off of growth velocity are among the preceding symptoms and signs.

Addison Disease

Symptoms may suggest anorexia nervosa, but the presence of lethargy and fatigue accompanied by hyperpigmentation of the skin should alert the physician to this possibility.

Other Causes

♦ Chronic Debilitating Disease

Various chronic diseases may affect menarche. Among the more common disorders are Crohn disease, chronic liver disease, and celiac disease.

Autoimmune Disorders

Rarely, the ovary may be affected by the production of antibodies directed against it, resulting in amenorrhea. There may also be associated adrenal or parathyroid antibodies.

Malnutrition

From any cause.

SECONDARY AMENORRHEA

♦ Physiologic Causes

Anovulatory Cycles

Menstrual irregularity is common during the first few years after menarche. Delays between periods may range up to 6 months.

Pregnancy

Pregnancy must always be considered, especially in the sexually active adolescent. A urine test for pregnancy is a quick screening method.

Hypothalamic-Pituitary Causes

♦ Psychogenic Factors

Emotional factors are common causes of secondary amenorrhea. Depression from moves, family disruption, separation from home, and so forth may be associated with menstrual failure.

♦ Strenuous Exercise

Amenorrhea is common in highly trained athletes.

♦ Anorexia Nervosa

"Crash" Diets

Malnutrition

From any cause.

Trauma

The hypothalamic-pituitary axis may have been damaged by a traumatic event, including infection.

Pseudocyesis

There may be all the signs of pregnancy without positive results of a pregnancy test or enlargement of the uterus as seen on ultrasonogram.

Tumors

Tumors are a rare cause of secondary amenorrhea. The presence of galactorrhea, however, should suggest a pituitary tumor.

Hyperprolactinemia

A prolactinoma may be responsible.

Pituitary Failure (Sheehan Syndrome)

Hypopituitarism may result from infarction of the pituitary gland.

Gonadal Disorders

◆ Hyperandrogenic Chronic Anovulation (Polycystic Ovary Disease)

One half of the women with this syndrome present with amenorrhea. Infertility is a more common initial complaint. Obesity, virilization, and hirsutism are common. The LH/FSH ratio is greater than 2.5:1.

Ovarian Neoplasms

Granulosa cell tumors may keep estrogen levels constantly high, preventing sloughing of the endometrium. Androgen producing tumors produce increasing signs of virilization.

Chemotherapy/Irradiation

The gonads may be damaged by cytotoxic drugs and irradiation.

Premature Ovarian Failure

This is an unusual cause of secondary amenorrhea. Premenopausal symptoms may be present.

Autoimmune Disease

Antibodies directed against the ovary may be responsible for the development of amenorrhea. Other endocrine glands may also be affected.

Gonadal Dysgenesis

Secondary amenorrhea may occur with sex chromosome abnormalities including mosacisim and mixed gonadal dysgenesis.

Endocrine Disorders

Thyroid Disorders

Hyperthyroidism is much more likely than hypothyroidism to be associated with amenorrhea.

Adrenal Disorders

Hypoadrenocorticism (Addison disease) and excessive production of corticosteroids (as in Cushing syndrome) are uncommon causes of amenorrhea.

Miscellaneous Causes

♦ Systemic Illness

Chronic, severe, and debilitating illnesses often may be associated with cessation of menstrual periods. Autoimmune hepatitis is particularly noteworthy in this regard.

♦ Oral Contraceptives

Amenorrhea may follow cessation of oral contraceptives, particularly in young women who began taking these hormones before normal hypothalamic rhythm had been established.

Drugs

Amenorrhea may be the result of intake of various drugs including anabolic steroids, opiates, amphetamines, and phenothiazines.

Obesity

The cause of amenorrhea in obese adolescents has not been well defined. In some cases, depression over a poor body image may affect hypothalamic centers.

Uterine Infections

Severe infections of the endometrial cavity may result in scarring or the formation of synechiae.

Chiari-Frommel Syndrome

This unusual and poorly explained disorder occurs in the postpartum period and is characterized by amenorrhea and persistent galactorrhea. Affected women are usually moderately obese and slightly hirsute.

SUGGESTED READING

Baird DT. Amenorrhea. *Lancet* 1997;350:275–279.
Braverman PK, Sondheimer SJ. Menstrual disorders. *Pediatr Rev* 1997;18:17–25.
Warren MP. Evaluation of secondary amenorrhea. *J Clin Endocrinol Metab* 1996;81:437–442.

= 84 =

Abnormal Vaginal Bleeding

Vaginal bleeding may be the result of physiologic alterations or indicative of significant pathology. In the newborn period, withdrawal of maternal hormones is the most common cause; whereas, in adolescence, dysfunctional uterine bleeding accounts for most cases. Premenarchal children with vaginal bleeding almost never have functional causes and demand additional evaluation.

♦ **Most Common Causes of Abnormal Vaginal Bleeding**

Preadolescent	**Adolescent**
Vaginal Foreign Body	Dysfunctional Uterine Bleeding
Trauma	Coagulation Disorder
Infection (Streptococcus, Shigella)	Pregnancy and Complications

● **Causes Not to Forget**

Sexual Abuse	Urethral Prolapse
Lichen Sclerosis et Atrophicus	

NEONATAL MATERNAL HORMONES

Vaginal bleeding, usually spotty, is a relatively common phenomenon in newborns following withdrawal of maternal hormones. Estrogen effects such as hypertrophy of the labia minora and leukorrhea are almost universally present in newborn females.

PREADOLESCENT VAGINAL BLEEDING

♦ **Infections**

See the section on vulvovaginitis (Chapter 85, Vaginal Discharge and Vulvovaginitis). Because the vagina of the preadolescent is thin, infections may result in vaginal bleeding. Group A β-hemolytic streptococcal infection is the most common.

♦ **Foreign Bodies**

A foul smelling, bloody discharge should raise the possibility of a foreign body. Occasionally, material may be milked from the vagina by a rectal examination.

♦ **Trauma**

Vaginal lacerations may occur as a result of injuries, such as falls or by masturbation; but sexual abuse must always be considered.

● **Urethral Prolapse**

Careful perineal examination should disclose a mulberry-like hemorrhagic mass surrounding the urethral opening. This is more common in young African-American girls.

Excoriations

Pruritus may lead to scratching severe enough to cause bleeding of the vulvar mucosa.

● **Lichen Sclerosis et Atrophicus**

The vulva are generally involved in an hourglass configuration of atrophic skin. Pruritus is common and may lead to purpuric areas and bleeding.

Pinworms

Rarely, significant infestation of the vagina may cause vaginal irritation and bleeding.

Precocious Puberty

Functional vaginal bleeding may be the result of true sexual precocity. Other signs of sexual development should be noted.

Estrogen Ingestion

May also be found in some skin creams.

Sarcoma Botryoides

A rare malignant rhabdomyosarcoma that can involve the vagina, cervix, uterus, or bladder. A polypoid, grapelike mass is found on examination. This tumor is rarely found in the vagina beyond childhood.

Other Tumors

Rare causes include endodermal carcinoma, mesonephric carcinoma, and clear-cell adenocarcinoma. Beware in children of mothers who received diethylstilbestrol.

ADOLESCENT VAGINAL BLEEDING

♦ **Dysfunctional Uterine Bleeding (DUB)**

The vast majority of abnormal vaginal bleeding in adolescents is due to DUB, but other causes must always be considered. DUB is defined as bleeding that occurs in cycles less than 20 days or more than 40 days; lasts longer than 8 days; has blood loss more than 80 mL; or is associated with anemia. It occurs in the absence of other demonstrable pathologic condition or disease.

The cause is thought to be a failure of feedback resulting in estrogen stimulation of the endometrium unopposed by progesterone. Anovulatory cycles are common in the perimenarchal age group and the most common cause of DUB.

♦ Pregnancy

A pregnancy test should be performed in any teenager who has reached Tanner stage III despite denial of sexual activity. Twenty percent of pregnancies are associated with some bleeding, but incomplete or threatened abortions, ectopic pregnancy, molar pregnancy, or complications of legal or illegal abortions must always be considered.

♦ Bleeding Disorders

Consider this group strongly if anemia is present.

von Willebrand Disease

Thrombocytopenia

Thrombocytopenia may be hereditary or acquired.

Platelet Abnormalities

Glanzmann thrombasthenia is an example.

Clotting Factors

Factor IX deficiency is an example.

Leukemia

Medications

Contraceptives

Midcycle bleeding is relatively common with oral contraceptives. Breakthrough bleeding occurs with missed doses. Intrauterine devices should not be used in adolescents.

Other

Anticoagulants, gonadal and adrenal steroids, platelet inhibitors, reserpine, phenothiazines, monoamine oxidase inhibitors, morphine, and anticholinergic medications have been associated with bleeding.

Salicylates

Decreased platelet adhesiveness secondary to salicylates may result in prolonged or heavy menstrual periods.

Infection

Pelvic inflammatory disease may cause uterine bleeding as well as other causes of endometritis.

Hydatidiform Mole

Irregular bleeding may occur late in the first trimester of mole growth. Other symptoms include nausea and hyperemesis gravidarum. The uterus is generally larger than expected for gestational age. Grapelike material may be passed vaginally.

Uterine Leiomyomas

Uterine submucous leiomyomas are unusual in adolescents.

Cervical Problems

Infections

Chlamydia

Gonorrhea

Cervical friability or endometritis may lead to spotting in pelvic inflammatory disease.

Trichomonas

Cervical Polyp

Hemangioma

Cervical Friability

This may occur in an area of squamous metaplasia.

Vaginal Disorders

• Trauma

Vaginal lacerations may be secondary to sexual abuse, rape, or masturbation.

Foreign Bodies

Tampons, diaphragms, contraceptive sponges, and other materials retained in the vagina may lead to chronic irritation and bleeding, usually accompanied by a foul discharge.

Papillomavirus Infections

Warts are an increasingly common form of sexually transmitted disease and if extensive may be associated with bleeding.

Adenocarcinoma

Vaginal or cervical neoplasms of this type are distinctly rare.

Ovarian Disorders

Functional Ovarian Cysts

Most functional ovarian cysts are follicular and represent failures of ovulation.

Corpus Luteum Cyst

This cyst may mimic an ectopic pregnancy by presenting with amenorrhea and an adrenal mass followed by vaginal bleeding and abdominal pain on rupture of the cyst.

Ovarian Tumors

Careful palpation for abdominal masses should be performed.

Polycystic Ovary Disease

Amenorrhea is a much more common problem, but a significant amount of functional uterine bleeding occurs. Obesity, hirsutism, and virilization are other findings.

Hypothalamic Pituitary Gonadal Dysfunction

Chronic Illness

Chronic illness often causes amenorrhea but may be associated with abnormal frequency or amounts of bleeding. Diabetes mellitus, inflammatory bowel disease, and systemic lupus erythematosus are examples.

Other

Emotional stress, eating disorders, crash diets, obesity, and exercise generally result in amenorrhea, but abnormal bleeding may also occur.

Prolactinoma

Prolactinoma is the most common pituitary tumor associated with menstrual irregularities. The first sign is irregular bleeding followed by oligomenorrhea and then amenorrhea.

Adrenal Disorders

Addison Disease

Abnormal vaginal bleeding occurs in about one fourth of the cases.

Congenital Adrenal Hyperplasia

Abnormal bleeding may occur in late onset disease or in previously diagnosed patients who are noncompliant with replacement steroid medications.

Thyroid Disorders

Hyperthyroidism

Hypothyroidism

Excessive bleeding may be the first sign.

Miscellaneous

Endometriosis

Although cyclic or acyclic pain, bladder dysfunction, gastrointestinal distress, and dyspareunia are more common symptoms, irregular bleeding may be a presentation.

Diethylstilbestrol

Estrogens used in mothers to suppress abortion may have caused changes in the fetus that later can present as bleeding. Cervical adenosis occurs in as many as 35% of exposed female fetuses. Adenocarcinoma is much rarer.

• Lichen Sclerosis et Atrophicus

Generally, the thinning of the skin has an hourglass distribution involving the labia. Occasionally, the thin skin may be traumatized because of associated pruritus and may lead to areas of purpura and occasionally bleeding.

SUGGESTED READING

Altchek A. Finding the cause of genital bleeding in prepubertal girls. *Contemp Pediatr* 1996;13:80–92.
Baldwin DD, Landa HM. Pediatric gynecology: evaluation and treatment. *Contemp Pediatr* 1995;12:35–60.
Braverman PK, Sondheimer SJ. Menstrual disorders. *Pediatr Rev* 1997;18:17–25.
Cowan BD, Morrison JC. Management of abnormal genital bleeding in girls and women. *N Engl J Med* 1991;324:1710–1715.
Hillard PA. Abnormal uterine bleeding in adolescents. *Contemp Pediatr* 1995;12:79–90.
Yanovski JA, Nelson LM, Willis ED, Cutler GB. Repeated, childhood vaginal bleeding is not always precocious puberty. *Pediatrics* 1992;89:149–151.

85

Vaginal Discharge and Vulvovaginitis

The most common gynecologic complaint in childhood is a vaginal discharge or irritation and pruritus of the vulvar area. Normal physiologic leukorrhea of the premenarchal adolescent must be differentiated from pathologic conditions such as irritative and infectious causes of vulvovaginitis.

The most common cause of vulvovaginitis is a nonspecific bacterial infection, and most of these are the result of either poor hygiene, obesity, tight clothing, or nonabsorbent underwear. Nonspecific means that a mixture of organisms, particularly coliform bacteria, are cultured from the vagina. This type of infection often follows a primary irritative problem with the secondary introduction of bacteria from the anal area. Specific bacterial infections such as streptococcal or gonococcal, among others, may also be found. The presence of a bloody vaginal discharge, particularly if malodorous, strongly indicates the presence of a foreign body. A careful history may suggest causes of irritation.

♦ **Most Common Causes of Vulvovaginitis**

Prepubertal	**Pubertal**
Nonspecific Vulvovaginitis	Nonspecific Vulvovaginitis
Poor Hygiene	Poor Hygiene
Group A β-Hemolytic Streptococcus	*Candida*
Vaginal Foreign Body	*Trichomonas*
	Retained Tampon

PHYSIOLOGIC LEUKORRHEA

The discharge is clear to whitish and mucoid; it is nonirritating and reflects the response of the cervix to rising estrogen levels. On Gram stain many epithelial cells but no bacteria are found.

♦ **Neonatal Leukorrhea**

Most newborn female infants have a thick discharge as a result of maternal estrogen effect.

♦ **Pubertal Leukorrhea**

Onset of the discharge is usually a few months before menarche.

Precocious Puberty

A whitish discharge may herald the onset of puberty earlier than expected.

IRRITATION

◆ Foreign Body

If the foreign material remains in the vagina long enough, the discharge will become malodorous and bloody. Wads of toilet paper are the most frequent foreign bodies found in prepubertal children and forgotten tampons in postpubertal adolescents.

◆ Chemicals

Bubble bath, various soaps, colored toilet paper, and feminine deodorant sprays may be irritating to the perineal area.

◆ Tight Undergarments

Particularly synthetic fabrics such as nylon that do not absorb secretions may cause irritation or promote bacterial or fungal overgrowth.

◆ Obesity

Trapping of urine, resulting in reflux into the vagina, may cause a chronic irritation.

Masturbation

Excoriations or irritation from masturbatory activity may lead to secondary infection.

Rhus Dermatitis

Poison ivy may be responsible, from the resin carried on hands or clothing.

Neurodermatitis; Atopic Dermatitis; Seborrheic Dermatitis

Pruritus leading to scratching may lead to lichenification, continuing the itch-scratch-itch cycle, and may predispose to secondary infection.

Drug Reactions

Local and, rarely, systemic reactions to drugs may produce a discharge. Drugs such as Mycolog, used for "diaper dermatitis," may produce local sensitization to its many ingredients.

Psoriasis

Local irritation may be the result of "napkin psoriasis."

"Sandbox" Vaginitis

Little girls sitting and playing in sand or dirt may develop irritation from particulate matter trapped in the vagina.

Sexual Abuse

Chronic irritation may be the result of unsuspected sexual molestation.

Scabies

Lichen Sclerosis et Atrophicus

An ivory white, atrophic, hourglass appearance in the perineum should suggest this diagnosis. Pruritus is frequently present.

INFECTION

♦ Nonspecific Vaginitis

This disorder most likely represents a mixed infection with coliforms, streptococci, *Haemophilus vaginalis,* and other bacteria; it is the most common cause of pathologic vaginal discharge in prepubertal children. The discharge is usually gray and malodorous but is generally nonirritating and nonpruritic.

♦ Moniliasis

Predisposing factors include removal of normal flora by systemic antibiotics, increased heat and moisture in the perineum due to tightfitting undergarments, diabetes mellitus, and oral contraceptives. The vulvae are erythematous, pruritic, and irritated, and a white, cheesy discharge is present.

♦ Trichomoniasis

Postmenarchal girls are those usually affected. The discharge is frothy and profuse with local erythema.

♦ Group A β-Hemolytic Streptococcal Infection

The infection may or may not be associated with a pharyngeal streptococcal infection.

Gonococcal Infection

The vaginal discharge is thick and purulent; dysuria is often present. Although it is most common in the postpubertal age group, young children may be infected as well.

Chlamydia

This organism must be considered in any nonspecific discharge.

Shigella

Most affected children do not have pain, pruritus, or dysuria; almost one half have a bloody discharge. Diarrhea is uncommon.

Other Bacteria

Streptococcus pneumoniae, Neisseria meningitidis, Staphylococcus aureus, Haemophilus influenzae, and Yersinia have also been implicated. *Gardnerella vaginalis* is more likely to be found in an adolescent who presents with a profuse, pruritic, and often foul smelling vaginal discharge, but is probably not a primary cause of infection.

Condyloma Acuminata

Venereal warts may extend into the vagina and may be associated with a discharge.

Herpes Simplex

Grouped vesicles and ulcers should suggest this diagnosis.

Pinworms

The tiny ubiquitous threadlike worms do not in themselves cause a vulvovaginitis, but the associated pruritus causes scratching and the transferral of bacteria from the perineum to the vulva.

Mycoplasma hominus

Consider this diagnosis if routine cultures are negative.

Syphilis

Chancres or luetic condylomata are possible causes.

Diphtheria

The infection may be primary but is usually secondary to nasopharyngeal infection. A thick, whitish gray adherent membrane may be seen.

DISCHARGE ASSOCIATED WITH SYSTEMIC ILLNESS

Several systemic illnesses may be associated with a vaginal discharge.

Scarlet Fever

Varicella

Kawasaki Disease

Measles

Typhoid

Smallpox

ANATOMIC ABNORMALITIES

Abnormalities may introduce bacteria or allow bacterial overgrowth.

Rectovaginal Fistula

Labial Agglutination

Fusion of the labia may trap urine or secretions in the vagina, resulting in secondary infection.

Aberrant Urethral Orifices

Constant dribbling of urine should be a clue to this diagnosis.

Urethral Prolapse

This problem is acute; a bloody discharge is present. A periurethral mulberry-like purplish mass is found on inspection.

MISCELLANEOUS CAUSES

Tumors

Sarcoma botryoides is the most common, albeit rare, malignant neoplasm of the lower genitourinary tract in infants and children. The discharge is frequently bloody, and a polypoid mass is found in the vagina.

Vaginal Polyps

SUGGESTED READING

Altchek A. Vaginal discharges. In: Stockman JA III, ed. *Difficult diagnosis in pediatrics.* Philadelphia: WB Saunders, 1990:383–389.

Murphy TV, Nelson JD. Shigella vaginitis in 38 prepubertal patients. *Pediatrics* 1979;63:511–516.

Vandeven AM, Emans SJ. Vulvovaginitis in the child and adolescent. *Pediatr Rev* 1993;14:141–147.

86

Scrotal Swelling

In order to separate the causes of scrotal swelling, it is helpful to determine the following: painful or nonpainful; acute onset or gradual; location; associated symptoms, such as dysuria or discharge; and whether there has been a change in size of the testis. The acute onset of painful swelling necessitates the rapid differentiation of testicular torsion from epididymo-orchitis. Clinical distinction of these disorders is often difficult. A radionuclide testicular scan or color Doppler ultrasonography may be helpful adjunctive diagnostic procedures, but the consequences of delaying surgical exploration in testicular torsion are too severe should these tests not give a clear answer.

Testicular tumors usually present as nonpainful masses. An old adage states that testicular masses are generally malignant, whereas extratesticular ones are usually benign.

♦ Most Common Causes of Scrotal Swelling

Painless	Painful
Hydrocele	Testicular Torsion
Hernia	Torsion of Appendix Testis
Varicocele	Epididymitis

• Causes Not to Forget

Testicular Tumor	Henoch-Schönlein Purpura
Insect Bite	Contact Dermatitis

ANATOMIC ABNORMALITIES

♦ Hydrocele

The mass, which does not change in shape or size with crying or straining, is painless, soft, and fluid filled; it is not reducible, and it transilluminates easily. Hydroceles may occur following trauma or may be associated with and obscure testicular tumors. A communicating hydrocele may change size, particularly when the child is recumbent.

♦ Hernia

The bulge may or may not extend into the scrotum. The testis should be palpable below the mass. Coughing or straining may increase the size of the swelling.

♦ Testicular Torsion

The onset of pain associated with torsion is usually acute. The scrotal skin quickly becomes edematous and discolored. Nausea, vomiting, and fever are frequent. Elevation of the testis does not relieve the pain.

♦ Torsion of Testicular Appendix

The onset of testicular pain is more gradual and less intense than in testicular torsion. A pea-sized mass may be palpable on the upper pole of the testis. The scrotum may be edematous in a small area overlying the mass.

♦ Varicocele

This disorder has been estimated to occur in 10% of boys during puberty. The scrotal mass feels like a bag of worms and represents tortuous dilation of pampiniform plexus veins. The swelling is without symptoms. The most common varicocele is on the left side and is known as primary. A right-sided varicocele is usually due to mechanical venous obstruction in the lower abdomen or pelvis and the cause should be determined. The right-sided lesions do not disappear on lying down, while the left-sided ones do.

Spermatocele

These are small, usually nontender cysts that develop from epididymal tubules and are superior and posterior to but distinct from the testis. The cysts are often bilateral and multiple.

INFECTIOUS CAUSES

♦ Epididymitis

The pain is slower in onset than in testicular torsion, from which this condition must be separated. An enlarged, tender epididymis may be palpated distinct from the testis. The scrotum may be red and parchment-like but is not edematous. Elevation of the testis and epididymis relieves pain. The cremasteric reflex remains intact.

Epididymitis may result from retrograde infection up the urethra, the organisms most responsible being *N. gonorrhoeae* and *Chlamydia*. Reflux of infected urine is another mode of infection with *E. coli* usually responsible. A third route is systemic disease. Fever, chills, dysuria, a urethral discharge, and inguinal pain are common. This infection is uncommon before puberty unless a urinary tract infection is present or urethral instrumentation has been performed.

Orchitis

Testicular pain, scrotal swelling, chills, and often rectal pain are present. The pain is often relieved with testicular elevation. Orchitis is rarely found in prepubertal boys. The most common cause is mumps virus; coxsackievirus, Echovirus, varicella, Epstein-Barr, *Mycobacterium tuberculosis,* and gonorrheal infections are rarer causes.

Scrotal Cellulitis

Swelling, pain, and edema may be associated with spreading infection of the skin of the scrotum and perineum.

NEOPLASIA

• Testicular Tumors

These tumors make up 1% of all cancers in males. The most common sign is painless, indurated, unilateral testicular enlargement. The masses are generally firm and nontender to palpation. Some tumors are associated with sexual precocity or gynecomastia. Although testicular tumors are rare in children, painless testicular enlargement should not be ignored. A hydrocele occurs frequently with the tumor.

Testicular Leukemia

The usual presenting sign is a painless swelling later in the course of leukemia. Testicular relapse is the second most common type of extramedullary relapse.

MISCELLANEOUS CAUSES

Edema

Any disorder causing generalized edema may be associated with marked scrotal swelling.

• Insect Bites

Never underestimate a bite as the cause of a swollen, erythematous scrotum. Pruritus rather than pain should be clue. Part of the scrotum is generally affected.

• Contact Dermatitis

The scrotum may be swollen as the result of a contact dermatitis. Poison ivy is best known.

Idiopathic Scrotal Edema

This unexplained, uncommon disorder may be confused with more serious causes of scrotal swelling. Affected children are otherwise well when they develop bilateral or unilateral, nontender but erythematous swelling of the scrotum. The problem resolves in 48 hours. It is uncommon after puberty.

• Henoch-Schönlein Purpura

Intense swelling of the scrotum may suggest testicular torsion, but the enlargement is bilateral. The purpuric rash may appear later in its typical distribution.

Trauma

The history of the trauma is important. The scrotum may be ecchymotic and swollen.

Traumatic Hematocele and Hydrocele

Blood or fluid in the scrotal sac may be the result of trauma.

Familial Mediterranean Fever

Underrecognized cause. The swelling is usually unilateral, red, and painful. The swelling lasts 1 to 3 days.

Healed Meconium Peritonitis

Scrotal masses are usually noted at birth. The problem may be secondary to an intrauterine volvulus, intussusception, intestinal atresia or stenosis, or meconium ileus (cystic fibrosis). Intraperitoneal calcifications are present on radiographs.

Cysts or Angiomas

Crohn Disease

Extraintestinal manifestations of Crohn disease may affect the scrotum, e.g., cutaneous granulomas, so called "metastatic" Crohn disease.

Arterio-Venous Malformations

Adrenal Hemorrhage in Neonates

Blood may collect in the scrotum of neonates who have had adrenal hemorrhage.

Sarcoidosis

A rare presenting sign of sarcoidosis in adolescence may be a paratesticular mass. Perihilar adenopathy is usually present.

Fat Necrosis

Hypertriglyceridemia

Other features may include episodic abdominal pain, eruptive xanthomas, and hepatosplenomegaly.

Elephantiasis

Scrotal swelling may follow disruption of lymphatic drainage by the parasite responsible for filariasis.

SUGGESTED READING

Gedalia A, Mordehai J, Mares AJ. Acute scrotal involvement in children with familial Mediterranean fever. *AJDC* 1992;146:1419–1420.

Kapphahn C. Male reproductive health: part 1. Painful scrotal masses. *Adolesc Health Update* 1992;4:1–5.

Kapphahn C. Male reproductive health: part 2. Painless scrotal masses. *Adolesc Health Update* 1992;5:1–8.

Klein BL, Ochsenschlager DW. Scrotal masses in children and adolescents: a review for the emergency physician. *Pediatr Emerg Care* 1993;9:351–361.

Skoog SJ, Roberts KP, Goldstein M, Pryor JL. The adolescent varicocele: what's new with an old problem in young patients? *Pediatrics* 1997;100:112–122.

Stillwell TJ, Kramer SA. Intermittent testicular torsion. *Pediatrics* 1986;77:908–911.

SECTION XII

Back

87

Back Pain

Back pain in a child lasting more than 1 to 2 weeks requires careful evaluation because this symptom is usually the result of a serious underlying disorder. Included in serious underlying disorders should be psychogenic back pain, which is often difficult to manage. In the past, unlike adults, children were thought to uncommonly have back pain related to psychogenic causes; this may be changing (1). Children with acute or short-lived back pain are more likely to have muscle and ligamentous strain or pain associated with systemic viral infection.

History should include the location, duration, radiation, and character of the pain, as well as illness or activity preceding its onset. Interference with normal daily and recreational activities should be determined. Examination should seek other signs such as abnormalities in gait or in the configuration of the back (subtle changes in contour may offer localizing clues) or tenderness on palpation. The skin overlying the spine should be carefully inspected for dimples, tufts of hair, hemangiomas, and other cutaneous changes, any of which may denote developmental defects. The lesions causing back pain may also produce neurologic changes in the extremities or bladder or bowel dysfunction. Signs of neuromuscular disease should also be sought.

♦ Most Common Causes of Back Pain

Hyperlordotic Mechanical Back Pain
Ligamentous or Muscle Strain
Spondylolisthesis
Myalgias

Psychogenic
Spondylolysis
Scheuermann Disease

● Causes Not to Forget

Herniated Disc
Spinal Dysraphism
Urinary Tract Infection

Spinal Cord Tumors
Diskitis

TRAUMA

♦ Lordotic Mechanical Back Pain

Reputed to be a common cause in adolescent athletes (2). The pain is only in the lumbar area, with variable increase with hyperextension or hyperflexion testing, but with inability to fully flex the spine forward. Kyphosis of the thoracic spine is present in compensation for the decreased forward mobility of the lumbar spine. Some have suggested contractures at the facet joints as the site of pain.

♦ **Ligamentous or Muscle Strain**

History of a fall, unusual exercise, or other forms of trauma should be sought. There may be a localized tenderness and a paravertebral muscle spasm. Strain is probably the most common cause of back pain, but it should be short-lived.

● **Prolapse of Intervertebral Disc**

This is an uncommon lesion in children. There is almost always a history of injury. The lower lumbar area is usually involved; pain may be local or radiate to the legs. An abnormal straight-leg-raising test is the most common physical finding.

Slipped Vertebral Apophysis

May occur after strenuous activity or heavy lifting. Signs are those of a herniated disc. A small bone fragment, the edge of the ring apophysis, may be seen within the spinal canal on imaging studies. The lower lumbar spine is the most common site.

INFECTIONS

♦ **Myalgias**

Muscle pain may be associated with a multitude of viral and bacterial infections. Aches are not limited to the paravertebral muscles.

● **Urinary Tract Infection**

Back pain may be the primary complaint; a urine culture should be done.

Referred Pain

In addition to urinary tract infections, other infections must be considered including pneumonia, appendicitis, pancreatitis, and cholecystitis.

● **Diskitis**

Aching pain in the lower back radiates to the flanks, abdomen, and lower extremities. The young child may refuse to walk. Illness may be associated with low-grade fever, irritability, and lethargy. Back motion is limited.

Osteomyelitis of Vertebra

Localized tenderness is present at a specific level. The spine is held rigid because of muscle spasm. Systemic signs are often absent.

Iliac Osteomyelitis, Sacroiliac Joint Infection

These are frequently confused with appendicitis or septic arthritis of the hip.

Tuberculosis

This is a less common cause of back pain today. Dull local pain is present over the involved vertebrae; there may be a localized swelling. Destruction of vertebrae may cause pressure on the spinal nerves. The gait is stiff; the back is held rigid.

Spinal Epidural Abscess

There are generally exquisite pain and tenderness on palpation over the site of the abscess, as well as rapidly developing signs of spinal cord dysfunction such as paraparesis, loss of bladder and bowel control, and sensory changes.

Brucellosis

Small abscesses may develop in the vertebrae. This disorder is generally associated with widespread lymphadenopathy and hepatosplenomegaly; it is transmitted from animals including cows, goats, and pigs.

Acute Transverse Myelopathy

This rare disorder is preceded by an upper respiratory infection. Back pain may be an early sign, but progressive weakness develops in 1 or 2 days.

NEOPLASTIC DISORDERS

Benign Tumors

Osteoid Osteoma

The onset of pain is gradual; it is worse at night and is often rapidly relieved by aspirin. Palpation discloses localized tenderness. Radiographs reveal a small translucent area with surrounding dense bone.

Benign Osteoblastoma

Symptoms are similar to those of osteoid osteoma, but the lesion is larger with less adjacent bone density seen on radiograph films.

Eosinophilic Granuloma

Usually only one vertebra is involved with collapse, but intervertebral disc spaces are maintained. The condition may be asymptomatic, or there may be backache and postural change.

Aneurysmal Bone Cyst

A cystic expansile lesion in a vertebra may cause neurologic symptoms.

Neurenteric Cysts

Signs of cord dysfunction are present.

Malignant Tumors

• **Spinal Cord Tumors**

Symptoms may be subacute or chronic. Gliomas are most common, followed by neurofibromas, teratomas, and lipomas. Developmental defects may be associated with cutaneous changes. There are signs of cord compression with changes in gait, bladder and bowel dysfunction, localized tenderness, and scoliosis. A deformity of the foot such as cavus or cavovarus is a frequent presenting complaint.

Ewing Sarcoma

Osteogenic Sarcoma

Metastatic Tumors

Neuroblastoma

Wilms' Tumor

Leukemia and Lymphoma

Pain may be fleeting and is not localized. Rarely, spinal cord compression may occur producing typical signs of spinal cord tumors.

BONY ABNORMALITIES

♦ **Scheuermann Disease (Vertebral Osteochondrosis)**

This disease produces a round-back deformity. Several vertebrae may be wedged anteriorly. The pathophysiologic mechanism is thought to be prolapse of the nucleus pulposis into the vertebrae body, possibly due to osteoporosis. Pain is common and usually located over the apex of the kyphosis.

♦ **Spondylolisthesis**

Pain is caused by anterior displacement of vertebrae; usually the fifth lumbar slides forward on the first sacral. Sciatica, increased lumbar lordosis, and tight hamstrings are often present.

♦ **Spondylolysis**

The defect in the pars interarticularis without vertebral slipping is probably the result of a stress fracture. Low-back pain, sometimes with radiation down the leg, is common. The pain is increased by activity.

Occult Fractures

Trauma, sometimes minor, may result in fractures of the pars interarticularis or the transverse or spinous processes. These fractures may not be seen on plain radiographs.

Osteoporosis

Fractures are more likely to occur in osteoporotic bones present in disorders such as Cushing syndrome, osteogenesis imperfecta, homocystinuria, Turner syndrome, malabsorption, and immobilization. Idiopathic juvenile osteoporosis has its onset between 8 and 14 years of age and is self-limited.

Scoliosis

This is almost always a painless disorder. When back pain is present an underlying problem should be sought such as infection, diskitis, or tumor.

♦ PSYCHOGENIC PAIN

Back pain may be associated with reaction to stressful situations. This cause should always be considered if the patient's affect is inconsistent with symptoms or if findings are unexplainable. A careful history must be obtained. As a cause of back pain, psychogenic causes seem to be on the rise (1).

MISCELLANEOUS CAUSES

Sickle Cell Disease

Painful crises may be associated with back pain.

Juvenile Rheumatoid Arthritis

Occasionally, cervical pain may be a presenting complaint.

Anklyosing Spondylitis

Affected children are usually boys; arthritis in hips or knees and loss of mobility of the back may be findings.

Chronic Hemolytic Anemias

Signs of cord compression may result from extramedullary hematopoiesis in the extradural space.

Calcification of Intervertebral Discs

Back pain is localized, with loss of mobility due to muscle spasm. The cause is unknown. Fluffy calcification in the disc space on radiograph films may not appear for 1 to 2 weeks following onset of pain.

• Spinal Dysraphism

Lesions, such as fibrous bands, lipomas, etc., may cause a tethered cord and result in back pain in addition to neurologic findings in the lower extremities and bladder problems. Clues to an underlying problem should be sought by close examination of the skin over the spine for cutaneous abnormalities.

Diastematomyelia

A developmental defect causes a cleft in the cord by bone, cartilage, or fibrous septum. Cutaneous abnormalities over the affected area may be apparent. Low-back pain is aggravated by cough or sneeze. Bladder dysfunction or slowly progressive weakness of the legs are earlier signs than back pain.

Arteriovenous Malformation of Cord

Symptoms are usually slow to develop. Low-back pain is common, with progressive gait and bladder or bowel dysfunction. There may be a cutaneous angioma over the cord lesion.

Limb Girdle Muscular Dystrophy

This is not a single disease entity but a group of dystrophies and myopathies, usually with an autosomal recessive inheritance pattern. First symptoms usually appear during the second decade; an early sign is difficulty in climbing stairs or rising from the floor. Low-back pain may be the source of either complaint. Pseudo-hypertrophy is sometimes present. Deep tendon reflexes are difficult to elicit.

Paroxysmal Cold Hemoglobinuria

Most commonly seen after viral infections. After cold exposure the child experiences back or abdominal pain, followed by chills, fever, and hemoglobinuria.

Multiple Epiphyseal Dysplasia

The most prominent symptoms are painful joints (usually the hips, knees, and ankles) with some decreased mobility. Back pain is frequent. The gait may be waddling.

REFERENCES

1. Combs JA, Caskey PM. Back pain in children and adolescents: a retrospective review of 648 patients. *South Med J* 1997;90:789–792.
2. Micheli LJ, Wood R. Back pain in young athletes: significant differences from adults in causes and patterns. *Arch Pediatr Adolesc Med* 1995;149:15–18.

SUGGESTED READING

Dyment PG. Low back pain in adolescents. *Pediatr Ann* 1991;20:170–178.
McIntire SC. Back pain. In: Gartner JC Jr, Zitelli BJ, eds. *Common & chronic symptoms in pediatrics.* St. Louis: Mosby, 1997:15–31.
Payne WK III, Ogilvie JW. Back pain in children and adolescents. *Pediatr Clin North Am* 1996;43:899–917.
Sponsellar PD. Back pain in children. *Curr Opinion Pediatr* 1994;6:99–103.
Thompson GH. Back pain in children. *J Bone Joint Surg* 1993;75-A:928–938.

88

Scoliosis

Scoliosis is defined as a lateral curvature of the spine from its normal straight position. A rotational deformity of the spine is present as well. Many children have an inconsequential curvature of less than 10° to 15°. True scoliosis is worrisome because of the possibility of progression during growth to a degree that might affect cardiopulmonary function. Scoliosis is described by the direction of the convexity of the curve. The most common pattern in idiopathic scoliosis is a right thoracic and a left lumbar scoliosis.

The prevalence of scoliosis with curves of more than 10° in adolescents has been estimated to be 2% to 3%. Idiopathic scoliosis comprises 60% to 80% of cases. Although most children who have idiopathic scoliosis require no therapy, close follow-up is recommended in order to detect undue progression of the curvature. Scoliosis in an adolescent is not necessarily idiopathic; it may be a sign of an occult neuromuscular disorder or other pathologic conditions.

The age at which scoliosis is noted is of importance in determining possible causes, as is the rapidity of development. Painful scoliosis should never be considered idiopathic in the adolescent. An adolescent with left thoracic kyphosis should be evaluated for underlying pathology. Delayed developmental milestones may suggest a neuromuscular cause.

The following classification divides the causes of scoliosis into nonstructural and structural. Nonstructural curves produce no rotary deformity on forward flexion or on lying down. Structural curves imply a fixed deformity.

♦ Most Common Causes of Scoliosis

Idiopathic	Neurofibromatosis
Congenital Vertebral Defect	Neuromuscular Disorder
Leg Length Discrepancy	

NONSTRUCTURAL CAUSES

♦ Primary Postural Scoliosis

This condition is seen most commonly in children between 10 and 15 years of age. The shoulders may be rounded or one hip may seem more prominent than the other. The apparent curvature disappears on forward flexion or on lying down.

♦ **Secondary Postural Scoliosis**

The curvature is a result of other conditions, such as leg length discrepancy. The curve disappears on forward flexion.

Hysterical Scoliosis

In this unusual type, the scoliosis is not present on forward flexion.

STRUCTURAL CAUSES

Idiopathic Scoliosis

The cause is probably genetic in 90% of cases.

Infantile Scoliosis

This type is noted in the first 3 years of life; it is rare in the United States and more common in boys than girls. In most cases, the curvature lessens with age.

Juvenile Scoliosis

This type is defined as that appearing in the 4- to 10-year-old age group. Boys and girls are equally affected.

♦ **Adolescent Scoliosis**

This is the most common type occurring in children older than 10 years of age. Girls outnumber boys 5 to 7 to 1. The condition generally goes unnoticed until the adolescent growth spurt.

♦ **Congenital Scoliosis**

Scoliosis may be associated with vertebral anomalies such as hemivertebrae, wedge vertebrae, congenital bars, or failure of vertebrae segmentation. Other significant congenital defects, such as of the heart or genitourinary system, or other bony abnormalities may be present. These disorders may be complicated by diastematomyelia, spinal lipomas, and other defects.

♦ **Neurofibromatosis**

This disorder accounts for approximately 2% of cases of scoliosis; in one half of these, a slowly progressive curve similar to the idiopathic variety develops. More significant, however, is the type with a short, sharply angular curve in the thoracic spine. Café au lait spots and axillary freckling are important cutaneous clues.

Neuromuscular Origin

Neuropathies

♦ Cerebral Palsy

Structural scoliosis occurs in 15% to 25% of children with cerebral palsy, more commonly in the more severely affected, especially those with spastic quadriplegia.

♦ Myelomeningocele

This lesion may be obvious or occult. Overlying skin defects, lower extremity weakness, neurologic changes, and bladder and bowel difficulties may be present.

♦ Spinal Cord Injury

Scoliosis will develop in almost one half of the patients with cord injuries.

Syringomyelia

Scoliosis may be a presenting sign before sensory changes are noted.

Diastematomyelia

There may be cutaneous defects or changes over the site of the bony abnormality.

Friedreich Ataxia

Ataxia develops in the first or second decade; deep tendon reflexes are hypoactive. Pes cavus and kyphoscoliosis develop in almost all patients.

Charcot-Marie-Tooth Disease

Atrophy of the peroneal muscles gives a stork leg appearance. Progressive weakness affects the lower and, later, the upper extremities.

Juvenile Spinal Muscle Atrophy

Onset of weakness ranges from early childhood to late adolescence. Signs of this disorder are often mistaken for muscular dystrophy.

Poliomyelitis

This disease is now an uncommon cause. Deformity occurs a year or two after the acute illness.

Myopathies

Duchenne-Type Muscular Dystrophy

Scoliosis occurs later, particularly when the patient is confined to a wheelchair.

Nemaline Myopathy

Limb-Girdle Muscular Dystrophy

Onset of symptoms is later than in the Duchenne type. Proximal muscle weakness is greater than distal.

Arthrogryposis

Multiple contractures are present at birth. Anterior horn cell loss may create muscle imbalance, leading to scoliosis.

Mesenchymal Origin

Marfan Syndrome

Almost 50% of affected children develop scoliosis in infancy or early childhood. Dislocated lens, spiderlike fingers and extremities, and a high arched palate are features.

Ehlers-Danlos Syndrome

Hyperlaxity of joints and skin is characteristic.

Congenital Laxity of Joints

Skin hyperelasticity is not part of this disorder.

Trauma

Direct Vertebral Trauma

Fractures or wedging of vertebral bodies or nerve root irritation may cause scoliosis.

Irradiation

Destruction of the vertebral growth plates, especially in treatment of Wilms' tumor, produces curvature later.

Extravertebral Trauma

Severe trunk burns or thoracic surgery may result in scoliosis.

Tumors

Intraspinal Tumors

Various types of tumors may result in scoliosis. Sensory and motor changes in the lower extremities and bladder and bowel incontinence may also occur.

Osteoid Osteoma

Vertebral body tumors may cause paraspinal muscle spasm and resultant scoliosis. Pain is often worse at night and is relieved by aspirin.

Miscellaneous Causes

Vertebral Body Infection

Scoliosis may be associated with osteomyelitis, diskitis, and tuberculous involvement of the spine.

Rickets

Scoliosis may develop late if the condition is untreated. Epiphyseal enlargement, bowing of long bones, growth retardation, apathy, and muscle weakness are among the features.

Osteogenesis Imperfecta

Collapse of vertebrae following fractures may result in scoliosis.

Scheuermann Disease

This disease causes the adolescent round back deformity; it rarely causes scoliosis.

Achondroplasia

Of affected children, 25% will develop scoliosis in late childhood.

Klippel-Feil Syndrome

Short neck with decreased movement is typical; cervicothoracic scoliosis may also be present.

Sprengel Deformity

Congenital high scapula is almost always associated with cervical or thoracic spine abnormalities.

Cleidocranial Dyostosis

This disorder features hypoplastic or absent clavicles, large head with delayed closure of the fontanel, and a narrow chest.

Hyperphosphatasia

This condition is characterized by fever, pain, and bone fragility with frequent fractures. Stature is short, limb bones are thickened, and sclerae are bluish.

Hypervitaminosis A

Features include dry skin, thickened bones, and often increased intracranial pressure.

Hypothyroidism

Congenital Indifference to Pain

Juvenile Rheumatoid Arthritis

Mucopolysaccharidoses

In type VII, progressive scoliosis may be the initial presenting sign. Hepatosplenomegaly, short neck, and cloudy corneae develop gradually. Type VI (Maroteaux-Lamy) also has scoliosis as a clinical feature.

Syndromes Associated with Scoliosis

Scoliosis has been described in a number of malformation syndromes (1); other features of these syndromes are more striking than the scoliosis.

Aarskog Syndrome	Basal Cell Nevus Syndrome
Camptomelic Dwarfism	Coffin-Lowry Syndrome
Cohen Syndrome	Conradi-Hunermann Syndrome
Cri du Chat Syndrome	Diastrophic Dwarfism
Fetal Trimethadione Syndrome	Freeman-Sheldon Syndrome
Hallermann-Streiff Syndrome	Klinefelter Syndrome
Larsen Syndrome	Metaphyseal Dysplasia (Pyle Disease)
Noonan Syndrome	Prader-Willi Syndrome
Proteus Syndrome	Rett Syndrome
Rubinstein-Taybi Syndrome	Seckel Syndrome (Bird-Headed Dwarfism)
Stickler Syndrome	Turner Syndrome
XXXXY Karyotype	XXY Karyotype

TRANSIENT STRUCTURAL SCOLIOSIS

Inflammation

A lateral curvature can be produced by irritation from empyema or a perinephric abscess.

Torticollis

Sciatic Scoliosis

Pressure of an intervertebral disk on nerve roots may produce a scoliosis.

REFERENCE

1. Jones KL. *Smith's Recognizable Patterns of Human Malformation,* 5th ed. Philadelphia: WB Saunders, 1997.

SUGGESTED READING

Boachie-Adjei O, Lonner B. Spinal deformity. *Pediatr Clin North Am* 1996;43:883–897.
US Preventive Services Task Force. Screening for adolescent idiopathic scoliosis. *JAMA* 1993;269:2664–2666.

89

Kyphosis and Lordosis

Curvature of the spine may occur in anterior and posterior directions as well as laterally as in scoliosis (see Chapter 88, Scoliosis). Most children with kyphosis, a posterior curvature of the spine, or lordosis, an anterior curvature of the spine, have postural deformities. Pathologic or fixed deformities, however, may result from various disorders, many of which are listed here. Lordosis is normal in young children but should no longer be present by mid-childhood.

KYPHOSIS

♦ Poor posture

Poor posture accounts for most cases of kyphosis, especially in adolescence when concern about appearance is most prevalent. Obviously, postural kyphosis is not fixed and can easily be corrected. The problem is finding the appropriate method of encouragement or exercises to maintain an appropriate appearance.

♦ Scheuermann Disease (Juvenile Kyphosis)

This poorly understood disorder usually develops about the time of puberty. The posture is poor, and a round back deformity is apparent. Fatigue and discomfort in the area of kyphosis are common and increased on standing. Full correction cannot voluntarily be obtained. One or more of the thoracic vertebrae have a wedged-shaped appearance on radiographs due to diminished anterior height. The cause is unknown. Lumbar lordosis is often accentuated.

♦ Congenital Kyphosis

The kyphosis is noted in infancy and usually progresses with age, especially after the child begins to walk and stand. The cause, a structural abnormality of the spine, is apparent on radiographic examination. This deformity is painless in childhood but may become painful during adolescence and adulthood. Compression of the spinal cord may occur.

♦ Neuromuscular Problems

Spinal deformities may be caused by almost any neuromuscular disorder in a growing child. Important causes include cerebral palsy, post traumatic paralysis, spinal muscular atrophy, myotonic dystrophy, and poliomyelitis.

Myelomeningocele

Kyphotic defects may be present at birth secondary to vertebral disruption or may develop later associated with muscle weakness.

Infection

Destruction of vertebrae from infectious causes may lead to kyphosis, or spasm of paravertebral musculature may be responsible for the abnormality. Tuberculosis is the archetypical cause but is much less common today than previously. Tuberculous spondylitis (Pott disease) may affect any level of the spine and is often insidious in onset.

Skeletal Dysplasias

A host of skeletal disorders may involve the vertebral column and produce kyphosis. A radiographic skeletal survey will help to differentiate the various types.

Spondyloepiphyseal Dysplasia

Mucopolysaccharidoses

Kyphosis is especially likely to be a finding in Hurler syndrome (type I), Morquio syndrome (type IV), Maroteaux-Lamy syndrome (type VI), and type VII.

Diastrophic Dwarfism

Diaphyseal Dysplasia (Engelmann Disease)

Kniest Dwarfism

Achrondroplasia

Cleidocranial Dystosis

Cockayne Syndrome

Neurofibromatosis

Noonan Syndrome

Metabolic and Endocrine Disorders

Hypothyroidism

Gaucher Disease

Ehlers-Danlos Syndrome

Marfan Syndrome

Homocystinuria

Osteogenesis Imperfecta

Juvenile Osteoporosis

Tumors

Benign or malignant tumors, either primary or metastatic, may cause a kyphotic deformity. Intraspinal tumors must always be considered.

Iatrogenic Kyphosis

Radiation Therapy

Damage to vertebral growth plates may follow radiation therapy, resulting in kyphosis.

Surgery

Surgical removal of parts of the vertebral column may lead to kyphosis.

Miscellaneous

Familial Dysautonomia

Scoliosis and kyphosis are common. Other symptoms and signs predominate including unexplained fever, aspiration, and other signs of autonomic nervous system dysfunction.

LORDOSIS

♦ Physiologic Lordosis

An exaggerated lumbar lordosis is common in toddlers.

♦ Compensatory Posture

A compensatory lumbar lordosis frequently accompanies kyphotic disorders such as Scheuermann disease.

♦ Pes Planus

Lordosis may be an adaptive mechanism for individuals with flat feet to keep a stable stance.

♦ Neuromuscular Disorders

Lumbar lordosis is prominent and progressive in muscular dystrophy and often accompanies cerebral palsy, spinal injuries with paralysis, and poliomyelitis.

♦ Spondylolisthesis

A slipping forward of the vertebral column at the lumbosacral junction can be secondary to congenital sacral defects or the result of trauma or of developmental or acquired bone defects. Poor posture and an increased lumbar lordosis may be the only complaints. Backache, often with radiation down the legs, occurs in the second and third decades.

Bilateral Flexion Contractures of the Hips

An increased pelvic inclination, the result of hip flexion contractures, will produce a compensatory lumbar lordosis. Flexion contractures may occur in juvenile rheumatoid arthritis, other hip dysplasias, and cerebral palsy.

Myelomeningocele

Lordosis is the most common spinal deformity in this disorder and is compensatory in nature.

Inflammatory Processes

Spasm of paravertebral muscles from inflammatory processes in the spine may cause an accentuated lordosis. In diskitis, an inflammation of the intervertebral disc space, symptoms of backache, pain radiating to the legs, and, occasionally, lower extremity muscle weakness are common.

Skeletal Dysplasias

Achondroplasia

Lumbar lordosis is exaggerated in this disorder because of fixed flexion of the hips and some thoracolumbar kyphosis.

Cleidocranial Dysostosis

Major features include a large head with a delayed closure of the anterior fontanel and hypoplastic clavicles.

Spondyloepiphyseal Dysplasias

SUGGESTED READING

Boachie-Adjei O, Lonner B. Spinal deformity. *Pediatr Clin North Am* 1996;43:883–897.

SECTION XIII

Extremities

90
Leg Pain

Leg aches are common in children. Fortunately, in most cases the episodes are short lived and the cause is benign, probably related to trauma or exercise. Should the limb pain continue or become increasingly severe or recurrent, an investigation for an underlying disorder is mandatory. In adolescents, psychogenic causes or somatization becomes important in the differential diagnosis of limb pain.

Many of the disorders listed in Chapter 91, Limp, and Chapter 92, Arthritis, may produce leg pain and they are not repeated here. The primary purpose of this chapter is to suggest possible causes for the kind of leg pain that is often referred to as "growing pains."

The physician is often faced with a dilemma of how far to proceed with the diagnostic evaluation. The leg pain associated with most disorders in this chapter can be differentiated from growing pains by careful evaluation including history and physical examination, with special attention to pain location and systemic symptoms, and a few laboratory studies such as radiographs, blood count, and sedimentation rate.

◆ Most Common Causes of Leg Pain

Trauma	"Growing" Pains
Hypermobility Syndrome	Somatization
Viral Myositis	Stress Fracture
Sickle Cell Disease	

● Causes Not to Forget

Osteoid Osteoma	Fibromyalgia

◆ IDIOPATHIC LEG PAIN (GROWING PAINS)

Leg pain is often attributed to this rather nebulous entity. As many as 10% to 20% of children may complain of vague leg pain on a recurrent basis, sometimes in association with headaches and abdominal pain. Various criteria have been suggested for differentiation of this symptom complex from serious underlying disorders. The pains are usually intermittent and bilateral and located deep in the legs, most commonly in the thigh or calf. Joint pain is rare and points to other diagnoses. Although the pains may occur at any time of the day or night, they typically occur only at night, either when the child is falling asleep or actually wakening the child from sleep; usually they last $\frac{1}{2}$ to 1 hour and may respond to rubbing, heat, or analgesics. Systemic signs and symptoms are absent, and radiographic findings and the sedimentation rate are normal.

The etiology has still not been determined, but most researchers agree that the pain is not due to "growth;" excessive exercise or trauma, hidden food allergy or emotional factors have been suggested.

TRAUMA

Trauma is probably the most common cause of leg pain. Often, superficial clues such as bruises are present, or there may be a history of an episode of physical trauma.

♦ **Muscle or Bone Bruises**

♦ **Fractures**

The prototype in this category may be the stress fracture produced by running on a hard surface for a prolonged period. The pain is localized rather than diffuse and bilateral. Initial radiographs may be normal.

Pathologic Fractures

Bone cysts or areas of fibrous dysplasia may make the bone susceptible to fracture from minimal trauma.

Osteoporosis

Fractures are more likely to occur in osteoporotic bone. Causes include Cushing syndrome, osteogenesis imperfecta, homocystinuria, Turner syndrome, malabsorption, and immobilization. Idiopathic juvenile osteoporosis has its onset between 8 and 14 years of age and is self-limited.

♦ **Muscle Injections**

LEUKEMIA AND LYMPHOMA

Leg pain, the result of leukemic infiltrate in the bone, may be an early symptom of leukemia or lymphoma. Systemic signs such as fever, weight loss, and adenopathy may not be present. Occasionally, radiolucent lines in the metaphyseal areas may be seen.

BONE TUMORS

Malignant Tumors

Characteristically, the pain is persistent and of increasing severity. Osteogenic sarcoma and Ewing tumor are the most common. Radiographs should be obtained in any child complaining of localized bone pain.

Benign Tumors

Benign neoplasms are more likely to be painless unless they are associated with a pathologic fracture or the result of some mechanical difficulty. These are two notable exceptions.

- **Osteoid Osteoma**

    The pain associated with this tumor is characteristically worse at night than during the day and is usually relieved by aspirin. On radiographic examination a small radiolucent nidus is found surrounded by a rim of sclerotic bone.

    Benign Osteoblastoma

    This lesion is larger than the osteoid osteoma, the nature of the pain is not so well defined, and the surrounding bone is less sclerotic.

Metastatic Tumors

Neuroblastoma is one of the more common metastatic bone tumors that may produce leg pain.

INFECTION AND INFLAMMATION

♦ Myositis

Pyogenic infection of muscle or inflammation as a result of a systemic infection, such as the severe calf tenderness associated with influenza, may produce leg pain with significant tenderness and weakness.

Osteomyelitis

Infection in the bone is usually localized and is associated with tenderness and swelling over the lesion, but not always with systemic signs. A bone scan rather than radiographs are much more likely to reveal early changes.

Tuberculosis

Limb pain without systemic symptoms may be a presenting complaint.

Syphilis

The great mimic may produce a periostitis with severe pain and pseudoparalysis, particularly in infants with congenital infections.

Trichinosis

Severe muscle pain is one of the characteristic findings, as well as fever, periorbital edema, and eosinophilia.

MISCELLANEOUS CAUSES

♦ Hypermobility Syndrome

Children with evidence of hypermobility may present with leg and joint aches without other obvious causes.

◆ Somatization (Psychogenic Rheumatism)

The leg pain is usually out of proportion to the physical findings. The children gradually become dysfunctional and may withdraw from activities and school.

● Fibromyalgia (Fibromyositis)

A chronic, and, usually, diffuse muscle tenderness in specific, and discrete anatomical points. Fatigue, headache, and other complaints are common.

Patellofemoral Pain Syndrome

Generally seen in adolescents. The pain is aggravated by climbing stairs. The medial patellar undersurface is tender to palpation. Pain is reproduced by movement of the patella over the knee.

Intermittent Nocturnal Leg Cramps

Cramping is thought to be the result of vigorous daytime play. The parents may be instructed to palpate the calf for muscle tightness to make the diagnosis.

Shin Splints (Anterior and Posterior Compartment Syndromes)

Hypertrophy or swelling of muscles of the lower leg will lead to muscle cramping and pain on sudden resumption of excessive exercise.

Reflex Sympathetic Dystrophy

The cause may not be post traumatic as found in adults. The child, usually an adolescent stops using an extremity, which may become swollen, cool and painful to touch. Psychogenic overlay is usually found.

◆ Sickle Cell Disease

This disorder should be considered in black children with painful extremities and anemia.

Acute Poststreptococcal Polymyalgia

Diffuse and exquisite tenderness of skeletal muscles without concomitant arthritis or elevated muscle enzymes may follow a streptococcal infection.

Hypervitaminosis A

The excessive intake of vitamin A may result in bone pain as well as symptoms of increased intracranial pressure.

Gaucher Disease

Bone lesions may suggest osteomyelitis in the early stages because of the severe pain, tenderness, swelling, erythema, and heat. The spleen is usually enlarged, and the skin develops a yellowish color.

Foods

Several observers have reported unexplained leg pains that seem to be related to the ingestion of potatoes, tomatoes, eggplants, and peppers.

Spinal Cord Tumor

Radicular or back pain are common presentations.

Renal Tubular Acidosis

In adolescents and adults osteomalacia with bone pain and pathologic fractures is a cardinal sign of distal renal tubular acidosis. Growth retardation may be the only early finding.

Chemical Preservatives

Inhalation of smoke from the burning of outdoor grade lumber may cause muscle aches, pains, and cramps as well as rashes, hair loss, seizures, red eyes, and other symptoms.

Ehlers-Danlos Syndrome

Leg cramps, particularly of the calves, are frequent. Types with the most hypermobility have more symptoms of pain.

Multiple Epiphyseal Dysplasia

Painful joints, sometimes enlarged in size, are a leading symptom. The hips, knees, or ankles are most commonly affected, and there may be some restriction in mobility. Back pain is common; the gait may be waddling. Radiographs show irregular, small, flat, or fragmented epiphyseal ossification centers.

Stickler Syndrome (Hereditary Artho-Ophthalmopathy)

Features may include a marfanoid habitus with large joints and hyperextensible knees, elbows, and finger joints. The joints are sometimes painful; morning stiffness is common. The midface is flat, the chin is small, and clefting is common. Congenital myopia is common; conductive hearing loss may be present. Inheritance pattern is autosomal dominant.

Melorheostosis

This rare disorder is characterized by longitudinal thickening of the shaft of long bones, usually of one limb. The pain may be severe, and overlying skin is often tense, shiny, and indurated.

Engelmann Disease (Diaphyseal Dysplasia)

This is another rare disorder characterized by symmetric enlargement and sclerosis of the shafts of the major long bones and changes in the skull as well. Affected children usually present with difficulty in walking because of limb pain.

Scurvy

This disorder is rarely seen in North America. Subperiosteal hemorrhages produce exquisite tenderness in the limbs.

Pseudoxanthoma Elasticum

A rare, autosomal recessive (AR) disorder, in which alterations in elastic tissues of vessels may lead to gastrointestinal bleeding and episodes similar to intermittent claudication. Skin changes occur after the second decade and give a plucked chicken-enlike appearance in localized areas.

Caffey Disease (Infantile Cortical Hyperostosis)

Although onset of symptoms in this uncommon disorder is usually before 6 months of age, failure to recognize early signs may suggest osteomyelitis in older infants with involvement of the lower extremities.

Idiopathic Periosteal Hyperostosis with Dysproteinemia (Goldbloom Syndrome)

This rare disorder of bone pain associated with fever, is characterized by radiologic evidence of periostitis and hypergammaglobulinemia. The long bones are primarily affected, but the mandible, facial bones, metatarsals, and metacarpals may also be involved.

SUGGESTED READING

Orlowski JP, Mercer RD. Osteoid osteoma in children and young adults. *Pediatrics* 1977;59:526–532.
Sherry DD. Limb pain in childhood. *Pediatr Rev* 1990;12:39–46.
Szer IS. Are those limb pains "growing" pains? *Contemp Pediatr* 1989;6:143–148.
Szer IS. Musculoskeletal pain syndromes that affect adolescents. *Arch Pediatr Adolesc Med* 1996;150:740–747.

91
Limp

Fortunately, the cause of limp in most children is fairly straightforward. The origin of the limp may range from the foot to the spine, or even the abdomen. A thorough history and physical examination usually reveal the origin of the problem. The type of gait responsible for the limp should be observed by having the child walk unencumbered by clothing in a hallway; the gait may suggest a foot, knee, or hip problem. The presence of systemic symptoms usually indicates a more complex problem than simple trauma. The extremities should be carefully palpated; changes in temperature, coloration, and evidence of swelling should be noted. All joints should be put through range of motion to elicit possible subtle manifestations in other areas. Refusal to walk may be an extreme form of the processes below.

It is important to remember that pain may be referred. A painful knee may result from hip disease. A child with hip complaints may have an intra-abdominal or a spinal disorder. Signs of trauma responsible for a painful limp may be subtle. An unusual or new activity for instance, hitting a bucket of golf balls or raking pine needles may result in toxic synovitis of the hip. A sudden twisting motion may produce the notorious incomplete, undisplaced "toddler's fracture" of the tibia, which is inapparent on initial radiographs.

The following classification of disorders associated with limp in childhood has been modified from an approach by Salter (1). Painful and nonpainful causes of limp are the two main categories.

◆ Most Common Causes of Limp

Painful
Trauma: Sprain, Bruise, Fractures
Foreign Body (Foot); Plantar Wart
Toxic Synovitis
Patellofemoral Pain Syndrome

Nonpainful
Leg Length Discrepancy
Legg-Calvé-Perthes Disease
Hypermobility Syndrome
Muscle Weakness
Slipped Capital Femoral Epiphysis

PAINFUL CAUSES OF LIMP

Trauma

◆ Local Superficial Lesions

Sometimes the cause is so obvious that it may be overlooked. Skin irritation from a tight shoe or a shoe defect, lacerations or foreign bodies in the foot, or plantar warts may be the cause.

♦ **Muscle Bruising**

There is usually a history of trauma; purpura of the skin may be present. Tenderness of affected muscle is usual.

♦ **Ligamentous Strains and Sprains**

Ankle and knee injuries are common and may mimic fractures. Joints are often swollen and sometimes bruised.

♦ **Fractures**

Fractures must be considered in any painful limp. Careful palpation of the extremity may localize the fracture site. Stress fractures may occur in joggers or children involved in athletics; the pain may not be severe. "Toddler fracture" is an undisplaced, often spiral fracture; radiologic confirmation may be lacking early on. It occurs typically in the tibia. Limp may be the presenting sign in a case of child abuse.

Tendon Disorders

Achilles tendonitis is characterized by sudden acute pain in the tendon; there is pain on palpation, but plantar flexion is usually strong. Rupture of the Achilles tendon, in which there is a lack of forceful plantar flexion, is uncommon before adulthood.

Child Abuse

There may be muscle bruising, sprains, or fractures. The history may not fit the injury; there may be other evidence of abuse present.

Injections

Limp is typically seen in toddlers after booster DPT injections. Gluteal injections may irritate the sciatic nerve; the large muscle mass of the thighs is the preferred injection site to avoid this problem.

Subluxation of Patella

Adolescent girls are most commonly affected; the knee suddenly gives way, followed by swelling of the joint. The patella is usually not displaced at the time of examination for the acute problem, but can be subluxed easily.

Spondylolysis and Spondylolisthesis

The former is a stress fracture of the pars interarticularis portion of the posterior vertebral arch, while the latter is a forward displacement of the vertebral column. Spondylolisthesis may follow spondylolysis. These problems tend to be more common in children between 10 and 15 years of age, and present with back pain, often referred to the buttock or leg, and sometimes a limp.

Herniated Nucleus Pulposis

Inflammatory Conditions

♦ **Toxic Synovitis**

The hip is the most common site by far. This condition follows trauma or viral infection; fever and systemic signs are usually minimal or absent. There is pain on abduction and internal rotation of the hip. It may predispose to Legg-Calvé-Perthes disease.

Henoch-Schönlein Purpura

A petechial or purpuric rash is characteristic; abdominal pain; arthritis, nephritis, and tissue swelling may be other features.

Lyme Disease

A chronic, recurrent monoarticular arthritis is most common as a joint manifestation.

Juvenile Rheumatoid Arthritis

There are many different presentations; one or many joints may be involved. This is a diagnosis of exclusion; pain is usually not exquisite.

Systemic Lupus Erythematosus

Arthritis or arthralgias and muscle weakness are common. There may be other clues, including rashes, and evidence of serositis.

Acute Rheumatic Fever

Migratory joint pain or swelling is typical. Diagnosis must be based on the Jones criteria. Pain is usually out of proportion to physical findings.

Dermatomyositis

Weakness is more pronounced in proximal muscles than distal; there is often pain on palpation of muscles, as well as erythematous scaling papules over elbows, knees, and knuckles.

Serum Sickness

Findings may include urticaria, arthralgias or arthritis, fever, and lymphadenopathy. The disorder is most commonly associated with drug use.

Inflammatory Bowel Disease

Arthritis or arthralgias may be associated.

Polyarteritis Nodosa

There may be diffuse symptoms, secondary to vasculitis of medium-sized and small arteries

Autoimmune Hepatitis

Arthritis or arthralgia with jaundice and hepatosplenomegaly are common.

Infections

Osteomyelitis

Usually, localized pain, fever, and an elevated sedimentation rate are present. At times osteomyelitis may mimic septic arthritis. The infection may be in the pelvis or vertebral column rather than the bones of the lower extremity.

Septic Arthritis

Onset is usually acute; the infection is generally monarticular and very painful. Gonococcal arthritis may be migratory.

Acute Myositis

This disorder follows a viral illness, usually influenza. There is severe pain in the calves; creatine kinase levels are elevated.

Pyomyositis

This is an uncommon localized muscle infection, usually caused by *Staphylococcus aureus.*

Diskitis and Intervertebral Disc Infection

Back pain is usual; pain may be referred to the hips. The child may refuse to walk.

Epidural Abscess

Exquisite back pain, with sensory changes in the lower extremities, is typical.

Acute Appendicitis

Psoas irritation may alter gait.

Retroperitoneal Masses

Pain from infection or inflammation may be referred to the hip. The abdomen should be palpated carefully for masses.

Acute Iliac Adenitis

Suppuration of lymph nodes may irritate the hip capsule, with resultant limp. Careful palpation along the ileum may detect the swelling associated with the adenitis.

Aseptic Necrosis and Osteochondritis

Osgood-Schlätter Disease

The tibial tuberosity is painful. Limping may occur after heavy exercise; usually boys 11 to 15 years of age are affected.

Legg-Calvé-Perthes Disease

The femoral epiphysis is involved; the condition may be totally asymptomatic; it is most common in boys 4 to 8 years of age.

♦ Patello-Femoral Pain Syndrome

Formerly referred to as chondromalacia patella, in which scoring of the cartilaginous surface of the patella produces a grating sensation when the patella is moved back and forth over the knee joint. Pain is worse after exercise and on stair climbing.

Freiberg Disease

The head of the second metatarsal is involved; there is pain on palpation. It is more common in girls 12 to 15 years of age.

Köhler Disease

Osteochondrosis of the tarsal navicular bone causes a mild limp; it is seen usually in boys 3 to 6 years of age.

Sever Disease

Calcaneal apophysitis, with pain on heel palpation, is seen primarily in boys 8 to 12 years of age.

Osteochondritis Dissecans

The knee is most commonly involved; there is a history of locking of the joint, as well as intermittent swelling.

Larsen-Johansson Disease

There is pain and tenderness over the lower pole of the patella, with swelling of the adjacent soft tissues. Boys between 10 and 14 years of age are most commonly affected. Limp with inability to kneel and run is typical.

Sinding-Larsen Disease

Avulsion of patellar ligament may occur, especially in cerebral palsy.

Neoplasms

Leukemia

Leg pain and limp may be presenting signs, both of which may suggest arthritis.

Benign Bone Tumors

Osteoid osteoma, eosinophilic granuloma, and fibrous dysplasia may cause limp.

Malignant Bone Tumors

Osteogenic sarcoma, Ewing sarcoma, and metastatic neuroblastoma are examples.

Spinal Neoplasms

These tumors may cause back pain, leg pain, weakness, and limp.

♦ Hematologic Conditions

Sickle Cell Anemia

The hand-foot syndrome in toddlers may be secondary to bone infarction. The symmetric swelling is painful.

Hemophilia

Hemarthrosis is usually obvious.

Phlebitis

There is tenderness of involved veins with local swelling.

Scurvy

Limp is secondary to periosteal hemorrhage.

Hypervitaminosis A

Bone pain may occur with intoxication. Signs of pseudotumor cerebri may be present.

Miscellaneous Causes

Hypermobility Syndrome

Children with this disorder have hyperextensible joints. Painful symptoms may be mistaken for rheumatoid arthritis.

Tarsal Coalition

Fusion of the tarsal bones leads to painful flatfeet, the onset of which is usually at adolescence.

NONPAINFUL CAUSES OF LIMP

Neurologic Disorders

Flaccid Paralysis

Limp is due to weak muscle groups. Poliomyelitis was the most common cause prior to routine vaccination programs.

Spastic Paralysis

Jerky gait is accentuated on running. Cerebral palsy is the most common cause. Increased muscle tone and hyperreflexia are other features.

Peripheral Neuropathy

Included in the causes are nerve damage from misuse of a car restraint.

Ataxia

Causes may be drugs, infection, or heredity. The gait is unsteady and broad based.

Involvement of Spine

Intraspinal masses, diastematomyelia, lesions of the cauda equina, herniated disk, and spondylolisthesis may cause limp. A careful neurologic examination is mandatory. The lumbar area should be examined carefully for suggestions of spinal dysraphism. There may be a subcutaneous mass, a hairy patch, port wine stain, or sinus tract.

Muscle Disorders

Muscular Dystrophy

Limp is secondary to muscle weakness; there may be pseudohypertrophy of calf muscles. Numerous other primary muscle disorders with weakness may produce an abnormal gait.

Arthrogryposis

The etiology is unclear; it may be neurogenic or muscular. There is a lack of full muscular extension due to contractures.

Joint Disorders

Stiffness or Contractures

These disorders may be seen in several inherited diseases, such as mucopolysaccharidoses.

Instability

Severe hyperextensibility of joints may also be a cause. Joint instability may occur with Ehlers-Danlos syndrome or severe pes planus.

Developmental Dysplasia of the Hip

May produce a waddling gait. Results of the Trendelenburg test are positive.

Bony Deformities

♦ Leg Length Discrepancies

Any child with a limp should have leg lengths compared.

♦ Slipped Capital Femoral Epiphysis

Onset in most cases is insidious; adolescents 11 to 15 years of age, often obese, are those most often affected. The limp may be painful.

♦ Legg-Calvé-Perthes Disease

The limp may or may not be painful.

Coxa Vara

In this congenital condition, the head of the femur is at a more acute angle; the gait is waddling.

Knock Knees

Severe knock knees may cause an unsteady gait.

Blount Disease

Unilateral or bilateral bowing of tibia and beaking of proximal tibial epiphysis on radiographs are findings.

Torsional Deformities of Lower Extremities

Congenital Vertical Talus

The plantar surface has a rocker bottom appearance.

Epiphyseal Dysplasias

Symptoms may mimic those of Legg-Calvé-Perthes disease. Hereditary multiple epiphyseal dysplasia, Gaucher disease, hypothyroidism, and sickle cell disease should be considered.

Postmeningococcal Skeletal Dystrophy

Symmetrical epiphyseal-metaphyseal lesions and asymmetrical destruction of major epiphyses may follow sepsis and DIC, especially with meningococcal infections. Months to years later these children may present with a limp, bowlegs, asymmetric limbs, and short stature.

Functional States

Hysteria

This cause is uncommon in young children.

Mimicry

The limp is likely to occur intermittently or to vary in form.

REFERENCE

1. Salter RB. Gait disturbances and limp in childhood. In: Green M, Haggerty RJ, eds. *Ambulatory pediatrics.* Philadelphia: WB Saunders, 1968:232–236.

SUGGESTED READING

MacEwen GD, Dehne R. The limping child. *Pediatr Rev* 1991;12:268–274.
McIntire SC, Farrell JD. The limping child. In: Gartner JC Jr, Zitelli BJ, eds. *Common and chronic symptoms in pediatrics.* St. Louis: Mosby, 1997:63–79.
Renshaw TS. The child who has a limp. *Pediatr Rev* 1995;16:458–465.

92

Arthritis

Joint complaints are relatively common in children; fortunately, in most cases the problem is transient and is the result of trauma or exercise. Arthritis, defined as swelling of a joint or limitation of motion accompanied by heat, pain, and tenderness, is much less common than arthralgia (joint pain), or pain of the extremity not referable to the joint but severe enough to cause a limp (Chapter 91, Limp). Disorders with periarticular swelling may mimic arthritis; they generally cause symmetric involvement and are identified by other features of the disorder (e.g., Henoch-Schönlein syndrome).

The causes of arthritis are numerous. Of causes of monarticular disease, traumatic arthritis is still the most common, but septic arthritis is a serious disorder that must be diagnosed and treated early. Painful monarticular arthritis must be considered as possible septic arthritis until proven otherwise. Acute rheumatic fever is now uncommon in the United States, but the incidence of juvenile rheumatoid arthritis (JRA) appears to be increasing. Unfortunately, the diagnosis of JRA is one of exclusion and requires the presence of swelling involving one or more joints for at least 6 weeks. These criteria create unsettling feelings in the physician who is evaluating the recent onset of joint swelling in a child. How extensive must the laboratory investigation be?

Many disorders that cause arthritis can be easily excluded from consideration. Others, such as the viral arthriditides, may be more common than realized; fortunately, these rarely are long lasting. The reactive arthriditides, such as with *Salmonella, Shigella,* or *Yersinia* infections, present interesting material for future investigation. Certain segments of the population such as those with the histocompatibility antigen HLA B27, seem to be prone to develop arthritis following certain environmental insults such as infection and as yet undetermined other factors.

♦ **Most Common Causes of Arthritis**

Traumatic	Transient Synovitis
Viral	Septic
Reactive	Lyme Disease
"Serum Sickness"	Juvenile Rheumatoid
Inflammatory Bowel Disease	Sickle Cell Disease
Leukemia	Osteomyelitis

RHEUMATIC DISEASES

◆ Juvenile Rheumatoid Arthritis

Criteria for the diagnosis of JRA include a chronic arthritis lasting more than 6 weeks in at least one joint and the exclusion of other possibilities. There are no confirmatory diagnostic tests. JRA has three general forms (a) systemic, characterized by prominent constitutional symptoms and, eventually, involvement of multiple joints; (b) polyarticular, with involvement of more than four joints, often symmetric in distribution and frequently affecting the hands, and with minor systemic manifestations; and (c) pauciarticular, with involvement of four or fewer joints. Systemic signs and symptoms are rare in this form, but iridocyclitis is not.

Acute Rheumatic Fever

Diagnosis is based on confirmation of a preceding streptococcal infection and the Jones criteria. The arthritis is typically migratory and lasts 3 to 5 days at most in each joint that becomes involved; the duration of arthritis in all joints does not exceed 1 month. The joints are usually exquisitely painful, occasionally have areas of erythema, and most frequently are not greatly swollen. The arthritis is not destructive.

Systemic Lupus Erythematosus (SLE)

Joint disease is the most common presentation of SLE. Fever, rashes or alopecia, weakness or fatigue, weight loss, photosensitivity, and neurologic complaints may be present. The antinuclear antibody titer is almost invariably elevated, but this finding is not specific for SLE.

Dermatomyositis

Symmetric, progressive muscle weakness is characteristic. The muscles may be tender to palpation. The classic skin rashes, scaly erythematous papules over the knuckles (Gottron papules), elbows, and kness, and a discoloration of the eyelids are found in three fourths of the cases. A few patients will have objective evidence of arthritis, particularly of the knees.

Scleroderma

Linear or Localized Scleroderma

Linear sclerotic areas of skin or multiple patches of sclerosis are found in this form, which is much more common than progressive systemic sclerosis. One third of patients will develop active synovitis at some time during the course of their disease, in either a polyarticular or pauciarticular distribution.

Progressive Systemic Sclerosis

In this form, skin symptoms are prominent and are characterized by a progressive tightening, usually symmetric in distribution. Raynaud phenomenon may precede the sclerosis; gastrointestinal disturbances and pulmonary, cardiac, and renal involvement develop. Arthritis is not common, but arthralgias and contractures of joints are often present.

Ankylosing Spondylitis

Back pain is a frequent presenting complaint. The sacroiliac and spinal apophyseal joints eventually become involved, but in children, initial involvement is often peripheral, asymmetric, and limited to a few large joints such as the hips, knees, and, rarely, small joints. Affected boys outnumber girls by 10 to 1, and 90% of affected children have the histocompatibility locus B-27. In some cases, the clinical presentation is recurrent attacks of acute iridocyclitis.

Mixed Connective Tissue Disease

Signs and symptoms of this curious disorder may be identical to those in a number of other disorders. The arthritis affects multiple joints and commonly the small joints. Skin changes may be consistent with scleroderma; serositis, hepatosplenomegaly, lymphadenopathy, Raynaud phenomenon, and abnormal esophageal motility may be found.

Polyarteritis

Prominent findings include fever, myalgias, abdominal pain, bizarre skin rashes including unusual erythema multiforme, petechiae or purpura, and painful nodular swellings along the course of blood vessels in some patients. Urinary sediment abnormalities are often present. Arthritis is less frequent than arthralgias, and the arthritis may be migratory. Hypertension and seizures are common.

OTHER RELATED CONDITIONS

♦ Inflammatory Bowel Disease

A peripheral arthritis involving a few large joints, of short duration, may be seen in about 10% of children with Crohn disease or ulcerative colitis. The arthritis may precede the bowel symptoms but usually does not.

Mucocutaneous Lymph Node Syndrome (Kawasaki Disease)

Criteria for diagnosis of this disorder include fever lasting more than 5 days, a polymorphous rash, conjunctival injection, cracking of the lips, pharyngitis, and cervical adenopathy. Arthralgias or arthritis may be found. Arthritis may develop late in the febrile stage that usually lasts 2 to 4 weeks.

Psoriatic Arthritis

Pauciarticular arthritis, especially involving the distal interphalangeal joints, is occasionally present in children with psoriasis. The arthritis may precede the skin disorder. There are few systemic symptoms.

Sarcoidosis

The most consistent features of childhood sarcoidosis are fever, weight loss, anorexia, dyspnea, cough, and lymphadenopathy. The arthritis is often monarticular at onset and relatively painless. A papular skin rash or uveitis should suggest this possibility.

Chronic Active Hepatitis

Arthritis or arthralgia may be confined to a single joint, but often several joints are involved, usually the large ones. Anorexia, weight loss, and jaundice are other features.

Sjögren Syndrome

This syndrome may present in other rheumatic disorders, particularly rheumatoid arthritis. The triad of characteristic findings is keratoconjunctivitis sicca (dry eyes), xerostomia (dry mouth), and salivary gland enlargement.

Reiter Disease

An episode of diarrhea frequently precedes onset of arthritis with significant swelling of joints (particularly those of the lower extremity), conjunctivitis, and urethritis.

Stevens-Johnson Syndrome

This hypersensitivity reaction characterized by erythema multiforme-like lesions, often progressing to bullae and extensive mucocutaneous lesions, can be triggered by drugs, infections, and, sometimes, other connective tissue disorders. Arthritis may be part of the clinical picture.

Behçet Syndrome

The primary symptoms of this rare disorder include recurrent aphthous stomatitis, genital ulceration, and iritis. Skin lesions (particularly pustular and ulcerative ones), erythema multiforme, and erythema nodosum are seen along with an arthritis, which is usually pauciarticular.

Giant Cell Arteritis

Early symptoms include fever, weakness, arthralgias or frank arthritis, myalgias, cough, and skin rashes.

Wegener Granulomatosis

Arthritis and arthralgias are usually overshadowed by evidence of upper and lower respiratory tract necrotizing granulomas and renal vasculitis.

ARTHRITIS ASSOCIATED WITH INFECTIONS

♦ Bacterial Infections

An important cause of arthritis that needs immediate attention is septic arthritis caused by various bacteria. In over 90% of the cases, involvement is monarticular, and usually the joint is exquisitely painful. Among the more common pathogens are *Staphylococcus, Streptococcus,* and *Neisseria gonorrhoeae. Haemophilus influenzae* b was common before routine immunization.

♦ Viral Infections

Arthritis has been reported to occur in a large number of viral infections including rubella (after immunization as well), mumps, EBV, adenovirus, parvovirus B19, and varicella. The joint symptoms usually last less than 6 weeks and are often pauciarticular. Infections with hepatitis A and B viruses may have as a prodrome a serum sicknesslike syndrome with urticaria and the swelling of multiple joints.

♦ Lyme Disease

The arthritis is sudden in onset, monarticular or oligoarticular and occasionally migratory. The knees are most commonly involved. The arthritis may last 1 day to 3 months and sometimes recurs for years.

♦ Reactive Arthritis

Children with invasive bacterial infections, such as meningococcal illnesses, *H. influenzae* type b, meningitis, and *N. gonorrhoeae* may develop a nonsuppurative arthritis involving multiple joints later in the course of antibiotic therapy or up to a few weeks after completion of therapy. Immune complexes have been found in both blood and synovial fluid in some cases.

Acute infections such as pharyngitis, scarlet fever, and bacteremias may also be associated with synovitis involving single joints, multiple joints, or even migratory in nature. Poststreptococcal reactive arthritis may mimic acute septic arthritis, when it is monarticular. The distinction between this condition and rheumatic fever is not always clear.

Various gastrointestinal infections, including *Salmonella, Shigella, Brucella, Yersinia,* and *Campylobacter* have been implicated. Persons with the histocompatibility antigen HLA B27 seem particularly predisposed.

♦ Osteomyelitis

Osteomyelitis occurring near a joint may produce a sympathetic effusion or a reactive, sterile arthritis. In young children, a septic arthritis may be produced by contiguous spread.

Human Immunodeficiency Virus

Mycoplasmal Infections

A migratory polyarthritis may occur, often with an urticarial rash. Pneumonia is common. One half of the cases have effusion. Recovery occurs when the respiratory infection clears.

Fungal Infections

Usually the infections involve bone before invading contiguous joints. Arthritis has been described with coccidioidomycosis, cryptococcosis, histoplasmosis, actinomycosis, and blastomycosis.

Mycobacterial Infections

The arthritis is usually monarticular but may be polyarticular. Systemic signs may be minimal and results of the skin test are negative in the first 6 weeks of illness.

Parasitic Infestations

A pauciarticular, self-limited arthritis has been described with *Giardia lamblia* infestation.

Syphilis

Miscellaneous Infections

A psoas abscess or retroperitoneal lymph node infection may stimulate a reactive arthritis of the hip joint.

Toxic Shock Syndrome

Hypotension, rash, and multiple other signs overshadow the arthritis.

Rat-Bite Fever (Haverhill)

This uncommon disorder is characterized by the abrupt onset of fever and chills about 1 week after exposure to the streptobacillary organism. A generalized rash, of various types, with involvement of the hands and feet is common. Pustules, vesicles, and petechiae may be present. Arthritis occurs in about one half of cases, occasionally migratory in nature.

NEOPLASTIC DISORDERS

♦ Leukemia

In some series, up to 10% of children who present to a rheumatologist for arthritis have leukemia. The arthritis is usually polyarticular but may be migratory; it is monarticular in 5% of the cases. Severe joint pain is frequent, and the rheumatoid factor may be present. Hematologic abnormalities may offer a clue, particularly anemia and thrombocytopenia.

Lymphoma

Neuroblastoma

Multicentric Reticulohistiocytosis

Clinical signs include papulonodular, wartlike skin lesions. The arthritis is potentially destructive.

TRAUMA

♦ Joint Injury

Direct trauma to a joint is the most common cause of monarticular arthritis.

♦ Transient Synovitis

This is a frequent cause of limp and hip pain in young children. The synovitis is probably secondary to any of a number of factors including trauma or viral infections.

♦ ALLERGIC REACTIONS

A hypersensitivity arthritis or "serum sickness" may result in the swelling of multiple joints lasting from a few days to several weeks. The joint swelling may be associated with edema of the hands and feet or periorbital area. Urticarial or erythema multiforme rashes are common. Although true serum sickness is now rare due to improved biologicals that no longer use horse serum, drugs and viruses cause a syndrome so serum sicknesslike as to justify the persistence of the term.

IMMUNOLOGIC CAUSES

Subacute Bacterial Endocarditis

Ventriculojugular Shunt Infections

Chronic infections, especially with coagulase negative staphylococci, may induce the formation of immune complexes with arthritis and nephritis.

Immunodeficiency Syndromes

Up to 20% of children with hypogammaglobulinemia or agammaglobulinemia may develop a chronic polyarthritis mimicking JRA.

Complement Deficiency

A polyarticular arthritis has been described with a hypomorphic variant of C3 associated with chronic glomerulonephritis.

METABOLIC AND ENDOCRINE DISORDERS

Gout

This is an unusual cause of arthritis in children.

Hyperlipoproteinemia

Type II and Type IV disorders may be associated with an oligoarticular arthritis, but usually in adults.

Gaucher Disease

Arthritis is rare, but bone pain may result from infiltration of the bone marrow with storage cells.

Lipogranulomatosis

Lumpy masses over the joints develop in infancy along with a hoarse cry, restricted joint movement, and recurrent infections; early death is common.

Thyroid Disorders

Joint swelling has been described both in hypothyroidism and hyperthyroidism but is an unusual manifestation.

Mucopolysaccharidoses

Restricted joint motion and swelling may occur in these disorders, which should be obvious from dysmorphic features.

Fabry Disease (Angiokeratoma Corporis Diffusum)

Nodular angiectases of the skin are noted at about 10 years of age. Attacks of burning pain of the hands and feet are often the presenting complaint.

Hyperparathyroidism

Primary Hyperoxaluria (Oxalosis)

This is a rare cause of acute arthritis. Renal findings with hematuria, nephrolithiasis, and renal failure are more common presentations.

HEREDITARY DISORDERS

A number of inherited disorders may be associated with joint symptoms, although many feature arthralgias, bony prominence, or intermittent swelling rather than a florid arthritis.

◆ **Sickle Cell Disease**

The hand-foot syndrome, painful swelling of the hands and feet, is seen in young children with SS hemoglobin. Avascular necrosis due to sickling may produce painful attacks in older children as well, but usually in other areas (e.g., hips); children with SC disease are at particular risk.

Hemophilia

Clinical signs of hemarthrosis may mimic an acute arthritis.

Familial Mediterranean Fever

This uncommon but striking disorder is characterized by acute, recurrent attacks of fever, serositis, and arthritis. The fever lasts 24 to 48 hours and is accompanied by peritonitis, pleuritis, synovitis, and often an erysipelas-like erythema. The joint involvement tends to be monarticular.

Marfan Syndrome

Ehlers-Danlos Syndrome

The joint hyperextensibility may lead to dislocations and traumatic effusions.

Homocystinuria

Affected children have a marfanoid habitus, but the joints tend to have a restricted rather than hyperextensible mobility.

Stickler Syndrome (Hereditary Arthroophthalmopathy)

The large joints may be prominent, and joint pains may be present. Generally, affected children have flat facies, depressed nasal bridge, deafness, myopia, and hypotonia. The joints tend to be hyperextensible.

MIMICS OF ARTHRITIS

Periarticular Cellulitis

May mimic a septic arthritis.

Hypermobility Syndrome

Children with joint hypermobility commonly present with leg and joint aches, sometimes with joint effusions, mimicking arthritis.

Patellofemoral Pain Syndrome

This relatively common cause of knee pain rarely may produce effusions; it may be a familial trait or occur after trauma.

Subluxation of Patella

Characterized by the sudden onset of pain and leg instability. A joint effusion may follow the subluxation, which has usually resolved by the time the adolescent is examined. Check for excessive lateral mobility of the patella.

Osteochrondritis Dissecans

An effusion may accompany the punched-out bone disorder.

Henoch-Schönlein Purpura

This relatively common vasculitis of unknown etiology is often categorized with the rheumatic diseases. The rash—purpuric, petechial or, occasionally, urticarial—is characteristic and is most prominent on the lower extremities, although it sometimes occurs on the arms and face, and rarely on the trunk. Arthralgia with periarticular swelling, involving a few joints, occurs in about 40% of the cases. Abdominal pain, nephritis, hypertension, and unusual areas of edema are frequently found.

Idiopathic Chondrolysis

Pain and limp in adolescence, with progressive loss of articular cartilage and loss of hip mobility, are characteristic features.

Popliteal (Baker) Cysts

The swelling, although popliteal, may cause knee pain and appear to be an arthritis. The synovial outpouching may follow a chronic arthritis.

Carpal Tarsal Osteolysis

This rare disease results in gradual disintegration of the carpal and tarsal bones. Other joints may be involved as well, with a clinical picture simulating that of rheumatoid arthritis.

Hypertrophic Osteoarthropathy

Arthralgia and occasionally a polyarthritis may precede the appearance of clubbing of the fingers.

Tietze Syndrome

The cause of the pain and swelling of costochondral junctions is unknown.

MISCELLANEOUS CAUSES

Cystic Fibrosis

Recurrent painful joint swelling has been reported in children with cystic fibrosis. Usually one or a few joints are involved during each short lived episode.

Thorn-Induced Arthritis

Unusual bacterial pathogens may be introduced into a joint by penetration with a thorn.

Whipple Disease

This rare disorder is characterized by diarrhea, malabsorption with steatorrhea, progressive weight loss, anemia, increased skin pigmentation, and joint symptoms, either arthralgias or arthritis. A Gram positive organism has been found on intestinal mucosal biopsies.

Villonodular Synovitis

This uncommon lesion produces masses of nodular synovium, resulting in a swollen joint. Aspirated synovial fluid is often dark and bloody or serosanguineous. Usually only one joint is affected.

Neuropathic Arthropathy

Swollen, tender, warm joints may result following recurrent episodes of inapparent trauma secondary to lack of sensory innervation (Charcot joint).

PSYCHOGENIC PAIN

Children may complain of joint pain as part of a conversion reaction. The joints are not swollen, hot, or erythematous, and the sedimentation rate is normal.

SUGGESTED READING

Birdi N, Allen U, D'Astous J. Poststreptococcal reactive arthritis mimicking acute septic arthritis: A hospital-based study. *J Pediatr Orthopaed* 1995;15:661–665.
Nocton JJ, Miller LC, Tucker LB, Schaller JG. Human parvovirus B-19 associated arthritis in children. *J Pediatr* 1993;122:186–190.
Schaller JG. Juvenile rheumatoid arthritis. *Pediatr Rev* 1997;18:337–349.

93

Fragile Bones/Recurrent Fractures

Young children, subjected to the same skeletal forces that would lead to soft-tissue injury in an adult (e.g., strain), may suffer a fracture, particularly around the epiphysis, because this area in growing children is weaker than ligaments or tendons. Nevertheless, the injury reflects an applied force, so physicians caring for children must be acutely aware of the possibility of child abuse in any child with a bone fracture. Rarely, other underlying problems with bone fragility are responsible. Most of these disorders can be separated by a careful history, and a physical and radiologic examination.

TRAUMA

◆ Child Abuse

The suspicion of abuse must always be entertained in children with trauma or fractures, particularly if the alleged history does not seem to fit the findings. Other manifestations such as failure to thrive, cutaneous lesions, poor hygiene, should be noted. One should always consider whether the explanation of the accidental trauma is plausible in light of the child's age and clinical findings.

◆ Accidents

The "accident prone" child may be unlucky enough to have repeated fractures.

DISORDERS WITH OSTEOPOROSIS

Osteogenesis Imperfecta

Undoubtedly many variants of osteogenesis imperfecta exist, but four general syndromes are often proposed. Be aware of the subtle forms, particularly type IV.

Type I

This is a dominantly inherited syndrome with osteoporosis leading to bone fragility. The sclerae are distinctly blue and hearing loss is common in the patient or the family. Other features include joint hypermobility, skeletal deformities, and easy bruisability. Fractures may be present at birth or begin at any time during infancy or childhood. Most patients are short in stature. The bones are usually slender, but otherwise relatively unremarkable. The family history is a key to diagnosis.

Type II

This autosomal recessive disorder is characterized by extreme bone fragility. Intrauterine or early infant death usually occurs. Wormian bones of the skull and significant deformities of the limbs are present. The skin is frequently fragile as well.

Type III

This is also an autosomal recessive variety characterized by severe bone fragility with multiple fractures and resultant severe, progressive deformities of the limbs and bones. The sclerae become progressively less blue with age. Growth failure is significant.

Type IV

A dominantly inherited osteopenic type with variable severity. The sclerae are not abnormally blue after early infancy. The incidence of hearing loss is low. Postnatal short stature is common as is bowing of the legs.

Exogenous Corticosteroids

Osteoporosis with bone fragility is a well-recognized complication of steroid therapy.

Immobilization Osteoporosis

Bone reabsorption continues in face of reduction of bone cell formation of matrix. When activity is resumed fractures may result. Children with paralytic disorders such as myelomeningocele, poliomyelitis, cerebral palsy, and arthrogryposis are particularly prone to fractures.

Rickets

Type I (Vitamin D Deficiency)

Osteoporosis may lead to fragile bones although other features of vitamin D deficiency rickets are usually more obvious. The deficiency may be the result of a lack of sunlight exposure, dietary lack, vitamin D malabsorption, liver disease, anticonvulsant drugs, renal disease, and vitamin D dependency.

Type II (Primary Phosphate Deficiency)

A host of disorders with different mechanisms resulting in phosphate deficiency may be seen. Disorders with renal tubule reabsorption problems include Fanconi syndrome (e.g., cystinosis, tyrosinosis, Lowe syndrome, etc.); renal tubular acidosis; genetic primary hypophosphatemia and hypophosphatemia associated with "nonendocrine" tumors. Phosphate deficiency or malabsorption may occur with parenteral hyperalimentation, low phosphate feeding in premature infants, and secondary to gastrointestinal binding with aluminum hydroxide.

Cushing Syndrome

Adrenocortical excess often leads to osteoporosis and fractures, particularly vertebral compressions.

Hyperparathyroidism

Hypercalcemic symptoms, anorexia, weakness, constipation, and polyuria overshadow bony problems. Bone pain, particularly in the back and lower extremities, is probably the result of microfractures. Pathologic fractures of long bones and vertebral compression may also occur. Radiographs show diffuse demineralization as well as localized areas of subperiosteal resorption.

Idiopathic Osteoporosis

The usual onset of this uncommon disorder is between 8 and 14 years of age. Fractures of the vertebrae and metaphyseal areas of long bones are most common. The disorder is self-limited and improves during adolescence. Low calcitriol has been found in some patients.

Protein Calorie Malnutrition

Osteopenia may result from severe malnourishment with resultant fragile bones. Diminished formation of collagen matrix as well as calcium deficiency may be operative.

Scurvy

Lack of vitamin C results in osteopenia with loss of trabecular structure and thinning of the cortices. Periosteal hemorrhages and submetaphyseal rarefaction are characteristic.

Copper Deficiency

Distorted bones, the result of osteopenia, are rarely due to a copper deficiency. Chronic intestinal malabsorption and Menke syndrome may be causes.

Homocystinuria

Osteoporosis leading to compression deformity of the vertebrae is a major manifestation of this inborn error. Dislocated lenses, thromboembolic phenomenon, and mental retardation are other features.

Primary Hyperphosphatasia

This rare disorder is characterized by proliferation of poorly mineralized subperiosteal osteoid. Bone thickening, pain, fractures, and deformity often result. The serum alkaline phosphatase is significantly high.

Osteoectasia

An autosomal recessive disorder characterized by small stature, large skull, progressive bowing of the legs and arms with pain, tenderness, and muscle weakness. The calvarium is thickened and tubular bones are expanded but demineralized.

Congenital Cutis Laxa and Osteoporosis

One case of apparent autosomal recessive inheritance has been described. The osteoporosis was incapacitating with multiple fractures.

DISORDERS WITH OSTEOSCLEROSIS

Osteopetrosis

Dense, marblelike bone is the classic radiologic appearance of this autosomal recessive disorder. Despite the density, the bone is brittle. The bone marrow is crowded out resulting in progressive anemia, thrombocytopenia, and propensity to infection. Sight and hearing are lost due to narrowing of cranial nerve foramina.

Pyknodysostosis

This rare disorder features short stature and craniofacial disproportion. The cranial sutures are widened and the fontanel remains open. The entire skeleton is dense.

Dysosteosclerosis

This rare autosomal recessive disorder includes short stature, failure to erupt permanent teeth, optic atrophy from sclerosis of the base of the skull, and other cranial nerve involvement. The bones are dense with vertebral platyspondyly and phalangeal tuft resorption.

MISCELLANEOUS DISORDERS

Bone Cysts and Tumors

Bone fragility occurs with a number of bony lesions, benign and malignant.

Polyostotic Fibrous Dysplasia

Pathologic fractures are prone to occur in the structurally unsound bone. McCune-Albright syndrome should be considered if hyperpigmented patches of skin and signs of endocrinopathy are present.

Trichorhinophalangeal Syndrome

Fractures are more frequent in this inherited disorder that features a pear shaped, bulbous nose, a long philtrum, a thin upper lip, and thin scalp hair. Multiple exostoses are common.

Primary Oxalosis

This rare inborn error results in widespread deposition of calcium oxalate crystals throughout the body. Symptoms usually begin before age 5, with nephrolithiasis and resulting urinary tract problems. Pathologic bone fractures occur later through cystic areas.

Pyle Disease

Significant flaring occurs at the metaphyses of tubular bones. Severe genu valgum develops early in life. There is an increased tendency to fractures of long bones.

Dyskeratosis Congenita

Skin findings predominate in this rare disorder that affects mostly males. Atrophy and pigmentation give the skin a reticulated pattern. Nail dystrophy occurs during childhood. The teeth are defective with early decay, and the hair is thin. Aplastic anemia develops in a significant number of young males.

Disseminated Nonossifying Fibromas with Café au lait spots (Jaffe-Campanacci Syndrome)

A rare disorder in which lytic lesions of long bones may lead to pathologic fractures.

Hallerman-Streiff Syndrome

In one family, two children who appeared to have this syndrome had intrauterine fractures.

SUGGESTED READING

Brunner R, Doderlein L. Pathologic fractures in patients with cerebral palsy. *J Pediatr Orthop B* 1996;5:232–238.

Carrie Fassler AL, Bonjour JP. Osteoporosis as a pediatric problem. *Pediatr Clin N Amer* 1995;42:811–824.

Steiner RD, Pepin M, Byers PH. Studies of collagen synthesis and structure in the differentiation of child abuse from osteogenesis imperfecta. *J Pediatr* 1996;128:542–547.

=====94=====
Asymmetry/Hemihypertrophy

Asymmetry of body parts exists in everyone to a minor degree. The left leg is usually longer than the right, and the right arm longer than the left; fortunately, this asymmetry is usually not noticeable. True, readily apparent asymmetry is unusual.

The following classification divides asymmetry into two types: hemihypertrophy (plasia) and hemidystrophy. In some cases, it may be difficult to tell whether one side is hypertrophic or the other is atrophic. In many of the disorders associated with asymmetry, the presence of other signs and symptoms provides diagnostic clues. Particularly noteworthy, however, is the association of congenital hemihypertrophy with tumors, especially Wilms' tumor and adrenocortical neoplasms.

HEMIHYPERTROPHY

♦ Idiopathic

Overgrowth of body parts may be localized to one area or involve an entire half of the body, or portions of the body on both sides may be affected. There is considerable variability in the severity of the deformity. Occurrence seems to be sporadic, although affected siblings have been described. Other associated abnormalities have been described in a significant number of cases, including mental retardation in as many as 25%, pigmented skin lesions, hemangiomas, and genitourinary anomalies. A distressing association of hemihypertrophy with neoplasms has also been described, most commonly Wilms' tumor, but also adrenocortical tumors and, less frequently, hepatoblastomas.

♦ Disturbances of Bone Growth

Longstanding Hyperemia

Overgrowth of a part may result from increased blood flow to growing bone. Causes may include arteriovenous fistulas, chronic osteitis, tuberculosis, arthritis, healing fractures, and neoplasms. Children with asymmetric chronic arthritis may have overgrowth of an extremity if the arthritis begins before age 7 years, and premature closure of an epiphysis if the arthritis begins after age 7 years.

Neurofibromatosis

This relatively common inherited disorder is characterized by multiple café au lait spots and later by the appearance of neurofibromas. A wide array of associated deformities and tumors may occur, including hemihypertrophy as well as bony reduction deformities.

Hemihypertrophy Associated with Soft-Tissue Abnormalities

Lymphedema

An extremity may appear hypertrophied because it is edematous (see Chapter 11, Edema).

Klippel-Trenaunay-Weber Syndrome

Hemihypertrophy may be associated with cutaneous hemangiomas, varicose veins, other cutaneous defects, visceromegaly, and a host of other anomalies.

Cutis Marmorata Telangiectatica

The skin has a reticulated vascular pattern.

Epidermal Nevus Syndrome

Hemihypertrophy may occur with peculiar linear or swirled, macular or verrucous skin lesions.

Hemihypertrophy Associated with Dysmorphogenic Syndromes

Beckwith-Wiedemann Syndrome

Important features of this disorder are postnatal somatic gigantism, macroglossia, omphalocele or umbilical hernia, transitory neonatal hypoglycemia, ear lobe grooves, and, in about 10%, hemihypertrophy. Wilms' tumor and other tumors have been described.

Russell-Silver Syndrome

Key features include prenatal growth deficiency, triangular facies, and clinodactyly of the fifth fingers. Hemihypertrophy has been described in some cases.

Langer-Giedion Syndrome

Exostoses, asymmetry, sparse hair, hypoplastic alar cartilage, protuberant ears, brachyclinodactyly, and mild mental retardation may be present.

Proteus Syndrome

Accelerated growth, macrocephaly, macrodactyly, thickening of plantar and palmar surfaces, epidermal nevi and other cutaneous changes are features of this syndrome. The hypertrophy increases over time. The "Elephant man" probably was affected with this disorder rather than neurofibromatosis.

Hypomelanosis of Ito

Hemihypertrophy has been described in association with this syndrome featuring swirls or patches of cutaneous hypopigmentation.

Multiple Pterygium Syndrome

Rarely, children with this disorder may have asymmetrical involvement, with one side or extremity larger than the other.

Hemihypertrophy, Macrodactyly, and Connective Tissue Nevi

A single case has been described.

HEMIDYSTROPHIES

Disturbances of Bone

Hypoplastic Bones

Short femora or tibiae are the most common.

Coxa Vara

Decreased angle of the head of the femur on the femoral shaft may give the impression of a shortened leg.

Developmental Dysplasia of the Hip

The dislocated leg appears to be shorter.

Multiple Exostoses

Bowing of the extremity secondary to exostosis gives an asymmetric appearance.

Epiphyseal Trauma

Interference with bone growth secondary to injury to the epiphysis will result in a shortened limb.

Conradi-Hunermann Syndrome

Shortening of an extremity may result from punctate mineralization in epiphyses. Scoliosis is common; the facies may be flattened, hair sparse, skin coarse, and cataracts present.

Ollier Disease

Masses of hyaline cartilage occur asymmetrically, leading to decreased growth of affected bones.

Maffucci Syndrome

Multiple hemangiomata appear after birth along with enchondromata, resulting in asymmetric retarded growth of bones.

Femoral Hypoplasia-Unusual Facies Syndrome

Most often both femurs are shortened.

Postmeningococcal Skeletal Dystrophy

Epiphyseal and metaphyseal damage may follow sepsis and DIC, especially with meningococcemia, resulting in asymmetry.

Linear Scleroderma

Bone growth may be retarded in areas of localized scleroderma.

Neurologic Insults

Asymmetric development of parts of the body may follow various neurologic insults.

Cerebral Palsy

Poliomyelitis

Meningomyelocele

Sturge-Weber Syndrome

Atrophy of one limb may occur contralateral to the leptomeningeal angioma.

Spinal Dysraphism

Strokes

Children who are predisposed to strokes (e.g., MELAS, coagulopathies, sickle cell disease) may have decreased bone growth on the affected side of the body.

Chromosomal Abnormality

Hemiatrophy has been observed in triploid and diploid mosaics. Other features include a very low birth weight, developmental retardation, and coloboma of the iris.

Congenital Torticollis

Asymmetry of the face will develop in children whose torticollis is not detected in early infancy.

SUGGESTED READING

Craft WW, Parker L, Stiller C, Cole M. Screening for Wilms' tumour in patients with aniridia, Beckwith Syndrome, or hemihypertrophy. *Med Pediatr Oncol* 1995;24:31–34.

Jaffe KM, Cohen MM Jr, Lemire RJ. Malformations of the limbs. In: Kelly VC, ed. *Practice of pediatrics*, vol. 10. Hagerstown: Harper & Row, 1987:1–45.

95

Muscle Weakness

Evaluation of muscle weakness in children presents an interesting challenge. A few disorders account for most cases seen in the average pediatric practice. However, when the diagnosis is not obvious, the cause may be any of numerous rare and unusual conditions with long and confusing names.

Diagnostic considerations include age at onset of the weakness; whether it occurred abruptly or developed slowly; whether there are associated systemic signs or symptoms; and, of course, whether there is a family history. It is also important to determine whether the weakness is static or progressive; whether it is focal or diffuse; and whether it is episodic or constant.

Results of the neurologic examination may indicate a specific anatomic site of the lesion. Upper motor neuron disease is suggested by increased muscle tone, increased deep tendon reflexes, clonus, presence of long tract signs, such as the Babinski response, and persistence of infantile reflexes. If the site of the disorder is a focus in the cerebral cortex, one-sided weakness, often with sensory loss is usually seen. Mental retardation may be part of the clinical picture. In spinal cord disease, the weakness is usually bilateral. Anterior horn cell disease is likely to be associated with decreased muscle tone, profound weakness, hyporeflexia, muscle atrophy and fasciculations, and the absence of sensory changes. Peripheral nerve disorders produce weakness, more pronounced distally, with sensory changes; deep tendon reflexes are usually absent or diminished. In myopathies, the weakness is usually proximal, and the deep tendon reflexes are reduced in proportion to the weakness; sensory changes are not part of the picture.

Weakness must be differentiated from other conditions such as ataxia, hypotonia, vertigo, and incoordination. In the following classification, disorders causing weakness are grouped according to mode of onset; however, there may be some overlap among categories.

♦ Causes to Consider

Down Syndrome	Werdnig-Hoffmann Disease
Prader-Willi Syndrome	Conversion Reaction
Guillain-Barré Syndrome	Hypokalemia
Dermatomyositis	Duchenne Muscular Dystrophy
Myasthenia Gravis	Acute Infectious Myositis

DISORDERS WITH ACUTE ONSET

◆ Acute Infectious Myositis

This disorder is most commonly associated with influenzal infections. Calf and thigh pain are often severe and overshadow the weakness. Muscle enzyme levels are elevated; myoglobinuria may be a finding. Bacterial myositis is relatively uncommon and is more likely to be unilateral.

◆ Guillain-Barré Syndrome

Etiology is varied. Development of distal paresthesias, often with muscle pain, may be sudden or gradual, followed by a progressive ascending muscle weakness, almost always symmetric. Deep tendon reflexes are lost. Cranial nerve involvement occurs in less than one half of the cases. It often occurs 1 to 3 weeks after a nonspecific respiratory or gastrointestinal tract illness. Specific infectious agents incriminated include cytomegalovirus, Epstein-Barr virus, enterovirus, mycoplasma, and *Campylobacter jejuni* as well as after immunization. Occasionally, the onset may be more insidious.

Trauma

Weakness or paralysis may follow trauma to the head, spine, nerve roots, muscles, or peripheral nerves.

◆ Hypokalemia

Loss of potassium from the gastrointestinal tract or kidneys, increased loss associated with drug therapy, or by iatrogenic induction may result in profound weakness. An ileus is often present.

Organophosphate Poisoning

Weakness is overshadowed by other symptoms including salivation, sweating, and tearing; coughing, choking, and dyspnea; vomiting, diarrhea, and abdominal cramps; anxiety, seizures, and confusion; and numerous other signs.

Atropine Poisoning

Mucous membranes are dry, and pupils are dilated; erythema of skin, fever, restlessness, and confusion are common.

Herpes Zoster

Weakness may occur in the distribution of the involved peripheral nerve, along with the cutaneous vesicles.

Infectious Mononucleosis

Generalized or focal areas of weakness may occur.

Botulism

Common presenting signs are diplopia, photophobia, and blurred vision, followed by difficulty in swallowing and weakness. In infants, constipation may be the first symptom, followed by decreased feeding and ptosis.

Tick Paralysis

The first symptoms may be some irritability and anorexia followed by an ascending weakness. Although the onset of weakness is often rapid, at times the weakness may develop over weeks. Always check the nuchal and occipital skin for the presence of a tick. Removal of the tick is curative, although sometimes more slowly than expected.

♦ Conversion Reaction

Hysterical weakness may be a reaction to rape, sexual abuse, or other stressful situations. The reflexes are normal and sensation is intact or altered in non-anatomical patterns.

Acute Demyelinating Encephalomyelitis

Must be differentiated from multiple sclerosis, which it closely resembles.

Brachial Plexus Neuropathy

The acute onset is characterized by pain, weakness, and muscle wasting of the upper extremity. It is usually seen in young adults. The cause is unknown. The neuropathy in infants is present at birth and usually associated with a difficult delivery.

Multiple Sclerosis

Very uncommon under age 10. Unlike acute demyelinating encephalomyelitis (ADEM), it has a remitting and relapsing course. Gait disturbances, because of leg weakness, are common.

Epidural Abscess

Fever, back pain, and lower extremity weakness are typical; paralysis may occur rapidly if the problem goes untreated.

Transverse Myelitis

Back pain with the rapid onset of a flaccid paralysis is characteristic.

Myoglobinuria

Etiology is varied. Usually sudden onset of muscle pain with weakness occurs, followed by the passage of dark urine.

Polyarteritis Nodosa

Affected children generally have fever, abdominal pain, muscle pain and tenderness, arthritis, and nodular skin lesions, often purpuric.

Anterior Spinal Artery Occlusion

The occlusion may be a result of trauma or local infection, a hypercoagulable state, or embolism. If occlusion occurs in the lumbar spine, weakness of the lower extremities, loss of deep tendon reflexes, and bladder difficulties occur.

Septic Arthritis/Osteomyelitis

A pseudoparalysis may occur in the involved extremity.

Acute Central Cervical Cord Syndrome

This syndrome is produced by minor trauma to the cervical spine. It is characterized by more motor impairment of the upper than lower extremities; flaccid upper extremities with decreased or absent DTRs, while the lower extremities are spastic with increased reflexes.

Poliomyelitis

This disorder was formerly a common and important cause of flaccid weakness. There is usually a prodrome of fever, headache, vomiting, and diarrhea, followed by back pain, muscle tenderness, drowsiness, irritability, and stiff neck.

Diphtheria Toxin

Early signs include palatal paralysis, resulting in a nasal voice, difficulty in swallowing, and blurred vision, followed by other signs of cranial nerve involvement, loss of reflexes, and a neuropathy.

ACUTE ONSET-EPISODIC

Hypokalemic Periodic Paralysis

Periodic attacks of weakness may be hereditary or associated with chronic renal disease, hyperthyroidism, or aldosteronism; the ingestion of excessive amounts of licorice has also been implicated. In the familial form, attacks most often begin in adolescence. Quadriplegia and areflexia without pain may occur. Duration of weakness is a few hours to 2 days.

Hyperkalemic Periodic Paralysis

Attacks usually begin in the first decade; they may occur daily or several times a day but are less severe than in the hypokalemic form. Calf muscles may be enlarged. Weakness of facial muscles and myotonia are common.

Sodium Responsive Periodic Paralysis

Onset is during the first decade. Attacks are severe, with quadriplegia and bulbar muscle involvement. Each episode may last 2 to 3 weeks, but oral or intravenous sodium chloride has been found effective.

Periodic Paralysis with Cardiac Dysrhythmias

Onset is during the first or second decade; attacks may occur at monthly intervals; they are of moderate severity; and they last 1 to 2 days.

Paroxysmal Paralytic Myoglobinuria

Onset is usually before 20 years of age. Recurrent attacks of muscle cramps with weakness and excretion of myoglobin in the urine are characteristic.

Acute Intermittent Porphyria

Attacks generally involve abdominal pain, disturbances of consciousness, apparent psychosis, seizures, and a rapidly progressing peripheral neuropathy. Urine is burgundy red. Onset is rare before puberty.

Aldosteronism

Muscle weakness may be episodic and can progress to paralysis. The lower extremities are more severely affected than the upper ones. Weakness is the result of potassium depletion. Other symptoms include polydipsia, polyuria, and hypertension.

Hyperthyroidism

There may be episodic muscle weakness associated with hypokalemia.

McArdle Disease (Glycogen Storage Disease, Type V)

Muscle weakness, stiffness, and painful cramps occur only after moderately severe exercise and they disappear with rest. Inheritance pattern is autosomal recessive.

Paramyotonia Congenita

Weakness is aggravated by cold and exercise. Findings on neurologic examination are normal except for percussion myotonia of the tongue or thenar eminence. Speech may be dysarthric after the ingestion of ice cream. Inheritance pattern is autosomal dominant.

Thiamine-Responsive Pyruvate Dehydrogenase Complex Deficiency

SUBACUTE ONSET

♦ Guillain-Barré Syndrome

The onset may at times be insidious.

♦ Dermatomyositis

Symptoms are similar to those of polymyositis, but skin changes or discoloration of the upper eyelids, a facial butterfly erythema, or more commonly, erythematous papules over knees, elbows, and knuckles may also be findings.

Polymyositis

Onset can be sudden or chronic. There is a proximal muscle weakness of the pelvic and shoulder girdles. Muscles commonly ache and are tender to palpation. Muscle enzyme levels are increased; dysphagia and neck weakness are common.

Systemic Lupus Erythematosus

Muscle weakness is rarely an initial complaint. Arthritis, fever, rashes, and evidence of nephritis are common.

Heavy Metal Poisoning

Lead

Signs of peripheral neuropathy such as footdrop may precede evidence of encephalopathy. Weakness may be symmetric.

Mercury (Acrodynia)

Hypotonia is often severe. Affected children are very irritable, with photophobia, absent reflexes, weakness, erythema, tremors, and increased sweating and salivation.

Arsenic

Following acute ingestion, gastrointestinal symptoms predominate. If the child survives, painful paresthesias, followed by symmetric weakness, occur within 1 to 6 weeks.

Thallium

Acute ingestion results in profound weakness, first with paresthesias, followed later by hair loss.

Gold and Zinc

Gold and zinc poisoning are rare causes of weakness.

Renal Disease

In chronic renal disorders with potassium loss, muscle weakness may be a symptom.

Brain Tumors

Cerebral hemisphere tumors produce a unilateral progressive spastic paraplegia.

Cat-Scratch Disease

If they occur, neurologic symptoms appear days to weeks after the initial adenitis. Fever, headache, weakness, and paralysis may be present. Encephalitis is more common, however. Osteolytic lesions may be present.

Steroid Myopathy

Excess production as in Cushing syndrome or more commonly from exogenous (iatrogenic) treatment may result in progressive muscle weakness, particularly proximally.

Brainstem Tumors

These tumors generally produce, among other symptoms, a progressive, symmetric spastic paraplegia or quadriplegia.

Spinal Cord Tumors

Spinal cord tumors may produce a flaccid weakness at the level of the lesion and a spastic weakness below. Extramedullary tumors may be associated with back pain, weakness, and, in some cases, bladder or bowel dysfunction. Intramedullary tumors are painless and result in a symmetric weakness.

Hyperparathyroidism

Proximal muscle weakness and wasting, hypotonia and discomfort on movement with increased or decreased deep tendon reflexes, and muscle cramps have been described in hypercalcemia.

Hypopituitarism

Weakness and muscle atrophy may be part of the clinical picture.

Kocher-Debré-Sémélaigne Syndrome

Affected children appear to have well-developed musculature but are weak. The condition is secondary to hypothyroidism.

Hyperthyroid Myopathy

Rarely, proximal muscle weakness may be the initial symptom.

Neoplasia

Asymmetric weakness may be secondary to infiltrates of peripheral nerves or compression of nerves from tumors such as Hodgkin disease. In occult malignancies, myopathy may be a presenting sign.

Thiamine Deficiency

This is rare in childhood. Edema of the extremities, cardiomegaly, generalized hypotonia, and weakness may be present.

Scleroderma

Very rarely, weakness may occur without obvious skin changes.

CONGENITAL OR ONSET IN EARLY INFANCY

◆ Down Syndrome

◆ Prader-Willi Syndrome

Neonatal hypotonia may be severe. Hypogonadism, small penis, decreased reflexes, and retardation occur. Later, hyperphagia leads to obesity. Affected children are short in stature.

◆ Werdnig-Hoffmann Disease

This disorder is also called infantile spinal muscular atrophy; it is the most common cause of severe hypotonia and progressive weakness during the first year of life. Diminished or absent reflexes, fasciculations of the tongue, and diaphragmatic breathing may be present. Inheritance pattern is autosomal recessive.

◆ Myasthenia Gravis

Onset in about one third of cases is at birth. Ptosis, difficulty in sucking, and respiratory difficulties may be present.

Cerebral Palsy

This disorder has a mixture of neurologic findings, the result of insults to the central nervous system causing spastic or flaccid weakness, poor coordination, lack of balance, and abnormal posturing.

Hydrocephalus

May cause weakness or spasticity.

Benign Congenital Hypotonia

The etiology is poorly understood. Many cases probably represent primary muscle disease; there is a tendency to improve with age.

Congenital Laxity of Ligaments

If laxity is severe, the child may appear weak.

Myotonic Dystrophy

Weakness and muscular wasting may begin at any age. Infants have difficulty in swallowing and delay in achieving developmental milestones. Maternal myotonia may be disclosed by shaking hands with her. Ptosis of eyelids and atrophy of facial muscles may occur early; cataracts, balding, and testicular atrophy occur later. The myopathy is associated with myotonia.

Tay-Sachs Disease

Affected infants appear normal until 4 to 6 months of age, when diminished muscle tone becomes evident. Loss of developmental milestones, progressive weakness, and decreased vision or blindness with a macular cherry red spot are typical. Hyperacusis, myoclonic seizures, and generalized seizures occur. Affected infants are usually of Eastern European Jewish ancestry; inheritance pattern is autosomal recessive.

Pompe Disease (Glycogen Storage Disease, Type II)

The metabolic defect is a deficiency of acid maltase. Significant hypotonia and weakness are present from early infancy. The tongue becomes enlarged; cardiomegaly develops; and swallowing and respiratory difficulties become major problems. Death occurs in early infancy.

Arthrogryposis Multiplex Congenita

Multiple contractures of arms and legs are present at birth. There are various types, some with decreased anterior horn cells.

Lowe Syndrome

Significant hypotonia, cataracts, growth failure, severe retardation with proteinuria, aminoaciduria, and acidosis are findings. Inheritance pattern is sex-linked recessive.

Myopathies

Over the past two decades, a number of primary muscle disorders have been described. In all forms, symptoms may be similar, but characteristic findings on muscle biopsy allow differentiation.

Central Core Disease

Hypotonia and weakness are evident in infancy; motor milestones are delayed. Osteoarticular problems, including dislocated hips, kyphoscoliosis, and flatfeet, are common.

Nemaline Myopathy

Weakness and hypotonia may be present at birth or appear much later. Affected children have a long, thin face and slender body build. There is gross motor weakness, but fine motor ability is undisturbed. Reflexes are variably affected. Inheritance pattern is autosomal dominant or recessive.

Myotubular Myopathy

Weakness and hypotonia may be present at birth or appear later. Most patients have facial weakness or extraocular movement problems. Deep tendon reflexes are normal or absent.

Mitochondrial Myopathies

This form probably represents a mixed bag of disorders. In some cases, a hypermetabolic state occurs, with weakness, hyporeflexia, profuse sweating, dyspnea, palpitations, polydipsia, polyuria, polyphagia, and unexplained rises in body temperature.

Canavan Disease

Symptoms appear in the first 6 months of life. Developmental failure, hypotonia, and moderate to severe head enlargement are early signs; spasticity and blindness occur later.

Gaucher Disease

The infantile form is characterized by a severe neurologic deficit with generalized hypotonia, opisthotonos, rigidity, dysphagia, laryngeal spasms, and mental and motor deterioration. Splenomegaly is followed by hepatomegaly.

Krabbe Disease (Globoid Leukodystrophy)

Psychomotor development is normal until 4 to 6 months of age, when progressive deterioration begins. Hypotonia is followed by progressive spasticity. Inheritance pattern is autosomal recessive.

Generalized Gangliosidosis

Psychomotor retardation appears early in infancy. Hypotonia, facial and peripheral edema, frontal bossing, lowset ears, alveolar ridge hypertrophy, and hepatomegaly followed by splenomegaly are characteristic.

Dejerine-Sottas Disease (Progressive Hypertrophic Interstitial Neuropathy)

Delayed development is usually noted in early infancy. There is progressive weakness, especially in the lower extremities; sensory involvement results in ataxia. Nystagmus is common, as are muscle cramps. Palpation discloses peripheral nerve enlargement.

Congenital Hypomyelination Neuropathy

Symptoms are similar to those of Dejerine-Sottas disease but are more severe. Deep tendon reflexes are absent.

Hyperlysinemia

Mental and physical retardation occurs with hypotonia and laxity of ligaments.

Atonic Diplegia

Nonprogressive, generalized muscle weakness is characteristic. The cause is unknown. Leg weakness is usually more pronounced than arm weakness. Reflexes most frequently are hypoactive but may be normal.

Congenital Choreoathetosis and Congenital Ataxia

Affected infants may have significant hypotonia and weakness during the first year of life. Ataxia and posturing should be noticeable.

Glycogen Storage Disease, Type III

The onset of symptoms is in the first 6 months of life, with failure to thrive, hepatosplenomegaly, and liver failure with cirrhosis. Retarded muscular development and weakness with hypotonia may also be findings.

Congenital Hemiplegia

Congenital hemiplegia may be the result of acquired injuries to the brain, frequently causing porencephaly. A genetic form of porencephaly has been described.

Lysinuric Protein Intolerance

This rare autosomal recessive disorder also features hepatosplenomegaly and osteoporosis.

Megalencephaly, Muscle Weakness, and Myoliposis

A number of children with these features were found to have a carnitine deficient myopathy. May be part of the spectrum of Ruvalcaba-Myhre-Smith syndrome.

ONSET IN LATE INFANCY OR EARLY CHILDHOOD

♦ Duchenne-Type Muscular Dystrophy

Onset of symptoms is between 2 and 4 years of age. Affected children are often late in beginning to walk, with steady progression of weakness. Calf muscles appear enlarged. Reflexes are decreased or absent. Two thirds of the cases are hereditary (sex-linked recessive); one third are sporadic. Muscle enzyme levels are elevated.

Emotional Deprivation

Weakness and hypotonia may also appear earlier in infancy. Growth rate may be diminished. A change in environment brings about improvement.

Vitamin E Deficiency

Malabsorption of vitamin E leading to prolonged deficiency results in multiple neurologic signs. Hyporeflexia is the initial warning.

Craniovertebral Anomalies

Spastic weakness with increased deep tendon reflexes is characteristic.

Basilar Impression

The cervical spine invaginates into the base of the cranium. Abnormalities of the cervical vertebrae, such as the Klippel-Feil syndrome, may have this problem. Occipital headaches, lower cranial nerve palsies, nystagmus, and spastic paraplegia or quadriplegia may be seen.

Occipitalization of Atlas; Atlantoaxial Dislocation; Separated Odontoid Process of Axis

There may be neck pain, ataxia, and posterior column deficits with numbness and pain in the arms and legs. The odontoid may compress the posterior vertebral artery giving rise to cranial nerve abnormalities as well.

Ataxia Telangiectasia

Ataxia develops during the first 2 years of life. Progressive ataxia, choreoathetosis, oculocutaneous telangiectasia, and recurrent sinopulmonary infections develop after the ataxia. Hypotonia and weakness occur in later stages.

Sulfatide Lipidosis (Metachromatic Leukodystrophy)

Onset of symptoms is by the end of the first year of life. Progressive weakness, hypotonia, and mental deterioration develop. Swallowing difficulties, optic atrophy, third or fourth cranial nerve palsies, nystagmus, and ataxia are prominent. There are three forms: infantile, juvenile, and adult. Inheritance pattern is autosomal dominant.

Subacute Necrotizing Encephalomyelitis

Onset of symptoms usually begins at less than 2 years of age. Feeding difficulties, vomiting, progressive hypotonia and weakness, asthmalike attacks, nystagmus, and normal or increased deep tendon reflexes are found.

Giant Axonal Neuropathy

Symptoms begin at 2 to 3 years of age, with clumsy gait and progressive weakness. Kinky hair is common; reflexes are absent.

Chediak-Higashi Syndrome

Features include defective pigmentation of hair and skin with pancytopenia, increased susceptibility to infections, and later, lymphatic malignancies. Mental retardation, seizures, and muscle weakness are common.

Refsum Disease

This disease is characterized by ichthyosis, hearing deficit, ataxia, and a polyneuritis with distal weakness.

Familial Spastic Paraplegia

Progressive spasticity and weakness of the lower extremities without sensory changes begin in the first or second decade.

Late Infantile Acid Maltase Deficiency

Slow or regressing motor development, hip weakness, calf muscle hypertrophy, and toe walking from Achilles tendon contracture are found.

Infantile Neuroaxonal Dystrophy

Onset of symptoms is late in infancy, with progressive weakness, muscle atrophy, and hypotonia. Urinary retention, nystagmus, and blindness develop. Inheritance pattern is autosomal recessive.

Kugelberg-Welander Disease (Juvenile Spinal Muscular Atrophy)

Onset may be in childhood to adolescence. Proximal weakness and atrophy begin first in the legs. This slowly progressive disease is often mistaken for muscular dystrophy. Reflexes are diminished or absent.

Abetalipoproteinemia

Early in infancy, steatorrhea and abdominal distension develop; growth rate is retarded. By 7 to 8 years of age, ataxia and muscle weakness are present. Later visual acuity is lost, and retinitis pigmentosa and nystagmus develop. Ptosis and weak extraocular movements are present; deep tendon reflexes are absent, and loss of position and vibration sensation occurs. Inheritance pattern is autosomal recessive.

Tangier Disease

Hepatosplenomegaly and significant orangish yellow tonsillar enlargement with a variable peripheral neuropathy are present. Inheritance pattern is autosomal recessive.

Diaphyseal Dysplasia (Engelmann Disease)

Leg weakness and pain are characteristics of this hereditary bone disorder.

ONSET IN LATE CHILDHOOD OR ADOLESCENCE

◆ Myasthenia Gravis

Progressive fatigability is typical. Younger children have generalized muscle weakness and partial or complete external ophthalmoplegia. Ptosis is common. Repetitive movements bring out weakness.

Diastematomyelia/Spinal Dysraphism

Foot abnormalities, such as severe pes cavus, are common. Spastic weakness of lower legs, bladder dysfunction and muscular atrophy develop. There may be cutaneous abnormalities over the spine.

Charcot-Marie-Tooth Disease (Progressive Neuropathic [Peroneal] Muscular Atrophy)

Footdrop is often the first symptom; pes equinus deformity develops later. Reflexes are often absent; lower leg muscular atrophy is characteristic. Symptoms usually become apparent late in the second decade.

Limb Girdle Muscular Dystrophy

Slowly progressive weakness begins between 4 and 15 years of age. Pseudohypertrophy of calves and low-back pain may be clues. Inheritance pattern is autosomal recessive.

Facioscapulohumeral Dystrophy

Onset of weakness is usually between 12 and 20 years, often with orbicularis oris, neck, and pectoral muscle weakness, and winging of the scapulae. Inheritance pattern is autosomal dominant.

Adrenomyeloneuropathy

An X-linked disorder that presents with slow onset of Addison disease symptoms, including weakness, spasticity, and sensory disturbances in the legs.

Carnitine Deficiency

This disorder produces progressive muscle weakness and liver enzyme abnormalities. Myopathic facies and ptosis are present. Onset is usually before 10 years of age.

Amyotrophic Lateral Sclerosis

This disorder is rare in childhood. Muscle weakness and wasting, fasciculations, spasticity, and hyperactive reflexes are findings.

Uremia

Is a rare cause of weakness in childhood. Peripheral neuropathy is characterized by dysesthesias, especially burning sensations, followed by slowly progressive weakness.

Diabetic Neuropathy

This is an unlikely cause of weakness in children.

Syringomyelia

Progressive inability to feel pain or temperature sensations develops, followed by weakness with decreased or absent deep tendon reflexes.

Glycogen Storage Disease, Type III

Features include hepatomegaly, hypoglycemia, and mild growth failure with late onset of weakness.

Muscle Phosphofructokinase Deficiency

Motor development during the first decade is usually normal, but children have decreased exercise tolerance. They may complain of muscle stiffness and weakness and may have muscle cramps.

Late-Onset X-Linked Muscular Dystrophy (Becker)

The clinical picture resembles that in Duchenne-type muscular dystrophy, but onset is later (in the second decade), and progression is slower. Pseudohypertrophy and Gower sign are present. Severity of disease seems to be consistent in affected families.

SUGGESTED READING

Lewis DW, Berman PH. Progressive weakness in infancy and childhood. *Pediatr Rev* 1987;8:200–208.
Patterson MC, Gomez MR. Muscle disease in children: a practical approach. *Pediatr Rev* 1990;12:73–82.
Swaiman KF. *Pediatric neurology, principles and practice,* 2nd ed. St. Louis: Mosby, 1994.

96

Muscular Hypertrophy

Muscular hypertrophy is not a common sign or complaint in the pediatric age group. Although adolescents may develop hypertrophied muscles with exercise, in younger children this condition is unusual.

The causes of muscular hypertrophy have been divided into three categories: generalized, localized, and apparent. In the last group, loss of adipose or nearby muscle tissue creates the appearance of muscular hypertrophy.

GENERALIZED HYPERTROPHY

- ### Anabolic Steroids

  Adolescents, both male and female, abuse anabolic steroids.

- ### Beckwith-Wiedemann Syndrome

  In the neonatal period macroglossia and an omphalocele or umbilical hernia are quite noticeable. Hypoglycemia is common. The infants may be large at birth or grow rapidly, thereafter. The viscera are large as well.

Adrenogenital Syndrome (Congenital Adrenal Hyperplasia)

21-hydroxylase deficiency is the most common enzymatic defect. There is nearly always an excessive production of adrenal androgens. Girls show progressive virilization. The children grow rapidly and have increased muscle mass as well.

Virilizing Adrenal Tumors

In both boys and girls, the musculature is well developed, and linear growth is rapid. Girls become hirsute and virilized. The prepubertal boy has enlarged genitalia without testicular development.

Kocher-Debré-Sémélaigne Syndrome

Muscular hypertrophy may occur in longstanding untreated hypothyroidism, either congenital, acquired, or induced. The hypertrophy is reversible on treatment of the hypothyroidism.

Acromegaly

Excessive secretion of growth hormone after epiphyseal closure results in generalized enlargement, particularly of distal parts of the body. Initially, there are generalized muscle hypertrophy and increased strength; however, muscle weakness occurs later.

Myotonia Congenita (Thomsen Disease)

Affected children have generalized muscular hypertrophy to the degree that they resemble body builders, but the muscles are weak. Relaxation of voluntary muscle contraction is delayed. Newborns may have sucking and feeding difficulties and, later, slow motor development. The muscular difficulties are generally not noted until childhood or adolescence when difficulty in releasing grasped objects or initiating movements becomes obvious.

Paramyotonia Congenita

In this disorder the myotonia is aggravated by cold; it is associated with mild weakness; and it is not progressive. Inheritance pattern is autosomal dominant.

Myotonic Chondrodystrophy (Schwartz-Jampel)

This unusual disorder is characterized by short stature, kyphoscoliosis, pectus carinatum, a small mouth with a pinched facial expression, myotonia, and muscular hypertrophy. Inheritance pattern is autosomal recessive.

Myhre Syndrome

In addition to muscular hypertrophy, the main features include short stature, mental retardation, blepharophimosis, decreased joint mobility, thick calvarium, broad ribs, hypoplastic iliac wings, and short tubular bones.

Generalized Muscle Enlargement, Severe Mental Retardation, and Central Nervous System Defects

This triad was described by DeLange in 1934. There is some question about whether this represents a single entity. The infants described had hypertonia and microcephaly with severe central nervous system defects including porencephaly.

LOCALIZED HYPERTROPHY (CALVES)

♦ Duchenne-Type Muscular Dystrophy

This is the classic condition with calf pseudohypertrophy. The child may walk later than expected, but an abnormal gait is not noted until 3 or 4 years of age. The muscle weakness is progressive and initially most prominent in the hip girdle and later the shoulder girdle. The quadriceps, infraspinatus, and deltoid muscle groups may be enlarged as well.

X-Linked Muscular Dystrophy (Becker)

The clinical picture resembles that in the Duchenne-type, but the signs develop later and progress slower with an onset often in the second decade.

Autosomal Recessive Pseudohypertrophic Muscular Dystrophy

Features of proximal muscle weakness and calf hypertrophy occur in both sexes. The onset is between 2 and 14 years of age.

Limb-Girdle Muscular Dystrophy

Muscle weakness develops in one or both groups of girdle muscles. Calf muscle hypertrophy occurs in a few cases.

Hyperkalemic Periodic Paralysis

Attacks of muscle weakness lasting 1 to 2 hours typically occur after exertion. The paralysis usually develops over a period of 30 to 40 minutes. The calf muscle may be enlarged. Inheritance pattern is autosomal dominant.

Late Infantile Acid Maltase Deficiency

In addition to calf muscle hypertrophy, hip weakness, slow or regressive motor development, atonic anal sphincter, and Achilles tendon contractures may be found.

Phosphoglucomutase Deficiency

The deficiency results in calf hypertrophy, mild generalized weakness, regression of motor development, and toe walking.

APPARENT HYPERTROPHY

Lipodystrophy

Due to the loss of adipose tissue, the muscles in involved areas appear enlarged because of prominent muscle outline and veins.

Partial Lipodystrophy

Insidious loss of subcutaneous tissue from the face is first noted at about 5 years of age. The loss progresses to the neck, upper trunk, and arms but rarely to the lower extremities.

Total Lipodystrophy

In this form, there is actually an increase in muscle mass. The abdomen is prominent, and the liver is enlarged. Diabetes resistance to insulin therapy generally develops.

Kugelberg-Welander Disease

In the juvenile form, an abnormal gait develops between the ages of 2 and 17 years because of hip and thigh muscle weakness. Atrophy begins in the quadriceps and then involves the shoulder girdle. The calf muscles appear hypertrophied because of the severity of the quadriceps atrophy.

97

Bow Legs and Knock Knees

Most infants have some degree of bowing of the legs as a result of intrauterine position. This physiologic phenomenon is responsible for the bowing seen in most infants. The bowing will often give way to knock knees as the infant passes through the toddler stage. Pathologic conditions associated with bow legs have characteristic clinical or radiographic features that allow easy differentiation. Similarly, most children with knock knees are passing through a developmental phase, usually between 2 and 6 years of age, in which the condition is normal.

It should be noted that the Latin term "genu varum" is commonly but incorrectly used to refer to bow legs. Genu varum actually refers to knock knees, and genu valgum to bow legs (1). To avoid confusion, use of the straightforward descriptive terms is recommended.

BOW LEGS

♦ Physiologic Bowing

Most newborn infants have some degree of bowing, the result of intrauterine position with the legs crossed and flexed. The bowing will not begin to correct until some time after weight-bearing begins, usually at 6 to 12 months of age. A second form develops during the second year of life and is more common in black children. Most of these children also resolve their bowing spontaneously.

• Rickets

Rickets, either vitamin D deficient or vitamin D resistant, is often blamed for the physiologic bowing. Radiographic examination should be performed if the bowing increases with age rather than improving, or if the separation of the medial femoral condyles is excessive (5 cm or more when the medial malleoli are touching and the patellae are facing forward).

• Tibia Vara (Blount Disease)

This rather uncommon disorder results from a growth disturbance of the medial aspect of the proximal tibial epiphysis. It usually occurs in early walkers and is bilateral in 50% to 75% of cases. The bowing increases rather than decreases with age. There is an adolescent form in which bowing does not develop until 8 to 13 years of age and is unilateral in most cases.

Asymmetric Growth Disturbance (Post Traumatic)

Various types of injury to the distal femoral or proximal tibial epiphyses may result in subsequent bowing. Causes include trauma and osteomyelitis.

Familial Form

The bowing occurs in the lower third of the tibia so that the ankles seem to curve sharply inward.

Bowing with Internal Tibial Torsion

Physiologic bowing often accentuates the appearance of internal tibial torsion.

Rheumatoid Arthritis

Some children with rheumatoid arthritis will develop bowing of the legs, although many more have knock knees.

Achondroplasia

Hypochondroplasia

In this mild short-limbed dwarfism with normal head size, the bowing is mild, and there is also ligamentous laxity.

Hypophosphatasia

Resembles rickets, but the alkaline phosphatase is low.

Osteogenesis Imperfecta

Bowing occurs in all four types of osteogenesis imperfecta.

Metaphyseal Dysostosis

Short stature and bow legs are apparent by 2 years of age. Radiographic changes in the metaphyses confirm the diagnosis.

Enchondromatosis (Ollier Disease)

This bone disorder of unknown cause is characterized by radiolucencies in the metaphyses and diaphyses of long bones, resulting in asymmetric limited growth.

Multiple Epiphyseal Dysplasia

Short stature and irregular mottled epiphyses on radiographs are findings in this rare disorder. The legs may be bowed or have a knock-kneed appearance. Inheritance pattern is autosomal dominant.

Cartilage Hair Hypoplasia

This is a metaphyseal chondrodysplasia with features of short stature, fine sparse hair, and short limbs and hands. Mild bowing of the legs may be present.

Postmeningococcal Skeletal Dystrophy

Epiphyseal and metaphyseal damage may follow sepsis and DIC, especially with meningococcemia.

Weismann-Netter Syndrome

A rare skeletal dysplasia that may present in childhood with bowing, a delay in ambulation, or short stature, the latter becoming apparent during the adolescent growth spurt. Radiographic findings include characteristic bowing at the junction of the lower and middle thirds of the diaphysis of the tibiae and fibulae.

KNOCK KNEES

♦ Physiologic Knock Knees

Many children between 2 and 6 years of age pass through a knock-kneed phase. The natural history is one of improvement, usually by age 5; if it persists past age 8, the condition will not correct spontaneously. Obesity accentuates the problem.

♦ Flatfoot

Pronation of the foot will result in a knock-kneed appearance.

Trauma

An injury to the distal femoral epiphysis or proximal tibial epiphysis may result in knock knees or bow legs. Causes include trauma, osteomyelitis, and rickets. A unilateral knock knee is almost always pathologic.

Adolescent Knock Knees

Adolescents with knock knees are generally large in height, body build, and weight. The medial distal femoral condyles are higher than the lateral. The problem does not resolve spontaneously but rather tends to worsen with age.

Rheumatoid Arthritis

Children with juvenile rheumatoid arthritis are more likely to become knock kneed than bowlegged.

Renal Rickets

Early signs may be growth failure and knock knees. Other symptoms include pallor, polydipsia, and polyuria.

Vitamin D Resistant Rickets

The presenting symptom is usually a limb deformity, either bow legs or knock knees.

Coxa Vara

This chronic hip disorder can result in the development of a knock-knee deformity.

Chondroectodermal Dysplasia (Ellis-van Creveld Syndrome)

In this disorder, inherited as an autosomal recessive trait, features include sparse hair, defective nails and dentition, cardiac defects, dwarfism, and polydactyly.

Congenital Dislocation of the Patella

Permanent dislocation of the patella laterally will create a knock-kneed stance.

Diaphyseal Dysplasia (Camurati-Engelmann Disease)

The shafts of the femur and tibia become progressively thickened. The gait is often waddling, the limbs are thin, and leg pain is present even in infancy.

Diastrophic Dwarfism

This short-limbed dwarfism is characterized by severe club foot, limited flexion of some joints, a proximal thumb, and soft cystic masses in the auricles. Micrognathia and cleft palate may be present.

Morquio Syndrome

This is a mucopolysaccharidosis with features of short trunk, severe knock knees, short flat nose, wide mouth, and pectus carinatum.

Maroteaux-Lamy Syndrome (Mucopolysaccharidosis VI)

Coarse facies, growth deficiency, stiff joints, corneal opacities, and lumbar kyphosis are also common.

Multiple Epiphyseal Dysplasia Syndrome

Slow growth is noted in early childhood. The gait is waddling, and joints are stiff. Radiographs reveal small, irregular epiphyses.

Spondyloepiphyseal Dysplasia

Shortened trunk, kyphosis, short neck, and, eventually, stiff joints are features. Inheritance is sex-linked recessive.

Homocystinuria

In this aminoaciduria, affected children have a marfanoid appearance. Dislocated lenses, malar flush, mental deficiency, and arterial and venous thromboses are common.

REFERENCE

1. Houston CS, Swischuk LE. Varus and valgus—no wonder they are confused. *N Engl J Med* 1980; 302:471–472.

SUGGESTED READING

Greene WB. Genu varum and genu valgum in children: differential diagnosis and guidelines for evaluation. *Compr Ther* 1996;22:22–29.

Heath CH, Staheli LT. Normal limits of knee angle in white children—genu varum and genu valgum. *J Pediatr Orthop* 1993;13:259–262.

MacMahon EB, Casmines DB, Irani RN. Physiological bowing in children: an analysis of the pendulum mechanism. *J Pediatr Orthop* 1995;4:100–105.

98

Toeing In

In the evaluation of the relatively common parental concern about toeing in, examination of the child should begin at the toes and move up to the hip. This chapter presents the most likely causes grouped by the anatomic location of the underlying problem.

FOOT PROBLEMS

♦ Metatarsus Adductus

This deformity of the forefoot is most likely a result of forefoot position *in utero*. The medial deviation of the forefoot should be apparent at birth. The forefoot can be abducted and is not fixed. The adduction may be compounded by the sleeping position; for example, the infant may lie prone with the feet turned in.

Metatarsus adductus is the most common cause of toeing in in infants. Generally, the in-toeing corrects spontaneously.

♦ Metatarsus Varus

This is a congenital subluxation of the tarsometatarsal joint, with adduction of the metatarsals. It is the result of compression of the forefoot in adduction, *in utero*. A deep vertical crease is present on the medial side of the foot at the tarsometatarsal joint. Unlike metatarsus adductus, the adduction cannot be corrected by abducting using the pressure of the thumb. Serial casting is required, as early as possible after birth, to assure optimum results in correction.

♦ Talipes Equinovarus

In mild clubfoot, the forefoot adduction may be more severe than the eversion and equinus deformities.

Pronated Feet (Flatfeet)

The child with pes planus tends to stand with the feet in a valgus position, with the heel everted and the forefoot turned out. Because this position is not the most stable for walking or running, the child will toe-in to shift the center of gravity toward the center of the foot.

LEG PROBLEMS

♦ Internal Tibial Torsion

Internal tibial torsion is purported to be a common cause of in toeing. It is most likely the result of intrauterine positioning and is accentuated by infants sleeping prone. The simplest clinical examination for tibial torsion is comparison of the relative positions of the medial and lateral malleoli while the child sits with legs extended and the patellae pointing straight ahead. Normally the medial malleolus sits anterior to the lateral malleolus in the transmalleolar axis. Fortunately, the torsion corrects with time. Dennis-Browne splints, used so frequently in the past, are not necessary.

Knock Knees

Knock-kneed children toe-in in order to shift the body's center of gravity medially.

Tibia Vara (Blount Disease)

Bilateral involvement produces bow legs, often with resulting toeing in.

Bow Legs

Children with developmental bowing of the legs also tend to toe-in when they walk.

HIP PROBLEMS

♦ Femoral Anteversion

In this condition the head of the femur assumes a more anteriorly directed angle as it sits in the acetabulum. Toeing in is the result of an effort to create a more stable hip during walking. On examination, with the legs extended and the pelvis flat, there are excessive internal rotation (80° or more) and limited external rotation (30° or less) of the hips. In most cases the cause of femoral anteversion is unknown, but it can be associated with developmental hip dysplasia, Legg-Calvé-Perthes disease, or congenital talipes equinovarus.

This entity accounts for almost all children with toeing in after age 3 years, especially girls.

Paralytic Conditions

Toeing in may be seen in conditions such as cerebral palsy, as a consequence of poliomyelitis, or with myelomeningocele.

Spasticity of Internal Rotators of the Hip

This may be a consequence of cerebral palsy.

Maldirection of the Acetabulum

If the acetabulum is directed anteriorly, the child will toe-in to swing the femoral head back into the hip joint for stability.

SUGGESTED READING

Craig CL, Goldberg MJ. Foot and leg problems. *Pediatr Rev* 1993;14:395–400.

99

Toeing Out

Toeing out is a much less common problem than toeing in. In most cases, the toeing out is probably a result of intrauterine position. In most children with toeing out there is no pathologic process; the toeing out is idiopathic and requires no therapy.

The causes of toeing out are briefly outlined according to the anatomic location of the underlying problem.

FOOT PROBLEMS

Talipes Calcaneovalgus

In this positional deformity, the foot is extremely dorsiflexed and everted, but it is flexible rather than rigid. With passive exercise in infancy, rapid correction is the rule.

Everted Flatfeet

Children with hypermobile, pronated feet may stand in a toeing out position, but when walking they tend to toe-in to improve the center of gravity.

Triceps Surae Muscle Contracture

Children with cerebral palsy may have toeing out at the foot because of spasticity affecting the triceps surae muscles (gastrocnemius and soleus). The foot is held in an equinus position.

Vertical Talus (Rocker-Bottom Foot)

Children with congenital vertical talus have severe flatfoot. The forefoot is abducted and dorsiflexed.

LEG PROBLEMS

External Tibial Torsion

The condition may be present at birth or acquired. The medial malleolus lies much more anterior to the lateral malleolus than the normal 5° to 15°. External tibial torsion may be a consequence of femoral anteversion, in which external rotation of the hip is restricted, or of contracture of the iliotibial band, in which the internal rotation of the hip is limited.

Congenital Absence or Hypoplasia of the Fibula

In this uncommon congenital abnormality, shortening of the peroneal and triceps surae muscles results in bowing of the tibia and equinovalgus position of the foot. The lateral malleolus is absent.

HIP PROBLEMS

Femoral Retroversion

This condition is much rarer than femoral anteversion. The retroverted position of the femoral head results in limited internal rotation and excessive external rotation of the hip.

Flaccid Paralysis of the Internal Rotators of the Hip

Physiologic Rotation in Newborns

Newborns whose intrauterine position was cross-legged have a relative external rotation contracture of the hips. When the legs are extended the toes will point out. Internal rotation at the hip is limited but improves rapidly with age.

Maldirection of the Acetabulum

The acetabulum may face posteriorly, resulting in outward turning of the leg.

SUGGESTED READING

Craig CL, Goldberg MJ. Foot and leg problems. *Pediatr Rev* 1993;14:395–400.

100

Toe Walking

Toe walking is not a common primary complaint in childhood. This peculiarity of gait, nevertheless, may indicate an underlying disorder. Even in so-called idiopathic toe walking, increasing evidence suggests that there may be underlying neurologic disorders (1). The association with delayed language development is particularly fascinating (2).

PHYSIOLOGIC CAUSES

◆ Normal Variant

Toe walking may be seen intermittently in toddlers for the first 3 to 6 months after they begin ambulation. Joint mobility, reflexes, and development are normal.

◆ Habit

Toe walking here tends to be intermittent. Dorsiflexion of the ankles is normal, as are patellar reflexes and muscle tone. The child can usually be persuaded to walk with the feet in the normal position.

◆ Idiopathic

Accumulating evidence suggests that children who toe walk without other physical findings may actually have underlying neuropathic processes. In addition, the incidence of language delay in children with toe walking is impressive.

Infantile Autism

Lack of interpersonal relationships, perseverations, and language delay are characteristic.

DISORDERS WITH A SHORTENED ACHILLES TENDON

◆ Spastic Cerebral Palsy

This disorder is the commonest cause of pathologic toe walking. Depending on the type of cerebral palsy the abnormal gait may either be unilateral or bilateral. Associated signs include hyperactive reflexes, limited dorsiflexion of the ankle, tightness of extremity movement, and usually a delay in motor development.

Congenital Short Tendocalcaneus

In this uncommon cause of toe walking, the ankle is held in talipes equinus position. The knees must be fully extended to allow standing with the feet flat. Reflexes, muscle tone, and development are normal.

Late Infantile Acid Maltase Deficiency

Only a few patients have been described; they were asymptomatic during the first year of life but then developed a slowly progressive weakness. Symptoms may mimic those of Duchenne-type muscular dystrophy. The gastrocnemius and deltoid muscles may be firm and rubbery; Gower sign is present. Toe walking is secondary to Achilles tendon contracture.

Phosphoglucomutase Deficiency (Thomsen Disease)

The Achilles tendon is shortened, and calf muscles are bulky. One patient described had multiple episodes of supraventricular tachycardia in early infancy.

Spinocerebellar Degeneration

An abnormal gait develops in school-aged children, who eventually develop spasticity in their lower limbs and increasing ataxia, especially involving the upper extremities.

DISORDERS WITH A SHORTENED EXTREMITY

Spinal Dysraphism

Lipoma of the cauda equina may be associated with enuresis, foot deformity, or leg shortening. Diastematomyelia should be considered if a cutaneous abnormality, such as a patch of hair, pigment, skin dimple, or sinus, is present over the spine. Talipes equinovarus or a shortened lower limb may be present with these deformities.

Unilateral Hip Dislocation

Toe walking occurs on the affected side to compensate for the relative shortening of the leg. The range of motion of the affected hip is abnormal, particularly in abduction. Results of Trendelenburg test are positive.

MUSCULAR DISORDERS

● Duchenne-Type Muscular Dystrophy

Toe walking may occur early. Because inheritance is sex-linked, only boys are affected. Pseudohypertrophy of the calves, the presence of Gower sign, and elevated creatinine kinase levels are findings.

Viral Myositis

The acute onset of calf and thigh pain associated with influenzal infections may result in toe walking during the illness.

Myotonic Dystrophy

Weakness and muscle wasting may begin at any age. Ptosis of eyelids and atrophy of facial muscles may occur early. Myotonia is characteristic.

Emery-Dreifuss Muscular Dystrophy

Onset is in the first decade. Initial features are toe walking, partial flexion of the elbows, and inability to fully flex the neck and spine. A distinct pattern of contractures in the absence of major weakness is the earliest clue to diagnosis.

Hemangioma of Gastrocnemius Muscle

A few cases of the late onset of toe walking with a hemangioma in the muscle have been described.

REFERENCES

1. Eastwood DM, Dennett X, Shield LK, Dickers DR. Muscle abnormalites in idiopathic toe walkers. *J Pediatr Orthop B* 1997;6:215–218.
2. Shulman LH, Sala DA, Chu MLY, McCaul PR, Sandler BJ. Developmental implications of idiopathic toe walking. *J Pediatr* 1997;130:541–546.

101
Flatfeet

Evaluation of flatfeet should begin with a determination of whether the condition is flexible or rigid. Most cases of flatfeet are a result of ligamentous laxity, producing a hypermobile flatfoot. Rigid flatfeet are uncommon and are usually easily distinguishable.

FLEXIBLE FLATFEET

♦ Newborn Fat Pad

Parents may mistake the presence of the normal pad of fat that occupies the medial arch of the foot in infancy for a flatfoot. The fat pad gradually disappears over the first 2 to 3 years of life. Absolutely no therapy is required, merely patient explanation to the concerned parent.

♦ Ligamentous Laxity (Hypermobile)

The degree of normal joint extensibility shows great variation and may reflect a familial trait. Most children and adults with flatfeet have hypermobile joints as a result of ligamentous laxity. In a non–weight-bearing posture a medial arch appears to be present; on standing, however, the arch disappears, and the foot may tend to pronate (a combination of abduction and eversion) because the ligaments stretch. The condition is rarely symptomatic in children and requires no treatment. Other joints can be demonstrated to be hyperextensible as well, and examination of other family members usually reveals flatfeet or other evidence of the laxity.

Syndromes with generalized joint laxity and hypermobility include the following.

Down

Marfan

Ehlers-Danlos

Accessory Navicular Bone

Presence of this accessory bone, manifested by bony prominence at the arch, results in the loss of the principal support of the arch. Pain may be localized over the medial aspect of the foot, often because of a bursitis over the prominence, and along the posterior tibial tendon.

Talipes Calcaneovalgus

In this positional deformity found in infants, the foot is held dorsiflexed, giving a flatfoot appearance. The foot is flexible, however, and the position can be corrected easily.

RIGID FLATFOOT

• Vertical Talus (Rocker-Bottom Foot)

Infants born with this rare anomaly have a severe rigid flatfoot with the appearance of a rocking chair bottom. The heel is pointed downward, and the forefoot is held dorsiflexed. The vertical talus deformity may be seen in arthrogryposis or with meningomyelocele or the trisomy 18 syndrome.

• Short Achilles Tendon

Due to spasticity of the triceps surae group of muscles, dorsiflexion of the ankle past 90° is not possible. Hyperactive reflexes and ankle clonus may be present. Toe walking is common. This condition is most commonly found in children with cerebral palsy and, less frequently, in those with spinal epidural tumors.

• Tarsal Coalition

Fusion of the tarsal bones occurs because of congenital bars, especially between the calcaneus and navicular. The principal feature on examination is lack of subtalar motion. Symptoms of foot pain with activity or walking do not usually occur until adolescence.

Low Insertion of the Soleus Muscle

Some children with tight heel cords may have an abnormally low insertion of the soleus muscle that can be palpated on examination.

SUGGESTED READING

Craig CL, Goldberg MJ. Foot and leg problems. *Pediatr Rev* 1993;14:395–400.
Meehan P. Other conditions of the foot. In: Morrissy RT, ed. *Lovell and Winter's pediatric orthopaedics*, 3rd ed. Philadelphia: JB Lippincott, 1990:991–998.

102

Raynaud Phenomenon, Acrocyanosis, and Other Color Changes

Intermittent episodes of color change in the extremities, usually associated with cold exposure or emotional stress, are called Raynaud phenomenon. The color change is triphasic: white, blue, and then red. Acrocyanosis refers to a persistent dusky discoloration of the hands and feet, which may be cold and sweaty as well; the pallor and discomfort characteristic of Raynaud phenomenon do not occur. Chilblains (perniosis) is a persistent reddish-blue discoloration associated with chronic exposure to a cold, damp environment. Erythromelalgia is a curious disorder of the extremities characterized by attacks of localized redness, congestion, burning pain and increased heat of the extremities. Differentiation of these conditions is important for the purposes of both prognosis and treatment.

ACROCYANOSIS

The duskiness may be transient after cold exposure or may persist throughout winter and, in some cases, summer as well. Slight hyperesthesias may occur. Trophic changes of the distal fingers and toes do not occur. The color change is always symmetric.

♦ Transient Acrocyanosis

This type is commonly seen in newborn infants.

♦ Recurrent Acrocyanosis

Adolescent girls are most frequently affected; there is often a familial history of the condition.

Ehlers-Danlos Syndrome

Affected children may have acrocyanosis in addition to the characteristic loose jointedness, skin stretchability and fragility, and easy bruising.

• Infectious Mononucleosis

Cold-induced acrocyanosis has been described. Cold agglutinins may be demonstrated in blood samples.

Sympathomimetic Drugs

Imipramine

Syndrome with Ethylmalonic Aciduria

A number of cases of children with this syndrome have been described. Onset of the disorder followed termination of breast feeding. The clinical phenotype is characterized by orthostatic acrocyanosis, relapsing petechiae, chronic diarrhea, progressive pyramidal signs, mental retardation, and changes of brain MRI. Significant persistent ethylmalonic aciduria is found.

CHILBLAIN (PERNIOSIS)

This disorder is characterized by a relatively persistent bluish or vivid red discoloration of the extremities; it is seen in damp cold climates and affects particularly young girls; it is not commonly described in the United States. Warmer or dryer weather may bring about improvement. The discoloration tends to blanch on pressure. There may be a doughy swelling, nodules, and severe pruritus or burning. Subepidermal bullae may develop in severe disease.

RAYNAUD PHENOMENON/DISEASE

Episodic attacks of color changes of the fingers or other acral areas, generally consisting of pallor followed by cyanosis and redness on warming, may be precipitated by cold exposure and, occasionally, emotional stress. For prognostic purposes it is important to differentiate primary Raynaud syndrome from Raynaud phenomenon. Use of an ophthalmoscope to view nailfold capillaries has proven most helpful. Children with systemic sclerosis and dermatomyositis demonstrate enlarged capillary loops and reduction in numbers of loops. Antinuclear antibodies, when present are an important marker for the future development of connective tissue diseases.

♦ Primary Raynaud Disease

Criteria for diagnosis include (a) episodes of Raynaud phenomenon brought on by cold or emotion; (b) bilateral involvement; (c) absence of extensive gangrene; (d) exclusion of any secondary causes; and (e) a history of symptoms for 2 or more years. It is most commonly seen in women; the hands and, less often, the feet are affected. In 25% of the cases, digital trophic changes may develop gradually. The primary disease was formerly thought to account for most cases of Raynaud phenomenon, but with more sophisticated diagnostic procedures uncovering the secondary form, a significantly lower percentage has the primary form. A familial form of this phenomenon has been described.

Secondary Raynaud Phenomenon

Numerous disorders have been implicated: a vasculitis associated with immune complex disorders, vasospasm, or poorly understood mechanisms of arterial obstruction. Involvement may not be symmetric.

Connective Tissue Disorders

Systemic Lupus Erythematosus

Arthralgias or arthritis, rashes, hair loss, and other systemic signs are clues.

♦ Scleroderma (Progressive Systemic Sclerosis)

Raynaud phenomenon occurs in most cases; in almost one half, the color change precedes other symptoms. Pain is common. The presence of digital ulcerations suggests this diagnosis.

Rheumatoid Arthritis

Joint findings usually predominate.

Morphea (Localized Scleroderma)

Raynaud phenomenon may occur, especially in linear scleroderma of the extremities.

Dermatomyositis

Muscle weakness, tenderness, and cutaneous changes are present.

CREST Syndrome

Calcinosis, Raynaud's phenomenon, esophageal dysmotility, sclerodactyly, and telangiectasias account for the acronym. There is some question as to whether this is a form of systemic sclerosis.

Periarteritis

Fever, malaise, and various rashes secondary to the vasculitis are found.

Mixed Connective Tissue Disease

Symptoms of various connective tissue disorders may be present.

Sjögren Syndrome

Arthritis, dryness of eyes and mouth, and recurrent parotid swelling are clues.

Blood Disorders

• Cold Agglutinins

These may occasionally be a cause in childhood, especially with viral infections and mycoplasma pneumonia. Intracapillary agglutination of red cells occurs in the acral areas of the body that are cooler. The process tends to be transient in infections but can be chronic when associated with malignancies. A hemolytic anemia may be present.

Cryoglobulinemia

A wide variety of disorders may be associated with monoclonal or polyclonal immunoglobulin proliferation, producing cold sensitivity, Raynaud phenomenon, and peripheral vascular occlusion precipitated by cold. Chronic infections, connective tissue diseases, and malignancies have been implicated. A low erythrocyte sedimentation rate and rouleaux formation on blood smear suggest this possibility or cold agglutinins as the cause.

Cryofibrinogenemia

A cold precipitable protein is present in the plasma but not in serum. Various causes include acute bronchiolitis in infants, pneumococcal pneumonia and meningitis, connective tissue disorders, and malignancies. Cold intolerance or thrombotic episodes in severe underlying disease may be presenting signs.

Paroxysmal Cold Hemoglobinuria

Most commonly seen after viral infections. After cold exposure the child experiences back or abdominal pain, followed by chills, fever, and hemoglobinuria. Raynaund phenomenon and urticaria may be present.

Thoracic Outlet Syndromes

Cervical ribs or pressure by the scalenus anticus muscle or even the clavicle may produce color changes in one extremity or a few digits secondary to traction or compression of the subclavian vessels or brachial plexus. Aggravation of symptoms by neck or shoulder motion may be used as a test.

Intoxications

Poisoning by lead, arsenic, or ergot may produce the phenomenon.

Occupational Trauma

This is obviously rare in children; it is seen in pianists, typists, pneumatic hammer operators, and so forth.

Chronic Occlusive Arterial Disease

Children are not affected; the disorders may include arteriosclerosis obliterans or thromboangiitis obliterans. Involvement is asymmetric in both, often with gangrene.

Miscellaneous Causes

Pheochromocytoma

Raynaud phenomenon may be seen; usual symptoms include nausea, vomiting, sweating, headaches, polyuria and polydipsia, hypertension, and weight loss.

Primary Pulmonary Hypertension

Raynaud phenomenon rarely may be part of an altered arterial reactivity.

Reflex Sympathetic Dystrophy

This uncommon phenomenon follows injury or surgery; vasospasm occurs later. Usually only one extremity is affected; the pain may be severe and burning.

Oral Contraceptives

ERYTHROMELALGIA

This uncommon disorder is characterized by episodic attacks of redness of the hands and feet. Primary and secondary types have been described, the latter mainly in adults with an underlying myeloproliferative disorder (polycythemia vera, thrombocythemia, and collagen vascular diseases). The primary, or early onset form, begins in childhood or adolescence and features episodes of redness that may occur spontaneously or be provoked by exercise and heat. A burning pain and increased heat are associated with the color change. The cause is unknown, although the disorder appears to be familial in some cases.

SUGGESTED READING

Cassidy JT, Petty RE. The scleroderma and related disorders. In: *Textbook of pediatric rheumatology,* 3rd ed. Philadelphia: WB Saunders, 1995:429–431.
Duffy CM, Laxer RM, Lee P, Ramsay C, Fritzler M, Silverman ED. Raynaud syndrome in childhood. *J Pediatr* 1989;114:73–78.
Kurzrock R, Cohen PR. Erythromelalgia: review of clinical characteristics and pathophysiology. *Am J Med* 1991;91:416–422.
Silver RM, Maricq HR. Childhood dermatomyositis: serial microvascular studies. *Pediatrics* 1989;83:278–283.

103
Digital Clubbing

Clubbing of the fingers is commonly found on physical examination in children with chronic hypoxemia, whether from lung disease or cyanotic congenital heart disease. Clubbing may be found with various disorders, however, most of which are not associated with hypoxemia.

The earliest sign of clubbing is the loss of the angle between the proximal nail bed and the soft tissue of the finger just beneath the cuticle. The best way to determine if clubbing is present is to appose the dorsal parts of the terminal phalanges of the corresponding fingers of each hand and note the presence of a diamond-shaped opening. If this space is reduced or filled in, as described by Schamroth, clubbing is present (1). The increased tissue beneath the cuticle of the nail gives a spongy feel on palpation. In severe clubbing the distal phalanx may be swollen as well giving a drumstick appearance to the digit.

Hypertrophic osteoarthropathy is most commonly seen in adults and includes clubbing of the fingers and toes, arthritis, and, sometimes, painful ossifying periosteitis of tubular bone. In adults, carcinoma of the lung is by far the most common cause. In children and adolescents, the development of new onset, painful clubbing should also raise the suspicion of underlying malignancy, particularly lymphoma. Keep in mind that asthma as a cause of clubbing is exceedingly rare.

PULMONARY CAUSES

♦ Cystic Fibrosis

It is important to examine the extremities of any child with asthma for the presence of clubbing. Its presence should suggest the possibility of cystic fibrosis rather than asthma.

Bronchiectasis

Pulmonary Abscess

Empyema

Neoplasms

Lymphoma and mesothelioma of the pleura have been described.

Tuberculosis

Interstitial Pneumonia

Chronic Pneumonia

Pulmonary Alveolar Proteinosis

CARDIAC

♦ **Cyanotic Congenital Heart Disease**

Coarctation of the Aorta

In limbs distal to the coarctation.

Subacute Bacterial Endocarditis

GASTROINTESTINAL

● **Crohn Disease**

Clubbing has been described in over one third of children with Crohn disease.

Ulcerative Colitis

Clubbing is less common than in Crohn disease, slightly over 10%.

Familial Polyposis

Celiac Disease

Chronic Colonic Amebiasis

HEPATIC DISORDERS

Biliary Cirrhosis/Atresia

Chronic Active Hepatitis

FAMILIAL

Other family members should be examined for clubbing in an asymptomatic child with this finding.

MALIGNANCY

Carcinoma of Nasopharynx

The most frequent association reported.

Osteosarcoma

Hodgkin Lymphoma

Periosteal Sarcoma

Mesothelioma of Pleura

Carcinoma of Thymus

MISCELLANEOUS CAUSES

Malnutrition and Kwashiorkor

Aquired Immune Deficiency Syndrome

Chronic Hypervitaminosis A

Thyrotoxicosis

Infantile-Onset Multisystem Inflammatory Disease

A rare disorder that features the neonatal onset of symptoms including an evanescent migratory urticarial-like rash, arthritis, fever, hepato-splenomegaly, and lymphadenopathy. Clubbing has been described in some patients.

Pachydermoperiostosis

This rare disorder is characterized by clubbing and bony changes as well as significant thickening of the skin of the face, forehead, and scalp.

REFERENCE

1. Lampe RM, Kagan A. Detection of clubbing-Schamroth's sign. *Clin Pediatr* 1982;21:125.

SUGGESTED READING

Paton JY, Bautista DB, Stabile MW, et al. Digital clubbing and pulmonary functional abnormalities in children with lung disorders. *Pediatr Pulmonol* 1991;10:25–29.
Staalman CR, Umans U. Hypertrophic osteoarthropathy in childhood malignancy. *Med Pediatr Oncol* 1993;21:676–679.

SECTION XIV

Nervous System

104

Seizures

Seizures are common in childhood; various studies have estimated that 4% to 8% of all children will have a seizure prior to reaching adulthood. A seizure is defined as a paroxysmal involuntary discharge of cortical neurons that may be manifested clinically by an impairment or loss of consciousness, abnormal motor activity, behavioral and emotional disturbances, or autonomic dysfunction (1). Epilepsy refers to recurrent seizures unrelated to fever or acute cerebral insult.

This chapter will not present the classification of seizure types, which can be found in standard pediatric textbooks and reference 1. Rather, the possible causes of seizures for each childhood age group are presented with the most common causes highlighted at the start of each section. A category of seizure mimics is also included; many of these disorders may be mistaken for seizures by parents and relatives. While it is important to attempt to determine the cause of seizures, it must be remembered that in most cases a cause will not be determined.

NEWBORN AND NEONATAL PERIOD

♦ Most Common Causes of Neonatal Seizures

Hypoxic-Ischemic Encephalopathy Intracranial Hemorrhage
Hypoglycemia Central Nervous System Infection
Developmental Defect of Brain Drug Withdrawal
Unknown

Seizures in the neonatal period are often difficult to diagnose; repetitive movements, including abnormal eye movements or sucking, may be subtle manifestations. It is often difficult to distinguish these movements from normal newborn activity.

♦ Hypoxic-Ischemic Encephalopathy

Hypoxic-ischemic encephalopathy is the most common cause of seizures in the newborn, more common than birth trauma. Hypoxia may also lead to intracranial hemorrhage.

♦ Intracranial Hemorrhage

Subdural Hemorrhage

A tense fontanel, retinal hemorrhages, and progressive enlargement of the head suggest a subdural hemorrhage.

Subarachnoid Hemorrhage

Spells of apnea and poor color are additional signs.

Intracerebral Hemorrhage

This type is more common in full-term infants born after prolonged, difficult labor.

Intraventricular Hemorrhage

Premature infants born by spontaneous deliveries are most commonly affected.

◆ Unknown Cause

In 25% to 33% of infants with seizures, no cause can be found.

Metabolic Derangements

◆ Hypoglycemia

Low blood sugar may be caused by many factors including perinatal stress, hyperviscosity, maternal diabetes, intrauterine growth retardation, galactosemia, and glycogen storage disease.

● Hypocalcemia

Seizures may be focal or tonic-clonic. In some series, hypocalcemia was the most common cause of neonatal seizures; those occurring after 3 or 4 days of life were commonly related to the high phosphate content of cow milk, when evaporated milk was the basis for infant formulas. Hypocalcemia may also be secondary to maternal hyperparathyroidism, idiopathic neonatal hypoparathyroidism, or DiGeorge syndrome. Infants of diabetic mothers have an increased incidence of hypocalcemia.

Hyponatremia

This condition may follow the administration of excessive intravenous fluid without adequate sodium to the mother or disorders causing inappropriate release of antidiuretic hormone.

Hypernatremia

Diarrhea with excessive water loss or poisonings in which salt is substituted for sugar in the feeding formula may be a cause. Salt poisoning has more severe sequelae than hypernatremic dehydration.

Metabolic Disorders: Aminoacidopathies, Organic Acidurias and Urea Cycle Defects

The early onset of lethargy, vomiting, and seizures indicates the possibility of one of these disorders; some are associated with elevated blood ammonia levels. Phenylketonuria, maple syrup urine disease, argininosuccinic acidemia, aciduria and citrullinemia are but a few. Other metabolic disorders to consider include nonketotic hyperglycinemia, the ketotic hyperglycinemias (including proprionic and methylmalonic acidemia), and isovaleric acidemia.

Galactosemia

The presence of jaundice, diarrhea, and vomiting requires a urine test for reducing substances. Galactosemia predisposes to *Escherichia coli* sepsis.

Hypomagnesemia

Tetany, convulsions, and hypocalcemia are characteristic.

♦ Central Nervous System Infection

Bacterial Meningitis

In the neonatal period almost any unusual change in the infant may be a sign of central nervous system infection or sepsis. An infant who has a seizure should have a lumbar puncture performed.

Viral Infection

Various congenital and acquired viruses may be responsible. Herpes simplex, rubella, cytomegalovirus or coxsackievirus infections are examples.

Other Infections

Syphilis

Neonatal Tetanus

Toxoplasmosis

Congenital Cerebral Malformation

♦ Cerebral Agenesis or Dysgenesis

Chromosomal abnormalities, teratogenic drugs taken by the mother, or fetal radiation exposure are possible causes.

Holoprosencephaly

Hypotelorism and microcephaly with midline facial defects may be present.

Porencephaly

This is a cystic area of absent cerebral tissue, the result of disruption of normal brain tissue, often following intracerebral hemorrhage, or faulty development of brain tissue.

Hydrocephalus

This problem is often associated with a myelomeningocele.

Drugs and Chemicals

♦ Withdrawal

Tremulousness, irritability, tachypnea, vomiting, diarrhea, sweating, and a shrill cry, especially in a premature infant or one who is small for gestational age, suggest this possibility. Drugs include heroin, methadone, barbiturates, and propoxyphene.

Toxic Reactions

Seizures may follow intravenous injections of drugs such as penicillin or even absorption of hexachlorophene from the skin. Inadvertent injection of caudal anesthetic into the infant's scalp during the delivery process is another cause.

Developmental Abnormalities

• Incontinentia Pigmenti

Seizures are common in this disorder, which is lethal to males *in utero*. Cutaneous changes include vesicles and verrucous lesions, often in a linear distribution, and later, pigmented swirls.

• Sturge-Weber Syndrome

A port-wine stain of the face, involving the area supplied by the ophthalmic branch of the trigeminal nerve, may be associated with ipsilateral cerebral angiomatosis leading to seizures.

• Tuberous Sclerosis

The earliest sign is the presence of hypopigmented macules on the skin.

Linear Sebaceous or Epidermal Nevus

Any linear macular or papular lesion on the skin, especially on the head, may indicate an underlying central nervous system abnormality.

Miscellaneous Disorders

Postmaturity

Postmature infants have an increased incidence of seizures for various reasons, including hypoglycemia.

Pre-eclamptic Toxemia

Maternal toxemia may be a cause.

Kernicterus

Jaundice, irritability, a shrill cry, and opisthotonos are features.

Hyperviscosity

Sludging in cerebral vessels and hypoglycemia may be responsible for seizures.

Pyridoxine Dependency or Deficiency

Seizures from this rare cause are treatable by pyridoxine. An intravenous test dose of vitamin B_6 may be given to an infant with seizures from no apparent cause.

Neonatal Adrenoleukodystrophy

Key features are hypotonia and intractable myoclonic seizures.

Cardiac Arrhythmias

Mimics of Seizures

Hyperekplexia

Also known as the stiff-baby or startle disease. A familial disorder with increased muscle tone, a pathologic startle response, and, occasionally, myoclonic jerks. May have apneic episodes and sudden infant death.

Benign Neonatal Sleep Myoclonus

These neonates have myoclonic jerks that cease with arousal. The jerks do not stop with restraint. There are no EEG changes.

INFANCY

♦ Most Common Causes of Seizures

Febrile	Idiopathic
Head Trauma	Hypoxic Episodes
Drug/Toxin	Unknown

♦ Febrile Seizures

Febrile seizures are by far the most common cause of seizures in children 6 months to 5 years of age. It is important to distinguish febrile seizures from seizures associated with fever. The criteria for febrile seizures include: (a) the seizure must occur with fever; (b) the seizure must be generalized, not focal; (c) the child must not have had previous nonfebrile seizures and must not have had abnormal neurologic findings or a history of central nervous system injury in the past; (d) the seizure is of short duration, less than 20 minutes; and (e) there must be no evidence of intracranial infection or other cause. The onset is generally between 6 months and 3 years of age.

♦ Intracranial Birth Injury

Seizures may begin after the neonatal period in infants who have sustained perinatal intracranial injuries.

Perinatal Hypoxia or Anoxia

Intracranial Hemorrhage

Congenital Cerebral Malformations

The onset of seizures may occur in infancy. Look for signs of physical abnormalities or developmental delays.

Infections

Bacterial Infections

Meningitis and cerebral abscesses are examples.

Viral Infections

Aseptic meningitis, meningoencephalitis, or encephalitis may cause seizures. Some congenital infections may not produce seizures until later. Human immunodeficiency virus infections may present with neurologic symptoms.

Other Infections

Cat-Scratch Disease

May present with a flurry of seizures that are difficult to control.

Roseola

The exact mechanism of seizures in roseola is not known; some are febrile seizures. The etiologic agent is herpesvirus 6.

● Shigella

The seizure may be toxin related.

Tuberculous Meningitis

Seizures are relatively late in the course.

Parasitic

Toxoplasmosis and, rarely, other parasites may be responsible. Cysticercosis, caused by the larval form of the pork tapeworm *Taenia solium,* is most commonly seen in immigrants from Mexico and Latin America. Seizures and signs of increased intracranial pressure are the most common manifestations in children.

Toxic Reactions

Exposure to various toxins may result in an encephalopathy with seizures.

- ### Heavy Metals

  Seizures may be a sign in lead, mercury, or thallium poisoning.

- ### Drugs

  Amphetamines, camphor, hexachloraphene, and scabicides have been implicated. The possibility of drug ingestion or exposure by inhalation, particularly of cocaine, must always be considered.

Ingestion of Other Toxic Substances

Organophosphates and hydrocarbons are examples.

Immunizations

Metabolic Causes

- ### Hypoglycemia

  Blood glucose levels should always be determined in children with seizures. Ketotic hypoglycemia is a poorly understood disorder that occurs most commonly around age 2 years after long fasts, especially if the children are ill.

- ### Hyponatremia

  Excessive water intake or the syndrome of inappropriate antidiuretic hormone secretion from various causes may cause hyponatremia. Water intoxication occurs when young infants are fed dilute formula or breast milk supplemented with water. All have increased vasopressin.

Hypernatremia

This disorder may occur in hypertonic dehydration during a gastroenteritis, in diabetes insipidus, or from solute overload (salt poisoning). The seizures occur most commonly during rehydration.

♦ Trauma

After Concussions

Post-traumatic seizures are common.

Subdural Hematoma

Child Abuse

External evidence of trauma may or may not be present. With shaking injuries, no external signs of trauma may be visible, but retinal hemorrhages are common.

Anoxic Episodes

Seizures may follow anoxic insults.

Inborn errors of metabolism

Seizures may develop in the neonatal period or later in infancy.

Aminoacidopathies

Organic Acidopathies

Urea Cycle Defects

Degenerative Diseases

Metachromatic leukodystrophy, Tay-Sachs disease, gangliosidoses and other storage diseases, Menkes syndrome and Lowe syndrome. All have other striking findings on examination.

Biotin-Responsive Multiple Carboxylase Deficiency

Other features include ataxia, periorificial dermatitis, and alopecia.

Neurocutaneous Disorders

Careful skin examination may reveal clues to underlying central nervous system disorders.

● Tuberous Sclerosis

This disorder is responsible for 10% to 15% of infantile spasms.

Incontinentia Pigmenti

Sturge-Weber Syndrome

Linear Sebaceous or Epidermal Nevus Syndrome

Neurofibromatosis

Miscellaneous Causes

Hypertensive Encephalopathy

If this occurs in young infants, consider renal causes, such as the infantile form of polycystic kidneys.

Intracranial Hemorrhage

Hemorrhage may occur in arteriovenous malformations, in severe thrombocytopenia, or rarely in coagulation disturbances.

Post Infections

A seizure focus may be the result of preceding bacterial meningitis or viral encephalitis.

Tumors

Convulsive Syncope

Pain or sudden fright may trigger cardiac asystole, which if longer than 10 seconds, may result in an anoxic seizure.

Cardiac Arrhythmias

Aicardi Syndrome

Infants have refractory seizures associated with absence of the corpus callosum, coloboma of the iris, and retinal lacunae. Occurs only in females.

♦ Unknown Causes

In a significant number of seizures the cause is of unknown etiology; some perhaps reflect a genetic predisposition.

CHILDHOOD

♦ Most Common Causes

Idiopathic	Head Injury
Central Nervous System Infection	Hypoxic Episode
Drug/Toxin	Hypoglycemia

♦ **Unknown Cause**

The seizure may be a one time event.

♦ **Idiopathic Seizures**

The most common cause in childhood epilepsy.

Infections

♦ **Meningitis**

Bacterial and, rarely, tuberculous infections may be associated with seizures.

♦ **Encephalitis**

Not only herpes simplex virus, but enteroviruses, Epstein-Barr virus, mumps, and other viruses may be responsible. Keep in mind mosquito transmitted viral infections.

Encephalopathy

Infectious diseases, such as shigellosis and legionnaires' disease, may produce an encephalopathy with seizures. Cat-scratch disease may present with seizures.

Human Immunodeficiency Virus Infection

Cerebral Abscess

● **Parasitic Infestations**

These are seen particularly in countries other than the United States. Cystercercosis must always be considered.

Tetanus

Genetic Predisposition

In as many as 4% to 8% of children with epilepsy, hereditary factors appear to be operative. Petit mal seizures are a common example.

♦ **Trauma**

Head Injury

Post-traumatic seizures may occur at the time of the injury or months to years later.

Anoxic Injury

Burn Encephalopathy

Seizures may occur within a few days of the burn.

Subdural Hematoma

Child abuse must be considered.

Epidural Hematoma

Beware of the lucid interval between injury and the rapid downhill course.

Previous Insult

Seizures may occur months to years following infection, trauma, or anoxia.

♦ **Toxic Reactions–Poisonings**

A host of drugs, chemicals, and metals may be responsible.

Drugs

Toxic reactions to acetylsalicylic acid, amphetamines, antihistamines, atropine, aminophylline, penicillin, narcotics and their congeners, steroids, or tricyclic anti-depressants may occur. Illicit drugs must also be considered, particularly cocaine.

Heavy Metals

Lead, mercury, or thallium poisoning may cause seizures.

Chemicals

Organophosphates, hydrocarbons, LSD, and phencyclidine are examples.

Vascular Causes

● **Hypertensive Encephalopathy**

Seizures may be a presenting sign of acute glomerulonephritis.

Subarachnoid Hemorrhage

Hemorrhage may result from a cerebral aneurysm. The neck is usually stiff.

Cerebral Embolization

Emboli may occur in young children with cyanotic congenital heart disease, but they may also occur in subacute bacterial endocarditis.

Vascular Thrombosis

Thromboses may occur in severe dehydration, sickle cell disease and syndromes such as MELAS (mitochondrial encephalopathy, lactic acidosis, and seizures/stroke).

Sickle Cell Disease

Vasculitis

The vasculitis associated with systemic lupus erythematosus, hemolytic-uremic syndrome, or, rarely, Henoch-Schönlein purpura may cause seizures.

Other Causes

Video Game-Related Seizures

Visual stimuli may precipitate seizures in susceptible individuals.

Tumors

Central nervous system tumors are an uncommon cause of seizures in this age group.

Metabolic Disorders

The causes listed for other age groups are less likely in childhood, but hyponatremia and hypoglycemia may be found.

Subacute Sclerosing Panencephalitis

Some years after rubeola infection, or rarely measles immunization, personality changes are noted; focal seizures and myoclonic jerks occur later.

Convulsive Syncope

Pain or sudden fright may trigger cardiac asystole, which if longer than 10 seconds may result in an anoxic seizure.

Arrhythmias

Syncope followed by hypoxic seizures may be seen in various cardiac arrhythmias, including the congenital long QT syndrome.

• Rett Syndrome

In this syndrome, slowly progressive neurologic deterioration is seen exclusively in girls. Onset is between 4 and 18 months with behavioral changes. Myoclonic seizures usually begin between 2 and 4 years of age. Choreoathetosis, ataxia, and hypotonia are other features.

Landau-Kleffner Syndrome

Usually seen in boys. Loss of language in a previously well child is characteristic. Various types of seizures follow.

Genetic Disorders with Progressive Myoclonic Epilepsy

Lafora Disease

First presents with generalized seizures and later myoclonic jerks. Mental deterioration is evident within 1 year of onset.

Myoclonic Epilepsy with Ragged-Red Fibers

Ceroid Lipofuscinosis

Juvenile Neuropathic Gaucher Disease

Juvenile Neuroxonal Dystrophy

Sialiosis Type 1

Reye Syndrome

The toxic encephalopathy follows a viral illness, often influenza or varicella. Vomiting precedes the central nervous system depression. Seizures are a late manifestation.

Mimics

See later text.

ADOLESCENCE

♦ Unknown Causes

In most seizures in this age group, the cause is unknown.

♦ Idiopathic Epilepsy

Accounts for most cases of recurrent seizures.

♦ Trauma

Various acute and post-traumatic causes account for a significant percentage of seizures in this age group.

♦ Juvenile Myoclonic Epilepsy (Janz Syndrome)

A relatively common cause of new onset seizures in this age group. Myoclonic jerks occur primarily on awakening in the morning. Generalized tonic clonic seizures occur later, particularly on sleep deprivation, anxiety, and stress.

Infection

Meningitis and encephalitis and abscesses are examples. Frontal sinusitis as a cause of frontal lobe abscess and seizures needs to be considered.

Genetic Predisposition

● **Drug Abuse**

Cocaine must always be considered.

Tumors

Tumors may account for as many as 2% of seizures in this age group.

Vascular Malformations

Other Causes

Causes listed in the preceding section, Childhood, may be responsible in this age group also.

SEIZURE MIMICS

♦ **Breath Holding**

Episodes occur most commonly between 6 and 36 months of age; they are triggered by a sudden fright or anger, whereas seizures are not. The child cries, holds his breath, and becomes cyanotic; a loss of consciousness and a few clonic twitches may follow. In pallid breath holding the child suddenly turns pale rather than blue and faints.

♦ **Syncope**

Simple fainting spells are short lived and not followed by a postictal period; there is no amnesia for the event as with a seizure.

♦ **Migraine**

Headache, visual complaints, nausea, and vomiting, along with a familial history of migraine, suggest this disorder.

♦ **Hyperventilation**

This phenomenon usually occurs in adolescents rather than young children. The extremities may become numb, with the fingers and toes in spasm; headache and shortness of breath are common.

♦ **Drugs**

Phenothiazines are notorious for producing the extrapyramidal tract symptoms including oculogyric crises, commonly mistaken for seizures. The child is, however, awake.

♦ **Myoclonic Jerks**

One or more sudden body muscle contractions, especially when falling asleep, may occur normally.

● **Gastroesophageal Reflux**

May cause laryngospasm, bradycardia, and apneic episodes in infants that may be mistaken for seizures.

Tics

Movements are repetitive and stereotyped and involve the same muscle groups.

Hair-Grooming Syncope Seizures

During hair grooming the child may experience a syncopal episode that may be followed by hypoxic-induced seizures. Unless hair grooming activity is asked, the parents may only report these as seizure episodes.

♦ **Pavor Nocturnus**

Night terrors sometimes are confused with seizures.

Hysteria

Preceding events allow easy distinction from seizures.

● **Malingering**

A feigned seizure can usually be readily distinguished from a genuine one, but adolescents with true seizures may feign attacks that are hard to distinguish from the real thing.

● **Spasmus Nutans**

There are often three components: head nodding, head tilt, and nystagmus; it occurs in young infants and disappears during sleep.

Cardiac Arrhythmias

Cardiac arrhythmias or severe aortic stenosis may be accompanied by fainting episodes. Long QT interval syndrome is a life-threatening disorder that may manifest as syncope.

● **Masturbation**

In young children masturbatory activity may simulate seizures. The children often rock back and forth, become flushed, and perspire; they resist interference during this activity.

- **Benign Paroxysmal Vertigo**

  Seen most commonly in toddlers, who suddenly stagger or fall. Nystagmus may be seen in some children with the attack that usually is brief.

Labyrinthitis

Attacks of vertigo may simulate epilepsy. In benign paroxysmal vertigo the attacks are sudden; the child is pale and frightened and attempts to hold onto anything close.

Shuddering Attacks

This benign disorder is characterized by rapid tremors involving the head and arms similar to shivering, but of longer duration. There are no EEG abnormalities.

Rage Attacks (Episodic Dyscontrol Syndrome)

A behavioral disorder in which the child loses control, usually after a confrontation.

- **Tetany**

  While hypocalcemia may cause seizures, it may also cause muscle twitching or tetany that simulates seizures. This may be the initial presentation of rickets. In adolescents, aggressive diuretic use may cause muscle twitching.

REFERENCE

1. Haslam RHA. Nonfebrile seizures. *Pediatr Rev* 1997;18:39–48.

SUGGESTED READING

Calciolari G, Perlman JM, Volpe JJ. Seizures in the neonatal intensive care unit of the 1980's. *Clin Pediatr* 1988;27:119–123.
Golden GS. Nonepileptic paroxysmal events in childhood. *Pediatr Clin North Am* 1992;39:715–725.
Graf WD, Chatrian G-E, Glass ST, Knauss TA. Video game-related seizures: a report of 10 patients and a review of the literature. *Pediatrics* 1994;93:551–556.
Holmes GL, Russman BS. Shuddering attacks. *Am J Dis Child* 1986;140:72–73.
Lewis DW, Frank LM. Hair-grooming syncope seizures. *Pediatrics* 1993;91:836–837.
Scher MS, Painter MJ. Controversies concerning neonatal seizures. *Pediatr Clin North Am* 1989;36:281–310.
Swaiman KF. *Pediatric neurology, principles and practice*, 2nd ed. St. Louis: CV Mosby, 1994.

105
Coma

Coma—the loss of consciousness and of responsiveness to environmental stimuli—is a distressing symptom that calls for immediate evaluation to determine the cause as well as prompt institution of measures to prevent permanent brain injury or death. Because the patient cannot respond, information about preceding events may not be available. Coma of sudden onset is most likely to be associated with trauma, poisonings, seizure disorders, or intracranial hemorrhage.

Various terms have been used in the past to describe levels of coma. The lack of common acceptance of the terms and disparity in use often created problems in the definition of the state of coma, not only for study purposes, but also with individual patients. The Glasgow Coma Scale, now in common use, gives quantitation to the level of the comatose state. This scale was devised for assessing acute traumatic head injury, however, and may be misleading when used in context of a slowly progressive process. Moreover, modification is required for application to infants.

◆ **Most Common Causes of Coma**

Head Trauma	Poisons/Toxins
Hypoglycemia	Hypoxemia
Encephalitis	Postictal State

In this chapter, the possible causes of coma are arranged according to the mnemonic.

AEIOU-TIPS

Alcohol Ingestion and **A**cidosis	**T**rauma
Epilepsy and **E**ncephalopathy	**I**nsulin Overdose and **I**nflammatory Disorders
Infection	orders
Opiates	**P**oisoning and **P**sychogenic Causes
Uremia	**S**hock

A group of relatively uncommon causes of coma is also included.

ALCOHOL INGESTION

Young children may accidentally ingest alcohol in amounts sufficient to cause stupor or coma; ingestion by older children and adolescents may be intentional. Important considerations in management include: (a) hypoglycemia as the primary cause of or an added insult in the comatose state resulting from alcohol ingestion; (b) the additive effects of alcohol and other drugs; (c) aspiration of stomach contents with resulting hypoxia and serious lung disease; and (d) methanol rather than ethanol ingestion.

ACIDOSIS AND METABOLIC PROBLEMS

Conditions that produce coma as a result of acidosis or metabolic problems are usually gradual rather than sudden in onset. The preceding clinical course supplies diagnostic clues.

● Diabetes Mellitus

Polyuria, polydipsia, weight loss, dehydration, and a fruity odor to the breath are signs of diabetic ketoacidosis.

Dehydration

Hypertonic or hypotonic dehydration may result in seizures and coma.

Hypercapnia

Respiratory failure occurring in primary lung or airway disease or with neurologic disturbances may cause the comatose state or add complications.

Hepatic Failure

Any severe, acute, or chronic liver disease may result in coma. Plasma ammonia nitrogen levels are usually elevated. Progressive stages are usually evident: mild depression, alterations in speech, and insomnia; drowsiness, inappropriate behavior, and loss of sphincter control; somnolence and confusion; and finally coma. Various precipitating factors include nitrogen overload, fluid and electrolyte abnormalities, infection and other stresses, and drugs. Beware of unintentional acetaminophen overdosage in young children with fever.

Fulminant Hepatitis

Wilson Disease

Alpha-1 Antitrypsin Deficiency

Cystic Fibrosis

Biliary Atresia

◆ Toxin Ingestion

Acetaminophen in particular has been implicated.

Reye Syndrome

This was an important, albeit now rare, cause of coma that usually followed a viral infection (influenza B or varicella). Generally around the fourth day of illness, as the child was recovering from the infection, the child began vomiting. Confusion and delirium preceded the increasing obtundation. Salicylates may have played a role in the syndrome.

♦ Hypoglycemia

See the Insulin Overdose and Hypoglycemia category.

♦ Hypoxia

Insufficient oxygen delivery to the brain may be a cause. Near drowning, carbon monoxide poisoning, congestive heart failure, and lung disorders must be considered.

Water Intoxication

Inappropriate antidiuretic hormone release may occur in a variety of disorders. Iatrogenic intravenous overload occasionally occurs. Rarely, the problem is of psychogenic origin. In infants it may result from overdilution of formula.

Electrolyte Disturbances

Hypernatremia

Hyponatremia

Calcium

Either hypocalcemia or hypercalcemia may occur.

Magnesium

Hypermagnesemia or hypomagnesemia may be a cause.

Uremia

The severity of coma is poorly correlated with serum urea nitrogen levels, other than as a threshold: central nervous system manifestations are rarely present with a urea nitrogen below 100 mg/dL.

Alkalosis

Metabolic or respiratory alkalosis may cause alterations in consciousness.

- **Inborn Errors of Metabolism**

In most of these disorders, onset of symptoms is early in life, with vomiting, seizures, and acidosis. Although all are uncommon, some are more prevalent than others.

Maple Syrup Urine Disease	Carbamyl Phosphatase Synthetase Deficiency
Methylmalonic Aciduria	Ornithine Transcarbamylase Deficiency
Ketotic Hyperglycinemia	Multiple Carboxylase Deficiency
Isovaleric Acidemia	Propionic Acidemia

Argininosuccinic Lyase Deficiency

The subacute form presents a Reye syndrome-like picture. Hepatomegaly is significant.

Medium-Chain Acyl-Co-A Dehydrogenase Deficiency

A Reye syndrome-like deficiency associated with hypoketotic hypoglycemia may follow a minor illness with diarrhea and vomiting.

Fatty Acid Disorders

Hypoglycemia and low levels of serum carnitine are common in these mitochondrial disorders.

Endocrine Disorders

Coma is a rare presentation of these disorders.

Addison Disease

Cushing Syndrome

Congenital Adrenal Hyperplasia (Adrenogenital Syndrome)

In the salt losing form, dehydration and hyponatremia may be presenting signs.

Pheochromocytoma

Hypertensive encephalopathy may occur.

Pseudohyperaldosteronism

Hepatic Porphyrias

Acute Intermittent Porphyria

Variegate Porphyria

◆ EPILEPSY

The postictal patient or the patient in status epilepticus may be comatose.

ENCEPHALOPATHY

Various metabolic and infectious insults may result in an encephalopathy presenting as coma. In many cases the insult may not be identifiable.

Toxic Encephalopathy

Shigella is a prime example of an extra-central nervous system infection that may be associated with seizures and altered consciousness.

INFECTION

Meningitis

A lumbar puncture should be performed on every comatose patient, although there may be a great dilemma when signs of increased intracranial pressure are present.

Bacterial Infection

Viral Infection

Mycoplasma Pneumoniae

Various neurologic findings, including coma, ataxia, seizures, and Guillain-Barré syndrome, among others, have been reported with this infection.

Fungal Infection

Protozoal Infestation

Mycobacterial Infection

◆ Encephalitis

Viruses (e.g., HSV, EBV, enterovirus, mumps), Rickettsial, and bacteria (cat-scratch disease) may be responsible. In cat-scratch disease lymphadenopathy may not be prominent.

Severe Systemic Infection

Stupor or coma may occur in severe infections such as pneumonia or pyelonephritis.

Postinfectious or Parainfectious Encephalomyelitis

An encephalomyelopathy may follow a viral illness, as a result of either direct invasion by the virus or an altered immunologic state.

Brain Abscess

Fever and headache precede the coma.

Subdural or Epidural Empyema

OPIATES

An overdose of narcotics, either illegal drugs or opiate congeners present in medications such as propoxyphene hydrochloride (Darvon) or diphenoxylate hydrochloride with atropine (Lomotil), may be responsible for coma. A trial dose of a narcotic antagonist may be diagnostic.

UREMIA

Other neurologic signs such as tremors, myoclonus, asterixis, convulsions, and a change in mental status usually precede coma. The severity of the coma does not correlate well with the elevation of the blood urea nitrogen, other than to note that central nervous system manifestations are unusual below a urea nitrogen of 100 mg/dL.

● **Hemolytic-Uremic Syndrome**

Children with this disorder may present with seizures and/or coma. An acute gastroenteritis is followed by pallor, lethargy, and, often, the presence of purpura.

TRAUMA AND OTHER PHYSICAL CAUSES

♦ **Blunt Trauma**

Concussions produce alterations of consciousness lasting less than 24 hours. A contusion of the brain produces greater periods of unresponsiveness and indicates bruising.

Subdural Hematoma

The bleeding may be of sudden onset or present for some time.

Epidural Hematoma

The classic picture is one of immediate loss of consciousness following the trauma and then a lucid period followed by a gradual onset of obtundation.

Heat Stroke

The body core temperature is generally greater than 106°F. Sweating has ceased and the skin feels hot and dry.

Significant Hypothermia

Excessive body cooling may result in coma.

Electric Shock

A period of cardiac asystole usually produces the coma.

Decompression Sickness

The formation of gaseous microemboli, usually nitrogen, in the "bends" may affect the brain.

Blood Loss

Blood loss may be a consequence of major trauma or may occur with minor trauma in association with clotting disorders.

◆ INSULIN OVERDOSE AND HYPOGLYCEMIA

Various disorders may produce hypoglycemia and consequent coma. Insulin overdose must always be considered as the cause in a known diabetic. However, infants and children are prone to develop hypoglycemia during fasting, especially with infections and in the newborn period. Determination of blood sugar is mandatory in the comatose child.

INFLAMMATORY DISORDERS

Coma may occur with cerebral involvement in systemic lupus erythematosus and polyarteritis nodosa.

◆ POISONING

Ingestion of a drug or toxin must always be considered as the cause of coma, especially if the onset of the illness producing the unresponsive state is acute. Phenothiazines, hydrocarbons, organophosphates, phencyclidines, salicylates, barbiturates and other sedatives, and antihistamines are the most common offenders. Lead poisoning with encephalopathy is usually characterized by a subacute course with vomiting, headache, and increasing lethargy.

PSYCHOGENIC CAUSES

Hysterical unresponsiveness is generally short lived. The history often provides diagnostic clues.

SHOCK

Shock or a shocklike state may be associated with many of the causes in this chapter.

MISCELLANEOUS CAUSES

• Intussusception

Curiously, young children with intussusception commonly have altered states of consciousness, which may draw attention away from the abdomen.

Vascular Disorders

Subarachnoid Hemorrhage

Trauma or rupture of an aneurysm may cause the bleeding. Although a stiff neck is present in most adults, this finding is not consistent in children.

Venous Thrombosis

Venous thrombosis may follow severe dehydration or a pyogenic infection of paranasal sinuses, middle ear, or mastoid. The presence of periorbital edema or scalp edema with dilated veins on the scalp and face is a clue.

Arterial Thrombosis

This cause is unusual in children. However, children with homocystinuria are prone to develop arterial thromboses; they have a marfanoid appearance with dislocated lenses and mental retardation.

Intracerebral and Intraventricular Hemorrhages

In newborns, these lesions may follow birth asphyxia or trauma; in older children, the cause is usually a disturbance of the clotting mechanisms.

Cerebral Emboli

Subacute bacterial endocarditis is the prototype; splinter hemorrhages, splenomegaly, and microscopic hematuria are suggestive findings.

Acute Infantile Hemiplegia

An acute seizure, followed by coma and hemiparesis, is characteristic.

Cardiac Disorders

Any disorder resulting in diminished blood supply to the brain may lead to the sudden onset of loss of consciousness.

Ventricular Fibrillation

Stokes-Adams Attacks

Heart block leads to unconsciousness.

Aortic Stenosis

Severe aortic stenosis may lead to attacks of unconsciousness secondary to diminished cardiac output.

Hypertension

Hypertensive encephalopathy may follow acute glomerulonephritis or may be associated with pheochromocytomas, familial dysautonomia, or drug ingestion.

Esophageal Foreign Body

May cause altered consciousness, perhaps as a result of excessive vagal response and brief hypoxia.

Neoplasia

Brain Tumors

The most common cause of a loss of consciousness in children with brain tumors is increased intracranial pressure. Other symptoms precede coma, except when a sudden hemorrhage into the tumor results in sudden increase in intracranial pressure or obstruction of cerebrospinal fluid outflow.

Metastatic Tumors

Wilms' and Ewing tumors may metastasize to the brain.

Meningeal Infiltration

This lesion may be present in acute leukemia.

SUGGESTED READING

Lockman LA. Impairment of consciousness. In: Swaiman KF, ed. *Pediatric neurology, principles and practice,* 2nd ed. St. Louis: Mosby, 1994:183–195.

106

Floppy Infant Syndrome

Hypotonia refers to a decrease in resistance to passive motion. It is important to remember, however, that a hypotonic individual does not always have muscle weakness. Down syndrome is an example of hypotonia without weakness. In this chapter, floppy is used as a descriptive term to encompass both hypotonic infants as well as those who have muscular weakness.

The floppy infant syndrome may be congenital or acquired. Hypotonic infants are much like rag dolls; if suspended over the palm of the hand, they literally droop around it. They slip through the examiner's hands when supported by the axillae. Signs of weakness or hypotonia include a weak cry, poor sucking reflex, and decreased body movement, as well as respiratory difficulty. Muscle weakness and hypotonia should always be considered in the differential diagnosis of neonatal respiratory distress.

Many disorders that may cause muscle weakness or hypotonia, especially with onset at later than 6 months of age, are listed in Chapter 95, Muscle Weakness, and are not repeated here. This chapter covers only those disorders that produce these signs in the first 6 months of life. It is helpful to separate central from peripheral causes of hypotonia. In causes with a central origin, other abnormalities are usually present, including lethargy, seizures, lack of visual tracking, and delayed development. Hypotonia in neonates generally has a central origin.

♦ **Most Common Causes of a Floppy Infant**

Hypoxic-Ischemic Encephalopathy
Down Syndrome
Werdnig-Hoffmann Disease
Neonatal Myasthenia

Birth Trauma
Benign Congenital Hypotonia
Prader-Willi Syndrome

TRAUMA

Infants with the following causes of hypotonia almost always have other signs of cerebrocortical dysfunction, including seizures.

♦ **Hypoxic-Ischemic Encephalopathy**

The most common cause of the floppy infant.

Cerebral Hemorrhage
Spinal Cord Injury

NEUROMUSCULAR DISORDERS

♦ Benign Congenital Hypotonia

This is a descriptive term used for hypotonic infants in whom no other cause for hypotonia is found. They are generally not weak.

Werdnig-Hoffmann Disease

Signs of this anterior horn cell disease may be present *in utero* with decreased fetal movement. The weakness becomes increasingly severe with age.

♦ Neonatal Myasthenia

This condition, which may be transient or persistent, is characterized by ptosis, weak cry, difficulty in swallowing, and generalized weakness.

Myotonic Dystrophy

Neonatal problems include difficulty in swallowing and in sucking, facial diplegia, ptosis, arthrogryposis, respiratory difficulty, and talipes equinovarus. Maternal hydramnios may have been noted. Often, it is the mother's handshake (demonstrating myotonia, the inability to release) that provides the strongest clinical clue to the diagnosis.

Congenital Myopathies

The many types are distinguishable by special stains of muscle biopsy material.

Central Core Disease

Nemaline Myopathy

Congenital Fiber-Type Disproportion

Myotubular Myopathy

Congenital Muscular Dystrophy

There is significant hypotonia with swallowing and sucking difficulties, ptosis, thin extremities, and joint contractures, which are often present at birth.

Atonic Paraplegia

Atonic cerebral palsy may be a cause.

Congenital Ataxia and Congenital Choreoathetosis

Infantile Neuroaxonal Dystrophy

Congenital Hypomyelination Neuropathy

Affected infants are hypotonic and inactive and have palpably enlarged nerves.

Polymyositis

This disorder is rare in infants.

Dejerine-Sottas Disease

Onset in infancy is rare. Weakness, hypotonia, delayed motor milestones, and areflexia are typical. Nerve biopsy is pathognomonic.

TOXINS AND DRUGS

Bilirubin

Hyperbilirubinemia may result in kernicterus. Early signs include hypotonia, lethargy, poor appetite, and decreased activity. The hypotonia is replaced by spasticity and opisthotonos in a few days to weeks.

Magnesium

Hypermagnesemia in newborns may result from magnesium sulfate given to their mothers during labor. Severely affected infants may be flaccid and cyanotic and require respiratory assistance.

Phenobarbital

Maternal therapy rarely results in neonatal depression with flaccidity.

Cocaine

Maternal cocaine use may be associated with neonatal hypotonia.

Botulism

Botulism must be considered in infants with sudden onset of hypotonia, lethargy, constipation, and poor feeding.

Fetal Warfarin Syndrome

Maternal therapy with warfarin during pregnancy may cause hypotonia, developmental delay, seizures, a hypoplastic nose, and stippling of the epiphyses on radiograph films.

Fetal Aminopterin Syndrome

Maternal exposure during pregnancy may result in a significantly abnormal phenotype, occasionally with hypotonia.

Aluminum Toxicity

Infants receiving aluminum containing phosphate binders may develop an osteodystrophy. Poor muscle tone, a ricketlike picture, and bulging fontanel may be found.

SYNDROMES WITH HYPOTONIA

♦ **Down Syndrome**

♦ **Prader-Willi Syndrome**

Hypotonia is a consistent feature of this syndrome, beginning *in utero*. Other signs, such as obesity, so prominent later in life, are not remarkable in infancy.

♦ **Achondroplasia**

Marfan Syndrome

Arachnodactyly and joint hyperextensibility are evident early in life. Hypotonia may be significant in some cases.

● **Cerebrohepatorenal Syndrome (Zellweger Syndrome)**

Large fontanels, high forehead, hepatomegaly, and redundant skinfolds of the neck are characteristic. In some affected infants, the appearance resembles that in Down syndrome. The cause of the high serum iron levels and excessive iron storage is unclear.

Familial Dysautonomia (Riley-Day Syndrome)

Additional findings include feeding difficulties, absent lacrimation and corneal reflexes, decreased or absent deep tendon reflexes, and absent fungiform papillae of tongue. Ashkenazi Jews are primarily affected.

Oculocerebrorenal Syndrome (Lowe Syndrome)

Williams Syndrome

This syndrome was previously called idiopathic hypercalcemia with supravalvular aortic stenosis and failure to thrive. Anteverted nose and a long philtrum are characteristic.

Trisomy 13 Syndrome

This chromosomal defect may cause hypotonia as well as numerous other abnormalities. Cleft lip or palate, microcephaly, cardiac defects, polydactyly, microphthalmia, and seizures are commonly present.

Cri du Chat Syndrome

Most affected infants are hypotonic. A catlike cry, hypertelorism, growth failure, downward slanting of the palpebral fissures, and microcephaly are prominent figures.

Short-Arm Deletion of Chromosome 4 (4p$^-$ Syndrome)

Typical features include ocular hypertelorism, a broad or beaked nose, microcephaly, cranial asymmetry, low set ears, and hypotonia.

Long-Arm Deletion of Chromosome 18 (18q⁻ Syndrome)

Midface flattening, microcephaly, hypotonia, long fingers, and ear abnormalities are usually present.

XXXXY Syndrome

Common findings include hypogenitalism, limited elbow pronation, low nasal bridge, and hypertelorism, as well as hypotonia in one third of the cases.

Marinesco-Sjögren Syndrome

This syndrome is characterized by cerebellar ataxia, cataracts, and weakness. Hypotonia may or may not be present.

Cohen Syndrome

Hypotonia and weakness occur early; obesity is noted later. Protruding maxillary incisors are part of the picture.

Stickler Syndrome

Flat facies, cleft palate, myopia, hypotonia, hyperextensible joints, and an arthropathy are characteristic.

Langer-Giedion Syndrome

Redundant or loose skin is noted in the neonatal period. The nose appears bulbous. Multiple bony exostoses occur.

Thanatophoric Dwarfism

Short-limbed dwarfism with feeble fetal activity, polyhydramnios, and hypotonia are characteristic. Affected infants die shortly after birth.

Coffin-Siris Syndrome

Growth failure, sparse hair, hypotonia, and absent fifth finger and toenails are among the more prominent features.

Gillespie Syndrome

The typical presentation is the discovery of fixed dilated pupils (secondary to partial aniridia) in a hypotonic infant.

Rieger Syndrome

A myotonic dystrophy of variable degree with iris dysplasia and dental abnormalities are features of this disorder inherited as an autosomal dominant trait.

Multiple Endocrine Adenomatosis Syndrome

Infants with the mucosal neuroma syndrome may be hypotonic at birth. Lingual neuromas may be present at birth or appear in the first few years.

INFECTION

Sepsis

Acquired infections may produce profound hypotonia and/or weakness.

Congenital Infections

The TORCH complex—Toxoplasmosis, rubella, cytomegalovirus, herpes simplex—and syphilis have been implicated. Poliomyelitis acquired *in utero* has also been described, but is exceedingly rare today. Human immunodeficiency virus infection must always be considered.

METABOLIC AND INHERITED INBORN ERRORS

Hypercalcemia

Hypocalcemia

Hypokalemia

Hypothyroidism

Infants are lethargic as well. Prolonged jaundice may be an early clue.

Osteogenesis Imperfecta (Autosomal Recessive Form)

Short-limbed growth deficiency, large fontanels with multiple wormian bones of skull, and multiple fractures of bones are features.

Congenital Joint Laxity and Ehlers-Danlos Syndrome

There is a wide variety in the expression of these disorders, but extreme hyperextensibility of joints may give the impression of hypotonia.

Adrenoleukodystrophy (Neonatal)

Hypotonia is significant and associated with the early onset of seizures.

Pompe Disease (Glycogen Storage Disease, Type II)

Cardiac and skeletal muscle is affected; a deficiency of acid maltase is the basic defect. Hypotonia and muscle weakness may be present in other glycogen storage diseases, but the onset is generally later.

Pseudodeficiency Rickets

The course is similar to that in early onset severe rickets, with growth failure, large fontanels, hypotonia, hypocalcemia, and in some cases, seizures. Inheritance pattern is autosomal recessive.

Glycoprotein-Deficient Carbohydrate Syndrome

Hypotonia, liver dysfunction, and inverted nipples are found in these infants with hypoalbuminemia and hypobetalipoproteinemia.

Generalized Gangliosidosis

Coarse features may suggest Hurler syndrome, but signs are evident at birth. Storage of ganglioside GM_1 occurs in liver, spleen, and brain. Inheritance pattern is autosomal recessive.

Carnitine Deficiency

This autosomal recessively inherited disorder may present with weakness at birth. Episodes of acute hepatic encephalopathy resembling Reye syndrome may occur.

Fucosidosis

Progressive developmental retardation with hypotonia begins early but is not evident at birth. Affected children later become hypertonic and develop cardiomegaly.

Mannosidosis

Affected infants may be hypotonic at birth. Hepatosplenomegaly, macroglossia, repeated infections, and lens opacities are other findings.

Infantile Thiamine Deficiency

Onset of symptoms is in the first 3 months of life if maternal intake of thiamine has been poor and exogenous sources are deficient. Anorexia, vomiting, lethargy, pallor, ptosis, edema of the extremities, and cardiac failure are characteristic.

Adenylate Deaminase Deficiency

It is not clear whether this muscle enzyme deficiency is primary or secondary.

Menkes Disease

These infants present with hypothermia, hypotonia, and myoclonic seizures. They have a characteristic pale, puffy facies with unruly (kinky) hair.

Copper Deficiency

Affected infants are pale and hypopigmented with hepatosplenomegaly.

Biotin Deficiency

Usually develops at age 3 to 6 months. Periorificial dermatitis, alopecia, conjunctivitis, irritability, and ataxia may also be present.

Hyperuricemia and Growth Retardation

This is an X-linked recessive disorder.

AMINO ACID AND ORGANIC ACID DISORDERS

Argininosuccinic Aciduria

Severe mental retardation occurs. Seizures, ataxia, and hypotonia may be noted; the hair tends to be fragile with nodes along the shaft.

Hyperlysinemia

Severe mental retardation with muscular hypotonia and ligament laxity is characteristic.

Pipecolatemia

Mental retardation, hepatomegaly, and hypotonia have been described.

Nonketotic Hyperglycinemia

Poor feeding, apneic episodes, and seizures occur in the neonatal period. Severe mental and developmental retardation develops in survivors.

Maple Syrup Urine Disease

Poor feeding, lethargy, and seizures begin early. Affected infants may be hypertonic or hypotonic.

Multiple Carboxylase Deficiency

Episodes of ketoacidosis, hyperglycemia, and hyperammonemia are brought on by ingestion of large amounts of protein. Vomiting, lethargy, and hypotonia are common.

MISCELLANEOUS CAUSES

Guillain-Barré Syndrome

Cerebellar Ataxia

Malformations of the Brain

Cerebellar hypoplasia is an example.

Kwashiorkor

Dietary Chloride Deficiency

Cases due to errors in formula production as well as breast milk chloride deficiency have been described. Key features also include failure to thrive and anorexia.

SUGGESTED READING

Jones KL. *Smith's recognizable patterns of human malformation*, 5th ed. Philadelphia: WB Saunders, 1997.
Miller VS, Delgado M, Iannaccone ST. Neonatal hypotonia. *Semin Neurol* 1993;13:73–82.
Swaiman KF. *Pediatric neurology: principles and practice*, 2nd ed. St. Louis: Mosby, 1994:227–233.

107

Ataxia

The ataxic gait is wide-based, characterized by unsteadiness, staggering, and lurching movements in any direction. When truncal muscles are primarily involved, ataxia is not as obvious. Because infants normally have poor balance and poorly controlled movements, the incoordination usually cannot be demonstrated until the end of the first year of life. In infants, muscular hypotonia associated with the ataxia may be the only finding.

The causes of ataxia may be grouped by mode of onset. Ataxia of short duration suggests toxic, infectious, or neoplastic causes. Slowly progressive ataxia may occur with posterior fossa tumors, but it may also be a sign of any of a large number of hereditary degenerative disorders. Nonprogressive, chronic ataxia is associated with congenital lesions. The classification of ataxia in this chapter is one suggested by Swaiman (1).

♦ Most Common Causes of Ataxia

Acute Cerebellar Ataxia following infections (e.g., Coxsackievirus, Rubeola, Varicella)
Drugs and Toxins (e.g., Alcohol, Barbiturates, Phenytoin)
Trauma
Tumors (Cerebellum and Brainstem)
Guillain-Barré Syndrome
Benign Paroxysmal Vertigo of Childhood

• Causes Not to Forget

Ataxia Telangiectasia   Vitamin E Deficiency

INFECTIONS

♦ Acute Cerebellar Ataxia

Profound truncal ataxia of sudden onset is typical; it is often preceded by a nonspecific illness occurring 2 to 3 weeks before. Tremors, hypotonia, scanning speech, photophobia, headache, and nystagmus may also be present; the deep tendon reflexes remain intact. Children 1 to 5 years of age seem most susceptible. An association with this disorder has been reported in various infections including ECHO virus, coxsackievirus, poliomyelitis, herpes simplex, varicella, Epstein-Barr virus, *Mycoplasma pneumoniae,* and legionellosis.

♦ Acute Febrile Polyneuritis (Guillain-Barré Syndrome)

Ataxia may occur during the course of this ascending polyneuropathy. The absence of deep tendon reflexes should make this disorder readily separable from acute cerebellar ataxia. The onset occurs 1 to 3 weeks after a nonspecific respiratory or gastrointestinal tract illness. Specific infections incriminated include cytomegalovirus, Epstein Barr virus, enterovirus, *M. pneumoniae,* and *Campylobacter jejuni.* The syndrome has also followed immunizations, especially influenza vaccine.

Ataxia During Acute Infections

Ataxia has been noted during the following infections.

Mumps	Poliomyelitis
Infectious Mononucleosis	Diphtheria
Coxsackievirus and ECHO Virus Infections	Rubeola
Varicella	Pertussis
M. pneumoniae	Scarlet Fever
Leptospirosis	Legionnaires Disease

Typhoid

Other bacterial enteritides may also cause ataxia.

Meningitis

Ataxia may occur during recovery from bacterial meningitis; occasionally it may precede the diagnosis of meningitis.

Human Immunodeficiency Virus Infection

Ataxia is one part of the progressive encephalopathy described in children with AIDS.

Cerebellar Abscess

This usually occurs in children with chronic middle ear infections. Bacteremia in children with cyanotic congenital heart disease is responsible for a minority.

Miller-Fisher Syndrome

This rare disorder is characterized by the acute onset of ophthalmoplegia, ataxia, and hyporeflexia. An antecedent URI may occur. Most individuals recover spontaneously without sequelae. It appears to be related to Guillain-Barré syndrome.

Acute Labyrinthitis

Acute onset of vertigo, nausea, and vomiting is typical. Ataxia may be present. Results of tests of labyrinthine function are abnormal.

Acute Viral Cerebellitis

Lyme Disease

Aseptic meningitis, encephalitis, chorea, cerebellar ataxia, cranial neuritis, and a host of other neurologic as well as systemic problems may occur.

Encephalitis

Ataxia has been described in a number of infectious encephalitides.

Tuberculosis

Central nervous system infection may result in increased intracranial pressure and cerebellar dysfunction.

Congenital Syphilis

Onset of central nervous system dysfunction occurs in late preschoolers or adolescents. Memory loss, personality changes, and academic failure are other signs. Stigmata of congenital syphilis are present.

Parasitic Disease

Cerebellar echinococcosis is a rare cause.

Kuru

This chronic slow virus infection may produce cerebellar disease in children. It is primarily found in New Guinea.

INGESTIONS AND TOXINS

Ataxia may occur with intoxication by various drugs and metals, whether deliberate, accidental, or iatrogenic. Some of the more common ones are listed.

♦ **Alcohol**

♦ **Anticonvulsants**

Phenytoin, phenobarbital, primidone, carbamazepine, and clonazepam have been implicated.

♦ **Antihistamines**

Tranquilizers (Diazepam)

Sedatives

Glue Sniffing

Lead, Thallium, Organic Mercurials

Gamma Benzene Hexachloride (Lindane)

DDT (Chlorophenothane)

5-Fluorouracil

Phencyclidine

TRAUMA

♦ Concussion

Acute cerebellar or, less commonly, frontal lobe edema may result in ataxia of short duration.

Posterior Fossa Subdural or Epidural Hematoma

Heat Stroke

Prolonged hyperthermia may cause cerebellar degeneration.

NEOPLASMS

♦ Posterior Fossa Tumors

This possibility must always be considered in any child with the gradual onset of ataxia, especially if headache, vomiting, and papilledema are present. Neck stiffness and head tilt may be other signs. A medulloblastoma may produce ataxia of a relatively abrupt onset.

Neuroblastoma/Ganglioneuroblastoma

Acute cerebellar ataxia may be a presenting symptom of an occult neuroblastoma. Opsoclonus (irregular, jerking eye movements) and myoclonic jerks of the body may also be present. The ataxia may persist after treatment.

♦ Brainstem Tumors

In addition to the ataxia, evidence of cranial nerve deficits is also present.

Cerebral Hemisphere Tumors

A small percentage of children with cerebral tumors may have ataxia; in these cases, the tumor is often clinically misdiagnosed as a posterior fossa mass.

Spinal Cord Tumors

Extramedullary tumors may produce ataxia along with weakness, spasticity, and sensory changes.

Paraneoplastic Syndrome with Hodgkin Disease

Although more common in adults, ataxia has been reported in a child with Hodgkin disease.

HEREDITARY DISORDERS

Friedreich Ataxia

Early signs include loss of vibratory and position senses. Distal muscle weakness becomes evident generally between 7 and 13 years of age. Deep tendon reflexes are absent. Pes cavus and kyphoscoliosis are common. Death by 20 years of age is the rule. Inheritance pattern is autosomal recessive.

● Ataxia Telangiectasia

Progressive cerebellar ataxia usually begins between 1 and 3 years of age. Telangiectatic lesions, most commonly affecting the conjunctivae and skin of the ear, appear later. Frequent sinopulmonary infections are typical. Deep tendon reflexes are decreased, and dysarthria is often present. Inheritance pattern is autosomal recessive.

Ataxia-Ocular Motor Apraxia

A slowly progressive syndrome that may be confused with ataxia telangiectasia, but has only neurological features.

Benign Familial Chorea of Early Onset

The gait is ataxic in this disorder inherited as an autosomal dominant trait.

Angelman Syndrome

Affected children have severe mental retardation, jerky movements, ataxic gait, and inappropriate laughter, leading to the term "happy puppet" syndrome.

Spinocerebellar Degeneration

An abnormal gait develops in school-aged children, who eventually develop spasticity in their lower limbs and increasing ataxia, especially involving the upper extremities. Affected children walk on their toes and have a broad based gait and pes cavus.

Roussy-Lévy Disease

This disorder may represent a mild and incomplete form of Friedreich ataxia; peroneal muscular atrophy also occurs.

Abetalipoproteinemia

The first sign is steatorrhea during the first year of life; progressive ataxia and muscle weakness develop later. Acanthocytes are found on peripheral blood smears.

Pelizaeus-Merzbacher Disease (Familial Centrolobar Sclerosis)

This sex-linked disorder is characterized by the gradual development of spasticity, ataxia, intention tremor, choreoathetosis, and intellectual deterioration. Nystagmus may be a finding in the first year of life.

Marinesco-Sjögren Syndrome

In this rare syndrome, inherited as an autosomal recessive trait, short stature, cataracts, and mental retardation are found.

Dentate Cerebellar Ataxia (Ramsay Hunt Syndrome)

Initial symptoms include generalized convulsions, myoclonic jerks, tremors, and ataxia. Coordinated movements become difficult to perform. Onset of this disorder inherited as an autosomal recessive trait is between 7 and 16 years of age.

Acute Intermittent Cerebellar Ataxia

In a number of families, the sudden onset of ataxia, intention tremors, and gait disturbances has been described.

Familial Calcification of Basal Ganglia

This disorder is characterized by convulsions, involuntary movements, and intellectual impairment.

Cockayne Syndrome

Ataxia, Retinitis Pigmentosa, Vestibular Abnormalities, and Intellectual Deterioration

Cerebellar Ataxia with Deafness, Anosmia, Absent Caloric Responses, Nonreactive Pupils, and Hyporeflexia

Familial Ataxia with Macular Degeneration

Familial Intention Tremor, Ataxia, and Lipofuscinosis

Hereditary Cerebellar Ataxia, Intellectual Retardation, Choreoathetosis, and Eunuchoidism

Hereditary Cerebellar Ataxia with Myotonia and Cataracts

Periodic Attacks of Vertigo, Diplopia, and Ataxia

Inheritance pattern is autosomal dominant.

Posterior and Lateral Column Difficulties, Nystagmus, and Muscle Atrophy

Gillespie Syndrome

Findings include partial aniridia, cerebellar ataxia, and mental retardation. Typical presentation is the finding of fixed dilated pupils in a hypotonic infant.

Progressive Cerebellar Ataxia and Epilepsy

Dejerine-Sottas Disease (Progressive Hypertrophic Interstitial Neuropathy)

The peripheral nerves are thickened and easily palpable. Pupillary irregularity, nystagmus, intention tremor, scanning speech, and scoliosis are features.

Biemond Posterior Column Ataxia

One family with ataxia secondary to progressive degeneration of the posterior columns of the spinal cord has been described.

Olivopontocerebellar Atrophy (Dejerine-Thomas Atrophy)

Onset of progressive ataxia, parkinsonian rigidity, resting tremors, and speech impairment is usually in adulthood. Both autosomal dominant and autosomal recessive types have been described.

CONGENITAL DISORDERS

Ataxic Cerebral Palsy

Various causes have been described including cerebellar malformations, perinatal brain damage, and acquired infections. An underlying cause should be sought.

Agenesis or Hypoplasia of the Cerebellum

Symptoms are usually noted during the first year of life; clumsiness and developmental delay may be seen.

Dandy-Walker Syndrome

Obstructive hydrocephalus is due to congenital atresia of the foramina of Luschka and of Magendie. The cerebellum atrophies as the fourth ventricle becomes enlarged. Hydrocephalus dominates the clinical picture.

Hydrocephalus

Progressive hydrocephalus may be associated with ataxic diplegia.

Arnold-Chiari Malformation

Displacement of the brainstem and cerebellar tonsils may be associated with ataxia.

Encephalocele

Cerebellar Dysplasia with Microgyria, Macrogyria, or Agyria

Basilar Impression (Platybasia)

Margins of the foramen magnum invaginate resulting in posterior displacement of the odontoid and compression of the spinal cord or brainstem. Other features include stiff neck, nystagmus, and cortical tract signs.

Craniovertebral Anomalies

Occipitalization of the atlas, separated odontoid process of the axis, and chronic atlantoaxial dislocation may all produce symptoms similar to those of platybasia, including spastic weakness, neck pain, ataxia, and numbness and pain in the extremities.

METABOLIC DISORDERS

● **Vitamin E Deficiency**

In chronic deficiency, as might occur in chronic intrahepatic or extrahepatic cholestatic disorders, a mild ataxia is a late finding. Hyporeflexia is the initial sign appearing between 1 and 4 years of age.

Niemann-Pick Disease (Type C)

Neurologic symptoms predominate in this form of the disease, which usually appears between 2 and 4 years of age with myoclonic or akinetic seizures and ataxia. A cherry-red macular spot is present.

Metachromatic Leukodystrophy

In the infantile type, ataxia begins between 1 and 2 years of age, followed by bulbar signs, hypotonia, and then spasticity. In the juvenile form, a previously normal child develops a gait disturbance, spasticity, and a progressively downhill course.

Hypoglycemia

The cerebellum may be damaged by frequent and severe episodes of hypoglycemia during the first year of life.

Maple Syrup Urine Disease

The intermittent variant occurs in infants and children who are otherwise normal but have attacks of acute ataxia, irritability, and, sometimes, coma.

Argininosuccinic Aciduria

Affected infants present with seizures, intermittent ataxia, hypotonia, hepatomegaly, and unusual kinky hair.

Hyperammonemia

Ornithine transcarboxylase deficiency is an example. Ataxia may accompany recurrent hyperammonemic encephalopathy.

Biotin Responsive Multiple Carboxylase Deficiency

Other features include seizures, hearing loss, developmental delay, periorificial dermatitis, alopecia, and eventually death.

Galactosemia

Tremors and ataxia may be seen in some infants. The urine should be checked for reducing substances.

Pyruvate Decarboxylase Deficiency

A progressive neurologic disease with variable symptoms, usually ataxia, weakness of ocular mobility and peripheral nerve disease. Acute episodes of weakness or ataxia may occur, often precipitated by fever or stress.

Hyperalaninemia

Sialidosis

Features include visual impairment, myoclonus, and intellectual deteroriation, as well as gait disturbances.

Tryptophanuria

Hyperalaninemia

GM 2 Gangliosidosis

Kearns-Sayre Syndrome

Characterized by progressive external ophthalmoplegia, pigmentary degeneration of the retina, heart block, and cerebellar dysfunction.

Neuronal Ceroid-Lipofuscinosis

Consists of a group of disorders with varying ages of onset.

Infantile Type (Haltia-Santavuori)

Onset is toward the end of the first year of life. In addition to ataxia, myoclonic seizures, blindness and intellectual deterioration are evident.

Late Infantile (Jansky-Bielschowsky)

Myclonic seizures begin between 2 and 4 years; progressive loss of visual acuity, ataxia, and dementia follow.

Kufs Disease

Problems begin in the second decade of life with cerebellar ataxia, spasticity, rigidity, choreoathetosis, and myoclonic epilepsy.

MERRF (Myoclonic Epilepsy and Ragged-Red Fibers)

After developing normally, affected individuals develop myoclonic epilepsy and progressive ataxia.

Leigh Disease (Subacute Necrotizing Encephalomyelopathy)

The onset is most often in infancy with feeding and swallowing problems, vomiting, and failure to thrive. Delayed motor development, seizures, hypotonia, ataxia, tremor, and nystagmus are prominent.

Juvenile Gaucher Disease

Progressive hepatosplenomegaly, intellectual deterioration, cerebellar ataxia, and spasticity are characteristic.

Refsum Disease

Prominent features include ataxia, ichthyosis, and retinitis pigmentosa.

Hartnup Disease

Intermittent attacks of ataxia may be accompanied by a pellagralike rash, mental changes, and double vision.

Neuronal Intranuclear Hyaline Inclusion Disease with Progressive Cerebellar Ataxia

A rapidly progressive fatal disease with progressively severe seizures and ataxia.

Cerebrotendinous Xanthomatosis

Ectopic xanthomas occur in the brain and lung as well as along the tendons. Other findings include spinal cord damage, mental impairment, and corneal opacities. Onset is as early as 10 years of age with progression throughout life.

HYSTERICAL ATAXIA

This cause can usually be differentiated by observation and a careful neurologic examination.

VASCULAR DISORDERS

Basilar Artery Migraine

Transient blindness, scotomata, formed hallucinations, vertigo, ataxia, loss of consciousness, and drop attacks may be part of this syndrome.

Cerebellar Embolism

Cerebellar Thrombosis

Arteriovenous Malformation

Von Hippel-Lindau Disease (Cerebelloretinal Angiomatosis)

Retinal angiomas enlarge during childhood and may cause visual problems later. Cerebellar angiomas produce signs of cerebellar dysfunction as they enlarge, but usually not until the third decade. Inheritance pattern is autosomal dominant.

Posterior Cerebellar Artery Disease

MISCELLANEOUS CAUSES

♦ **Benign Paroxysmal Vertigo of Childhood**

Attacks of ataxia and vertigo are self-limited, lasting minutes. The etiology is unknown.

Seizures

Children may develop sudden ataxia as a result of frequent transitory impairment of consciousness associated with repetitive minor motor seizures.

Systemic Lupus Erythematosus

Ataxia has been described in severe cases.

Tick Paralysis

Ataxia is an early sign, but impressive muscular weakness rapidly follows.

Multiple Sclerosis

This disorder is rare in children, but acute intermittent attacks of optic neuritis, ataxia, or regional paresthesias are strongly suggestive findings.

Hypothyroidism

Ataxia has been described in hypothyroid adults.

Rett Syndrome

A slowly progressive neurologic deterioration seen exclusively in girls. Onset is between 4 and 18 months with behavioral changes. Seizures occur later along with choreoathetosis, ataxia, and hypotonia.

Cerebello-Trigeminal-Dermal Dysplasia

Also known as the Gomez-Lopez-Hernandez syndrome. Features include craniosynostosis, ataxia, trigeminal anesthesia, scalp alopecia, midface hypoplasia, corneal opacities, mental retardation, and short stature.

REFERENCE

1. Swaiman KF. Cerebellar dysfunction and ataxia in childhood. In: Swaiman KF, ed. *Pediatric neurology: principles and practice,* 2nd ed. St. Louis: Mosby, 1994:261–269.

SUGGESTED READING

Gieron-Korthals MA, Westberry KR, Emmanuel PJ. Acute childhood ataxia: 10-year experience. *J Child Neurol* 1994;9:381–384.

108

Chorea

Chorea is a movement disorder characterized by random, brief, involuntary, and purposeless jerking movements. The movements may involve the trunk and face as well as the extremities. Chorea is usually grouped with other forms of movement disorders, known as dyskinesias, disorders featuring involuntary movements. Tics, tremors, dystonia, and myoclonus are other forms of dyskinesias.

Chorea is a relatively uncommon movement disorder in children. In this chapter the differential diagnosis is broken down into subgroups to assist in classification. Acute and chronic forms have not been separated.

◆ Most Common Causes of Chorea

Benign Familial Chorea
Cerebral Palsy
Systemic Lupus Erythematosus
Post-Pump Chorea
Wilson Disease

Sydenham Chorea
Drugs: Especially Phenytoin
Anoxic Encephalopathy
Kernicterus
Huntington Chorea (Juvenile Form)

CONGENITAL DISORDERS

◆ Cerebral Palsy

Choreiform movements are usually not detected until later in infancy when attempts at purposeful movements are made. Hypotonia is often present and more prominent early on than chorea.

Progressive Atrophy of Globus Pallidus

Choreiform movements are a consequence of atrophy of the pallidal system of the corpus striatum.

INFECTION RELATED

◆ Sydenham Chorea (St. Vitus Dance)

The chorea of rheumatic fever is the most common cause of acquired chorea, despite an apparently decreasing incidence of acute rheumatic fever in developed countries. Although the etiology is still unclear, this disorder seems to follow a streptococcal infection by weeks or months. Evidence of preceding streptococcal infection often is lacking at the time of onset of chorea. The abnormal movements most often begin insidiously and increase in severity over a few weeks. The entire episode rarely lasts more than 3 months. Early signs are often attributed to an emotional disorder. Affected children cannot control their movements and become hyperkinetic, emotionally labile, and often hypotonic. These problems cause interference with normal activities.

Encephalitis

Choreiform movements have been described in encephalitis associated with rubeola, mumps, and varicella and in St. Louis encephalitis.

Associated with Other Infections

Human Immunodeficiency Virus
Pertussis
Infectious Mononucleosis
Neurosyphilis

Lyme Disease
Typhoid Fever
Legionellosis
Diphtheria

♦ DRUGS AND TOXINS

Choreiform movements may occur in children taking the following.

Anticonvulsants
Antidepressants
Amphetamines
Calcium Channel Blockers
Scopolamine
Lithium

Antihistamines
Methylphenidate
Reserpine
Digoxin
Isoniazid
Theophylline

Neuroleptic Drugs

May produce dyskinesias. Haloperidol, phenothiazine, pimazole, metoclopramide, and thioridazine are best known.

Oral Contraceptives

An important cause to consider in adolescents.

Carbon Monoxide

Chorea may occasionally be seen in patients surviving acute or chronic poisoning.

Mercury

Phencyclidine

GENETIC DISORDERS

◆ Benign Familial Chorea of Early Onset

In this disorder, transmitted as an autosomal dominant trait, the early onset of chorea may interfere with motor development. The gait is ataxic. No abnormal results of laboratory tests have been found and there is no mental deterioration.

Familial Paroxysmal Choreoathetosis

This unusual disorder is characterized by the sudden onset of choreoathetosis lasting seconds to 4 hours without changes in consciousness. In most cases the movements last less than 1 minute. The episodes may be precipitated by exercise, fatigue, or the ingestion of coffee, tea, or alcohol. It is thought to be a form of reflex epilepsy and responds to anticonvulsants.

◆ Huntington Chorea

In this disorder, inherited as an autosomal dominant trait, the average age of onset is 35 years. In childhood onset, seizures may be an initial manifestation. The chorea is progressive and relentless with mental deterioration, hypotonia, and death after 5 to 18 years. Psychosis is also a prominent feature.

◆ Wilson Disease (Hepatolenticular Degeneration)

Hepatic symptoms are often prominent in children. Neurologic symptoms include abnormal posturing, muscle hypertonia, dystonia, chorea, athetotic movements, and tremors. Inheritance pattern is autosomal recessive.

Lesch-Nyhan Syndrome

Chorea, dystonia, tremor, and athetosis are findings in this sex-linked disorder. Self-mutilation often occurs; affected boys must be restrained from injuring themselves. Serum uric acid levels are elevated.

Ataxia Telangiectasia

Although truncal ataxia is the predominant feature, in some cases there is severe choreoathetosis.

Friedreich Ataxia

Affected children usually do not begin walking when expected. Ataxia, abnormal speech, and incoordination of hand movements occur later. Choreiform movements occasionally occur.

Dystonia Musculorum Deformans

Spasmodic dystonic movements, opisthotonos, and writhing, twisting movements are characteristic.

Incontinentia Pigmenti

Linear vesiculopustular lesions followed by the appearance of verrucose lesions and later pigmented swirling suggest this disorder.

Hallervorden-Spatz Disease

Choreoathetosis occurs in some cases. More prominent features are progressive rigidity and dementia. The inheritance pattern is autosomal recessive.

Pelizaeus-Merzbacher Disease (Familial Centrolobar Sclerosis)

In this sex-linked disorder, the development of spasticity, ataxia, intention tremor, choreoathetosis, and intellectual deterioration is gradual.

Abetalipoproteinemia

Steatorrhea begins during the first year of life. Progressive ataxia and muscle weakness develop later.

Fabry Disease (Angiokeratoma Corporis Diffusum)

Presenting signs of this sex-linked disorder may include weight loss, fever, joint and abdominal pain, and burning pains in the extremities. Punctate angiomas appear on the lower abdomen and scrotum in late childhood.

Familial Microcephaly, Retardation, and Chorea

Chorea with Curvilinear Bodies

Onset tends to be in childhood with severe chorea, seizures, and intellectual deterioration.

Porphyria

Acute intermittent porphyria usually begins at puberty with episodes of abdominal pain, vomiting, and diarrhea. Neurologic symptoms include seizures, peripheral neuropathy, and personality changes.

METABOLIC-ENDOCRINE DISORDERS

◆ Bilirubin Encephalopathy (Kernicterus)

Children who survive eventually develop choreoathetosis, often not evident until a few years later. The neonatal history is of great importance. Other features include deafness, mental retardation, and paralysis of upward gaze.

Metabolic Derangements

Hypocalcemia	Hypoglycemia
Hypomagnesemia	Hypernatremia
Thiamine Deficiency	Vitamin B_{12} Deficiency in Infants

Glutaric Acidemia, Type I

In addition to choreoathetosis, affected infants may have hypotonia, or hypertonicity, seizures, and dystonia. The onset may be acute or chronic.

Phenylketonuria

Some children may have twisting movements suggestive of chorea.

Endocrine Disorders

Addison Disease

Hypoparathyroidism

Tetany is the prominent finding.

Thyrotoxicosis

Short, rapid, uncoordinated jerks may be present.

NEOPLASMS

Chorea has been described in association with cerebellar tumors.

VASCULAR DISORDERS

Henoch-Schönlein Purpura

Sturge-Weber Syndrome

Chorea as a result of cerebral angiomatosis rarely occurs.

Cerebrovascular Accidents

Posthemiplegic chorea generally involves the affected leg or arm.

Moya Moya Syndrome

Chorea may be the initial presentation of this vascular abnormality of the brain.

TRAUMA

Burns

May cause an encephalopathy with choreiform movements.

◆ ANOXIA

Chorea, athetosis, or dystonia may follow anoxic encephalopathy, a result of cardiac arrest, near drowning, strangulation, and other insults to the brain.

DEGENERATIVE

Canavan Disease (Spongy Degeneration of Central Nervous System)

Symptoms begin between 2 and 4 months of age. Additional features include optic atrophy, hypotonia, and developmental failure. The head circumference usually increases by 6 months of age. Seizures and spasticity follow. Choreoathetotic movements are occasionally noted.

MISCELLANEOUS CAUSES

◆ Systemic Lupus Erythematosus

Chorea is rarely a presenting symptom; however, more cases with chorea are being reported.

Bronchopulmonary Dysplasia

Former premature infants with severe bronchopulmonary dysplasia may develop choreiform movements at 2 to 3 months of age.

◆ Post-Pump Chorea

Choreoathetoid movements develop within 2 weeks following cardiopulmonary bypass. Developmental delay is frequently associated.

Pregnancy

Chorea gravidarum may be a recrudescence of rheumatic chorea.

Polycythemia

Hyperkinetic Syndrome

Movements are sometimes mistaken for chorea.

Nevus Unius Lateralis

Central nervous system and bony abnormalities have been described in association with this skin disorder.

Rett Syndrome

A slowly progressive neurologic deterioration seen exclusively in girls. The onset is between 4 and 18 months with behavioral changes. Seizures occur later accompanied by choreoathetosis, ataxia, and hypotonia.

Polymyoclonus

These movements may be mistaken for choreiform movements. When accompanied by opsoclonus (dancing eyes and dancing feet), suspect the presence of a neuroblastoma.

SUGGESTED READING

Golden GS. Movement disorders: sorting the benign from the serious. *Contemp Pediatr* 1987:4:77–92.

Haddeers-Algra M, Boz AF, Matijn A, Prechtl HF. Infantile chorea in an infant with severe bronchopulmonary dysplasia: an EMG study. *Dev Med Child Neurol* 1994;36:177–182.

Holden KR, Sessions JC, Curé J, Whitcomb DS, Sade RM. Neurologic outcomes in children with postpump choreoathetosis. *J Pediatr* 1998;132:162–164.

Holinski-Feder E, Jedele KB, Hortnagel K, Albert A, Meindl A, Trenkwalder C. Large intergenerational variation in age of onset in two young patients with Huntington's disease presenting as dyskinesia. *Pediatrics* 1997;100:896–898.

Kiessling LS, Marcotte AC, Culpepper L. Antineuronal antibodies in movement disorders. *Pediatrics* 1993;92:39–43.

Kinast M, Erenberg G, Rothner AD. Paroxysmal choreoathetosis: report of five cases and review of literature. *Pediatrics* 1980;65:74–77.

Klawans HL, Brandabur MM. Chorea in childhood. *Pediatr Ann* 1993;22:41–50.

Pranzatelli MR. Movement disorders in childhood. *Pediatr Rev* 1996;17:388–394.

Swedo SE, Leonard HL, Schapiro MB, et al. Sydenham's chorea: physical and psychological symptoms of St. Vitus dance. *Pediatrics* 1993;91:706–713.

Wheeler PG, Weaver DD, Dobyns WB. Benign hereditary chorea. *Pediatr Neurol* 1993;9:337–340.

109

Delirium

Delirium is a frightening alteration in consciousness characterized by hallucinations, disorientation, and delusions. Normal thought processes are impaired, judgment is altered, and rational behavior is lost. The cause may be a metabolic derangement, an acute infection, or, in a distressing number of cases, drug abuse.

INFECTIONS

♦ Acute Systemic Infections

Children may become delirious during acute infections, from any class of organism. Bacterial sepsis, pneumococcal pneumonia, pyelonephritis, influenza, measles, and other viral disorders with exanthems and high fever are relatively common causes.

♦ Central Nervous System Infections

Children with meningitis, encephalitis, brain abscesses, and other central nervous system infections often are delirious.

Rocky Mountain Spotted Fever

Delirium with hallucinations may precede the appearance of the rash. At onset of the illness, symptoms include fever, headache, muscle aches, and shaking chills.

Malaria

Syphilis

Neurosyphilis is relatively uncommon in children.

Rabies

DRUGS AND TOXINS

♦ Alcohol

Acute intoxication and, less commonly, withdrawal from alcohol may cause delirious behavior.

♦ Antihistamine

♦ **Glucocorticoids**

Beware of unusual behavior as a manifestation of steroid "psychosis."

♦ **Amphetamines**

Tremor, dry mouth, tachycardia, hyperactivity, and occasionally, hypertension are signs.

Aminophylline

Cimetidine

Phenothiazines

● **Atropine; Scopolamine**

"Mad as a hatter, dry as a bone, blind as a bat."

Hallucinogenic Drugs

LSD, mescaline, and psilocybin produce vivid hallucinations. Tremors, dilated pupils, abdominal pain, and nausea may be present.

● **Phencyclidine ("Angel Dust")**

Affected children have tachycardia, hyperreflexia, visual hallucinations, and hypertension. Ataxia and nystagmus with small or normal-sized pupils suggest this ingestion.

● **Opiates; Cocaine**

Delirium may occur both in intoxication and withdrawl.

Marihuana; Hashish

Caffeine

Barbiturate Withdrawal

Benzodiazepine Withdrawal

Often accompanied by myoclonic jerks.

Salicylates

Camphor

Lead; Mercury; Arsenic

Organic Solvents

Organophosphates

METABOLIC DERANGEMENTS

● **Hypoglycemia**

Diabetic Ketoacidosis

Hyponatremia

Hyponatremia may occur in various disorders with inappropriate antidiuretic hormone secretion. Lethargy and seizures may be other signs.

Uremia

Fatigue, irritability, and difficulty in concentrating occur early; delirium generally appears later.

Acidosis

PSYCHOSES

Delirium and hallucinations are less commonly reported in children with affective disorders than in adults. Auditory hallucinations are characteristic, whereas visual hallucinations generally accompany delirium of organic etiology.

CENTRAL NERVOUS SYSTEM DISORDERS

◆ **Head Injury**

Delirious behavior may follow significant head injury.

Migraine

Visual hallucinations are relatively common, but less so than scotomata, transitory blindness, blurred vision, and hemianopsia. An acute confusional state can be seen as a form of complicated migraine.

Increased Intracranial Pressure

Headache and vomiting in the presence of papilledema suggest this problem.

Epilepsy

Olfactory and visual hallucinations may be part of a preconvulsive aura or occur in the postictal state.

Brain Tumor

Cerebral Thrombosis or Embolism

Cerebral Degenerative Disease

DIMINISHED CEREBRAL OXYGENATION

◆ **Hypoxia**

Any cause of hypoxemia may alter cerebral function producing hallucinations, disorientation, and other symptoms of delirium.

Acute Blood Loss

Severe Anemia

Congestive Heart Failure

MISCELLANEOUS CAUSES

Fatigue

Dehydration

Heat Stroke

● **Hepatic Failure**

Common initial symptoms are alterations in consciousness, including disorientation, restlessness, slurred speech, and delirium. Tremors and decerebrate and decorticate rigidity may follow.

Insect and Spider Bites

Potent toxins may be released by various biting insects and spiders.

Burn Encephalopathy

Chorea

Systemic Lupus Erythematosus

Cerebral vasculitis may be associated with psychotic behavior. It may be difficult to separate effects of steroid therapy from those due to the disease.

Porphyria

Attacks of psychotic behavior usually do not begin until late adolescence or early adulthood.

Pellagra

In severe vitamin deficiency delirium, tremors, spasticity, polyneuritis, and optic atrophy may overshadow the skin changes.

Hartnup Disease

This rare inherited disorder is characterized by a pellagra-like skin rash, cerebellar ataxia, and psychological disturbances. Attacks of these symptoms may be intermittent.

Reye Syndrome

Delirious behavior often rapidly follows vomiting and precedes stupor and coma.

110

Vertigo (Dizziness)

Vertigo is a subjective symptom in which the affected person feels as though he or his environment were moving, usually spinning. This complaint is not thought to be a common one in children, but may be due to the difficulty young children have in expressing this sensation. It may be difficult to distinguish vertigo from dizziness, a more inclusive descriptive term that includes vertigo as well as dysequilibrium, motion sickness, presyncope, and even psychological manifestations.

Studies of vertigo in childhood are distinctly uncommon, but in a thorough evaluation of this symptom in 42 children by Eviatar and Eviatar (1), a seizure focus was the cause in 25; psychosomatic vertigo, migraine, and vestibular neuronitis each accounted for 5 cases. Otitis media with effusion is the most common cause of vestibular disturbance in children, although seldom does it cause vertigo. Balance problems are more common than vertigo in serous otitis media. The presence or absence of hearing loss may help in narrowing the diagnostic choices.

The evaluation of this symptom is complex and requires specialized expertise.

♦ **Most Common Causes of Vertigo**

Vertiginous Seizures   Migraine: Includes Paroxysmal Vertigo
Vestibular Neuronitis   Psychosomatic Vertigo
Head Trauma

CENTRAL CAUSES

♦ **Vertiginous Seizures**

These seizures may be characterized by sudden attacks of vertigo alone, or sometimes with headache, nausea, vomiting, falling, and loss of consciousness, or combinations of these symptoms. The electroencephalogram (EEG) may show a temporal lobe abnormal focus, or the tracing may be diffusely abnormal.

♦ **Migraine (Basilar Artery)**

Vertigo may be an aura prior to the onset of migraine and sometimes persists during the other symptoms. Dizziness or true vertigo may occur with or without a headache. Basilar artery migraine often presents with dizziness.

♦ **Trauma**

Vertigo may be associated with temporal bone fractures, brain contusions, and, occasionally, cervical spine injuries. Fractures of the temporal bone usually cause hearing loss, tinnitus, and nystagmus; the vertigo appears a few days to weeks after the trauma. Trauma may also result in the development of a perilymphatic fistula. Depending on the area traumatized, hearing may or may not be lost.

Infection

Vertigo may accompany or follow meningitis, meningoencephalitis, or a brain abscess. The symptom of vertigo is generally less noticeable than other signs and symptoms of infection.

Demyelinating Disease

Dizziness or vertigo occurs at some time during the onset or course of multiple sclerosis in most cases.

Tumors

Cerebellopontine angle tumors, such as acoustic neuromas, or increased intracranial pressure may cause vertigo.

Vertebrobasilar Artery Ischemia

The most common symptom of this problem is dizziness. The attacks are recurrent and spontaneous and last 5 to 15 minutes. Other symptoms such as diplopia, difficulty in speaking, weakness, headache, and impaired consciousness may occur.

Vestibulocerebellar Ataxia

Postural vertigo may occur in this rare form of hereditary ataxia. Nystagmus is usually present. The vertigo may precede the onset of ataxia.

PERIPHERAL CAUSES

♦ **Vestibular Neuronitis**

Most patients have symptoms of a recent viral illness, usually an infection of the upper respiratory tract. The vertigo usually begins abruptly, often with nausea, but without hearing loss or central nervous system disturbance.

♦ **Benign Paroxysmal Vertigo**

This disorder occurs primarily in young children between 1 and 4 years of age, with recurrent, sudden, short-lived attacks of vertigo. The attacks disappear over a variable period of time. This disorder may represent a migraine equivalent, especially if there is a positive familial history. Classic migraine may follow in later life.

♦ **Paroxysmal Torticollis of Infancy**

This may be a variant of benign paroxysmal vertigo. Attacks are characterized by the head tilting to one side, with resistance to straightening. Vomiting, pallor, and agitation occur in some cases. The average duration is 2 to 3 days.

Middle Ear Disease
Acute Otitis Media

Vertigo or dizziness may be a secondary complaint.

Chronic Serous Otitis Media

The tympanic membrane is immobile and retracted.

Chronic Suppurative Otitis

Labyrinthitis occurs from spread of middle ear infection to the inner ear. Hearing is lost, and there is a history of chronic ear drainage.

External Auditory Canal

Children with complete obstruction of the canal and pressure on the tympanic membrane may have dizziness and decreased hearing.

Postural Vertigo

Most cases are due to inner ear disorders, but rarely it may be idiopathic in children. Vertigo is precipitated by changes in head position.

Labyrinthitis

Common viral infections such as mumps, influenza, measles, and the common cold may cause transient hearing loss and vertigo.

Perilymphatic Fistula

A rupture in the oval or round window allows fluid to leak into the middle ear. The injury may be caused by direct ear trauma or severe pressure changes. Hearing loss and tinnitus are present.

Herpes Zoster Oticus (Ramsay Hunt Syndrome)

Vesicles are found in the external auditory canal. Ear pain is usually severe.

Vascular Accidents
Hemorrhage

Inner ear bleeding with destruction of the vestibular labyrinth and cochlea may occur in leukemia and other blood dyscrasias.

Embolus

Thrombus

The arterial blood supply to the inner ear may be blocked; this may occur in collagen vascular diseases such as periarteritis nodosa.

Meniere Disease

This disorder is characterized by recurrent attacks of vertigo associated with hearing loss and often a sensation of fullness in the ear. As the attacks continue deafness may occur. It is rare before puberty and probably has many causes.

PSYCHOGENIC VERTIGO

Vertigo or dizziness may be a chronic or recurrent complaint in psychological disturbances. There may be other complaints or unusual behavior. Chronic headaches are common.

MISCELLANEOUS CAUSES

Hyperventilation

Dizziness commonly occurs during episodes of hyperventilation, along with headache, chest pain, anxiety, paresthesias of fingers and toes, and carpopedal spasm.

Hypoglycemia

Drugs

Vestibular damage may be caused by various drugs, resulting in balance problems. Common offenders include the aminoglycosides. Larger doses of aspirin and long-term therapy with large doses of phenytoin may also result in disturbances of vestibular function.

Cardiac Arrhythmias

Dizzy spells may be caused by a number of rhythm disturbances.

Hypertension

Dizziness may be a complaint in children with hypertension.

Pellagra

Syncope Associated

Dizziness rather than syncope may be present with any of the disorders reported in Chapter 62, Syncope.

REFERENCE

1. Eviatar L, Eviatar A. Vertigo in children: differential diagnosis and treatment. *Pediatrics* 1977;59:833–837.

SUGGESTED READING

Busis SN. Vertigo. In: Bluestone CD, Stool SE, Kenna MA, eds. *Pediatric otolaryngology,* 3rd ed. Philadelphia: WB Saunders, 1996:285–301.
Dunn DW. Dizziness: when is it vertigo? *Contemp Pediatr* 1987;4:67–88.
Evitar L. Dizziness in children. *Otolaryngol Clin North Am* 1994;27:557–571.
Tusa RJ, Saads AA Jr, Niparko JK. Dizziness in childhood. *J Child Neurol* 1994;9:261–274.

SECTION XV

Skin

111

Alopecia (Hair Loss)

Alopecia, derived from the Greek word for "fox mange," refers to hair loss. In the evaluation of alopecia in children with the complaint of hair loss it is important to determine whether the loss is congenital or acquired; whether it is diffuse or patchy; and whether there is associated scarring or preceding scalp disease.

The classification of conditions causing alopecia in this chapter has been modified from an approach used by Weston et al. (1). The first category represents the most common causes of alopecia found in children, which account for about 95% of the hair loss seen by the primary care physician. In the remaining categories, possible causes are grouped by characteristic patterns of hair loss.

The congenital diffuse alopecias contain several primary hair defects that can often be distinguished on microscopic examination of the hair shaft. A primary presenting complaint of these disorders is that the child's hair does not seem to grow. A relatively long list of malformation syndromes associated with hair abnormalities is also included in this category. Acquired diffuse hair loss usually results from an underlying systemic disorder; because most of these disorders are correctable, early diagnosis is of particular benefit.

MOST COMMON CAUSES OF HAIR LOSS

◆ Tinea Capitis

This disorder must always be considered as the cause of any alopecia. Broken hairs are usually present in the affected area. The scalp is often scaly, and the hair in the involved areas is dull. It is usually seen in prepubertal children.

◆ Alopecia Areata

This condition is characterized by the complete or almost complete loss of hair in circumscribed areas. The hair loss often begins suddenly. The scalp is smooth and not inflamed. Total loss of scalp or body hair may occur.

◆ Traumatic Alopecia

Various types of prolonged or recurrent pull or tension on the hair may lead to areas of alopecia. "Corn row" and ponytail hair styles and the use of hot combs are relatively common causes.

◆ Trichotillomania

Irregular areas of hair loss are the result of self-inflicted pulling; broken off hairs are readily apparent in the areas of alopecia. The scalp is usually normal in appearance.

◆ Telogen Effluvium

Various stressful circumstances may cause the abrupt, premature cessation of growth in certain normal hair bulbs. These hairs then enter an involutional phase, followed by the resting or telogen phase during which they may be shed. The period between the causative stress and the hair loss is 2 to 4 months. Rarely, more than 50% of the hair is lost. Various stressful situations that have been implicated are listed below.

Febrile Illnesses

High fevers associated with various illnesses, particularly pneumonia, influenza, and typhoid fever, may be followed by hair loss.

Physiologic Hair Loss in Newborns

Parturition

Severe Emotional Stress

Crash Diets

Traction

Surgery and Anesthesia

Drugs

Valproic acid; hypervitaminosis A; heparin; coumadin; propanolol.

Oral Contraceptives

Hypothyroidism or Hyperthyroidism

CONGENITAL, CIRCUMSCRIBED AREAS OF HAIR LOSS

Sebaceous Nevus (of Jadassohn) or Epidermal Nevus

There is no hair growth in the area of the yellowish tan plaquelike lesion of a sebaceous nevus whose surface resembles pigskin. The epidermal nevi tend to be verrucous rather than flat.

Aplasia Cutis Congenita

At birth affected areas appear as punched out, ulcerlike lesions. On occasion, an atrophic skin covering is present. The lesions generally heal in a scar devoid of hair.

Hair Follicle Hamartomas

Triangular Alopecia of the Frontal Scalp

Generally overlies the frontotemporal suture.

Incontinentia Pigmenti

Patchy alopecia, especially of the posterior scalp, may be found in 20% of the cases. The skin lesions are the main diagnostic clues. There may be a progression of lesions from linear bullae and vesicles, to verrucous looking lesions, to hyperpigmented streaks and swirls. Eye, teeth, and central nervous system abnormalities may occur.

Myotonic Dystrophy

Frontal baldness usually develops during childhood. Muscle myotonia, weakness, and an immobile facies are early clues.

Goltz Syndrome

Areas of hair loss, focal dermal hypoplasia (areas of atrophic skin with outpouchings of subcutaneous tissue), syndactyly of fingers and toes, strabismus, and dystrophic nails may be found.

Conradi-Hünermann Syndrome

Affected children have mild to moderate growth deficiency, low nasal bridge, flat facies, asymmetric short limbs, scoliosis, stippled epiphyses, and occasionally areas of alopecia.

ACQUIRED, CIRCUMSCRIBED AREAS OF HAIR LOSS WITH SCARRING

Following Infection

Kerion

Hypersensitivity reaction to tinea capitis may, if untreated, lead to scarring with hair loss. The hair invariably grows back, but the delay may be prolonged.

Pyoderma

Scalp infections if deep enough may destroy hair follicles.

Recurrent Herpes Simplex

Varicella

Dissecting Cellulitis; Folliculitis Decalvans

Destruction of hair follicles secondary to the inflammatory process leads to scarring.

Tuberculosis; Sarcoid; Leprosy

Localized areas of inflammation may result in alopecia.

Following Inflammation

Lupus Erythematosus

Both systemic and discoid lupus may cause patches of alopecia. In the systemic form scarring is not always present.

Morphea

Areas of localized scleroderma in the scalp result in atrophy of hair follicles.

Keratosis Follicularis

This disorder, transmitted as an autosomal trait, is characterized by the development of papules on the face, chest, back, and extremities. The lesions may coalesce to form scaly, greasy masses. Scalp involvement leads to hair loss. The buccal mucosa and nails are also involved.

Lichen Planus

Small, flat topped, polygonal papules first appear on the extremities and may become generalized. Scalp involvement may lead to scarring.

Porokeratosis of Mibelli

A plaquelike lesion surrounded by a keratotic ridge.

Following Trauma

Physical Trauma

Chronic traction, neurotic excoriations, or clumps of hair pulled out with force result in hair follicle disruption with scarring.

Chemical or Thermal Burns

Caustics, acids or alkalis, and phenol as well as burns may cause permanent hair loss.

Radiation Injuries

CONGENITAL, DIFFUSE ALOPECIA

● **Loose Anagen Syndrome**

The hair pulls out easily without pain. Parents complain that their child's hair rarely needs cutting. On microscopic examination the hair shaft bulb is misshapen. This may be a more common cause of thinning hair than previously recognized.

Hair Shaft Defects

Trichorrhexis Nodosa

Familial Form

An increase in hair fragility is the only finding. On microscopic examination the hair resembles two brooms that have been pushed together end to end. Excessive combing, permanent treatments, and the like provide the trauma. The condition is more common in blacks, especially adolescents.

Argininosuccinic Aciduria

The hair is stubby and fragile in affected infants, who are severely mentally retarded.

Pili Torti (Twisted Hair)

Classic Form

The hair appears normal at birth but by 2 or 3 years of age it looks brittle and spangled. The condition occasionally is associated with deafness.

Menkes Syndrome

In this severe X-linked neurodegenerative disorder, kinky short hair is characteristic. It often stands straight up.

Monilethrix (Beaded Hair)

This rare disorder, transmitted as an autosomal dominant trait, is characterized by breaking off of scalp hair.

Trichorrhexis Invaginata

On microscopic examination the hairs look like bamboo shoots. The disorder is associated with ichthyosis (Netherton syndrome).

Trichothiodystrophy

This is a rare syndrome with sparse, brittle hair. It may be found in association with other problems, such as cerebellar ataxia, short stature, mental retardation, hypogonadism, and ichthyosis, in varying combinations. The hair shaft shows alternating bright and dark zones under polarizing microscopy.

Congenital Hypothyroidism

Anhidrotic Ectodermal Dysplasia

The skin seems thin and wrinkled giving an aged appearance. A saddle nose, thick lips, and dental abnormalities accompany the hypotrichosis.

Hidrotic Ectodermal Dysplasia

Hypoplasia of hair with painfully thickened nails is typical.

Rothmund-Thomson Syndrome

Striking, irregular hyperpigmentation and depigmentation of the skin with telangiectactic lesions are characteristic. Alopecia, photosensitivity, and cataracts are common.

Progeria

This is a fascinating rare disorder producing premature aging.

Atrichia Congenita

Familial cases of sparse to absent hair have been reported.

Marinesco-Sjögren Syndrome

Main features are cerebellar ataxia, growth deficiency, cataracts, and weakness. Sparse hair has also been reported.

Cartilage-Hair Hypoplasia

Fine, sparse hair in patients with short stature, short limbs, short hands, and irregularly scalloped metaphyses on radiographs, and immune deficiency are findings.

Ellis-van Creveld Syndrome (Chondroectodermal Dysplasia)

A combination of hair and dental abnormalities occurs with shortened extremities; trunk size is normal. Polydactyly and congenital heart disease are also prominent features.

Trichorhinophalangeal Syndrome (Langer-Giedion Syndrome)

Sparse hair, a pear-shaped nose, and short metacarpals are the main physical findings.

Cockayne Syndrome

Growth deficiency becomes evident after 1 year of age. Mental retardation, an unsteady gait, tremors, deafness, sunken eyes, skin photosensitivity, joint movement limitations, and sparse hair create a striking picture.

Hallermann-Streiff Syndrome (Oculomandibulofacial Syndrome)

This syndrome is characterized by small stature, prominent forehead, congenital cataracts, a small, thin nose with "pinched" facies, hypoplastic teeth, and sparse hair.

Oculodentodigital Dysplasia

Microphthalmos, a thin nose with hypoplastic alae, enamel hypoplasia, fixed and flexed fifth fingers, and sparse, dry, slow growing hair are important features.

Crouston Syndrome

Physical findings include thick, dyskeratotic palms and soles; hyperpigmentation over knuckles, elbows, axillae, and pubic area; nail dysplasia; and hair abnormalities ranging from hypoplasia to alopecia.

Laurence-Moon-Biedl Syndrome

Hypotrichosis is seen occasionally in affected children; prominent findings include short stature, obesity, polydactyly, mental retardation, and hypogonadism.

Homocystinuria

The hair of children with this aminoaciduria may be sparse and light. A marfanoid slender build, subluxated lenses, malar flush, and venous thromboses are prominent features.

Werner Syndrome

This is a syndrome of premature aging that begins in adolescence.

Oral-Facial-Digital Syndrome Type I

Abnormalities include cleft soft palate, asymmetric shortening of digits, and webbing of buccal mucosa and alveolar ridges. Alopecia is a rare finding.

Seckel Syndrome

Individuals with this syndrome, originally called the "bird-headed dwarf" syndrome, may occasionally have sparse hair.

Dyskeratosis Congenita

Dystrophy of nails with chronic paronychiae develops first, followed by the appearance of mucous membrane blisters and reticular brown pigmentation of the skin. The hair may be sparse diffusely.

ACQUIRED DIFFUSE HAIR LOSS

Endocrine Disorders

Androgenetic Alopecia

Physiologic male pattern baldness may occur in adolescents.

Hypothyroidism

Diffuse thinning of scalp hair may occur with some patchy areas of alopecia.

Hypopituitarism

Scalp, eyebrow, and sexual hair is sparse. The skin is thin and prematurely wrinkled.

Hypoparathyroidism

Hair is thin and coarse and sheds easily; the loss may be complete or patchy. Muscle cramps, tetany, and convulsions are more impressive features.

Diabetes Mellitus

Chemicals and Drugs

- **Heavy Metals**

  Thallium, arsenic, and lead ingestion may cause hair loss. Arsenic may be inhaled via smoke from the burning of outdoor grade lumber treated with preservatives.

Antithyroid Drugs

Anabolic Steroid Use

Heparin; Coumarin

Antimetabolites

Trimethadione

Carbamazepine (Tegretol)

Nutritional Disorders

Hypervitaminosis A

Chronic ingestion may lead to hair loss, peeling of the skin, and bone pain.

Acrodermatitis Enteropathica

Zinc deficiency in affected children is associated with alopecia, irritability, diarrhea, and perioral and perianal as well as distal extremity rashes.

Marasmus and Kwashiorkor

The nutritional deficiency must be severe for hair loss to result.

Celiac Disease

Iron Deficiency

Thinning of hair may occur with chronic, severe iron deficiency anemia.

Rickets

Miscellaneous Causes

Seborrhea

Chronic involvement of the scalp with thick scales may lead to thinning of the hair. In young infants, hair loss is accompanied by hypopigmentation of the involved skin as well.

Atopic Dermatitis

Rubbing and scratching of the scalp may lead to hair thinning and loss.

Psoriasis

Heaped-up layers of silvery scale may lead to hair loss in involved areas.

Biotin Responsive Multiple Carboxylase Deficiency

Biotinidase deficiency results in seizures, ataxia, hearing loss, developmental delay periorificial dermatitis, alopecia, and eventually death.

REFERENCE

1. Weston WL, Lane AT, Morelli JG. *Color textbook of pediatric dermatology,* 2nd ed. St. Louis: Mosby, 1996:243–252.

SUGGESTED READING

Atton AV, Tunnessen WW Jr. Alopecia in children: the most common causes. *Pediatr Rev* 1990;12:25–30.

112

Hypertrichosis and Hirsutism

Hirsutism is the term usually used to denote an increase in body hair; however, it refers specifically to the excess growth of hair, in an adult male distribution pattern, which may be seen in women and children. Hypertrichosis is the correct term to describe a generalized or localized increase in body hair compared to other individuals of the same age, sex, and race.

Hirsutism results from an excess production of androgens from either adrenal or ovarian sources or from a constitutional increase in sensitivity of hair follicles, or possibly from both. Hypertrichosis refers to hair growth that is not androgen-dependent, and is most often of nonendocrine origin. In this chapter the causes of increased hair growth are divided into disorders with hypertrichosis and those with hirsutism.

HYPERTRICHOSIS

Generalized Hypertrichosis

♦ Genetic Trait

Certain races and certain families may have more hair.

♦ Drug-Induced Hypertrichosis

Glucocorticoids, diphenylhydantoin, diazoxide, minoxidil, and streptomycin are among the drugs that have been implicated. Hypertrichosis has been reported in the offspring of a mother treated with minoxidil throughout her pregnancy as well as in infants whose mothers consumed excessive alcohol.

Central Nervous System Disorders

Hypertrichosis has been reported following encephalitis and concussions, and in multiple sclerosis.

Starvation and Anorexia Nervosa

Hypothyroidism

Hair is increased, especially on the back and limbs.

Dermatomyositis

Generally, increased hair is seen on the legs and temples.

Epidermolysis Bullosa

Dysmorphogenic Syndromes

Hypertrichosis has been described in Bloom, Seckel, de Lange, Rubinstein-Taybi, Coffin-Siris, cerebro-oculofacioskeletal, Gorlin, leprechaunism, Marshall-Smith, trisomy 18, and partial trisomy 3q syndromes. Other syndromes reported with hypertrichosis include Hajdu-Cheney, Barber-Say, Weyer acrofacial-dysostosis, osteochondrodysplasia, and amaurosis congenita.

Metabolic Disorders

Mucopolysaccharidoses

GM1-Gangliosidosis

Porphyria

Children with congenital erythropoietic porphyria develop increased body hair, but other signs and symptoms such as red urine, significant photosensitivity with bullae formation and scarring, and, eventually, red to pink teeth are more prominent. Affected persons were the so-called werewolves of old.

Hypertrichosis Universalis Congenita (Ambras Syndrome)

An extremely rare disorder characterized by excessively long lanugo hair present at birth that increases during childhood. The hair is soft and silky. This is a familial disorder inherited as an autosomal dominant trait with varying expressivity. The hypertrichosis associated with gingival fibromatosis may represent the same genetic disorder.

Transient Congenital Hypertrichosis Universalis

A rare disorder with excessive hair present at birth that spares the face, hands, and feet. The hair disappears in infancy.

Acrodynia

Increased hair is an unusual feature in chronic mercury poisoning; it occurs primarily on the limbs.

Lipodystrophy

Children with congenital or generalized lipodystrophy tend to have increased body hair.

Localized Hypertrichosis

Trauma

Increased hair growth may occur at sites of trauma or chemical irritation.

788 SKIN

Nevi and Hamartomas

Localized hair growth may occur in various nevi or over spinal cord defects or other lesions.

HIRSUTISM

◆ Idiopathic Hirsutism

In most cases no cause for the hirsutism can be found. There may be a familial history. Support for the idiopathic appellation includes a history of normal menses, no deepening of the voice, and lack of frontal hairline recession. As more sensitive assay techniques for androgens are developed most patients will be shown to have an underlying abnormality of androgen metabolism.

◆ Obesity

Insulin resistance may occur in obese patients with subsequent elevation of androgens and menstrual irregularities as well as hirsutism.

◆ Iatrogenic Hirsutism

Among the exogenous causes are progestational agents, anabolic steroids, and testosterone. Systemic steroids and adrenocorticotropic hormones cause an increase in lanugo hair. Phenytoin, diazoxide, and minoxidil are also drugs that should be considered.

◆ Physiologic Hirsutism

Hirsutism without virilization may occur in precocious puberty, at puberty, and during pregnancy.

Adrenal Disorders

Congenital Adrenal Hyperplasia (Adrenogenital Syndrome)

Classic adrenogenital syndrome as well as compensated forms involving 11 and 21 hydroxylation and 3-B-hydroxysteroid dehydrogenase activity demonstrate hirsutism and other signs of virilization. In the last form, intermittent elevations of cortisol precursors may be missed.

Virilizing Tumors

Clitoral enlargement in girls and phallic enlargement in prepubertal boys are important clinical signs.

Cushing Syndrome

Other signs are more prominent including moon facies, truncal obesity, short stature, and hypertension.

Ovarian Disorders

Virilizing Ovarian Tumors

Arrhenoblastoma and granulosa-theca cell tumors are uncommon causes.

Stein-Leventhal Syndrome (Polycystic Ovary Syndrome)

Features include amenorrhea or dysfunctional uterine bleeding with infertility, with or without obesity, in association with polycystic ovaries. Other non-neoplastic causes of ovarian androgen production may present a spectrum of severity of clinical findings less obvious than the above.

Pure Gonadal Dysgenesis

Pituitary Disorders

Acromegaly associated with an eosinophilic pituitary tumor may be accompanied by diabetes and hirsutism.

Miscellaneous Causes

Achard-Thiers Syndrome

Obesity and facial hirsutism develop by 15 to 30 years of age. Hypertension and diabetes occur later.

Male Pseudohermaphroditism

SUGGESTED READING

Baumeister FAM, Schwarz HP, Stengel-Rutkowski S. Childhood hypertrichosis: diagnosis and management. *Arch Dis Child* 1995;72:457–459.

Emans SJ, Grace E, Fleischnick E, Mansfield MJ, Crigler JF Jr. Detection of late onset 21 hydroxylase deficiency congenital adrenal hyperplasia in adolescents. *Pediatrics* 1983;72:690–695.

Kustin J, Rebar RW. Hirsutism in young adolescent girls. *Pediatr Ann* 1986;15:522–528.

Lee IJ, Im SB, Kim D-K. Hypertrichosis universalis congenita: a separate entity, or the same disease as gingival fibromatosis? *Pediatr Dermatol* 1993;10:263–266.

113

Purpura (Petechiae and Ecchymoses)

Purpura is the name given to the discoloration of the skin or mucous membranes caused by extravasation of red blood cells; the areas of discoloration do not blanch on pressure. Petechiae are purpuric lesions that are 2 mm or less in diameter; purpuric lesions per se are defined as ranging in size from 2 mm to 1 cm; and, ecchymoses are purpuric lesions greater than 1 cm.

Purpuric lesions are generally the result of a defect in the circulating blood (platelets or coagulation factors) or the blood vessels. Petechiae and random purpuric lesions are characteristic of thrombocytopenias and thrombocytopathies (platelet dysfunction). Coagulation disturbances cause hemostatic problems in large vessels and usually produce ecchymoses rather than petechiae. Vascular disorders may produce either type of lesion, and often produce palpable purpuric lesions.

Fever with petechial or purpuric lesions deserves special mention. Although meningococcemia and other forms of sepsis are first thoughts, most children who present to an emergency room with fever and petechiae have benign, non-bacteremic illnesses (1). Only 1.9% of 411 children enrolled in the Mandl et al. (1) study had bacteremia or clinical sepsis. Viral illnesses and streptococcal pharyngitis probably account for most cases, particularly those with petechiae above the nipple line, who have been coughing (2). The list of infectious agents associated with petechial-purpuric lesions is extensive (3). A sick appearing child with petechiae or purpura should be treated as having sepsis, either bacterial, including meningococcal, or in some areas of the United States, rickettsial, including Rocky Mountain spotted fever. The immunocompromised child who develops purpuric lesions is a far different story. Pseudomonal and other bacterial and fungal infections become much more likely.

Although in this chapter the causes of purpuric lesions are divided into categories of thrombocytopenic, nonthrombocytopenic, vascular, and coagulation disorders, more than one defect may be involved. For instance, infections may cause purpura with or without thrombocytopenia, and thrombocytopenia and vascular damage may occur together. Causes of purpura in the neonatal period have been treated as a separate grouping.

NEONATAL PURPURA

♦ Most Common Causes of Neonatal Purpura

Trauma
Infection, Congenital (CMV)
Maternal Autoimmune Thrombocytopenia

Infection, Acquired (Sepsis)
Isoimmune Thrombocytopenia

◆ Trauma

Petechial and purpuric lesions are relatively common in newborns as a result of venous congestion and pressure points from delivery.

Infection

Infections of various types are a common cause of neonatal purpura. Thrombocytopenia or disseminated intravascular coagulation may or may not be associated.

◆ Bacterial Infection

Group B streptococci, *Escherichia coli, Listeria,* and other organisms have been implicated. *Pseudomonas* is an important cause in infants who are in intensive care units for a prolonged period.

Viral Infection

Infections may be congenital or acquired. Important congenital infections include cytomegalovirus infection, rubella, and herpes simplex; the last may be acquired, usually during passage through the birth canal. Parvovirus, mumps, and human immunodeficiency virus infections rarely are responsible.

Parasitic Infections

Toxoplasmosis may be associated with purpura.

Other Infections

Purpura may be a finding in syphilis.

Extramedullary Hematopoiesis

The appellation "blueberry muffin baby" was coined to describe neonates with purpuric appearing cutaneous lesions associated with congenital rubella syndrome. The lesions are not a result of intradermal hemorrhage, but rather of extramedullary hematopoiesis. Causes include the following.

◆ Congenital Infections

CMV is now the most common virus responsible. Others include rubella, parvovirus B19, and coxsackievirus B2.

Hematologic Dyscrasias

Severe anemia *in utero* may result in extramedullary hematopoiesis. Causes include severe Rh incompatibility, maternal-fetal ABO blood group incompatibility, spherocytosis, and twin-to-twin transfusion syndrome.

- ● **Neoplastic-Infiltrative Disorders**

  The lesions here are true metatases, not dermal erythropoiesis; however, the appearance may be similar. Disorders to consider include neuroblastoma, congenital leukemia, rhabdomyosarcoma, and Langerhans cell histiocytosis.

Immunologic Disorders

◆ Isoimmune Neonatal Thrombocytopenia

Maternal IgG antibody against fetal platelets crosses the placenta. The maternal platelet count is within normal limits.

◆ Maternal Auto-Antibody Disease

Maternal disorders associated with auto-antibody formation may cause thrombocytopenia in her offspring. Examples are maternal idiopathic thrombocytopenic purpura, systemic lupus erythematosus, and drug-induced autoimmune thrombocytopenia.

Heparin-Induced Immune Thrombocytopenia

Rarely, infants receiving low doses of heparin to keep intravenous lines open can develop this problem.

Erythroblastosis Fetalis

In severe disease the platelet count may be depressed.

Disseminated Intravascular Coagulation

Triggering mechanisms include infection, shock, severe respiratory distress syndrome (or any cause of severe hypoxia and acidosis), and necrotizing enterocolitis, among others.

Other Blood Clotting Defects

Hemorrhagic Disease of the Newborn

Occurrence is rare now that vitamin K is given at birth. The bleeding typically occurs on the second or third day of life and most commonly is from the gastrointestinal tract, not the skin. The late onset form presents between 3 and 8 weeks after birth, often with central nervous system bleeds.

Congenital Deficiencies of Coagulation Factors

Bleeding associated with these deficiencies generally does not take place in the first few weeks of life but has been reported in severe deficiencies, particularly those involving factors VIII and IX. Less commonly, bleeding has been reported with von Willebrand disease and deficiencies of factors V, VII, X, XI, and XIII.

Protein C and S Deficiencies

Infants who are homozygous for these deficiencies have severe bleeding problems in the newborn period, with diffuse purpuric and ecchymotic lesions that may evolve into hemorrhagic bullae and areas of necrosis. These deficiencies are the most common cause of purpura fulminans in the neonatal period.

Platelet Production/Function Defects with Other Abnormalities

Thrombocytopenia with Absent Radii (TAR) Syndrome

The thrombocytopenia tends to improve after the first year of age.

Wiskott-Aldrich Syndrome

Thrombocytopenia and eczema usually develop later, as do the recurrent infections.

Trisomy 13 and 18 Syndromes

Hermansky-Pudlak Syndrome

Albinism with thrombocytopenia.

Miscellaneous Causes

Maternal Drug Ingestion

Maternal warfarin therapy and chronic maternal ingestion of anticonvulsants such as barbiturates and phenytoins, may be associated with low levels of vitamin K in the newborn.

Necrotizing Enterocolitis

Thrombocytopenia may be associated.

Congenital Leukemia

Giant Hemangioma

Purpuric lesions are a consequence of platelet trapping, known as the Kasabach-Merritt syndrome. The vascular lesions may be tufted angiomas or kaposiform hemangioendotheliomas rather than true hemangiomas.

Renal Vein Thrombosis

Congenital Thyrotoxicosis

Phototherapy-Induced Purpura

An unusual occurrence in neonates undergoing phototherapy. Circulating porphyrins may be the underlying cause.

PURPURA BEYOND THE NEONATAL PERIOD

♦ Most Common Causes of Purpuric Lesions

Trauma	Infections, Viral
Streptococcal Pharyngitis	Drugs
Bacteremia and Sepsis	Idiopathic Thrombocytopenic Purpura
Henoch-Schönlein Purpura	von Willebrand Disease
Acute Leukemia	Autoimmune Disorders

Purpura Secondary to Platelet Disorders

Disorders with Thrombocytopenia

♦ Idiopathic Thrombocytopenic Purpura

This condition may be chronic or develop abruptly. A viral illness often precedes the appearance of the petechiae. The bone marrow contains an abundance of megakaryocytes.

♦ Infection

Various infections may cause purpura with or without thrombocytopenia, including meningococcemia, other bacterial septicemias, and some viral infections.

Acquired Immune Deficiency Syndrome

Isolated thrombocytopenia and petechiae may be the presenting sign in infants. In older children the thrombocytopenia is overshadowed by opportunistic infections.

♦ Drugs

Sulfonamides, iodides, digitoxin, quinine, and quinidine may cause thrombocytopenia. Others may impair platelet function without causing thrombocytopenia (see the following). A list of drugs that may cause purpura in children may be found in reference 3.

♦ Autoimmune Disorders

Examples include systemic lupus erythematosus, acquired hemolytic anemia, and hyperthyroidism.

♦ Neoplastic Disorders

Leukemias, lymphomas, and other tumors may replace the bone marrow, with a resulting decrease in platelet production.

Disseminated Intravascular Coagulopathy (DIC)

In addition to thrombocytopenia, children with DIC have hypofibrinogenemia, reduced factors II, V, and VIII, and the presence of fibrin-split products in the serum. DIC has many precipitating causes including infections (bacterial, viral, rickettsial, and protozoal), malignancies, head injury, shock, and transfusion reactions.

● Hemolytic Uremic Syndrome

Hemolytic anemia, acute renal failure, and thrombocytopenia are the classic findings; it usually follows a gastroenteritis. This syndrome occurs chiefly in young children, although its signs may mimic those of thrombotic thrombocytopenic purpura in adults.

Aplastic Anemia

The condition may be idiopathic or drug-induced. The bone marrow may also be suppressed by radiation, drugs, and chemicals.

Disorders Producing Hypersplenism

Splenic enlargement may result in platelet trapping as seen in thalassemia major and Gaucher disease. Liver disorders causing portal hypertension may also induce thrombocytopenia.

Inherited Disorders with Decreased Platelet Production

Fanconi Anemia

Pancytopenia usually does not appear until 5 years of age or later. Various abnormalities may be found in affected children including short stature, hyperpigmentation, thumb abnormalities, strabismus, renal abnormalities, and microcephaly. Inheritance pattern is autosomal recessive.

TAR Syndrome

In this disorder, inherited as an autosomal recessive trait, the thrombocytopenia is of most concern during the first year of life.

Hermansky-Pudlak Syndrome

Affected children have albinism and thrombocytopenia.

Inherited Disorders with Increased Platelet Destruction

Wiskott-Aldrich Syndrome

This is a sex-linked disorder characterized by recurrent infections, an eczematoid rash, and thrombocytopenia.

May-Hegglin Anomaly

Giant platelets and inclusions in leukocytes are findings in this inherited blood defect. One third of patients have decreased platelets.

Bernard-Soulier Disease

This rare blood disorder is characterized by giant platelets, often decreased in number. Bleeding may be severe.

Miscellaneous Disorders

Iron-Deficiency Anemia

In severe cases iron deficiency may be associated with thrombocytopenia.

Osteopetrosis

Replacement of marrow by bone eventually leads to severe anemia and thrombocytopenia.

Giant Hemangioma

Platelets may be trapped in the hemangioma. The vascular lesion may be a tufted angioma or hemangioendothelioma rather than a true hemangioma.

Cyanotic Congenital Heart Disease

Associated with polycythemia.

MMR Immunization

Thrombocytopenia after MMR ranges from 1 in 25,000 for measles to 1 in 3,000 for rubella. Thrombocytopenia may recur after reimmunization with MMR.

NORMAL PLATELET COUNTS WITH ABNORMAL PLATELET FUNCTION

Drug-Induced Thrombocytopathies

◆ Aspirin

Small doses of aspirin may cause prolonged platelet effects.

Other Drugs

Penicillins, at high doses, antihistamines, phenothiazines, sulfonamides, antidepressants, and local anesthetics are among the offenders.

Uremia

Inherited Thrombocytopathies

Glanzmann Thrombasthenia

This disorder, inherited as an autosomal recessive trait, is characterized by mucosal and cutaneous bleeding from early life. The bleeding time is prolonged; clot retraction is absent or deficient.

Adenosine Diphosphate Storage Pool Disease

Mild purpura may occur in this rare disorder inherited as an autosomal-dominant trait.

Adenosine Diphosphate Release Disease

A mild bleeding tendency is present.

PURPURA SECONDARY TO VASCULAR DISORDERS (NONTHROMBOCYTOPENIC)

♦ Trauma

Trauma is the most common cause of purpura overall. The following should be considered.

Child Abuse

Unexplained or poorly explained bruising in a young child suggests abuse.

Raised Intravascular Pressure

Coughing, vomiting, or choking may cause petechiae on the head and neck.

Suction Purpura

The "hickey" on the neck is the best recognized form.

Factitious Lesions

Bruises unusual in shape and position in teenagers may be factitious.

Cupping and Coin Rubbing

In some cultures lesions caused by attempts to "bring out" the cause of illness may be the result of vacuum-induced (suction) purpura from cupping or rubbing the skin with coins.

Autoerythrocyte Sensitization

This disorder was originally thought to represent an unusual autosensitivity to the erythrocytes, resulting in purpuric areas. More recently, a psychogenic origin has been suggested; the lesions may be self-induced.

Vasculitis

♦ Infection

Petechiae may appear during infections without thrombocytopenia. Viral infections, particularly with coxsackieviruses A9 and B3 and echoviruses 9 and 4, may be associated with purpuric lesions. Petechiae of the head and neck may be found in streptococcal pharyngitis. Rocky Mountain spotted fever and atypical measles may also produce a vasculitis.

◆ Henoch-Schönlein Purpura

The lesions tend to be located on the lower extremities, almost never on the trunk. Abdominal pain, arthralgia with periarticular swelling, and nephritis each occur in about one half of the cases. The etiology is still unknown.

● Acute Hemorrhagic Edema of Infancy

A disorder much like Henoch-Schönlein purpura, but generally occurring in children less than 3 years of age. The purpuric lesions are acrally located, but have an unusual targetoid appearance.

Septic Emboli

Purpuric lesions may be a presenting sign in subacute bacterial endocarditis.

Drug-Induced Lesions

Ingestion of sulfonamides, penicillins, iodides, mercury, bismuth, and other substances may produce purpuric lesions. A vasculitis secondary to drug reactions has been described with a wide variety of drugs including penicillins, sulfonamides, hydantoin, and allopurinol. Palpable purpura should suggest vasculitis. Hemorrhagic vesicles and bullae may also appear.

Other Causes of Vasculitis

A host of disorders may be associated with vasculitis, creating palpable purpura especially in dependent areas. Lupus, Wegener granulomatosis, other connective tissue disorders, and diseases associated with immune complexes, complement, and immunoglobulin deposition should be sought.

Dysproteinemias

Abnormal plasma proteins, such as seen in hyperglobulinemias, cryoglobulinemias, or macroglobulinemias, may be associated with purpura.

Progressive Pigmentary Dermatosis (Schamberg Disease)

This disorder is characterized by the insidious onset and slow progression of grouped petechiae over the extremities, usually the lower. The lesions contain fresh and old petechiae, giving rise to various colors. Adolescents may be affected. It is a capillaritis.

Lichen Aureus

A rare skin condition with localized lichenoid papules and plaques, usually golden to rust colored, but sometimes purpuric appearing. The lower legs is the usual location. Other similar pigmented purpuric lesions include Majocchi disease and pigmented purpura of Gougerot and Blum.

Increased Vascular Permeability/Weakness

Corticosteroids

Easy bruising may be seen in patients on prolonged steroid therapy or, rarely, with Cushing syndrome.

Scurvy

This disorder is unusual in children in the United States. Perifollicular petechiae with swollen gums and painful limbs are suggestive findings.

Inherited Vascular Disorders

Ehlers-Danlos Syndrome

Various types have been described. Easy bruisability, skin hyperelasticity, and joint laxity may be seen.

Hereditary Hemorrhagic Telangiectasia

Telangiectatic lesions usually do not appear until late childhood. Epistaxis and gastrointestinal bleeding are more likely than cutaneous bleeding.

Marfan Syndrome

Bleeding problems are more likely to involve the large vessels, such as the aorta, with dissecting aneurysm.

Osteogenesis Imperfecta

Capillary fragility may lead to increased bleeding tendency.

COAGULATION DISTURBANCES

Clotting factor disorders are more likely to cause deep muscular or joint bleeding than superficial skin bleeding, although purpura may occur in any of these disorders (all are not listed).

♦ von Willebrand Disease

In this relatively common disorder, transmitted as an autosomal-dominant trait, there is a deficiency of a circulating plasma protein related to factor VIII. The most common presenting sign is excessive bleeding after dental extraction, tonsillectomy, or other surgical procedure. Petechiae may appear after ingestion of salicylates.

Factor VIII, IX, XI, or XII Deficiency

These disorders are characterized by a prolonged partial thromboplastin time (PTT) and a normal prothrombin time (PT).

Late Hemorrhagic Disease

Vitamin K deficiency states may occur in various disorders including diarrhea, cystic fibrosis, biliary atresia, alpha-1-antitrypsin deficiency, hepatitis, abetalipoproteinemia, celiac disease, and chronic warfarin exposure. Breast-fed infants occasionally develop late hemorrhagic disease.

Factor V, X, II (Prothrombin), or I (Fibrinogen) Deficiency

Both PTT and PT are prolonged.

Factor VII Deficiency

The PT is prolonged; the PTT is normal. Because factor VII has the shortest lifespan of the clotting factors produced by the liver, the coagulopathy of liver disease begins as factor VII deficiency.

Factor XIII Deficiency

Bleeding from the umbilical stump as the cord separates is the most common sign.

Protein C and S Deficiency

These proteins are important physiologic anticoagulants. Congenital deficiency leads to recurrent episodes of superficial thrombophlebitis, deep vein thrombosis, and pulmonary embolism.

OTHER

♦ Maculae Cerulae

Faint, grayish purpuric lesions of the lower abdomen and back may be caused by pubic lice, simulating purpuric lesions.

♦ Papular-Purpuric "Gloves and Socks" Syndrome

This unusual exanthem is suspected to be related to viral infections, most frequently parvovirus B19. Symmetric, intensely pruritic or painful edema and erythema of the hands and feet appears first and then the areas become covered with petechiae.

REFERENCES

1. Mandl KD, Stack AM, Fleisher GR. Incidence of bacteremia in infants and children with fever and petechiae. *J Pediatr* 1997;131:398–404.
2. Baker RC, Seguin JH, Leslie N, Gilchrist MJR, Myers MG. Fever and petechiae in children. *Pediatrics* 1989;84:1051–1055.
3. Baselga E, Drolet BA, Esterly NB. Purpura in infants and children. *J Am Acad Dermatol* 1997;37:673–705.

SUGGESTED READING

Greer FR. Vitamin K deficiency and hemorrhage in infancy. *Clin Perinatol* 1995;22:759–777.
Metzker A, Merlob P. Suction purpura. *Arch Dermatol* 1992;128:822–824.
Paller AS, Eramo LR, Farrell EE, Millard DD, Honig PJ, Cunningham BB. Purpuric phototherapy-induced eruption in transfused neonates: relation to transient porphyrinemia. *Pediatrics* 1997;100:360–364.
Pramanik AK. Bleeding disorders in neonates. *Pediatr Rev* 1992;13:163–173.
Vlacha V, Forman EN, Miron D, Peter G. Recurrent thrombocytopenic purpura after repeated measles-mumps-rubella vaccination. *Pediatrics* 1996;97:738–739.

114

Pruritus

Pruritus—from the Latin *prurire,* "to itch"—is a most annoying symptom. It is a subjective complaint of an uncomfortable skin sensation that leads to the response of scratching. Scratching often results in relief of this sensation, but the relief is only temporary.

Pruritus may or may not be associated with skin lesions that provide diagnostic clues. It is important to remember, however, that repeated scratching of the skin will cause excoriations, and if the scratching persists, lichenification or thickening of the skin will result.

Exogenous causes of pruritus such as contactants, parasitic infestations, and environmental factors (drying, high humidity, and excessive bathing) are the most common; the atopic person is especially susceptible. Psychogenic causes of pruritus are less common in children than in adults. Endogenous causes account for very few of the cases except perhaps for drug reactions, although, because of their lethality, neoplasia cannot be ignored as a possible cause.

When a thorough investigation fails to reveal an underlying cause for the pruritus, it may be said to be idiopathic, an unsettling diagnostic appellation.

♦ Most Common Causes of Pruritus

Atopic Dermatitis	Dry Skin
Contact Allergens (Poison Ivy, Nickel)	Contact Irritants (Soap, Chemicals)
Insect Bites/Infestations	Drugs
Cholestasis of Pregnancy	

EXOGENOUS CAUSES

♦ Contactants

Various substances, either irritants or allergens, may produce pruritus on contact with the skin; only a few examples are listed. In most cases, a rash occurs with the pruritus; typically it is localized and well-defined with sharp borders.

Irritants

Harsh soaps, bubble bath, saliva, citrus juices (especially on perioral skin), urine and feces (diaper dermatitis), chemicals (creosote), wool (especially in atopic children), and caterpillar contact may cause skin irritation.

Allergens

Poison ivy (plant dermatitis), jewelry (nickel), topical medications (especially anesthetics and antihistamines), clothing dyes, and cosmetics may cause allergic reactions.

Parasitic Infestations and Insect Bites

♦ Scabies

This infestation must be considered in the differential diagnosis of any pruritic rash of recent onset, especially if the characteristic distribution (hands, wrists, axillae, gluteal cleft, and genitalia) and papular, papulovesicular, or nodular lesions, as well as involvement of other family members, are found. Beware of "scabies in babies," in which the characteristic distribution may be absent, with involvement of the head.

♦ Papular Urticaria

Bites of insects, especially fleas and mosquitoes, may be followed by localized pruritus. In some cases, periods of intense pruritus are associated with many papules having a central punctum on an erythematous base. Papular urticaria is a hypersensitivity reaction to bites, with more severe reaction than an ordinary bite.

Pediculosis

Body lice may be difficult to see, but their egg sacs (nits) are stationary, attached to hairs.

Swimmers' Itch

The problem may develop following bathing in certain freshwater lakes that contain schistosomal cercariae. The eruption occurs on exposed parts.

Seabather's Eruption

A highly pruritic eruption that appears under swimwear after bathing in the ocean. The cause is larvae of a jellyfish.

Other Mites; Chiggers; Hookworm (Creeping Eruption)

Humans are often accidental hosts for these mites and larvae.

Foreign Bodies

Fiberglass is probably the best recognized and the most common, particularly if clothing is washed with materials containing fiberglass. Cactus spines and hair may also cause pruritus.

♦ **Environmental Factors**

Drying of Skin

Low humidity, especially in temperate climates, may be a factor, most commonly in the winter months when the heat is turned on.

Excessive Bathing

Removal of natural oils allows drying of the stratum corneum and resultant pruritus.

High Humidity

Retention of moisture in the skin may produce pruritus, which may be associated with miliaria rubra (prickly heat).

ENDOGENOUS CAUSES

♦ **Pregnancy**

Cholestasis associated with pregnancy is a relatively common cause of pruritus.

♦ **Drug Reactions**

A large number of drugs may produce pruritus, often without primary skin lesions. Occasionally, exposure to sunlight precipitates the itch. Among the more common offenders are aminophylline, aspirin, barbiturates, opiates, erythromycin, gold, griseofulvin, isoniazid, phenothiazines, and vitamin A.

● **Neurofibromatosis**

Individuals with this relatively common neurocutaneous disorder may be affected by an annoying pruritus.

Internal Malignancies and Lymphomas

This is the most worrisome group of disorders that may cause pruritus, although overall they make up a tiny percentage. The pruritus may precede other manifestations of neoplasia by months or even years; curiously, it may be localized as well as generalized.

Acquired Immunodeficiency Syndrome

Pruritus may be the presenting symptom or a major complaint of individuals.

Blood Dyscrasias

Polycythemia vera is a well-recognized cause of pruritus in adults but is rare in children. Iron deficiency has even been suggested as a cause.

Renal Disease

Retention of products usually excreted by the kidney may cause pruritus. The association of pruritus with uremia is well known. Uric acid and other products, as yet undetermined, may play a role.

Hepatobiliary Disorders

Pruritus may occur with or without jaundice. Cholestatic conditions such as familial cholestasis or biliary atresia and cholestasis secondary to drugs may produce itching. In acute hepatitis pruritus often precedes jaundice and may be associated with urticaria. Repeated scratching will produce excoriations and eczema.

Endocrine and Metabolic Causes

Hypothyroidism

The associated dry skin may be the cause of the pruritus.

Hyperthyroidism

This condition rarely is associated with itching.

Hypoparathyroidism

Diabetes Mellitus

Pruritus most commonly occurs on the lower extremities.

Carcinoid Tumors

Pruritus may rarely accompany flushing attacks.

Hypercalcemia

Immobilization as well as other causes of hypercalcemia may result in various symptoms including pruritus.

Autoimmune Disorders

Systemic Lupus Erythematosus

Juvenile Rheumatoid Arthritis

The characteristic rash is occasionally pruritic.

Parasitic Diseases

Trichinosis and hookworm infestations may be associated with itching.

Congenital Ectodermal Defects

Both the anhidrotic and hidrotic forms of ectodermal dysplasia may be associated with pruritus.

PSYCHOGENIC PRURITUS

Before a psychological origin is considered, a thorough search must be made for organic causes.

PRURITUS ASSOCIATED WITH SKIN DISORDERS

Pruritus may be a problem in many skin disorders. Only a few important conditions are listed.

◆ Atopic Dermatitis

This apparently hereditary condition of the skin is common. It was aptly described years ago as an "itch that rashes," because if the child could be prevented from scratching, no rash would appear. Several exogenous factors as well as stress may produce pruritus in the atopic child.

Infections

Pruritus may accompany fungal, candidal, bacterial, or viral skin infections.

Seborrheic Dermatitis

Pityriasis Rosea

Pruritus may occur in 5% to 10% of affected persons.

Psoriasis

Urticaria Pigmentosa (Mastocytosis)

Occasionally, pruritus without pigmented skin lesions may be present or precede the more typical lesions. Dermatographia in these cases may be intense.

◆ Urticaria

Urticarial skin lesions are pruritic (see Chapter 115, Urticaria).

Erythropoietic Protoporphyria

Burning pruritus may occur within a few minutes following exposure to sunlight. Erythema, urticarial wheals, or vesicles develop. A laboratory hallmark of this disorder is a high free erythrocyte protoporphyrin level.

Neurodermatitis

Repeated scratching of the skin may lead to the itch-scratch-itch cycle. Various stimuli trigger the phenomenon.

IDIOPATHIC PRURITUS

SUGGESTED READING

Denman ST. A review of pruritus. *J Am Acad Dermatol* 1986;14:375–392.
Liautaud B, Pape JW, DeHovitz JA, Thomas F, LaRoche AC, Verdier RI, Deschamps MM, Johnson WD. Pruritic skin lesions. A common initial presentation of acquired immunodeficiency syndrome. *Arch Dermatol* 1989;125:629–632.

115
Urticaria

Urticaria (hives) are easily recognizable, even by most laymen, because the lesions are such a common sign. It has been estimated that as many as 15% of the population may experience urticarial lesions at some time during their lives. The recognition of hives is one matter; finding the underlying cause is another. Most of the literature on this subject divides hives into two categories: acute and chronic. Acute hives last less than 6 weeks; chronic hives are present or recur for more than 6 weeks. In roughly three fourths of patients, particularly those with chronic hives, no definite etiology can be established.

Urticaria is characterized by the presence of wheals that come and go and are usually pruritic. Individual lesions usually last less than 4 hours, although they may persist for 24 to 48 hours. Longer lasting urticarial lesions should suggest a vasculitis, or hereditary angioedema. The wheals vary in size, ranging from a few millimeters to many centimeters. There are even giant urticarial lesions covering large areas. At times the central area of lesions may take on a dusky hue, suggesting targetlike lesions. These urticarial lesions should not be mistaken for erythema multiforme, a common mistake. There may or may not be other signs and symptoms associated with the appearance of urticaria. Careful investigation, however, may reveal characteristic features. Information about the duration of episodes and the pattern of occurrence is important. The hives may occur only in certain places such as home or school. There may be an association with certain activities such as food ingestion or exercise.

The pathogenic mechanisms are many and often poorly understood. Immunologic and non-immunologic mechanisms may be involved.

◆ DRUGS

Drug reactions are among the most commonly recognized causes of acute urticaria. Almost any drug is a potential offender, especially penicillins, non-steroidal anti-inflammatory agents, sulfas, sedatives, tranquilizers, analgesics, laxatives, hormones, and diuretics. Drugs such as penicillin may be present in trace amounts in foods, especially cow milk. There may be no clear history of exposure. Aspirin may be responsible for the exacerbation of chronic urticaria in as many as 20% to 40% of patients; the effects of aspirin may last for a few weeks rather than just a few days as is commonly thought.

◆ FOODS

Foods are another common cause, especially of acute urticaria. The causative factor may be food protein or an added preservative. Commonly incriminated foods are nuts, milk, fish, eggs, tomatoes, lobster, strawberries, yeasts, naturally occurring salicylates, citric acid, azo dyes, and benzoic acid. A food diary, as well as elimination and readdition diets, may be helpful in identifying the offending substance. Often more than one food may be the cause.

INFECTIONS AND INFESTATIONS

Transient urticaria may be associated with a variety of infections, sometimes as a prodromal feature. Included in this group are streptococcal infection, viral hepatitis (especially B), infectious mononucleosis, coxsackievirus, adenovirus, mycoplasmal infections, and parasitic infestations (trichinosis, giardiasis, or roundworms). Chronic focal bacterial infection (such as sinus, dental, genitourinary, or gastrointestinal), dermatophytosis, or candidiasis are probably uncommon causes of chronic urticaria despite popularity in the old literature. Giardiasis, malaria, and infestations with *Entamoeba histolytica* are also uncommon causes of chronic urticaria.

PHYSICAL FACTORS

The physical urticarias may account for as many as 15% of the causes of urticaria. A few of the conditions in this category deserve special mention.

♦ Dermatographia

Some reviewers estimate that dermatographia accounts for 8% to 9% of all cases of urticaria. Wheal and erythema follow minor stroking or pressure.

♦ Cholinergic Factors

From 5% to 7% of all cases of urticaria may be induced by heat, emotion, stress, or exercise. Wheals 1 to 3 mm across are surrounded by large erythematous flares.

Cold

Urticaria may be associated with cryoglobulin formation and immune complex disease, especially collagen-vascular diseases, although these are rare in children. An acquired form is characterized by the appearance of wheals in a cold exposed area after rewarming.

Pressure

This form occurs primarily in adolescents. Deep, painful swelling appears 4 to 6 hours following prolonged pressure.

Solar

In this uncommon form, pruritus, erythema, and wheals appear within a few minutes of sun exposure. The lesions are localized to exposed skin.

INHALANTS

Reactions are seen primarily in atopic persons with a history of allergic rhinitis and asthma in a seasonal occurrence pattern. Pollens, mold spores, animal danders, aerosols, and plant products may be responsible. Identification may be aided by skin tests.

INSECT AND ARTHROPOD BITES AND STINGS

These usually cause acute, transient episodes of urticaria. Bees, wasps, fleas, mites (especially *Sarcoptes scabei*), bedbugs, mosquitoes, scorpions, spiders, and jellyfish are included. Papular urticaria deserves special recognition. Some individuals develop intensely pruritic wheals with insect bites, particularly fleas. This represents a hypersensitivity reaction to the flea. Usually only one person in the family is affected, leading to difficulty convincing the parents that fleas are involved.

PENETRANTS AND CONTACTANTS

A wide variety of types of materials may be the cause of urticaria. Possibilities include foods, textiles, animal dander and saliva, plants, medicaments, chemicals, and cosmetics.

SYSTEMIC DISEASES

This group of disorders is an uncommon cause of urticaria in children. In adults lymphomas, visceral carcinomas, autoimmune thyroiditis, and hyperthyroidism are more prominent as causes. In children, juvenile rheumatoid arthritis, systemic lupus erythematosus, acute rheumatic fever, and Henoch-Schönlein purpura must be considered. Urticaria may be an early manifestation of these disorders or may be associated with other signs and symptoms. Urticaria pigmentosa is usually associated with pigmented macules or nodules; stroking these lesions causes them to become edematous. Hives, bullae, or erythema may occur in areas of skin free of the pigmented lesions.

PSYCHOGENIC URTICARIA

Unfortunately, chronic urticaria is often labeled as psychogenic in origin, usually because other causes cannot be found. Chronic pruritic lesions can cause psychological disturbances in almost anyone. Recent evidence indicates that psychological stress may exacerbate urticaria but rarely is the sole cause.

GENETIC DISORDERS

These conditions are rare causes of urticaria. Individuals with hereditary angioedema do not really develop hives. They may develop life-threatening swelling of soft tissues, especially after trauma. The swelling is diffuse and brawny, often of the extremities. Abdominal pain is a common accompanying feature.

Others in this group of inherited condition with urticarial lesions include familial cold urticaria, familial localized heat urticaria, vibratory angioedema, the heredofamilial syndrome of urticaria with deafness and amyloidosis (Muckle-Wells syndrome), and erythropoietic protoporphyria.

URTICARIAL VASCULITIS

Urticarial lesions tend to remain in the same areas, generally the extremities, for more than 24 to 72 hours. Malaise, arthralgias, fever, elevated sedimentation rates, and decreased serum complement levels are generally found. The clinical picture may suggest serum sickness.

SUGGESTED READING

Casale TB. Urticaria and angioedema. In: Oski FA, ed. *Principles and practice of pediatrics,* 2nd ed. Philadelphia: JB Lippincott, 1994:222–227.

Harris A, Twarog FJ, Geha RS. Chronic urticaria in childhood: natural course and etiology. *Ann Allergy* 1983;51:161–165.

Rosen FS. Urticaria, angioedema, and anaphylaxis. *Pediatr Rev* 1992;10:387–390.

Soter NA. Acute and chronic urticaria and angioedema. *J Am Acad Dermatol* 1991;25:146–154.

Weston WL, Badgett JT. Urticaria. *Pediatr Rev* 1998;19:240–244.

Weston WL, Lane AT, Morelli JG. *Color textbook of pediatric dermatology,* 2nd ed. St. Louis: Mosby, 1996:220–229.

Subject Index

813

Trichorhinophalangeal syndrome, alopecia in, 782
  deafness in, 222
  microcephaly in, 175
  recurrent fractures in, 662
Trisomy 13 syndrome, cataracts in, 262
  floppy infant syndrome in, 741
  microcephaly in, 172
Trisomy 18 syndrome, cataracts in, 262
  microcephaly in, 172
Trisomy 21 syndrome, macroglossia in, 305
Trisomy 9p syndrome, macrocephaly in, 165
Trisomy X, tall stature in, 27
Trypanosomiasis, and periorbital edema, 239
Trypsinogen deficiency, and edema, 78
Tryptophan malabsorption, and irritability, 57
Tuberculosis, and alopecia, 780
  ataxia in, 749
  and back pain, 615
  and cervical adenopathy, 68
  and cough, 377
  and failure to thrive, 21
  and fatigue, 48
  and fever of undetermined origin, 4
  and hepatomegaly, 471
  and hoarseness, 329
  and leg pain, 635
  orbital, and proptosis, 275
  and parotid gland swelling, 199
  pulmonary, and hemoptysis, 394
    and sweating, 129
  and pyuria, 549
  renal, dysuria in, 546
    and hematuria, 556
    and hypertension, 417
  and torticollis, 354
Tuberculous peritonitis, abdominal distension in, 436
  ascites in, 447
Tuberous sclerosis, and hypertension, 421
  and macrocephaly, 168
  and precocious puberty, 575
  and seizures, 716, 720
Tularemia, and fever of undetermined origin, 5
  and parotid gland swelling, 199
  and periorbital edema, 236
Turner syndrome, amenorrhea in, 587–588
  ascites in, 442
  cataracts in, 263
  delayed puberty in, 581
  edema in, 84
  obesity in, 43

Typhilitis, vomiting in, 497
Typhoid fever, body/urine odor in, 125
  fever of undetermined origin in, 4
Tyrosinemia, ascites in, 445
  breath odor in, 127
  diarrhea in, 515
  hereditary, jaundice in, 109
  irritability in, 57

U
Ulcer, and epistaxis, 294
  peptic, and abdominal pain, 450
    and hematemesis, 530, 531–532
    and vomiting, 494, 503, 506
  stress, and hematemesis, 532
Ulcerative colitis, abdominal distension in, 436
  anorexia in, 33
  digital clubbing in, 709
  failure to thrive in, 19
  fever of undetermined origin in, 5
  maternal, and diarrhea, 510
  and melena and hematochezia, 537
  melena and hematochezia in, 539
  vomiting in, 497
Upper respiratory tract infection, and cervical adenopathy, 67
  and cough, 376
  recurrent, and nasal obstruction, 298
  and torticollis, 353
Urachal cyst, and abdominal mass, 485
Urate crystals, and hematuria, 561
  and red urine, 563
Urea cycle, disorders of, and hepatomegaly, 463
  and seizures, 715
Uremia, breath odor in, 127
  coma in, 731, 734
  delirium in, 768
  epistaxis in, 295
  fatigue in, 51
  muscle weakness in, 682
  pallor in, 89
  vomiting in, 500
Ureteropelvic junction obstruction, intermittent, vomiting in, 507
Urethral diverticulum, and dysuria, 547
Urethral prolapse, and dysuria, 547
  and vaginal bleeding, 596
  and vulvovaginitis, 605

Urethral stricture, and dysuria, 547
  and pyuria, 551
Urethritis, dysuria in, 545
  and pyuria, 549
Urethroprostatitis, and hematuria, 556
Urinary calculi, and dysuria, 547
Urinary retention, and irritability, 60
Urinary tract, congenital abnormalities of, and hematuria, 557
  disorders of, and abdominal pain, 450
    and hematuria, 556–557
    and vomiting, 506
  obstruction of, perforation with, and ascites, 440
    and recurrent infections, 115
    and vomiting, 499, 504
  trauma to, and hematuria, 558–559
  tumor of, and pyuria, 551
Urinary tract infection. *See also* Cystitis; Pyelonephritis; Urethritis.
  and back pain, 614
  and body/urine odor, 125
  dysuria in, 545
  and enuresis, 570
  and failure to thrive, 15
  and fever of undetermined origin, 4
  and pyuria, 549
  and weight loss, 36
Urine, color changes in, 563–566
  odor of, unusual, 124–126
Urolithiasis, and hematuria, 559
Uropathy, obstructive, and failure to thrive, 16
Urticaria, 808–811
  and pruritus, 806
Urticaria pigmentosa, irritability in, 60
Urticarial vasculitis, 811
Usher syndrome, vision loss in, 287
Uterus, congenital absence of, and delayed puberty, 585
  enlargement of, and abdominal mass, 485
  infection of, and amenorrhea, 592
  leiomyomas of, and vaginal bleeding, 598
Uveitis, and vision loss, 288

V
Vaccinia, and periorbital edema, 236
Vaginal atresia, and amenorrhea, 587